Canine and Feline
Geriatric Oncology

Canine and Feline Geriatric Oncology

Honoring the Human–Animal Bond

Second Edition

Dr. Alice Villalobos
with Laurie Kaplan, MSC

WILEY Blackwell

Registered Office
John Wiley & Sons, Inc., 111 River Street, Hoboken, NJ 07030, USA

Editorial Office
111 River Street, Hoboken, NJ 07030, USA

For details of our global editorial offices, customer services, and more information about Wiley products visit us at www.wiley.com.

Wiley also publishes its books in a variety of electronic formats and by print-on-demand. Some content that appears in standard print versions of this book may not be available in other formats.

Library of Congress Cataloging-in-Publication Data
Names: Villalobos, Alice, author. | Kaplan, Laurie, MSC, author.
Title: Canine and feline geriatric oncology : honoring the human-animal bond / by Dr. Alice Villalobos with Laurie Kaplan.
Description: Second edition. | Hoboken, NJ : Wiley, 2018. | Includes bibliographical references and index. |
Identifiers: LCCN 2017026916 (print) | LCCN 2017027886 (ebook) | ISBN 9781119290407 (pdf) | ISBN 9781119290445 (epub) |
    ISBN 9781119290391 (cloth)
Subjects: LCSH: Dogs–Diseases. | Cats–Diseases. | Cancer in animals. | Veterinary geriatrics. | Veterinary oncology. | MESH:
    Neoplasms–veterinary | Dog Diseases | Cat Diseases | Aging–physiology | Bonding, Human-Pet
Classification: LCC SF992.C35 (ebook) | LCC SF992.C35 V55 2018 (print) | NLM SF 992.C35 | DDC 636.7/0898976994–dc23
    LC record available at https://lccn.loc.gov/2017026916

Cover images: Courtesy of Alice Villalobos
Cover design by Wiley

Set in 10.5/13pt TimesLtStd by Aptara Inc., New Delhi, India
Printed and bound in Singapore by Markono Print Media Pte Ltd

10 9 8 7 6 5 4 3 2 1

Contents

Foreword

The amount of information that applies to contemporary veterinary geriatric oncology is mounting at a frenetic pace. It is generated from the hard work of thousands of clinical researchers and authors of scientific publications in oncology, hematology, gerontology, radiation oncology, internal medicine, surgery, immunology, nutrition, sociology, epidemiology, and research in all related fields. This book draws from the texts and the milieu of references available. Instead of reprinting material, the author delivers applied knowledge to individual cases. For more in-depth detail, readers are referred most notably to the following general references used for this book, listed alphabetically by title:

- AAHA Guidelines on Managing Cancer in Dogs and Cats is an excellent summary. www.aaha.org/professional/resources/oncology.aspx 2016.
- AAHA/AAFP Pain Management Guidelines for Dogs and Cats: an Implementation Toolkit. www.aaha.org/professional/resources/pain_management.aspx 2015.
- AAHA/IAAHPC End of Life Care Guidelines and Implementation Toolkit: 2016.
- www.aaha.org/professional/resources/end_of_life_care_guidelines.aspx
- AVMA Animal Health Studies Database. Offers a centralized source for clinical trials.
- https://ebusiness.avma.org/aahsd/study_search.aspx
- AVMA Guidelines for Veterinary Hospice Care, 2015
- www.avma.org/KB/Policies/Pages/Guidelines-for-Veterinary-Hospice-Care.aspx
- *Being Mortal: Medicine and What Matters in the End*, by A. Gawande, Metropolitan Books, Henry Holt and Company, NY, 2014.
- *BSAVA Manual of Canine and Feline Oncology*, 2nd and 3rd edns, eds J.M. Dobson and D.B.X. Lascelles. Quedgeley, Gloucestershire, England: British Small Animal Veterinary Association, 2003 and 2011.
- *Cancer Control: Journal of the Moffitt Cancer Center*. Geriatric Oncology, Guest ed. L.Balducci. Vol. 1, No. 2, March 1994.
- *Cancer in Dogs and Cats: Medical and Surgical Management*, 2nd edn, by W.B. Morrison. Jackson, WY: Teton New Media, 2002.
- *Cellular and Molecular Immunology*, 8th edn, by A.K. Abbas, A.H. Lichtman, and S. Pillai. Saunders/Elsevier, 2014, 554 pp.
- *Clinical Oncology*, 3rd edn, by M.D. Abeloff, J.O. Armitage, J.E. Neiderhuber, M.B. Kastan, and W.G. McKenna. Philadelphia, PA: Churchill Livingstone, 2004.

- *Comprehensive Geriatric Oncology*, 2nd edn, eds L. Balducci, G.H. Lyman, W.B. Ershler, and M. Extermann. Oxon, UK: Taylor & Francis, 2004.
- *Feline Oncology*, by G. Ogilvie and A. Moore. Trenton, NJ: Veterinary Learning Systems, 2001.
- *Geriatrics and Gerontology of the Dog and Cat*, 2nd edn, by J.D. Hoskins. Philadelphia, PA: Saunders, 2004.
- *Hematology: Basic Principles and Practice*, 4th edn, by R. Hoffman, E.J. Benz, S.J. Shattil, B. Furie, H.J. Cohen, L.E. Silberstein, and P. McGlave. Philadelphia, PA: Churchill Livingstone, 2004.
- *Managing the Veterinary Cancer Patient*, by G. Ogilvie and A. Moore. Trenton, NJ: Veterinary Learning Systems, 1995.
- *Palliative Care: Transforming the Care of Serious Illness*, eds D.E. Meier, S.L. Issacs, and R.G. Hughes. San Francisco, CA: Jossey-Bass/Wiley, 2010, 452 pp.
- *Small Animal Clinical Oncology*, 3rd, 4th, and 5th edns, by S.J. Withrow, E.G. MacEwen, R. Page, and D.M. Vail. Philadelphia, PA: Saunders, 2001–2007, 2013, Elsevier.
- *Tumors in Domestic Animals*, 3rd edn, ed. J. Moulton. Berkeley, CA: University of California Press, 1990.
- *Tumors in Domestic Animals*, 4th edn, ed. D. Meuten. Ames, IA: Blackwell Publishing Professional, 2002.
- *Veterinary and Comparative Oncology*, journal eds. D. Argyle and D. Thamm, Wiley Blackwell, all issues.
- *Veterinary Cancer Medicine*, 2nd edn, eds G. Theilen and B. Madewell. Philadelphia, PA: Lea & Febiger,1987.
- *Veterinary Oncology Secrets*, by R. Rosenthal. Philadelphia, PA: Hanley & Belfus, 2001.
- *Zoobiquity: What Animals Can Teach Us About Health and the Science of Healing,* by B. Natterson-Horowitz and K. Bowers. Knopf, 2012.

Disclaimer: Geriatric patient oncology care and client communications are ultimately the attending doctor's responsibility. Author and publisher shall not be liable for any loss related to the use of information in this textbook. Readers are encouraged to check and verify doses and schedules and current information or consult with specialists. Some excellent resources available online include:

- www.vetcancersociety.org
- https://ebusiness.avma.org/aahsd/study_search.aspx (clinical trials database)
- http://www.lib.ncsu.edu/vetmed/boards/ACVIM/oncology: 2017 Residency reading list
- *How the Immune System Sees and Destroys Tumors*, Jeffrey S. Weber, MD, PhD, Moffitt Cancer Center, Tampa, Florida. https://www.youtube.com/watch?v=3hlGq-3F1uQ
- World Small Animal Veterinary Association, 2014. Guidelines for Recognition, Assessment and Treatment of Pain, *Journal of Small Animal Practice*. http://www.wsava.org/sites/default/files/jsap_0.pdf
- https://clinicaltrials.gov/ct2/results?term=oncology&Search=Search (information on five thousand – mostly NIH – clinical research studies
- http://pubmed.gov/ (full text biomedical articles dated back to 1966)

- www.oncology.medscape.com (provides current information on human oncology)
- www.VIN.com Veterinary Information Network (interactive exchange)
- www.veterinarypartner.com (VIN's client information resource)
- www.csuanimalcancercenter.org
- http://www.vsso.org/ (the Veterinary Society of Surgical Oncology)
- www.veterinaryoncologyconsults.com (clinician consults with Dr. Anthony Moore)
- http://csu-cvmbs.colostate.edu/vth/diagnostic-and-support/argus/pet-hospice/Pages/default.aspx (pet hospice resource)
- www.argusinstitute.colostate.edu (the Argus Institute for Families and Veterinary Medicine counseling support featuring a *Making Decisions* booklet)
- http://pet-loss.net/emotions.shtml (about pet loss grief by Moria Anderson Allen, M.Ed.)
- http://www.griefhealingblog.com/2010/09/is-pet-loss-comparable-to-loss-of-loved.html (is pet loss equivalent to loss of a loved one?)
- www.clinicaltrials.gov (clinical trials resource)
- www.petloss.com (grief support, rainbow bridge, and Monday candle ceremony)
- https://rainbowsbridge.com/Grief_Support_Center/Grief_Support_Home.htm (pet loss support)
- www.PetCureOncology.com (stereotactic radiation information from Neil Mauldin, DVM, ACVIM, ACVR)
- http://www.modianolab.org/cancer/cancer_lymphoma.shtml
- http://www.modianolab.org/cancer/cancer_osteosarcoma.shtml
- https://www.mycancergenome.org

Preface

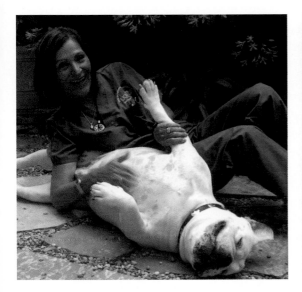

Dr. Alice Villalobos with Neo

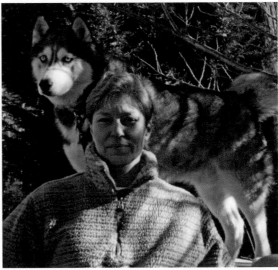

Laurie Kaplan with Bullet

Canine and Feline Geriatric Oncology distills out the most important useful information needed by veterinary practitioners and teams to deal with geriatric cancer patients and their carers. Veterinarians contact me daily to fill in the gaps left between the lines in their textbooks. When I was lecturing in Beijing, the head of oncology at the Agricultural University told me that she slept with my book for three months and that it helped her with her students, clients, and patients. During the World Veterinary Cancer Congress, in Brazil, an oncologist, who translated the First Edition, said that she knew my mind and another oncologist said, "We see our books walking, when we see you and Dr. Theilen." In Portugal, a surgeon told me that he had my textbook right next to his Ettinger! Drs. Mark Gendizer and Virginia Quelch said their staff uses the book often.

This Second Edition text draws from an overwhelming deluge of information that overloads practitioners in the rapidly growing field of oncology and end of life care. We have new technology and information from genomics, proteomics, metabolomics, immunogenomics, immuno-oncology (onco-immunology), and nutrigenomics. Researchers may use artificial intelligence to extract information and find the keys to open the gates of many cellular pathways and map the molecular biology of specific tumors. Data would be used to suggest which drugs and immunotherapies would be best to use for the cancer patient for precision therapy.

These technological keys are guiding better diagnostics, earlier detection of cancer, and the development of targeted therapies and immunotherapy. Bioengineering technology enhances the capabilities of radiation therapy, interventional therapy, and electrochemotherapy (electroporation) as new and improved weapons to battle cancer. Further advances in medical technology and research will allow us to extend the health and longevity of our geriatric oncology patients with combinations of newer, less toxic, targeted therapy such as small molecules and vaccine therapy from the growing field of immuno-oncology.

Tumors are organized into five large categories, according to tissue of origin: carcinomas, sarcomas, blood cancer, nervous system tumors, and miscellaneous/unknown. Tumors are also organized by location: skin, head and neck, chest, abdomen, and bone and blood (lymphoid). Sorting tumors with this perspective may assist practitioners with the initial decision-making process, to improve the diagnostic approach and expedite treatment plans.

This text is a unique reference for veterinary students, interns, residents, attending doctors, and nursing personnel challenged with the rigors of decision making and caring for geriatric oncology patients. It is a helpful resource for highly motivated pet owners. Its greatest contribution may be in the fields of end of life care (Pawspice), communication, attachment, the human–animal bond, decision making, bioethics, and philosophy. The H5M2 Quality of Life scale helps the veterinary team guide carers through the maze of decision making for their geriatric pets in Pawspice and hospice care.

Cases are presented that highlight issues in geriatric oncology and in the management of interpersonal relationships with various types of clients. This multilevel approach offers readers scientific subject matter, mixed with cases overlaid with situated knowledge harvested over many years of experience. Victory and frustration are inherent in the management of elderly oncology patients and readers are cautioned to recognize and avert compassion fatigue with uplifting self-care as a key wellness strategy.

This tour through geriatric oncology blends elements of attachment, the human–animal bond, end of life Pawspice, and hospice care with compassion. All facets of practice are woven into the reality of applying cancer therapy with empathy, adjusted for variable client preferences and financial situations. This is what veterinary teams do every day in practice. This book is a comprehensive resource for those learning how to do it better.

May this second edition help you negotiate the ebb and flow of emotions as senescent cancer patients and their deeply bonded families challenge and enrich your career.

Acknowledgements

This Second Edition of *Canine and Feline Geriatric Oncology* culminates my lifetime contribution to the veterinary profession. This book would not exist if it were not for the persistence of publisher-editor and book mentor Mr. Dave Rosenbaum. When Dave was with Iowa State Press, he and Bernie Rollin, PhD, coaxed me to step out of the "trenches" and take the time to write a much needed, different type of textbook. David insisted that the book be written in my own personal style. He awakened a sense of duty in me to give back to my profession. Dave asked me to share the wisdom and humility that 35 years in the trenches battling cancer had conferred upon me. Now it has been 45 years, and I am still in the trenches, soaring with hope for a new era in oncology. In the 1980s, we decreased FeLV infection and related lymphomas in cats by testing, elimination, quarantine, and vaccination. Thanks to brilliant research, we hope to help dogs with early detection and prevention of their most common cancers in the 2020s.

Thinking back to my roots, I thank my parents, siblings, and the good Sisters of St. Joseph of Carondelet for their teaching skills at St. John's Hyde Park and St. Mary's Academy in Los Angeles. I thank my botany teacher, Mr. Charles Luger, at El Camino Junior College. He replaced a stolen textbook and encouraged me to pursue my goals. I thank the late professor Julius Sumner Miller for his Einstein-like expertise in teaching college physics on a practical level. I thank Oscar Schalm and the amazing faculty at UC Davis Veterinary School in the late 1960s and 1970s. I thank my world class oncology mentor, Dr. Gordon Theilen, the first President of the Veterinary Cancer Society. This second edition is rededicated to him along with my beloved parents, Antonio and Alicia Villalobos.

I sincerely thank Dr. Frank Lux, who encouraged me to partner with him to open Coast Pet Clinic/Animal Cancer Center in 1974. Coast expanded rapidly into a 24-hour, 12 doctor, 70 staff member clinic, with four satellite cancer consultation clinics. I thank the late Dr. Bill Zontine, ACVR, who was my veterinary "dad" practice mentor. I am grateful for the friendship and encouragement of the late Drs. Greg MacEwen and Art Hurvitz, who inspired me with their brilliance and work at the Animal Medical Center in New York. I thank my founding colleagues, officers, and members of the Veterinary Cancer Society, who forged the specialty of oncology with unwavering dedication. I genuinely thank Dr. Sue Cotter of Tufts University and Angel Memorial for 45 years of friendship, guidance, and faith in me on and off the slopes. I thank the late Dr. Hal Snow, Drs. Jane Turrell and Alain Theon of UCD for their encouragement and enthusiasm in radiation oncology. I profoundly thank Ira Lifland, my best friend and unbelievably supportive husband since 1982. Ira fills my life with his love and intense multilevel support. In 1983, Ira, Hal, Jane, clients, and friends helped me build the first dedicated radiation therapy facility in private practice in the US after the banks declined to give me a loan for such an unheard of animal service adventure. These friends, along with my associates, interns, and the referring doctors of Southern California, helped me to pioneer one of the first comprehensive oncology services in private practice.

I thank Drs. Frank Lux, Curtis Willauer and Don Wood for their surgical oncology skills. I thank the following veterinary organizations for their energizing effect, while I learned, networked, and lectured at their meetings: VCS, American Association of Human-Animal Bond Veterinarians, Society for Veterinary Medical Ethics, ABROVET, ONCOVET, WVCC, AAHA, AVMA, ACVIM, NAVC, WVC, OVMA, CVMA, SCVMA, the late Dr. Bob Pensinger's Veterinary Post Graduate Institute, Sierra Veterinary Medical Association, and the National Academies of Practice.

I deeply thank my clients, John Peel and Laurel Hunt for nominating me for the 1999 Bustad Award, which ignited my career track into the science of the human–animal bond.

Thanks to editors Brian Hutchins, Marilyn Iturri, and Ken Niedziela at *Veterinary Practice News*, who managed my two columns: *Oncology Outlook, The Bond and Beyond*, and *Dr. Alice At Large*. I thank the legendary Dr. Robert Miller (RMM) for his mentorship and for starting the SVMA, which joyfully blended collegiality and skiing. I thank my mentors, Dr. Gordon Theieln of UC Davis, and the late Dr. Bill Zontine.

Thank you, Drs. Paul Pion, Jack Stephens, Robin Downing, Elizabeth Hodgkins, Frank McMillan, Curt Willauer, Chris Hutson, Kathleen Carson and Rachel Jones for your moral support, example, and inspiration. I thank all my career associates, interns, nurses, and staff who worked with me at Coast Pet Clinic/Animal Cancer Center, Pawspice and Animal Oncology Consultation Service. I will never forget the contributions of the late Peter Zippi, Brandi Romain, and Tammy Wood, RVT, who loved our patients.

I wholeheartedly thank Carreen Segal, RVT, my Pawspice partner. Carreen and I have worked side by side by for most of the past 35 years! Thank you, Roni Miyashiro, for your invaluable work as my assistant, and for management of our clinics for over 24 years! I thank our current power team: Miranda Becerra, Christine Lugo, Oner Orellana, Joyce Brown, and Daniel Williams, and our former staff RVTs: Gary Yumaico, Travis Bradley, Carol Merrigan, and Lisa Teague, and oncology assistants Bonnie McKinley, Beth Brussell, and Jennifer Dressler. I also thank Mao Mau LaBeet, Gus Nunez, Jose Alfaro, Lu Storier, and Wendy Triggs for their love, loyalty, and longtime devotion and service.

I joyously thank Leslie Neff, Larry Hoskinson, Linda Washburn, Margaret Norton, Maria and Wolfgang Petersen, Elisabeth Stone, and the entire amazing Peter Zippi Volunteer Club for caring and placement of over 15 thousand pets. The Peter Zippi Memorial Fund for Animals is a big part of my heart.

I thank Drs. Ira Gordon, Emi Ohashi, Leticia Gonzalez, Goksun Soysal, Tami Shearer, Dani McVety, Mary Gardner, Lide Doffermyre, Annie Forslun, and Kathy Cooney for our mentor–mentee relationships. I thank researchers and colleagues: Max Essex, Sue Cotter, Steve Withrow, Ted Valli, Guillermo Couto, Barb Kitchell, Jaime Modiano, Matthew Breen, VCS members and leaders, whose life work informs and inspires us. I thank Linda Hines, Chandi Duke Hefner, the UC Davis Global HealthShare® Initiative, and philanthropists worldwide who help humans, animals, and the environment in our One Health, one Medicine world.

Erica Judisch, of Wiley, twisted my arm and encouraged me to create this Second Edition, and I thank her persistence. My deepest appreciation goes to Laurie Kaplan, MSC, for editing the manuscript. Laurie contributed enormously to the First Edition by organizing my concepts, articles, lecture notes, and case studies into chapters. I am grateful for artwork provided by Andy Hoffman, Stephen Lewis, and David Perrot. Thanks go to Drs. Robson Pasquale, Annie Forslund, Kimberly Pope-Robinson, Sandi Grossman, and to Ellie Freedman, who contributed new sections for this text.

I thank the late Dr. Carl Osborne and the late Dr. Leo Bustad for emphasizing that compassion is essential in practice. Thank you, Dr. Robin Downing and the leaders of the International Veterinary Academy of Pain Management. I thank Dr. John Wright and members of the AAH-ABV for honoring the human–animal bond, the glue that holds us all together, and the SVME for centering me in bioethics. Special thanks to Dr. Dani McVety, for fleshing out my concept of "ethics fatigue" as separate from compassion fatigue for our profession to ponder. I thank colleagues who found their calling; to minister to end of life patients; to improve quality of life and palliative care; to provide Pawspice, hospice, and home euthanasia. Admiration and thanks go to the amazing leaders of the International Association of Animal Hospice and Palliative Care. Your collaborative efforts are fulfilling my dreams! And most importantly, I give heartfelt thanks to all pet carers who ask our profession to help their aging pets when threatened by cancer's fatal agenda.

Introduction

My people are destroyed from lack of knowledge.

Hosea 4:6

This book attempts to blend didactic oncology with end of life care for geriatric pets in a way that demystifies it for veterinarians and patient families. I accepted the provocative invitation to write this book in order to light a high-touch fuse for end of life care. This Second Edition rekindles the text, to fan the flames that now burn brightly in this arena. This book may serve as a torch or guiding beacon for veterinarians and staff to engage geriatric cancer patients as highly valued sentient beings. It may help prioritize honoring the humanity of the human–animal bond, as we deliver our modern medicine.

My career as a "trench oncologist" began in 1972 in battles and skirmishes against cancer at the forefront of the rapidly growing field of veterinary oncology. This work is intended to be a force for change, to fuse the art of our high-tech medicine with high-touch empathy and compassion.

Since cancer kills half of our aging patients, it is the single disease responsible for ending the life of millions of highly valued dogs and cats. Cancer breaks hearts in the companion animal community on a routine basis. The human–animal bond has emerged into a respected, life-enriching relationship in our contemporary society. The human–animal bond is validated and celebrated as a viable, healthy relationship, one that often takes a priority position in millions of people's daily routines, lifestyles, and economic choices. People purchase pet-friendly vehicles, motor homes, and homes so that their companion animals can share their lives and be with them as much as possible.

Pet owners are caregivers (carers). The word "family" is used broadly in this text to describe any situation that includes a pet. Family and carers can include singles, partners, and people with or without children who share the human–animal bond with pets. Carers have created the demand for dog parks, dog beaches, dog hiking paths, pet-friendly hotels, and pet service businesses, and a demand for more expertise in end of life care. While carers are at work or on vacation, they hire pet sitters to care for and entertain their animals. Doggie day care and high-end boarding facilities are geared toward quality care and pampering pets.

Today's enlightened carers willingly feel that they are their pet's parents and, figuratively (not legally) speaking, their guardians. Pet carers actively try to learn more about the emotions, thoughts, consciousness, and behavior of their pets. Carers are convinced that their pets think, have emotions, feel happy, sad, lonely, upset, stressed, and painful when injured or sick, and manifest grief when a companion animal or person dies. Carers want and need relief for their pet's ailments because their own quality of life is impacted negatively when a beloved pet is suffering. Pet carers need, demand,

and deserve compassion and understanding from their veterinarians, along with quality medicine and surgery.

When carers want something for their pets, they search the Internet and ask Siri, Google, or Bing. They seek services from specialty veterinarians, complementary and alternative treatments, and a wider growing attaché of pet care services (rehab, acupuncture, massage) to find comfort, help, and relief for their ailing pets.

Veterinarians contribute not only to the well-being and health of their patients; they have an equally large responsibility for supporting the well-being of the family. Until veterinarians fully appreciate this part of their role in society, they will continue to fall short of their obvious and central role in promoting the health and happiness of society through their pets. One of this book's two key themes is that veterinarians must reach out as much to pet carers as to the pet. Providing the best medicine is achieved when carers are educated to understand their pet's needs.

Pets age within a mere 10 years. Pet aging happens so quickly that most families are unaware that the routine activities of daily living may place too much demand on an older pet. Carers will often present their senior pets for examination when the pet is exhibiting only mild symptoms or non-specific preliminary signs of aging, illness, or cancer. Carers are concerned, but they do not understand the value of a thorough examination and screening tests for their aging pet with an increased risk for cancer. It is up to us to educate our clients.

Cancer often invades a pet's body insidiously, with only a few (if any) warning signs. When the diagnosis of cancer strikes a beloved pet, fear and anxiety fill the exam room. Unfortunately, these gripping emotions often fall on unwilling, deaf ears or they are dismissed impatiently by the attending doctor who is rushing from one exam room to the next in a busy practice. Much is left unsaid.

This book serves to reconstruct the initial steps when the veterinarian is working up or presenting the diagnosis of cancer. It can help that a first oncology consultation be a life-supporting and client-saving opportunity. This work can also help you understand how to keep your clients affectionately bonded to your practice, despite their pet's passing at your facility. Carers need to know that you care about what happens to their pets, and that you care about them.

In the past, an exam room scenario resembled an old Norman Rockwell painting or one of those beloved scenarios from a James Herriot book. Picture the wise Dr. Smith discussing Fido's cancer problem with Jane (the stay-at-home wife, one child in a stroller and another concerned child in hand). Jane explains Fido's problem to husband Joe at dinnertime, and Joe calls Dr. Smith to verify the gravity of the situation. The two men make the decision to put old Fido down. Times have certainly changed!

Today, the exam room scenario is often a single adult millennial, perhaps a man and his cat, consulting with a woman veterinarian. She explains a disease process and offers high-tech diagnostics and therapeutic procedures as options. Carers search the Internet and develop the confidence to assert themselves with their doctors, because they want to prolong their pet's life. This generates the need for further consultation, to answer a list of questions. Carers may not know how to inform their doctor that they are highly attached and willing to fulfill their sick pet's needs, to preserve the human–animal bond, even during the hospice setting while their pet declines at home.

Many pet carers have the willingness and ability to pursue diagnosis, staging, and therapy for their geriatric dog or cat, and will pursue referrals for specialty consultation and treatment. Others cannot afford costly diagnostics and treatment, or are philosophically against cancer therapy for their geriatric pet. However, many of these would fully want palliative care, hospice, and home euthanasia, if they knew about it.

Carers openly and proudly regard their geriatric pet as a family member who has loved them unconditionally for a long time. An older pet is often regarded as a "partner" or "best friend" or "family member" who helped their carers during difficult times. The human–animal bond is especially strong if the pet is a guide dog or involved in pet-assisted therapy, service work, agility, or show work. Many relationships with pets have outlived friendships, marriages, and helped ease the loss of family members.

It is up to the veterinarian to ask the client pointed questions to find out about the unique human–animal bond that they share with their geriatric pet with cancer. There is no doubt that veterinarians would be appreciated more by their clients if cancer could be detected earlier and treated with more forethought, expertise, and kindness.

The goal of this book is to provide readers with a useful decision-making tool. Like other resources, it spotlights the warning signs, and the most common forms of cancer in geriatric pets, and current treatment options. However, this text goes much farther. It unlocks the mystique about cancer, reveals pitfalls and adverse events that can be avoided, and arms readers with the ability to think through the variables and complexities of geriatric oncology. It gives examples of good communication skills in planning therapy based on the family's concerns, philosophy, and budget restrictions. This book introduces electrochemotherapy (electroporation) and yttrium-90 brachytherapy as novel options and provides the rationale for combinatorial palliative cancer care using various modalities such as metronomic chemotherapy, radiation therapy, immunotherapy, immunonutrition, and palliative end of life support to enhance and maintain a good quality of life. The book stresses the importance of quality of death, offering a protocol for peaceful passage. It also describes ways to provide emotional and grief support to the family during end of life care and after life. It offers colleagues another way to think about euthanasia as being truly a privilege to help our beloved patients peacefully transition, without feeling diminished. Last and very importantly, self-care strategies are presented to lift ourselves up to regain and sustain resilience so that we may continue our special calling for a fulfilled and loving career.

Veterinarians across the United States contact me daily to fill in the gaps left between the lines in their textbooks. This book tells what is often left unsaid in the exam room, and fills in the gaps left between the lines in textbooks about treating cancer. It is the only book dedicated to caring for geriatric oncology patients.

Part One

Chapter 1
Molecular Biology of Cancer and Aging

The roots of the problems of cancer and aging involve the molecular changes of aging priming aging (cellular senescence). These changes prime aging cells to be more susceptible to the effects of environmental carcinogens. These changes are only partly understood and may or may not be reversible.

Lodovico Balducci, MD

What Is Cancer? How Does It Start?

Hippocrates coined the name for malignant cancer from the Greek word for crab (*karkinos*), because tumors resembled the claws of a crab. Cancer is an insidious, nefarious, complex, obstinate, and disruptive disease. Cancer is an intricate set of biological aberrations that originate in the nucleus of cells that transform and progress with diverse heterogeneity, which is not completely understood. Cancer results in the uncontrolled and reckless growth of destructive cells that overwhelm the body as they accumulate. Cancer's immortal cells replicate relentlessly. They can use existing vessels or recruit cells to form new blood vessels via angiogenesis for nourishment. Cancer cells slip into the lymphatic and vascular systems and invade vital structures via metastasis to ultimately kill its host with its fatal agenda.

This chapter will attempt to describe the intricacies of cancer's malignant processes. Terms are defined and readers will be subjected to only a small taste of the alphabet soup milieu that drives the intracellular and extracellular microenvironment. As you read, keep in mind that this is an attempt to illustrate the essentials of a complex disruptive process and forgive or congratulate me if the text has oversimplified or exemplified cancer!

Normal cellular division creates a constant flow of injured genes. These defective genes are regularly corrected by innate repair mechanisms present in normal cellular function. Certain genetic point mutations become multifarious if they are not repaired. Genetic damage occurs in cells that lack coordinating signals necessary for self-repair. If genetically damaged cells escape innate detection and destruction and are allowed to live and replicate, cancer gets a foothold and then proceeds with its mechanistic drivers to grow and metastasize and disrupt vital functions.

Each of the trillions of cells that compose a body contains over one hundred thousand genes, arranged in chromosomes. The DNA that composes normal genes is called a "proto-oncogene." A proto-oncogene encodes all genetic information and regulates cell replication so that cells can replenish themselves normally in the bone marrow, intestine, skin, connective tissue, and organs when needed. Genes also regulate normal wound healing, hair growth, puberty, and gestation (Abeloff et al. 2004).

Canine and Feline Geriatric Oncology: Honoring the Human–Animal Bond, Second Edition. Alice Villalobos with Laurie Kaplan.
© 2018 John Wiley & Sons, Inc. Published 2018 by John Wiley & Sons, Inc.

About one in every million cell divisions undergoes a point mutation resulting in defective, aberrant, or altered genes that clone and initiate tumorigenesis. These genetic mutations can be seen by the immune system as copy errors and they are normally corrected by immunosurveillance. If the mutations are involved in the mechanism that controls repair, replication, proliferation, tumor suppression, or telomere (the terminal portion of genes, encoding programmed cell death) control, the defective genes are converted into oncogenes and their descendant cells take on a renegade behavior.

Cancer evolves on a cellular and sub-cellular level through three basic stages: initiation, promotion, and progression. *Initiation* involves exposure to carcinogens such as sun, tobacco smoke, alcohol, herbicides (2,4-D weed killer), insecticides, asbestos, free radicals, viruses, infections and so forth. This initial exposure may result in permanent damage "hits" to DNA. Initially this damage may not be a direct cause of cancer; however, continued exposure causes more gene "hits" and increases the risk of tumorigenesis. Tumor initiation and promotion is also seen in chemically induced tumors in experimental animals.

Promotion events are poorly understood. The *promoter* (an abnormal DNA base sequence in genes) stimulates cell division and results in the accumulation of cells that cause the formation of tumors. Aging, poor diet, obesity, toxins, smoke, and chemicals injure the stability of genes and are also considered potential promoters.

Progression to malignancy occurs when the tight controls that normally govern cell cycle progression are suppressed or break down. This results in the uncontrolled growth of abnormal immortal cells (cells that do not respond to normal cell death signals). Progression also involves the ability of cancer cells to initiate the formation of new capillaries (angiogenesis) to nurture growth. The most malignant cancer cells invade surrounding tissue, work their way into vessels and lymphatics and metastasize to distant parts of the body.

These events involve proteins that function by giving and receiving signals on the surface of the cell and along complex and intricate intracellular pathways in the process of cell-to-cell communication. Understanding the complexity and specifics of cell signaling and the alphabet soup that names the proteins and receptors can be overwhelming to the busy practitioner. There are basic families and systems of signaling that share certain pathways that aid and abet neoplastic changes. These basic mechanisms are fascinating and some have clinical relevance. Targeting aspects of these basic signaling mechanisms holds the key to promising therapeutics that will interfere with clonal evolution, progression, and relapse in cancer patients. Scientists attempt to manipulate the proteins that govern the intricate cell signals in ways to prevent, protect, and reverse cancer, especially in the senescent (Ihle 2004).

Tumor Suppressor Genes, Apoptosis, and Genomics

Tumor suppressor genes (*p53*) are responsible for repair of the hordes of copy errors and genetic damage that occurs during normal cell replication. When tumor suppressor genes malfunction, the risk of cancer rises. Tumorigenesis may also arise due to the loss of programmed cell death (apoptosis) signaling pathways. All normal cells have a certain life span dictated by telomere shortening after every division and suicide signaling. Suicide mechanisms to self-terminate can malfunction due to mutations of the signaling systems for apoptosis, causing cells to persist and become immortal. Scientists have identified the programmed death ligand 1 (PD-L1) gene, which promotes cancer by protecting cancer cells from T-cell mediated destruction. A ligand is a molecule on the cell surface that binds to another (usually larger) molecule. Researchers are very enthusiastic about using PD-L1 as a treatment target. Targeting PD-L1 and other tumor specific ligands is expected to provide great benefit in controlling aggressive and advanced cancer in patients in the future, with fewer adverse events.

Cell immortality is dangerous to the host. Armed with immortality and lack of suppression by tumor suppressor (*p53*) genes, these aberrant cells become malignant. They replicate and accumulate into clones of neoplastic cells. The clones undergo successive genetic changes that select for growth factors and chaotic replication. Malignant clones acquire the ability to create their own capillary blood supply (angiogenesis). These new capillaries provide nourishment and oxygen for new cell growth, thus allowing more abnormal cells to accumulate and create larger tumors. Tumors send their most vigorous, athletic scout cells into lymphatic vessels and capillaries. These resilient scout cells are able to slip under the radar of the immune system using checkpoint inhibitors that protect them from being detected and recognized for destruction by the immune system. The cells travel and metastasize into immortal tumor clonogens (cell clones or tumor stem cells that are more resistant to treatment). Clonogens may appear anywhere in the body (Khanna 2004; Morrison 2002).

Because renegade cancer cells have minimal cell death, do not curb their telomeres, and bypass senescence, they continue to divide and replicate tumultuously without repairing. Cancer cells grow wildly without control since they lack the ability to terminate themselves through apoptosis. In frenzy, they push, crowd, and dissolve their way into the society of normal tissue cells causing mayhem. *The battle against cancer is often won or lost at this microscopic preclinical stage.*

Most scientists realize that the real and decisive battle against cancer is truly fought at this molecular and immune system level, long before the tumor has expanded and accumulated enough cells to be detected. At this early, preclinical stage, a healthy, militant immune surveillance system could identify and eliminate every renegade cancer cell. Unfortunately, aging is associated with a weakened immunosurveillance system, leaving our geriatric patients at greater risk for cancer. New technology may enhance the immune system to detect and destroy malignant cancer cells.

Cancer genomics helps researchers identify the biological drivers of particular cancers. By blocking the effects of these drivers, targeted therapy may be able to inhibit cancer progression. Many human cancers have a correlation between the presence of certain genomic aberrations and the clinical outcome of the tumor and/or the tumor's response to therapy. Therefore, many chromosome aberrations are of prognostic value and the information generated via machine data collaboration may be used by clinicians to determine the most appropriate therapy. It is inevitable that veterinary oncology will benefit enormously from data derived from genomics and that this era will see a huge shift in the ways in which companion animal cancer patients are evaluated and subsequently treated (Breen 2009).

Cancer and Aging

Cancer is a disease, but aging is not. Aging is the phenotype of the normal phenomenon of cellular senescence. Carcinogenesis is a nefarious multistep process that takes time. Aging animals provide that time as their life span increases. Cancer's multistep process, enhanced by a longer exposure to carcinogens, emerges as a major syndrome associated with aging. Basic molecular and genomic research proposes many reasons for the increased incidence of cancer in older animals. Aging is associated with a decline in antitumor defenses. Older animals have less resistance, less immune competence, less DNA repair, more damaged tumor suppressor genes (*p53*), reduced numbers and function of mitochondria, and defects in biological responses. Aging is associated with diminished functional reserve of multiple organ systems, sarcopenia (muscle loss) and an increase prevalence of chronic diseases, which may cause frailty and stress, causing the geriatric body to be more susceptible to cancer.

Certain proteins or cytokines such as interleukin-6 (IL-6), D-dimer, and C-reactive protein (CRP) are found to be elevated in the aging process. D-dimer is a product of fibrin lysis and CRP is an acute phase protein produced in the liver. These cytokines increase with inflammation and age-related conditions such as osteoarthritis. Cancer creates an immune challenge, which drives the activation and release of a cascade of cytokines including tumor necrosis factor (TNF-α, cachexin), which is responsible for creating the hypermetabolic state of cachexia. TNF-α, IL-6, D-dimer, and CRP also increase with cytokine signaling induced by inflammation, infection, cancer, thromboembolism, and acute illness.

These factors are likely to be responsible for the higher incidence and mortality rate from cancer in older and geriatric companion animals. Cancer cells proliferate with anarchy and defiance of the normal constraints that keep cell growth and division in check. Cancer instigates cytokine dysregulation and a domino effect as it disrupts the aging body.

Research hopes to provide new molecular and genomic detection and prevention methods to target and tackle the intricate cytokines and signaling steps of cancer as it evolves. The goal would be to "target" cancer out of existence at the precancerous stage, before it embarks on its fatal course. One day, we may be able to provide dogs and cats with immunoprophylaxis using preventative cancer vaccines, and chemoprophylaxis using tumor specific agents (Modiano 2016).

One Medicine and Cancer Awareness

Human and animal cancers and diseases often share a similar pathogenetic process. Companion animals are often good comparative models for human cancer. This concept fueled the "One Medicine" philosophy, which was strong in the late 1960s to 1970s. The One Medicine concept has reemerged in the last decade with universal vigor and it is universally supported by the CancerMoonShot2020 campaign. Client education regarding prevention and awareness of risk factors can help companion animals live longer and avoid some cancers. Educating pet owners about carcinogenesis, and the preliminary stages and early warning signs of cancer may help save millions of beloved pets. A well-informed clinician, using improved diagnostics in a timely fashion, can help clients with geriatric pets identify and treat cancer in its earliest stages, which may offset its devastation.

The most obvious tumors in elderly dogs and cats appear on the body surface, in the skin, in the subcutis layer below the skin, or fixed to the body wall. Cutaneous cancers may appear as tumors, ulcers, non-healing sores or petechiae (pinpoint blood blisters). They may appear as plaques or crusts on the ears, eyelids, and nose and in the non-pigmented skin of sun-exposed senior cats and dogs. The contemporary veterinarian will not suggest, "Let's wait and see if it grows." It is justifiable to examine every mass on a geriatric pet (other than obvious warts) with fine needle aspiration (FNA) cytology to determine whether the mass is truly a lipoma, inflammation, a mast cell tumor, or a malignant tumor. Read the section on cytology.

Epigenetics, Environmental Influences, Toxins, and Risk Factors

Epigenetics is the study of how genes are switched on and off. The multistep process of cancer development over time explains why we see more cancer in aging animals. One Medicine researchers view animals as sentinels that parallel human diseases and cancers that result from environmental exposure. Certain environmental factors have been found to cause inflammation and epigenetic changes that initiate and promote cancer. It may take many years for environmentally induced cancer to develop in people whereas the same exposure may take less time to cause cancer in companion animals. Overall, cancer risk increases with exposure, time and age. The most well-known environmental risk factors for cancer in people are smoking, snuff and betel nut chewing, obesity, lack of exercise, unhealthy eating habits, occupation, viruses, family history, alcohol, toxins, asbestos, ultra-violet light (tanning beds), sun, radiation exposure, prescription drugs, reproductive factors, pollution, and unknown causes (medicinenet.com/cancer/article.htm). Infection with human papilloma virus (HPV), human immunodeficiency virus (HIV), hepatitis B and C infections, and *Helicobactor pylori* are associated with cancer worldwide. Certain food additives such as preservatives, nitrates, chemicals, and aflatoxins are known to be carcinogenic. These carcinogens are associated with epigenetic changes causing gastrointestinal (GI), hepatic, and bladder cancer in humans and are presumed to create similar risk for exposed companion animals as they age.

Certain dogs and cats also have additional breed predispositions to environmental toxins. For instance, Scottish Terriers are 20 times more susceptible to bladder cancer than other breeds of dogs and are at greatest risk if exposed to 2,4-D lawn herbicides (Raghavan et al. 2004). Cancer is promoted in the skin by solar radiation in white cats and dogs. They develop squamous cell carcinoma (SCC) because the non-pigmented skin of the feline face and canine ventrum is highly susceptible to "hits" that result in mutations from solar exposure. Cancer is promoted in the lymph nodes by toxins and retroviruses, and iatrogenically by local inflammation and neoplastic transformation resulting from adjuvanted feline leukemia virus (FeLV), rabies virus vaccines, and other injections (Ford 2004; Macy 2004).

Cats ingesting particulate residue from cigarette smoke contaminating their fur are at greater risk for developing oral and GI cancer (Snyder, Bertone, and Moore 2001). Cats exposed to smokers lick carcinogens deposited on their coats and thus are at increased risk for oral squamous cell carcinoma. Cats exposed to smokers are also at greater risk for lymphoma of the GI tract. Lymphoid tissue, reproductive organ tissue, and growth plates may be more susceptible to epigenetic changes and mutagenesis by their inherent nature. Lymphoid cells may undergo genetic damage through mechanisms triggered by environmental radiation and toxins. Exposure to 2,4-D weed killer is associated with greater risk of lymphoma in dogs. Obviously, there are many more environmental factors in modern living that may influence epigenetic changes and the multistep genetic mutations that transition into cancer's development that threatens the lives of dogs and cats as they age.

Risk factors related to size, breed, and age play a role in development of bone cancer (osteosarcoma), which most frequently appears in the growth plates of the long bones of late middle-age to senior large breed and geriatric giant breed dogs, while being rare in small dogs and cats. Reproductive tissue is at risk of developing cancer over time. Mammary tissue is sensitive to hormonal influence in female dogs of most but not all breeds as most are protected from breast cancer if their ovaries were removed by 2 years of age. Some publications speculate that sex hormones may have a protective role due to an increased incidence of cancer in dogs neutered at young ages versus intact dogs (Hart et al. 2014).

Immuno-Oncology or Onco-Immunology

There is tremendous research interest in immune checkpoint pathways in the growing arena of "Immuno-Oncology" or "Onco-Immunology." Research has revealed how the T-cell immune response receptors, given the name programed death-1 (PD-1) receptors, that normally should detect and destroy tumors cells, are suppressed by dual ligands called PD-L1 and PD-L2, which are on the surface of cancer cells. Scientists found that cancer cells also suppress and downregulate the T-cell's cytotoxic mediators that should destroy them and that cancer cells create an immunosuppressive microenvironment (www.discoverthepd1pathway.com). This One Medicine immuno-oncology information has prompted the development of targeted therapy agents to stop the PD-L1 and PD-L2 ligands from connecting with PD-1 checkpoints and allow T-cells to continue immunosurveillance. The ability to use checkpoint inhibitors to gain information on efficacy and adverse events in clinical trials in veterinary medicine will bring benefit to humans and companion animals in the battle against cancer (Nass and Gorby 2015).

Retroviral and Infectious Disease in Cancer

Retrovirus infections, such as FeLV and feline immunodeficiency virus (FIV), cause diseases related to immune suppression and lymphoma in cats and rank as the main cause of infectious morbidity in cats. Papilloma virus causes self-limiting transmissible oral papillomas in young dogs. As yet, no virus has been found to cause other cancers in dogs.

Cancer is augmented by retroviruses that are found in many animal species, from mice to birds to cats to cattle to primates to humans. Retroviruses enter the body and cause mutations in susceptible cells. Cats have the feline sarcoma virus (FSV). FeLV and FIV both cause mutations in lymphocytes, immunosuppression, anemia, pancytopenia, leukemias, and lymphoid tumors. Thymic tumors and lymphadenopathy were seen in young to middle aged cats before the late 1980s and currently most lymphomas primarily affect the gut in older cats. FeLV also causes chronic wasting, abortions, and fading kitten syndrome (Theilen, Madewell, and Gardner 1987; Pedersen et al. 1987).

A large survey found the prevalence of FeLV and FIV each at 3% in the cat population (Little 2005). Some cats survive into their geriatric years while remaining retrovirus infected. Both FeLV and FIV attack the immune system, causing a drop in the number and activity of T-cells. This results in opportunistic infections, anemia, and weight loss similar to acquired immune deficiency syndrome (AIDS) in humans with HIV. Testing and vaccines are available for cats at risk. The FIV vaccine currently available obfuscates detection of truly infected cats due to false positive results following vaccination. Kittens of vaccinated queens test positive up to 3 months of age due to passive transfer of antibodies (MacDonald et al. 2004).

Canine lymphoma occurs in 83% of all canine hematopoietic (blood-related) malignancies and makes up 7–24% of all canine cancers (Vail, Pinkerton, and Young 2013). It is not associated with a virus or an acquired immune deficiency syndrome. Boxers are more likely to have T-cell lymphoma, whereas Rottweilers are more prone to B-cell lymphoma than other breeds (Lurie, Lucroy, and Griffey 2004). Infection with *Helicobacter* may stimulate immune responses that may promote GI lymphoma in humans. The increased incidence of lymphoma found in Golden Retrievers may hypothetically be related to infection with *Bartonella* and stimulation of specific immune responses. However, more research relating infectious disease to cancer in companion animals requires extensive epidemiologic studies and sophisticated testing.

All animals have a specific gut microbiota that operates in balance. Dysbiosis is a state of altered microbial community that disrupts the symbiotic relationship and causes or contributes to disease or dysfunction. Polymerase chain reaction (PCR) gene amplification and research technology may verify the hypothesis that certain infectious diseases and variations in the gut microbiome content may contribute to tumorigenesis. Although evidence is emerging in this area, more research is necessary to elucidate the role of the gut microbiota in pancreatic, laryngeal, and gallbladder cancers in addition to colorectal cancer in humans (Kelly et al. 2016). No doubt that companion animal cancer patients will benefit from this very interesting research in dysbiosis, which may also shed light on the microbiota's relationship to cancer malnutrition and cancer cachexia.

Endocrine Influences in Tumorigenesis

Endocrine, autocrine, and sex hormones also play a role in tumorigenesis when stimulatory signals occupy the normal cell membrane receptors of target tissues. Altered tissue growth factor genes can also promote cells toward transformation. Dysregulation of normal growth regulatory pathways, ligand binding, and constitutive activation of transmembrane tyrosine kinase receptor activity all promote carcinogenesis.

A practical example of this altered microenvironment is the carcinogenic effect of progesterone on the mammary tissue of intact female dogs and cats. Many but not all breeds of intact dogs are at risk for developing mammary tumors as they age. The risk is minimal with early ovariohysterectomy (OVH) and reduced if OVH is by $2^1/_2$ years in dogs. Carcinomas can be iatrogenically initiated in mammary tissue with progesterone therapy in cats. Testosterone plays a similar causative role for perianal tumors in intact male dogs. However, sex hormones may confer a protective effect against hemangiosarcoma and OSA, as speculated by publications that find a decreased rate of these tumors in intact dogs (Hart et al. 2014).

Feline Injection Site Sarcoma (FISS)

Adjuvanted vaccines containing killed FeLV and rabies virus with aluminum hydroxide were implicated to act as carcinogenic promoters of normal inflammatory oncogenes in some genetically predisposed cats in the early 1990s. Localized postvaccinal panniculitis that progressed to persistent inflammatory reactions caused malignant transformation at vaccine sites, initiating promitogenic (pro cell division) signaling and genetic mutations and translocations. This genetic damage occurs in the C-myc oncogenes and C-kit oncogenes. They become activated and replace normal oncogenes, resulting in the unregulated stimulation of fibroblasts. If tumor suppressor genes (antioncogenes, antisense) such as the ubiquitous p53 genes are damaged, there is too little self-inhibition and autonomous cell death. Consequently, in a variable time period from 4 months to 15 years, vaccine-associated inflammation may ultimately direct mutation and mutagenesis of reactive fibroblasts that undergo the intricate phenomenon of transition into malignant high grade fibrosarcomas or other types of sarcomas. The location was most commonly in the interscapular region and the incidence is somewhere within 1/1,000 and 1/10,000 of vaccinated pet cats (Ford 2004; Macy 2004). FISS is deceptively invasive with a very high recurrence rate postsurgically. Cats that were treated with surgery, radiation, and chemotherapy and gained long term survival endured metastasis at a rate of 22%. The Vaccine-Associated Feline Sarcoma Task Force was formed in 1996 and worked with The American Association of Feline Practitioners to change vaccination practices and to address issues and disseminate information. It was disbanded in 2005. However, a survey in Canada did not find a decrease in FISS prevalence from 1992 to 2010 despite recommended changes in feline vaccination protocols. This raises the ethical debate for veterinarians to explain options to clients so that they may decide which product safety profile they would prefer to use for their cat (Wilcock, Wilcock, and Bottoms 2012).

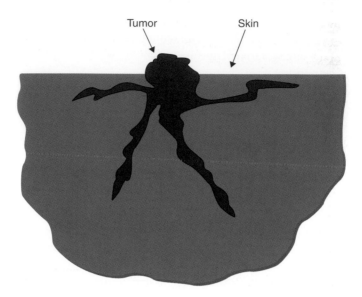

Figure 1.1.   This cartoon displays the octopus-like shape of a cancerous mass with its head and streaming tentacles that extend into the normal tissues.

How Cancer Kills

Cancer kills because of its freedom from regulatory constraints, which allows for its persistent unrestrained growth that develops resistance to treatment. Cancer overtakes its victims with its exponential cell kinetics. After only seven to eight doublings, the cells of a tumor will reach a critical volume that becomes incompatible with host survival. Cancer patients die due to the rapid exponential growth and metastasis of their tumors.

A tumor one cubic centimeter in diameter (about the size of a grape) contains one billion cells, of which 10% are blood vessel cells undergoing angiogenesis to feed and oxygenate the tumor cells that enables them to metastasize. Many tumors, especially soft tissue sarcomas, develop tentacles that use enzymes such as metalloproteinase to dissolve cell walls and invade adjacent normal tissues. They invade tissue along the fascial planes or by direct extension applying pressure to surrounding structures such as nerves, vessels, and organs. It is easy to visualize a cancerous mass as an octopus, with its palpable head and its streaming cells acting as the tentacles that insidiously reach into and invade normal tissues (Figure 1.1).

Cancer also kills by altering and stealing sugar and carbohydrate nutrition from its victims to feed its own troops of invading renegade cells. Cancer-induced weight loss is an involuntary cancer–host interaction resulting in cancer cachexia. Pets with thick fur coats and older geriatric dogs and cats with age-related sarcopenia and mild to moderate geriatric cachexia may camouflage the debilitating condition of cancer cachexia in its early stages.

Mechanisms of Metastasis

Metastases is the spread of cancer cells to new areas of the body. Metastatic lesions arise either by direct spread and invasion into areas immediate to the primary tumor and/or by cellular travel to distant locations, primarily to the lungs, liver, and spleen in animals and humans and including the bones in humans. The prognosis for metastatic cancer (generally called Stage IV cancer) is generally poor. The cancer cells that venture out into the circulatory system from primary or secondary tumors to metastasize can be thought of as the most outgoing and vigorously athletic cancer cells from a malignant tumor. Metastatic cells creep and slip into adjacent lymphatic and vascular channels. This creeping process is called diapedesis. These resilient cancer cells defy host immunosurveillance and travel via the lymphatics and circulatory system to distant locations in the body. Microscopically, scientists can see small clumps of cancer cells sending out "scout" cells that undergo diapedesis as they creep out of the primary tumor.

Cancer cells can destroy their surrounding stroma by dissolving the walls of their neighbor cells with a signaling system that regulates lysis by metalloproteinase enzymes. The cells squeeze through or between endothelial cells and pass into and creep along the walls of capillaries or vessels of the lymphatic system. These scout cells are the immortal "marathon runners" of the clone and are the most resistant to destruction. These "marathon" malignant cells must detach from the primary tumor and its extracellular matrix and defy normal death by *anoikis* (apoptosis due to loss of cellular contact). The initiation and execution of *anoikis* is mediated by different pathways, all of which terminally converge into the activation of caspases and downstream molecular pathways, culminating in the activation of endonucleases, DNA fragmentation, and cell death. The induction of the *anoikis* program occurs through the interplay of two apoptotic pathways, the intrinsic pathway, which is the perturbation of mitochondria, or the extrinsic pathway, which involves triggering cell surface death receptors (Paoli, Giannoni, and Chiarugi 2013). However, cancer cells defy the normal programed cell death pathway of *anoikis* as they take on immortal properties and become cancer stem cells, which are resistant to most conventional cancer therapies due their "stemness."

The marathon cancer cells escape their matrix and slip into the circulation system under the radar of the immune system and go on to lodge and create micrometastases in a new site with tougher, more resistant progeny cells. These cells react to the microenvironment signals that allow them to divide and survive with acquired immortal properties. Cancer cell signaling recruits endothelial cells for neoangiogenesis and they grow and accumulate into a detectable metastatic mass (Khanna 2004).

In part, the ability of a neoplasm to grow exponentially is due to the fact that metastases can further metastasize. This biological phenomenon can be used to explain to pet owners why metastatic lesions found in the lungs, liver, bone marrow, or brain are more resistant to the previously used first line chemotherapy and radiation therapy treatments.

The "liquid biopsy" is a new test that can detect metastatic cancer cells in the blood using a chip device that captures cancer cells with antibodies attached to carbon nanotubes. In the future, "liquid biopsy" tests may be able to diagnose cancers at earlier stages and yield their genomic information to customize treatment based on the specific markers of the patient's cancer (Khorsravi et al. 2016). New advances in precision based immunotherapy may be able to halt the neoplastic process during the development of metastasis (www.CancerMoonShot2020.com).

Angiogenesis

Angiogenesis is a normal regulated process that takes place during wound healing, gestation, and growth. We would all look like Frankenstein if we did not heal properly. The microenvironment of cancer cells allows signals for pathological neoangiogenesis. Cancer cells create new blood vessels and capillaries to feed and bring oxygen to their progeny of growing renegade cells. One mechanism may involve recruiting angioblasts and circulating endothelial precursor cells (EPCs) as with hemangiosarcoma and other solid tumors (Lamerato-Koziki et al. 2005). However, "inducing angiogenesis" is not an essential hallmark of all cancers. Some non-angiogenic tumors use or co-opt and exploit preexisting vessels and newly formed ones to feed themselves as they grow and metastasize. This finding adds more complexity and raises the question of the relative importance of angiogenesis versus preexisting vessels in the high proportion of cancers containing both. It is hard to pinpoint how much angiogenesis and how much pre-existing vessels are contributing to tumor growth. These findings are therefore seriously questioning the idea that all tumors will respond to antiangiogenesis therapy (Pezzella et al. 2015).

Without angiogenesis, most tumors cannot enlarge beyond a few millimeters or become large enough to be detected on radiographs and imaging scans. This is why antiangiogenesis agents are intriguing to use. This approach is especially kinder and gentler for geriatric cancer patients because there is a low adverse event profile when prescribed as metronomic chemotherapy. However, since not all tumors depend on angiogenesis, it would be great to have a diagnostic test that can differentiate as to which patients will benefit from metronomic therapy aimed at inhibiting angiogenesis.

Why Are There So Many Kinds of Cancer?

Researchers recognize at least 200 types of cancer – that is approximately as many cancers as there are types of tissue in the body. Each individual's cancer is different in terms of its prognosis and treatment. Its properties depend on the type of tissue from which it arose and on which tissues it subsequently invades. The names and terminology for various cancers are generally based on the cell of origin. Each type of cancer has its own name with specific unique variations, characterizations, and behavior. This information forms the premise for most practicing oncologists in that if we can name a cancer, we can diagnose it and stage it and understand and predict its biologic behavior in a specific patient. Geriatric patients have one more layer of complexity due to the aging process and associated comorbidities. Cancer can be classified into five basic groups: carcinomas, sarcomas, blood cancer, central nervous system (CNS) cancer, and cancers of miscellaneous or unknown origin (Table 1.1).

Tissue biopsy and/or fine needle aspiration (FNA) cytology provide the cell morphology or structural characteristics that enable us to determine the cell type of a specific tumor for diagnosis. Intricate tests that examine the DNA array of tumors and that stain cells for certain protein markers are needed to identify the genetic phenotype of cells that are microscopically and morphologically indistinguishable from one another, such as T-cell and B-cell lymphomas.

The nomenclature that is used in oncology and pathology has its origins in Latin and Greek. Pathologists will change terminology and classifications from time to time. The words and acronyms describing the molecular biology of tumors and the mechanisms of targeted drug action used in the field of oncology and tumor immunology represent by far the largest alphabet soup and the most confusing terminology in medicine.

An understanding of oncology requires familiarity with tumor tissue origins and with the names and various biological behaviors of each cancer, based on its general tissue type. The biopsy report specifies the type of cancer and this is synonymous with its diagnosis. Staging the cancer tells us something about the size of the primary tumor, whether it is localized or has infiltrated local lymph nodes or regional nodes, and if it is metastatic to distant locations in the body.

Table 1.1.   Common Terminologies and Abbreviations for Basic Types of Cancer Based on Tissue of Origin

General Tissue of Origin	Specific Tissue of Origin	Basic Cancer Type (Terminology/Abbreviations)
	CARCINOMA (CA)	
Skin/epidermis (ectoderm)	Squamous cell: skin, tonsil, respiratory	Squamous cell carcinoma (SCC)
	Basal cell	Basal cell carcinoma (BCC)
	Wax glands	Adenocarcinoma (AC)
	Sweat glands	Sebaceous gland AC; ceruminous gland AC
		Apocrine gland AC
	Anal sac	Anal sac AC
	Reproductive tissue	
	Breast	Breast cancer (MGAC)
	Prostate	Prostatic AC
	Uterus	Uterine AC
Glandular tissue with ducts or tubes (endoderm)	Testes (may produce sex hormones)	Sertoli or interstitial (Leydig) cell carcinoma
	Ovaries (may produce sex hormones)	Ovarian granulosa cell tumor
	Respiratory tract	Respiratory AC
	Gastrointestinal tract	Intestinal AC
	Hepatobiliary: liver, bile duct	Hepatocellular (HC), cholangiocellular carcinoma (CC)
	Kidney	Renal cell AC (RCC)
	Bladder	Transitional cell carcinoma (TCC)
		Endocrine tumors
Hormone-producing ductless glands (may produce paraneoplastic syndromes)	Thyroid gland	Thyroid AC
	Adrenal gland	Pheochromocytoma, adrenal AC
	Pituitary gland	Pituitary AC
	Pancreas	Pancreatic AC
	Heart	Heart base tumor (HBT)
	SARCOMA (SA)	
	Fibrous connective tissue	Fibrosarcoma (FSA)
	Vascular: endothelial cells, angioblasts	Hemangiosarcoma (HSA)
Connective tissue (mesenchymal)	Vascular: pericytes	Hemangiopericytoma (HPCT)
	Skeletal muscle	Rhabdomyosarcoma (RMS)
	Smooth muscle	Leiomyosarcoma (LMS)
	Peripheral nerve	Schwannoma (neurofibrosarcoma) (nerve sheath tumor) (NTS)
	Bone and joint	Osteosarcoma (OSA); synovial cell sarcoma
	Plasma cells	Multiple myeloma; IgM macroglobulinemia
Combination of epidermal and neuroendocrine tissue	Melanocytes containing melanin granules	Malignant melanoma, melanosarcoma (MM)
Allergy cells in skin; gut	Mast cells containing vasoactive chemicals	Mast cell tumor (MCT) Mastocytoma, mastosarcoma

(continued)

Table 1.1.   (*Continued*)

General Tissue of Origin	Specific Tissue of Origin	Basic Cancer Type (Terminology/Abbreviations)
BLOOD CANCERS		
Blood-forming cells	Hematopoietic cells	Leukemias
	Lymphoid cells (in cats +/− retrovirus)	Lymphomas (T-cell, B-cell) (lymphosarcoma) (LSA)
	Lymphoid cells	Cutaneous lymphoma (T-cell, B-cell) (epi- or non-epitheliotrophic) (CL)
	Hemangioblasts/angioblasts (Pluripotent stem cells of bone marrow)	Hemangiosarcoma
CENTRAL NERVOUS SYSTEM (CNS)		
	Brain	Brain tumors
		Meningioma
Central nervous system (Neuroendoderm)		Glial, ependymal, neuronal, and embryonal tumors
	Pineal gland	Pituitary tumor
	Choroid plexus	Choroid plexus carcinoma
	Spinal cord	Spinal tumors
MISCELLANEOUS OR UNKNOWN CELL OF ORIGIN		
	Dendritic cells (Histiocytes)	Histiocytosis
	Macrophages	Malignant (MH); systemic (SH); cutaneous (CH)
	Pleomorphic, bizarre fibroblast-like and/or histiocyte-like cells with spindle and round cell characteristics	Malignant fibrous histiosarcoma (MFH) (solitary or multicentric)
Unknown cell types of the immune system	Histiocytic round cells	Transmissible venereal tumor (TVT)
	Pleomorphic atypical lymphoid cells	Pulmonary lymphomatoid granulomatosis (PLG)
	Monocytes	Unknown
	Langerhans cells	Unknown
	Plasma cells that produce IgG or lambda light chains in the cytoplasm	Plasmacytoma, reticulum cell sarcoma, Merkel cell tumor of neuroendocrine origin, atypical histiocytoma, cutaneous plasma cell tumor
Mesoderm (mixed epithelial/mesenchymal)	Epithelial lining cells of coelomic cavities	Mesothelioma
Thymic epithelium	Thymus	Thymoma (infiltrated with mature lymphocytes)

Imaging helps us to acquire more diagnostic details for staging purposes and surgical or radiation treatment planning. The biopsy report also allows the histologic grading of tumors (I, II, III), and states if it is well, moderate, or poorly differentiated, in the hope that this will help the clinician predict their biological behavior. Naming, staging, and grading are considered essential in order to make decisions and plan cancer treatment. However, in veterinary medicine, some patients' carers do want advice, even if they cannot afford staging.

Diagnostic Molecular Technology

Genomics tools have developed rapidly since the publication of the complete canine genome sequence in 2005 by researchers at the Broad Institute of MIT and Harvard (www.broad.mit.edu/mammals/dog). In combination with resources allowing wider access to tumor tissue and the ability to conduct clinical trials, the stage is set for rapid advancement of knowledge about canine diversity, disease genes and pathways, aging, cancer susceptibility, and importantly lymphoma. One Medicine researchers know that dogs are a great lymphoma model because they share many significant similarities with human non-Hodgkin lymphoma and learning more will benefit dogs and humans (Richards and Suter 2015).

Some malignancies grow so rapidly that they are difficult to classify by cell type. They are called "un" or "de" differentiated. In such cases, immunohistochemical stains can help to classify cells for diagnostic and subsequent therapeutic purposes. All cancers have a gene signature and new technology assays will reveal their identity. The pathologist will offer these stains when necessary. It is a good idea to pursue the newer sophisticated genomics diagnostic testing such as that offered by Innogenics™, which will advance the accuracy of diagnostics and help determine if a tumor has a high or low metastatic potential and provide information to improve treatment planning and prognosis. The Innogenics Enlight™ assay technology offers personalized biomarker and genomic information with treatment options for dogs (www.innogenics.org).

When applicable, tumor markers can be used to identify certain types of neoplastic cells. Tumor markers, which are generally specific antigens, may be found in tissue samples and in serology samples from the patient. Pathologists can now identify certain growth factors and receptors in tumor tissue that can be used for the development of therapeutic strategy as well as to determine disease prognosis. Markers found in blood are commonly used in human cancer patients following treatment to monitor for recurrence. Markers may be positive when a tumor is clinically undetectable but they may also rise due to other factors. This situation places clinicians in a quandary. If the clinician cannot locate the tumor, should he or she interpret rising positive markers as recurrence or as background cross-reactivity? This conundrum frustrates decision making for attending doctors and all concerned. Ruling out other causes and good clinical judgment should prevail.

Our profession has the availability of exciting new tests such as the mast cell tumor (MCT) panel and genetic profile testing. The MCT panel runs all the special stains for MCT markers. Early indications suggest that a panel of markers like the MCT panel may be helpful in predicting the biological behavior of a patient's initial tumor. Following tumor markers sequentially may enable early detection of microscopic recurrence. With this information, however, comes the responsibility of ethical and practical decision making. The clinician must deal with the inherent lack of specificity of some tumor markers and still make the call to treat or not to treat the patient for suspected recurrence (see Chapter 8). This quandary places a huge responsibility on clinicians. Should we treat to be safe rather than sorry? Should the considerations be modified for aging pets?

New technology using gene arrays (maps) will enhance our ability to know the molecular details of specific tumors. Soon oncologists will be able to characterize cancers further by genetic markers and mechanisms that may express one growth factor over another or a certain enzyme or cytokine. This information will benefit cancer patients with improved modes for targeted therapy. Detailed testing with gene arrays may be affordable and routinely available for veterinary patients in coming years. Practitioners will need to comprehend the gross terminology in the field of oncology and stay abreast of the ever-increasing ability and advantages of delving into the molecular structures and functions involved in neoplasia with emerging technology and therapy.

We may change our approach to cancer and treatment philosophy in the future. With new diagnostics and treatment options such as: antiangiogenesis agents, nanoparticles, gene therapy, targeted therapy, stealth antibody therapy, and checkpoint inhibitors, we may soon be able to address cancer on general terms and ambush its basic molecular mechanisms. In the future, we may be able to prevent common cancers such as lymphoma, hemangiosarcoma, and osteosarcoma in dogs with prophylactic vaccine cocktails. We may one day abandon the conventional standard approach to crisis oncology that dictates us to ask, "What is it? Where is it? Now let's cut it out, irradiate it, or poison it."

Aberrations in oncogenic pathways are the fundamental underpinnings of cancer phenotypes. These are shared between human and canine lymphomas in many cases. As more targeted therapies become available, understanding which genes are dysregulated and which are "Achilles heels" for a particular type of cancer becomes increasingly important.

What Are Sarcomas, Carcinomas, and Adenocarcinomas?

Sarcomas are malignancies that originate in connective tissue. Soft tissue sarcomas (STSs) arise from connective tissue other than bone. STSs are tumors that originate in the connective tissue found in skin, muscle, vasculature, and fibrous tissue. These tumors belong to a large group of tumors and are often treated similarly (Table 1.2). Because people can see and feel the entire body surface of their pet animals, family members or the groomer initially discover many STSs.

Sarcomas of bone are osteosarcoma, chondrosarcoma, synovial cell sarcoma, and tumors arising from any other bone constituent. In addition, any other tumor type including metastatic adenocarcinomas may infiltrate bone. Pet owners often misunderstand the basic concept of metastasis to the bone. They may say, "My father died of bone cancer, now my dog has it," when in fact, the father had metastatic prostate cancer that invaded the pelvic bone. The same is true for metastatic breast cancer in women. Clients tell us that their mother or sister died of lung or bone cancer, but it was actually metastatic breast cancer. Animals do not have as high an incidence of bone invasion from metastatic cancer as humans do. Most likely, either animal cancer patients do not survive long enough for the metastasis to occur or their bones are endowed with some unknown sanctuary mechanism. Bone cancer in dogs is an identical model for bone cancer in humans. The study of molecular mechanisms of mutation and sarcomagenesis in multiple species may result in prevention therapies (C3O, 2016, http://bit.ly/2cur1M2).

Table 1.2.   Soft Tissue Sarcomas of Clinical Significance in Dogs

Mast cell tumor	Malignant melanoma
Nerve sheath tumor (Schwannoma)	Hemangiopericytoma
Fibrosarcoma	Hemangiosarcoma
Neurofibrosarcoma	Plasmacytoma
Myxofibrosarcoma	Rhabdo(myo)sarcoma
Myxosarcoma	Malignant fibrous histiocytoma
Fibroma (invasive)	Liposarcoma
Synovial cell sarcoma	Reticulum cell sarcoma

Blood Cancer

Blood is a connective tissue and sarcomas of hematopoietic cells are commonly referred to as blood cancer or leukemias and lymphomas. They are further classified as to the type of leukemia by the cell of origin: lymphoblastic, chronic lymphocytic, myelogenous, acute myelogenous, granulocytic, multiple myeloma, plasma cell, erythrocytic, and so forth. There are numerous types of non-Hodgkins lymphomas (NHL) in dogs and cats and they sadly cause high mortality. The World Health Organization (WHO) system of classification for canine NHL is currently used with an 83% accuracy amongst 17 pathologists (Valli et al. 2011).

As clinicians, we are familiar with large cell, blastic, cleaved cell, small cell, T-cell, B-cell lymphoma in dogs. It is helpful to differentiate lymphomas by immunophenotyping during the workup phase in dogs. This would provide a more accurate expectation of response and overall prognosis, since T-cell lymphomas, which are more common in Boxers, are more resistant to standard treatment. Feline lymphomas are classified according to the National Cancer Institute working formulation (Valli et al. 2000). The *Veterinary and Comparative Oncology Journal* published Volume 14 as a supplement devoted exclusively to canine and feline lymphoma in August 2016, with an editorial by D.J. Argyle and F. Pecceu. This special supplement issue brought together key publications on lymphoma and serves as an excellent reference.

Carcinomas and Adenocarcinomas in Dogs and Cats

The terms "carcinoma" (CA) and "adenocarcinoma" (AC) generally apply to cancer that arises in the epithelial tissues of skin and body organs. People often use "carcinoma" synonymously with "cancer" because 80–90% of human cancer cases are carcinomas. ACs originate in abnormal gland cells that are in the lining or inner surface of a cavity or organ. Adenomas are benign tumors of gland cells that, over time, may transition into malignant tumors. ACs and adenomas may originate in any part of the body. The skin and delicate mucous membranes are commonly affected in senior pets. Dogs are prone to develop sebaceous, apocrine (anal sac), perianal, ceruminous, salivary, and sweat gland tumors, while cats are prone to basal cell tumors.

Breast cancer, which is sex hormone related, is commonly encountered in intact female dogs or in dogs spayed after $2^1/_2$ years of age. It is less common in cats. Squamous cell carcinoma (SCC) that appears in lightly pigmented facial skin of cats and in the glabrous skin of lightly pigmented dogs is solar induced. However, SCC also appears in the oral cavity, tongue, tonsils, esophagus, nasal and paranasal sinuses, respiratory tract, and nail beds. Some reports have associated tonsillar SCC in dogs with environmental pollution and oral SCC and GI lymphoma in cats with exposure to coat-associated carcinogens from cigarette smoke.

ACs in the abdomen may originate from glands such as the liver, colon, intestine, stomach (gastrinoma), kidney, bladder, pancreas, prostate, and adrenal. Widespread dissemination of cancer in the abdomen and throughout the rest of the body is often termed as "carcinomatosis." The term may also include other tissue types. AC may also originate from any gland in the neuroendocrine or reproductive system such as the thyroid glands, pancreas, adrenal glands, pituitary gland, ovaries, uterus, testicles, and prostate. These tumors often cause paraneoplastic syndromes related to their cell products. Anal sac AC is well known for causing malignant hypercalcemia. However, other malignancies, especially lymphoma, may also cause this potentially life-threatening paraneoplastic syndrome.

Nasal AC in pets may extend past the ethmoid plate into the brain. Primary CNS brain tumors are very pleomorphic. Only choroid plexus tumors of the brainstem, which are poorly responsive to treatment, are classified as carcinomas. AC may appear in the ciliary body in the eye and occasionally in the glands of the eyelids.

Aortic body (heart base tumors, chemodectoma) and bronchogenic AC originate in the chest cavity. Bronchogenic AC is often found as a round solitary mass in the caudal chest. If it is located in the distal lung lobe without nodal metastases, affected dogs may have good survival times following lobectomy. Cats rarely have primary lung cancer, but when they do, it is generally found to be SCC, which may metastasize to the digits and resist treatment.

Mesotheliomas originate from the epithelial lining of the pleura, pericardium, and peritoneum. They originate in the chest and abdominal cavity, causing malignant effusions. In humans, mesotheliomas are associated with asbestos inhalation. They are rare in dogs and cats – most mesotheliomas diagnosed in pets are actually ACs.

Pulmonary lymphomatoid granuloma (PLG) is a rare condition categorized as a precancer that may confuse the clinician. It occurs in middle-aged dogs, appears as massive pulmonary involvement with very large nodules, and infiltrates similarly to an end stage AC or sarcoma. It is important to distinguish this disease from AC as most cases of PLG respond nicely to treatment and have a favorable prognosis despite the enormity of the lesions.

Some malignant tumors have cells that are so undifferentiated or "dedifferentiated" that the pathologist can only report them as anaplastic carcinomas with no indication of the cell type of origin. This was the case with Alfie, the author's $11\frac{1}{2}$-year-old Australian Shepherd. Ultrasound-guided FNA cytology of Alfie's mass revealed two populations of bizarre cells appearing to be both carcinoma and sarcoma. The histopathologic diagnosis was undifferentiated carcinoma with no definite gland of origin. Direct visualization at exploratory laparotomy disclosed that Alfie's carcinoma was hepatic in origin.

The biological behavior of most ACs is aggressive with a persistent tendency for metastasis. Most ACs expand to a detectable size by outward growth (like an onion) and by direct extension into local tissue. The cells use matrix metalloproteinase enzymes to dissolve neighboring cell walls for local invasion. Through diapedesis, AC cells gain entry into lymphatic and capillary vessels and then disseminate throughout the body.

Locoregional recurrence and lymph node invasion are common, followed by widespread metastasis (Figure 1.2). Metastatic AC generally appears as nodular cell clones in the lungs, liver and other abdominal structures, brain, and eyes. AC may further metastasize to bone and dermis (Figure 1.3). On rare occasions, AC may metastasize to the digits in cats. German Shepherd dogs may develop a rare form of renal AC, classified as cystadenocarcinoma, which causes the bizarre formation of multiple benign fibrous nodules in the skin.

ACs are commonly visualized as fluffy, or milliary, infiltrates or nodules in chest X-rays of pets in advanced stage disease. Some pets develop pulmonary effusion and hemoptysis (coughing up blood). Nasal cancer patients exhibit chronic unilateral nasal discharge and/or frank hemorrhage (epistaxis). Some dogs and cats develop occult disease with warning signs of coughing, gagging, exercise intolerance, or dyspnea due to pulmonary compromise from the metastatic disease process.

What Can Be Done to Halt Cancer in Pets?

Until recently, the overall goals of research and therapy in veterinary cancer medicine have been twofold: firstly, to cure or palliate existing cancer while leaving the patient with a good quality of

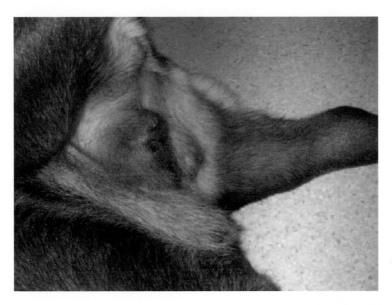

Figure 1.2.   This large primary mammary gland adenocarcinoma caused edema and swelling of Bear Brown's perineum and legs.

life and, secondly, to prevent cancer cells from colonizing in the body. However, with the Cancer-MoonShot2020 tremendous optimism has been revived in the potential benefits of immunotherapy. Scientists are finding ways to awaken or to relieve suppression of the immune system's job to detect and destroy cancer cells. They also have developed technology to "train" the immune surveillance system of the body to kill cancer cells at any stage of disease, including advanced stage patients that are considered terminal.

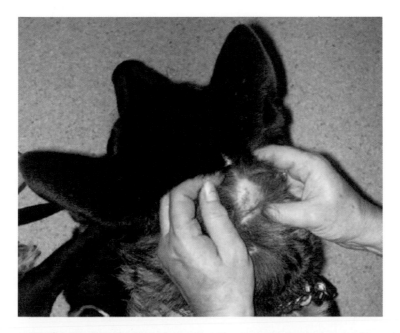

Figure 1.3.   12-year-old F/S Akita, Bear Brown, with a metastatic mammary gland adenocarcinoma lesion in the skin of her dorsal neck.

Proposed ways to win the battle against cancer also include chemoprevention and nutritional concepts such as "starving the cancer cells while feeding the patient." Another approach is to use supplements that support the immune system and microenvironment on a preventative basis. Some supplements may have antineoplastic or protective effects in helping the liver to function and detoxify. Some act as antioxidants that scavenge free radicals. The terms immunonutrition and chemoprevention are used when discussing this approach by this author.

Future therapies for cancer may control it through medications that will cripple its aberrant angiogenesis capabilities or cripple its ability to create lytic enzymes and cytokines. For example, "targeted" gene therapy, such as the small molecule protein kinase inhibitors, may become the norm. Inhibitors of angiogenesis such as Avastin® block vascular endothelial growth factor (VEGF) by injection. Oral metronomic chemotherapy and multitargeted tyrosine kinase inhibitors such as masitinib, toceranib, dasatinib, AngioStop®, etc., that have antiangiogenic activity will be included in combinatorial protocols. Drugs that inhibit metalloproteinase enzymes prevent cancer cells from dissolving neighbor cell walls to slow invasive behavior. Some of these agents may be given for permanent maintenance therapy or used in chemoprevention protocols.

Innovative treatments such as precision or personalized therapy, with vaccines or specific gene therapy, may be used to control cancer by correcting replication defects. In gene therapy, special genes are transfected into bacterial, viral or cellular vectors and injected into the patient. These therapeutic genes then signal the cells of cancer patients to produce specific proteins that will, it is hoped, suppress or destroy the tumor. In antiangiogenesis gene therapy, proteins such as endostatin and angiostatin may be used to arrest the angiogenesis process. Gene therapy may offer several ways to fight back at the microscopic level where cell-to-cell signaling in the neoplastic battlefield is most crucial. Researchers are also studying the use of stem cells in cancer therapy to help replace bone marrow and organs that may have been destroyed by treatment or by the neoplastic invasion.

It is quite possible that, in the near future, the use of surgery to "cut and slash" at tumors, chemotherapy to "poison" cancer cells (along with trillions of healthy cells innocently undergoing cell division), or radiation therapy to "burn" cancer cells (along with millions of innocent normal bystander cells) will become methods of the past.

One approach that uses natural or synthetic substances to prevent cancer by interrupting mutation, oncogenesis, angiogenesis, and metastasis is called "chemoprevention" or "chemoprophylaxis" by mainstream conventional medicine (Bergman 1999). An example of chemoprevention for women at high risk for recurrent breast cancer would be the use of antiestrogen medications such as tamoxifen and raloxifene (Love 2000). Another example of chemoprevention is the use of calcium supplements to decrease the risk of colorectal cancer in humans (Popchain 2004). Research will identify more helpful compounds that may protect or offer support for geriatric pets against cancer. The use of metformin to enhance the efficacy of chemotherapy by suppressing the multiple drug resistance gene (MDR1) is an example of repositioning existing drugs and placing them in combinatorial protocols. (MacDonald et al. 2015)

There are millions of microscopic skirmishes between immune cells and cancer cells in a body on a daily basis. Macrophages, NK (Natural Killer) cells, and cytotoxic T-cells operate by signal cell transduction. Much of this action takes place on cell membranes while the intracellular signaling systems are affected. The body's surveillance cells and tumor suppressor genes (especially *p53*) work for the immune system and can eliminate renegade cancer cells if they are activated, trained, or empowered and if they can avoid being suppressed by tumor cell ligands. It is at this cellular microenvironment level, the microscopic proteomic, metabolomic field, where the true battle against cancer is won or lost. It is here that the battle should be fought, not when a tumor is already established.

Nutritional and holistic treatment promotes prevention and balance with the use of a healthy diet and supplementation with natural substances such as fatty acids, antioxidants, supplements, and nutraceuticals. The agents used are known or believed to operate at the cell surface signaling level to work on the immune system and/or to protect or detoxify various organs and systems to prevent or lower the risk of cancer. Data regarding the efficacy of large-scale trials is available online from ClinicalTrials.com.

A significant segment of the pet-owning community is drawn toward nutrition and holistic medicine for the prevention and/or ancillary treatment of cancer in aging pets. These methods are popular with the people who believe in them; however, Western medicine remains skeptical as few controlled clinical studies can verify claims. Holistic, alternative, and complementary medicine and its many branches of nurturing therapies may have a positive contribution to make in the overall care and well-being of the cancer patient. The holistic approach attempts to care for the entire patient and enhance the quality of life by decreasing uncomfortable symptoms and feelings, seeking to balance the body's systems including emotions, and supporting the immune system. Holistic medicine also actively addresses the nutrition of patients on a preventative and therapeutic basis. There are various types of alternative and holistic medicine including acupuncture, chiropractic, massage therapy, homeopathy, and herbal medicine. Some approaches are under justifiable scrutiny by the watchful and the skeptical, but clinicians should be aware that when faced with advanced and aggressive cancer, the pet carer is often compelled to seek information beyond his or her local veterinarian's scope or comfort zone. It is estimated that 8–10% of human cancer patients whose diagnosis has been confirmed by tissue biopsy decline mainstream therapy (Love 2000). This may be true for pet owners as well. This is viewed as potentially harmful to the patient if the pet owner foregoes the opportunity for curative conventional therapy.

The quest to self-educate with information from the Internet may confuse worried caregivers initially. However, eventually their quest and your consultation and recommendations will empower them with the information needed for comprehensive, personal decision making for their pets. Ultimately, practitioners may use the best from both worlds by combining and interdigitating the most successful conventional treatments with the most supportive complementary treatments to palliatively extend a dear pet's life. This blending and delivery of many different types of medical knowledge is called "integrative medicine." Taking an integrative approach to help their geriatric pet with cancer will most likely be welcomed by your clients.

Much Is Left Unsaid and Unaddressed

Cancer is the grim reaper of geriatric pets. Cancer colonizes from genetic error and environmental insult through the steps of initiation, promotion, and progression. When cancer becomes clinically obvious in a geriatric oncology pet, the battle to save that pet's life will require skill (both interpersonal and medical) and luck. The decisions made at the onset of clinical detection often dictate the ultimate fate of that pet. Those decisions include not only clinicopathological considerations of the patient but also considerations of emotional and psychosocial sensitivities of the family. These issues may exist with any geriatric oncology case presenting at early, middle, and advanced stages of disease.

This book illuminates emotional and decision-making issues in geriatric oncology that are often left unaddressed in textbooks. It will also clearly outline the information that each pet owner should acquire from a consultation with the primary veterinarian and then, on a more specialized level, from their referral veterinarian. There is a cry for help to the veterinary profession from deeply bonded pet owners because many of their needs, including clear clinician-to-client communication, emotional support, pet pain control, and end of life care issues, such as when to enter a hospice, are not handled properly.

Too often, vital interactive information is lost or forgotten in the hurry through exam rooms. Attending doctors, staff, and carers leave much unsaid that needs to be said. Veterinarians who learn to mindfully listen to their clients, and understand attachment, and how the human–animal bond factors into the geriatric pet–cancer equation, will gain a tremendous potential for enriching their practice. Veterinarians, who devote time to compassionately transfer vital "soft" information to their care-giving clients, truly serve the needs and expectations of the companion animal community in our society.

Ageism

Ageism, or bias against old people and old animals that limits medical options to extend life, is not uncommon in our modern society. Shelters are always getting old animals that people do not want any longer or cannot afford. You may not know that your client might be afraid that you will not help their geriatric pet because of its old age. Of course, ageism undermines our ethical duty to always act in the best interests of the patient, geriatric or not! Finessing complex cases with fastidious care will avoid many complications, especially in patients with comorbidities and advanced disease.

As doctors and healers, we need to have the discussion that offers the option of Pawspice, akin to human palliative medicine, which treats the primary cancer in kinder gentler ways and addresses symptoms. The use of metronomic chemotherapy is a kinder, gentler, and effective approach that may benefit cancer patients without the adverse events related to standard chemotherapy (Mutsaers 2014). We must also recognize when further treatment is futile and offer clients the option of true hospice, which is palliative comfort care that does not treat the cancer. When our patients show signs that they are actively starting to die, we need to emphasize the value and the purpose of the hospice vigil and assist the family in decision making for euthanasia. These principles will help ease the bumpy road that is end of life.

Physiologic and Chronologic Aging Variability

There is no straightforward method for defining the age at which dogs and cats become "senior" or "geriatric." Of the two species, dog aging is more difficult to pin down due to genetic variability, breed longevity, environmental influences, body weight, and whether or not the dog is obese. Overfeeding and obesity have been shown to reduce the longevity of dogs by 2 years. This may be true for obese cats as well. One study found that almost 30% of our nation's senior dogs were overweight. By 12 years of age, only 5% of dogs were overweight, and 16% were underweight (Donoghue 1991). The ravages of age interacting with the molecular events and genetic mutations that generate cancer may be potentially reversible with treatment.

Clients often ask, "How can I estimate my pet's age in comparison with human aging?" A 1-year-old medium-sized dog has accelerated maturation and is comparable to a 15-year-old teenager. During the middle years, the aging process slows down, adding only 4 years per 1 human year. During the last 25% of a pet's life, aging accelerates.

"Senior" is a term that softens the concept of aging and flows well into "geriatric." "Senior" prepares pet owners to witness the comparatively accelerated aging of their beloved companion animals. The term "senior" is commonly used to describe dogs over the age of 7 years and cats over the age of 9 years.

I propose that large dogs be considered senior after 5 years of age and giant breed dogs be considered senior after $4^{1}/_{2}$ years of age. Using the term "senior" to describe dogs and cats that have reached 60% of their life expectancy seems reasonable.

"Geriatric" is defined as the state of being in the last 25% of one's life expectancy (Abeloff et al. 2004). The term "geriatric" is commonly and arbitrarily used to describe dogs and cats over 8 years of age, even though cats and small breed dogs live longer than large and giant breed dogs. The life expectancy for cats and small dogs (less than 20 pounds) is 9 to 13 years. The life expectancy for medium-sized dogs weighing 21–50 pounds is $9–11^{1}/_{2}$ years. Large dogs weighing 51–90 pounds have a life expectancy of $7^{1}/_{2}–10^{1}/_{2}$ years. Giant breed dogs weighing over 90 pounds have the shortest life expectancy, only 6–9 years.

For this text, all cats, and dogs weighing under 90 pounds, that are over 8 years of age, and all giant breed dogs over 5 years of age, are considered geriatric. Clients are enlightened when they see comparable aging tables showing the variations between animals and humans by species and weight. A combination of several comparable aging charts for pet cats and dogs stratified by weight was prepared for this text to illustrate the ranges of opinion (Table 1.3).

We often encounter exceptions to the rule when we see chronologically old pets that are physiologically youthful. Some geriatric animals are not afflicted with the usual arthritis, spondylosis, nuclear sclerosis, visual and hearing deficits, muscle loss, and cognitive dysfunction of their counterparts. This vitality may be the best reason, next to financial limitations, that explains why geriatric medicine is applied on a somewhat arbitrary basis from one clinician to the next.

The clinician who fails to recommend health screening for a senior or geriatric pet because the pet is physiologically youthful deprives that patient of the potential benefits of an early diagnosis of cancer. The synergism of cancer with aging involves the molecular changes of aging that prime senescent cells to the effects of environmental carcinogens (Balducci 1994). We must individualize our management approach to suggest preventative screening for early detection of cancer in our geriatric patients. A protocol composed of personalized therapy utilizing guidance from cancer genomics testing and combinatorial modalities may best control cancer while maintaining a good quality of life for each geriatric patient.

Incidence

There are currently more than 170 million pets in the United States and each year more than one million dogs are treated for cancer (www.nap.edu21830). Cancer kills 50% of all dogs over the age of 10 and one in four dogs under the age of 10. Cancer kills one-third of the feline population.

A 1998 Gallup Poll found that 39% of the 58 million dogs that were in the general population were "senior" and that 47% of the senior group was considered "geriatric." The US dog population increased from 65 million to 80 million between the first and second editions of this text. Now we can estimate that the senior dog population increased from 25.35 million to 32 million and that the geriatric dog population increased from 12 million to 15 million. Since half of dogs over the age of 10 develop cancer, this translates into 6–7.5 million canine cancer patients that our relatively small profession may potentially encounter in the US. Osteosarcoma was diagnosed in 8,000 dogs in the US each year before 2005 (Eldredge and Bonham 2005). However, current estimates note an increase to 10,000–12,000 dogs diagnosed with bone cancer per year in the US. Bladder cancer accounts for

Table 1.3.   **Comparative Aging Chart for Cats and Dogs**

Chronologic Age	Human Age Equivalent for Feline	Canine by Weight				
		0–20# 0–9kg	21–50# 10–23kg	51–90# 24–41kg	91–120# 42–54kg	>120# >54kg
		Human Age Equivalent for Canine in Years				
3 months	5	5	5	5	5	>5
6 months	8–10	10	10	10	10	>10
9 months	12	11	11	13	15	>15
1 YEAR	15–24	12–15	14	16	20	>20
2	21–24	19	21–24	23	26	>26
3	25–42	25–28	25–29	24–34	28–39	>39*–40
4	29–32	32	32–34	35–42	43–49	>49*
5	33–48	32–36	36–39	43–49	40–58	>59*
6	37–40	40	40–44	44–49	49–69	>69*
7	41–44	44	47–49	50–55	62–79	>79*
8	45–57	48	50–54	56–63	64–89	>89*
9	49–52	52–53	56–59	61–68	71–99	>99*
10	52–56	56–57	60–64	68–73	79–87	
11	56–60	60–63	65–69	72–76	88–95	
12	61–66	64–67	69–74	77–83	96–102	
13	66–70	68–70	74–79	84–88	103–108	
14	71–74	72–73	78–84	88–94	109–114	
15	75–80	76	83–89	94–99	115–122	
16	80–84	80	87–94	99–104	123+	
17	85–89	84	92	104–108		
18	90–94	88	96	109–114		
19	95–98	92	101	115–120		
20	99–102	96	105	120–123		
21	102–105	99	109			
22	105–108	102	113			
23	?	104	117	**GERIATRIC**		
24	?	107				
25	?	109				
26	?	112				
27	–					

Source: This table is a compilation of several comparative aging charts by William Fortney, DVM, Director of Community Care at Kansas State University School of Medicine; Ron Kurtus, School for Champions, 2005; Fred Metzger, DVM, ABVP, State College, PA, for Senior Care Vet. Ec. Supplement, 1998; Alice Mills, DVM; and Feline Medicine, DVM, Best Practices, 2002. The table was adapted by Villalobos to reflect patient population 12-17-16.

Note: Physiological differences exist between cats and dogs when using their chronologic age. In dogs, the breed, size, and weight create further differences between chronologic and physiologic aging. This table is a compilation of aging tables showing comparable aging for cats as well as for small, medium, large, and giant dogs per standard weight. Overweight and obese dogs have a greater comparable age and shorter life span than normal-weight dogs.

*Information from William Fortney.

2% of all canine tumors and can affect up to 20,000 pets each year, with Scottish Terriers being at 19 times greater risk (www.nap.edu21830). It can be estimated that as many as 2.5 million dogs may die from hemangiosarcoma overall (Lamerato-Koziki et al. 2005). Pet cats in the US increased from 77.6 million to 90 million. The estimated prevalence of cancer-related death in the geriatric cat population is approximately 32%. It is plain to see that there is an increasing demand for expertise in canine and feline geriatric oncology and compassionate end of life care is upon our profession. This trend is worldwide.

Preventable Tumors in Geriatric Pets

As companion animals age, they develop many of the same types of tumors that are found in humans. Since pets do not smoke cigarettes, they do not often get lung cancer. There is epidemiologic research from Tufts University and Amherst College, however, showing that cats exposed to carcinogenic cigarette smoke are at greater risk of developing certain cancers. Their surveys found that smoking for 3–5 years in the presence of cats increases their risk for oral and lingual SCC and for GI lymphoma by three to five times. Cats consume coat-associated carcinogens in the form of smoke particles that settle on their fur. It has been shown that smoking stimulates COX-2 in mucus membranes as a mechanism of carcinogenesis. A few reports claim that dogs living in cities where air pollution is heavy may be at a higher risk for tonsillar SCC.

The most preventable cancers in dogs are mammary, ovarian and uterine, testicular, and perianal. Female dogs spayed before the first heat period are protected from reproductive organ cancer for life. Male dogs neutered under 4 years of age are spared testicular and perianal tumors (some of which are malignant).

Another preventable cancer that afflicts the skin of dogs and cats is solar-induced skin cancer. Any unpigmented skin that is exposed to an excess of sun undergoes "field cancerization." The entire field of exposed skin is more prone to develop actinic SCC or cutaneous hemangiosarcoma. Application of daily sunscreen, keeping pets in the shade, or keeping them indoors during the heat of the day will deter skin cancer. Lesions appear as pets age due to the cumulative genetic damage from solar exposure and field cancerization.

The future may bring us tumor prevention vaccines for common malignancies in companion dogs and cats. If these vaccines can reduce the incidence of hemangiosarcoma from one in five Golden Retrievers down to one in sixty or reduce the incidence of lymphoma from one in eight to one in eighty Golden Retrievers, that would demonstrate excellent prevention efficacy (Modiano, World Veterinary Cancer Congress, Brazil, 2016).

Summary

Understanding theoretical cancer biology, genomics, immuno–oncology, and senescence is essential for the contemporary veterinarian who treats geriatric cancer patients. The increasing association of cancer with senescence places our aging pet population at greater risk for the many manifestations of neoplasia. How cancer, and its treatment, impacts and affects the geriatric oncology patient is paramount when offering options. Managing cancer in the oldest portion of our diverse pet population is only anecdotal at this time. Because pets are living longer and the human–animal bond, as a celebrated relationship, has created extremely devoted pet caregivers, there is an increasing demand and need for more information and expertise in veterinary geriatric oncology. Caring for geriatric oncology patients is an arena where academic know-how must be blended with good clinical judgment, compassion, and honor for the human–animal bond.

Soon new applications against cancer will involve improved diagnostics, combinatorial therapeutics along with the early and routine use of immunoprophylaxis, chemoprophylaxis, and gene therapy.

The genetic codes for dogs and cats are available for imaginative and hypothetical research. It may soon be possible to correct breed-related predispositions to certain cancers. Perhaps some day we will be able to perform genetic adjustments for pets at risk for cancer. Perhaps, through gene therapy, we will be able to prevent mast cell cancer for Boxers, Bulldogs, and related breeds and reduce the cancer risk for lymphoma and sarcomas in cats and Golden Retrievers. Perhaps we can reprogram large and giant dog breeds to sidestep osteosarcoma and hemangiosarcoma. Frankly, I look forward to the day when the eradication of animal cancer will put my Animal Oncology Consultation Service and Pawspice practices out of business!

> Medical genetics is rapidly developing. I suspect someone looking at the new edition of Ettinger and Feldman a hundred years from now will laugh at what we all had to say. We must remain alert to growth and changing paradigms in medicine.

> *Stephen Ettinger, DVM, ACVIM*

References

Abeloff, M.D., J.O. Armitage, J.E. Niederhuber, M.B. Kastan, and W.G. McKenna. 2004. *Clinical oncology*, 3rd edn. Philadelphia, PA: Churchill Livingstone.

Balducci, L. 1994. Do we need geriatric oncology? *Cancer Control: Journal of the Moffitt Cancer Center* 1 (2):91–94.

Bergman, P.J. 1999. Differentiation and chemoprevention: Fact or fiction? *17th Annual ACVIM Forum Proceedings*, pp. 388–390.

Breen, M. 2009. Update on genomics in veterinary oncology. *Top Companion Animal Medicine* August; 24 (3):113–121, doi: 10.1053/j.tcam.2009.03.002.

CancerMoonShot2020.org, 2016.

Clinical Trials.com. www.clinicaltrials.com. Search for tumor type and drug.

C3O. 2016. *Consortium for Canine Comparative Oncology Proceedings* (http://bit.ly/2cur1M2).

Donoghue, S. 1991. Providing proper nutrition for dogs at different stages of the life cycle. *Veterinary Medicine* July.

Eldredge, D.M., and M.H. Bonham. 2005. *Cancer and your pet: The complete guide to the latest research, treatments and options*. Sterling, VA: Capital Books, Inc.

Ettinger, S. 2005. An interview with Dr. Stephen Ettinger. *Veterinary Medicine*, pp. 88–90.

Ford, R. 2004. Vaccine protocols: Change is in the wind. *Merial Symposium Booklet, 141st AVMA Annual Convention Notes*, pp. 40–46.

Hart, B.L., L.A. Hart, A.P. Thigpen, and N.H. Willits. 2014. Long-term health effects of neutering dogs: Comparison of Labrador Retrievers with Golden Retrievers. *PlosOne*.

Ihle, J.K. 2004. "Intracellular signaling." In *Clinical oncology*, 3rd edn, eds M.D. Abeloff, J.O. Armitage, J.E. Niederhuber, M.B. Kastan, and W.G. McKenna, pp. 19–45. Philadelphia, PA: Churchill Livingstone.

Kelly, D.L., D.E. Lyon, S.L. Yoon, and A.L. Horgas. 2016. The microbiome and cancer: Implications for oncology nursing science. *Cancer Nursing* 39 (3):E56–E62.

Khanna, C. 2004. Advances in our understanding of cancer: Explanations for your clients. *Merial Symposium Booklet, 141st AVMA Annual Convention Notes*.

Khorsravi, F., P.J. Trainor, C. Lambert, G. Kloecker, E. Wickstrom, S.N. Rai, and B. Panchapakesan. 2016. Static micro-array isolation, dynamic time series classification, capture and enumeration of spiked breast cancer cells in blood: The nanotube-CTC chip. *Nanotechnology* 27 (44): 44LT03. doi: 10.1088/0957-4484/27/44/44LT03.

Lamerato-Koziki, A.R., K. Helm, S.C. Helfand, and J.F. Modiano. 2005. Innovations in the diagnosis of canine hemangiosarcoma. Personal Communication, *VCS NL* 29 (1).

Little, S. 2005. Feline retrovirus testing and management update. *DVM News*, July, p. 70.

Love, S.M. 2000. *Dr. Susan Love's breast book*, 3rd edn. Cambridge, MA: Perseus Publishing.

Lurie, D.M., M.D. Lucroy, and S.M. Griffey. 2004. T-cell-derived malignant lymphoma in the Boxer breed. *Veterinary and Comparative Oncology* 2 (3):171–175.

MacDonald, K., J.K. Levy, S.J. Tucker, and P.C. Crawford. 2004. Effects of passive transfer of immunity on results of diagnostic tests for antibodies against feline immunodeficiency virus in kittens born to vaccinated queens. *JAVMA* 223 (10):1554–1561.

MacDonald, V., Gaunt, V., Arnason, T., Davies, G., Harkness, T., 2015. Validation of adjunct use of metformin in reversing multiple drug resistance (MDR) biomarkers in canine lymphoma. *VCS Proceedings*, p. 59.

Macy, D.W. 2004. The big, the bad, the ugly: Fibrosarcomas. *Merial Symposium Booklet, 141st AVMA Annual Convention Notes*, pp. 47–53.

Modiano, J.F. 2016. Innovations in cancer treatment and prevention with immunoprophylaxis and chemo-prophylaxis. *3rd World Veterinary Cancer Congress Proceedings*, Brazil.

Morrison, W.B. 2002. *Cancer in dogs and cats: Medical and surgical management*. Jackson, WY: Teton New Media.

Mutsaers, A.J. 2014 State of the art: Metronomic chemotherapy: Theory and practice, *VCS Proceedings*, p. 36.

Nass, S.J. and Gorby, H. 2015. *The role of clinical studies for pets with naturally occurring tumors in Translational Cancer Research: Workshop Summary*, 83 pp. North West Washington, DC: National Academies Press. (www.nap.edu21830).

Paolo, P., E. Giannoni, and P. Chiarugi. 2013. Anoikis molecular pathways and its role in cancer progression. *Biochimica et Biophysica Acta (BBA) – Molecular Cell Research* 1833 (12):3481–3498.

Pederson, N.C., E.W. Ho, M.L. Brown, et al. 1987. Isolation of T-lymphotropic virus from domestic cats with an immunodeficiency-like syndrome. *Science* 235:790–793.

Pezzella, F., A.L. Harris, M. Tavassoli, K.C. Gatter. 2015. Blood vessels and cancer much more than just angiogenesis. *Cell Death Discovery*, Editorial, Article No. 15064, doi:10.1038/cddiscovery.2015.64.

Popchain, M.B. 2004. *What your doctor may not tell you about colorectal cancer*. New York: Warner Books.

Raghavan, M., D.W. Knapp, M.H. Dawson, P.L. Bonney, and L.T. Glickman. 2004. Herbicide exposure and the risk of transitional cell carcinoma of the urinary bladder in Scottish Terriers. *JAVMA* 224 (8):1290–1297.

Richards, K.L., and S.E. Suter. 2015. Man's best friend: What can pet dogs teach us about non-Hodgkin lymohoma? *Immunology Review* 263 (1):173–191.

Snyder, L.A., E.R. Bertone, and A.S. Moore. 2001. Environmental tobacco smoke exposure and p53 expression in feline lymphoma. *Veterinary Cancer Society Proceedings*, p. 5.

Theilen, G.H., B.R. Madewell, and M.B. Gardner. 1987. "Hematopoietic neoplasms, sarcomas and related neoplasms." In *Veterinary cancer medicine*, eds G.H. Theilen and B.R. Madewell, pp. 345–381. Philadelphia, PA: Lea & Febiger.

Vail, D.M, M.E. Pinkerton, and K.M. Young. 2013, Hematopoietic tumors. In *Withrow and MacEwen's Small Animal Clinical Oncology*, eds S.J. Withrow, D.M. Vail, and R.L. Page, pp. 608–637. St. Louis, MO: Elsevier Heath Sciences.

Valli, V.E., R.M. Jacobs, A. Norris, C.G. Couto, W.B. Morrison, D. McCaw, et al. 2000. The histologic classification of 602 cases of feline lymphoproliferative disease using the National Cancer Institute working formulation. *JV Diagnostic Investigation* 12:295–306.

Valli, V.E., M. San Myint, A. Barthel, D. Bienzle, J. Caswell, F. Colbatzky, et al. 2011. Classification of canine malignant lymphomas according to the World Health Organization Criteria. *Veterinary Pathology* 48:198–211. doi: 10.1177/0300985810379428.

Wilcock, B., A. Wilcock, and K. Bottoms. 2012. Feline postvaccinal sarcoma: 20 years later. *Canadian Vet Journal* 53 (4): 430–434.

Suggested Reading

Abbas, A.K., A.H. Lichtman, and S. Pillai. 2014. *Cellular and molecular immunology*, 8th edn. Saunders/
    Elsevier, p. 554.
AVMA Animal Health Studies Database (AAHSD), https://ebusiness.avma.org/aahsd/study/_search.aspx.
IMB Watson Oncology Genomics, http://www.ibm.com/watson/health/oncology/genomics/.
National Cancer Institute, http://ccr.nci.nih.gov/resource/onemedicine.
https://www.mycancergenome.org/ This is an excellent information source for cancer molecular genomics.
Veterinary Cancer Society, http://www.veterinarycancersociety.org.
Veterinary Cooperative Oncology Group, www.vcog.org.

Chapter 2

Caring for Geriatric Cancer Patients: The Concept of Pawspice and What Is Needed Aside from Medical Care

More and more, the older cancer patient has become the majority of cancer patients.

Lodovico Balducci, MD

Age Brings More Complexity and Susceptibility

Treating cancer in geriatric pets is more complex than any other discipline in veterinary medicine due to the comorbidities associated with senescence and the need for expertise in oncology, communication skills, and compassion. Geriatric pets come to us with a smorgasbord of diagnostic dilemmas that may need a wide range of specialty care including a philosophy that embraces end of life care. In fact, End of Life should be considered a separate and distinct 5th stage of life because it requires unique medical expertise and communication skills.

The concept of Pawspice embraces treatment of the geriatric patient's cancer with a kinder and gentler approach, and simultaneously focuses on quality of life with top priority. The aging pet's skeletal system and organ systems undergo compromise with arthritis and exposure to general toxins, age, obesity, and the impact of other organ failures. For example, heart disease has a negative impact on renal vascular flow and function and may add risk during sedation for diagnostic procedures and anesthesia for surgical tumor removal. Heart disease would exclude the use of Adriamycin due to its cardiotoxic effects. Renal disease would exclude the use of nephrotoxic chemotherapy. Various conventional modalities of therapy including surgery, chemotherapy and radiation therapy are often used in combination and/or in sequence to deal with specific types of cancer in dogs and cats (Table 2.1). Newer combinatorial therapies will include small molecules, checkpoint inhibitors, targeted agents, and multiple forms of immunotherapy, and so forth. Each of these modalities has their own set of adverse events, which must be considered and discussed during decision making.

Age is a condition, not a disease. Many veterinarians are complacent after diagnosing cancer in an old dog or cat past a certain chronological age. Instead of working with the pet carers and offering multiple options, some veterinarians are thinking about their euthanasia speech. This cold shoulder attitude is unfair to clients and their geriatric pets. Veterinarians and their professional staff must overcome the doldrums and get rid of the defeatist attitude and not abdicate end of life medical care and individualized precision oncology management for geriatric cancer patients. Think of End of Life as a distinct Stage of Life. It may come at any age but generally it is associated with the last 25% of

Canine and Feline Geriatric Oncology: Honoring the Human–Animal Bond, Second Edition. Alice Villalobos with Laurie Kaplan.
© 2018 John Wiley & Sons, Inc. Published 2018 by John Wiley & Sons, Inc.

Table 2.1. Frequently Recommended Treatment Modalities

Type of Cancer	Surgery (Sx)	Chemotherapy (CTx)	Radiation Therapy (RTx)	Adjuvant or Specialized Therapy
Mast cell	*	*	*	H-2 blockers
Skin cancer, SCC	*	+/−	*	Cryotherapy, ECT/EP Laser therapy
Lymphoma/leukemia	−/+	*	−/+	MoAb, vaccines
Breast cancer	*	*	−/+	Vaccine
Anal, sweat AC	*	*	*	Ck calcium, ECT/EP
STS	*	*	* SRS	Targeted therapy
FVAS	*	*	*	Gene therapy
OSA	*	*	Samarium *	Limb-sparing, vaccines
Head/neck	*	*	*	Brachytherapy, ECT/EP
M. melanoma	*	*	*	Vaccines, ECT/EP
Oral cancer	*	*	*	Brachytherapy, ECT/EP
Nasal cancer	−/+	+/−	*	Post RTx Sx
Brain tumors	+/−	*	*	Steroids, Vaccines
Endocrine tumors	*	*	+/−	Iodine 131 for thyroid cancer
Abdominal tumors	*	*	−/+ SRS	Second-look Sx
Bladder/prostate	−/+	*	−/+	Piroxicam
Hemangiosarcoma (HSAs)	*	*	−	Antiangiogenic therapy Chemoprophylaxis, BLT
Liver cancer	*	*	−	Percutaneous ethanol
Thyroid tumors	+/−	*	Iodine 131 +/−	injection (PEI).
Intestinal AC	*	+/−	−	Downstage with CTx/RTx
Colorectal AC	*	*	−/+	Before Sx: NeoAdjuvant
Lung cancer or metastatic disease	−/+	*	−/+ SRS	Targeted therapy, vaccines Nebulized liposomes

Note: The most frequently recommended treatment modalities used in combination and/or in sequence for the most common types of cancer in dogs and cats. SRS: stereotactic radiosurgery, ECT: electrochemotherapy, EP: electroporation, BLT: bispecific ligand-targeted toxin (Borgatti et al. 2015)

Key:
* Yes
− No
+/− Often
−/+ Seldom

life span. End of life may be a slow decline but it may be threatened or hastened with the ravages of cancer. It may last a short time but it may also last for months and occasionally stretch into years of unexpected good quality time. End of life care requires its own unique medicine and skill set. Atul Gawande, MD, in his insightful book, *Being Mortal* (2014), encourages physicians to ask end of life patients: What are your priorities, goals, fears, and what tradeoffs are you willing to make? We can ask these same questions of our Pawspice clients (carers) so that we can better serve them and their beloved geriatric pets afflicted with cancer.

People have preconceived notions about cancer. Carers, who want to protect their older pets, worry about potential adverse events such as toxic effects that may cause vomiting, diarrhea, lethargy and bone marrow suppression, and other complications. Apart from Veterinary Cooperative Oncology Group (VCOG) papers, adverse events are selectively and heterogeneously reported. This may overestimate the benefits of a treatment relative to its harms (Giuffrida 2016). Aside from those clients who come in self-educated by searching the Internet, many caregivers have little to no knowledge about cancer. Many people hold myths and misunderstandings about cancer and the wide range of available treatments options. Personal biases and ingrained feelings regarding cancer may cause procrastination toward diagnosis and treatment, especially in geriatric pets. One client declined to treat her dog for early stage cutaneous multifocal mast cell tumors with oral prednisone and chlorambucil because her grandfather, a retired veterinarian, was against it.

There are also cost concerns. The CancerMoonShot2020 is a global coalition organized by Dr. Patrick Soon-Shiong to rethink how cancer is treated by using the body's own immune system and re-training it to detect and destroy cancer cells. Its 2016 launch was headed by Vice President Joe Biden, who is also looking into "financial toxicity," the other toxic side effect faced by families paying for cancer care. One in three cancer patient families in the US borrows money to pay their bills and is 2.6 times more prone to bankruptcy. A pet owner often tries to explain the financial impact of their pet's illness on their budget. It is important for veterinarians to listen to their clients and to understand that this financial and emotional stress is very real and that they must work hard to recommend and support affordable treatment options.

Each member of the veterinary staff needs to dispel his or her negative notions about cancer. The entire profession must prepare to meet the medical and surgical challenges ahead to help care for the growing number of geriatric cancer patients. By adopting a more contemporary and integrative outlook regarding cancer care, veterinarians and their nursing staff can be successful in meeting the increasing demands for improved geriatric oncology case management.

Aging and senescence are associated with immune system compromise, accumulation of free radicals, and deposition of immunoglobulin in tissues that injure the functional integrity of various organs. This is most evident in old, older, and aged pets as they develop degenerative, hepatic, and renal disease. A list of changes in body systems associated with senescence has been adapted with permission from Dr. Robert Hamlin (1988) (Table 2.2).

Many geriatric pets have pre-existing endocrine disease such as hypothyroidism, Cushing's disease, or diabetes. Many geriatric animals, especially overweight cats on dry food diets, have been fed a less-than-ideal diet their entire lifetime. The multifaceted geriatric companion dog or cat with all its comorbidities becomes our most complex and medically demanding patient when cancer strikes. The attending doctor and family must set realistic goals depending on the geriatric oncology patient's physiologic age as well as chronologic age. We enter our geriatric cancer patients into Pawspice to help the family understand that their pet is nearing the end of life. In many cases, quality of life, comfort, and palliation may take precedence over radical curative intent (Kitchell 1988).

Geriatric cancer patients, burdened with comorbidities, often need interventional help. Diagnostics and treatment may require pain control, sedation, anesthesia, surgery, chemotherapy, radiation therapy, immunotherapy, or rehabilitation therapy. Treating the geriatric cancer patient with the philosophy of "do no harm" is a weighty medical and surgical challenge. Unfortunately, this therapeutic goal is lofty and cannot always be achieved, even with the best doctors, specialists, and medical equipment and the know-how. We are unable to make promises that our efforts to help a geriatric oncology patient will not backfire with an adverse reaction.

The human–animal bond is intensified during the special period that the family spends caring for their geriatric cancer pet. Witnessing the debilitating changes of aging and cancer marks an understanding and acceptance of one's own mortality. Seeing an old friend become feeble or experience a bad reaction hurts the inner spirit. Tears and memories come to the surface during medication, feeding, and cleaning times. Goodbyes are said every day with glances toward the resting pet, during walks, and when the pet is being tucked in at night. It is a sad time for the caregivers who are pondering

2

Table 2.2. Changes in Body Systems with Aging/Senescence

Musculoskeletal	Loss of flexibility
	Loss of muscle mass
	Decreased response to stress
	Loss, graying, and dullness of hair
	Hyperkeratinization of pads
	Brittle claws
	Thick, non-compliant dehydrated skin
	Granulation and fragmentation of collagen
	Hyperplasia of sebaceous and apocrine glands
	Sebum becomes waxier and rancid
	Splitting and fragmentation of cartilage
	Arthritis, painful joints
Gastrointestinal	Dental calculus and periodontal disease
	Decreased salivary secretions
	Esophageal muscular tone decreases
	Constriction of lower esophageal sphincter
	Decreased HCl results in emesis, flatulence, diarrhea
	Fatty liver, nodular hyperplasia, cirrhosis
	Diminished output of pancreatic enzymes
	Decreased absorption of lipids and fats from GI tract due to villous atrophy
Respiratory	Chronic bronchitis
	Decreased volume and increased viscosity of mucous
	Ciliary paralysis and above leads to retention of materials
	Increased histamine release and reduction in cyclic AMP leads to bronchoconstriction, decreased protective airway reflexes
	Weakening of respiratory muscles
Cardiovascular	Fibrosis
	Tracheal collapse
	Decreased oxygen diffusion
Renal Changes	Decreased glomerular filtration rate and renal perfusion, decreased tubular mass
	Thickened capillary walls of glomerular tufts
	Ischemic atrophy and fibrosis of peritubular tissue
	Hypertension, increased vascular resistance
	Diminished response to ADH
	Decreased output of erythropoietin
	Accelerated death of RBCs due to uremia
Urogenital	Loss of sphincter tone
	Chronic cystitis, increased frequency of urinary tract infections
	Pendulous prepuce due to Sertoli cell secretion of estrogen
	Relative androgen deficiency, ovarian involution
Endocrine	Decrease in hormonal secretion from most glands
	Decreased receptor density for thyroxin
Central Nervous System	Decreased neurotransmitters
	Deafness, blindness, loss of tactile sense
	Cognitive dysfunction syndrome
	Behavioral changes
	Behavioral changes with cognitive dysfunction syndrome
	Disorientation

Table 2.2. *(Continued)*

	Reduced social interaction
	Forgetfulness with house training
	Sleep disturbances
	Altered and variable levels of activity
Molecular, Immune System	Decreased T-cell population
	Decreased tumor suppressor and repair gene activity
	Increased rate of neoplasia
	Thymic involution

Source: Adapted from Geriatric Medicine I, 1988, Veterinary Post Graduate Institute, Santa Cruz, CA, with permission from Drs. Robert L. Hamlin and Robert R. Pensinger, 2005.

whether they are doing the right thing by tending to their geriatric cancer pet even though the cancer is expected to ultimately win.

Surgery, radiation therapy, and chemotherapy are modalities for cancer care that are most effective. However, geriatric cancer patients are potentially at greater risk for harm and adverse events before they may realize a benefit. Geriatric patients are not predictable in their responses and reactions to procedures such as dietary changes, anesthesia, surgery, drugs, pain medication, chemotherapy, radiation therapy, or complimentary therapy.

Clients need to be made aware of the potential adverse events before they agree to a treatment plan. Clear communication is essential. You might tell clients, "We are not treating a machine that needs replacement parts. Our geriatric oncology patient is an aging body with variable organ and tissue responses and sensitivities. If the geriatric oncology patient has a reaction to a drug or a slow recovery from surgery, we feel badly about it. Do not blame yourself or us. We need to stay on the same side, holding hands together as a strong, supportive team to help your old pal live longer with a good quality of life. So, let's talk about the options for treatment or palliation and the potential risks and benefits. After that, we can decide together whether or not you are willing to take the risks needed to reap the benefits that we might be able to win."

The Bond Grows Stronger with Age

Living with and caring for a geriatric pet creates a human–animal bond that is often intensified when cancer strikes. Because of the long duration of the relationship, a dog or cat may have a particular meaning to the owner or one of the family members because of an extenuating circumstance. If the pet provided devotion, comfort, and companionship through an illness, divorce, or the loss of a loved one, the human–animal bond is stronger. Some caregivers have a spiritual attachment with a particular pet.

Some feel that their pet is their last link to a deceased parent or loved one, and so they hold on dearly to that pet's life. The thought of losing this special pet may rekindle the heartache and loss that was experienced when a loved one died. I call this loss "tears of the ages" because pet loss may bring back the feelings that compile all our losses.

When a pet provides a sense of security, stability, or support, the human–animal bond may be a paramount consideration for the family. A pet may serve as a surrogate, in the role of child, partner, best friend, confidant, or other family member. Some pet loss heartbreaks will be harder than others. For many, the first loss is the hardest.

The long duration of the relationship is not the only criterion for a strong bond between a person and his or her geriatric pet. In the last 15 years, we have provided a greater number of oncology consultations for pets that were adopted or rescued as seniors than ever before. We have found that the attachment and The Bond that caregivers share with a new but aging arrival in their lives is often filled with compassion for the pet's endurance of an abusive or neglectful past. They feel a strong commitment to nurture the older pet. They want to provide good health care and make the remainder of the pet's life the best it can be. For these reasons and more, many pet caregivers are willing to engage in the battle against cancer for their geriatric pets.

Noodles's Case (She Needed to Outlive Mom)

Noodles, a 16-year-old F/S Pug, was adopted at age 10 by Robin Birnbaum. Noodles was diagnosed with metastatic mast cell cancer, which extended along the skin of her mammary glands and involved her axillary and inguinal lymph nodes. Robin's 80-year-old mom routinely called her after every appointment to ask how things went with Noodles. Robin's mom had been battling lymphoma for 11 years and she had recently been told that she only had 2 or 3 weeks to live. Robin said that she thought her mom felt a deep kinship with Noodles ("They were both old ladies with terminal cancer"), linking her own survival to Noodles'. During her chemotherapy treatments, Noodles became the poster dog and mascot for the local wellness community dog walk in Redondo Beach, CA. Robin carried Noodles for most of the walk due to Noodles' declining health (Figure 2.1). The mast cell tumors that were once in remission had returned and developed along her mammary lymphatic vessels.

We added lomustine to her chemotherapy protocol. This helped Noodles achieve a partial stable remission. When Noodles' platelet count dropped below 40,000, Robin's mom was especially concerned. Eight months went by. After Robin's mom passed away, Robin told me that

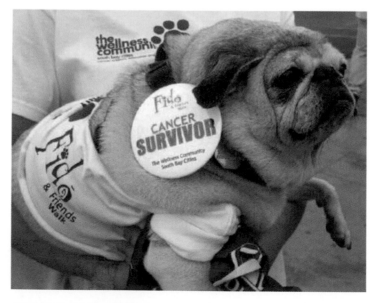

Figure 2.1.   16-year-old F/S Pug, Noodles Birnbaum, during difficult days with metastatic mast cell cancer. The cancer was resistant to initial treatment but responded to a change in protocol that incorporated lomustine. Noodles achieved a durable complete remission, which lasted 10 months.

she worried that Noodles would die before her mother. If Noodles had died, she said, it would have dashed her mother's will to live. Instead, Noodles went into a complete remission and delighted everyone with her longevity and vitality. Since the release of tyrosine kinase inhibitors (masitinib, toceranib) mast cell cancer patients have enjoyed more durable responses.

Geriatric oncology requires us to do much more for our clients than to merely understand treatment and provide good medical care. We must also be resourceful and compassionate to assist caregivers in decision making and comprehensive home care for the benefit of their pet and other family members. We need to provide emotional support to our heartbroken clients who are overwhelmed with feelings of anticipatory grief and depression.

Individualize Client Character

At each appointment, the veterinarian should take note of the love bond that exists between each individual client and their pet, not to judge but to appreciate and respect its power within the human–animal bond. Taking note of this relationship with a comprehensive focus gives each office visit intensity and purpose. This is no less important than the physical examination or the analysis of scientific data. This fact-finding interview will also help determine the best way to communicate with family members.

Some clients have strong personalities. They may be impatient if they need to wait to see you. Some may not want a detailed medical explanation. Most clients are used to having control of most aspects of their lives until cancer strikes their pet. They feel awful because they have no control over their pet's aging process or the cancer. A good approach to these issues would be to acknowledge them. Explain that we have no control over aging and that may be able to offer some help with the cancer. Point out the areas where they still have control, such as: pain control, supporting quality of life, and how and when their geriatric pet will pass, because you can assure the pet a quality death.

Other clients with more subdued, dependent personalities may slump into a depression and go blank. They may just stare at you while you are speaking and not be able to comprehend the necessary information that you are trying to give them for decision making. It would be ideal if the client could communicate this distress but they often do not. Offer to tape record the visit. This helps when you have a lot of information to give but one of the carers is not present or if there is upset. Remind your client that it is very easy to misunderstand or forget something that you are saying during the consult.

In addition, the diagnosis of cancer may be a more critical blow to the pet's survival or perceived treatability. This hits the carer, if their geriatric oncology patient has another worrisome concurrent morbidity such as incontinence or chronic kidney disease (CKD) or a neuropathy. The client may already be physically or emotionally stressed with the rigors of long-term or burdensome care for their compromised geriatric pet (Schoen 1991). The diagnosis of cancer on top of an age-related disability may be too stressful for family members to deal with at the moment.

All personality types and situations need information handouts or access to reliable online information to read in privacy at home. Clients may need a few days to absorb the information. Suggest veterinary college related information or VetPartners.com, which is the Veterinary Information Network (VIN) information source for pet owners. Suggest a consultation with an oncologist and a grief or pet loss counselor. Let clients know that you will collaborate and partner with them to help them make the best decisions regarding options to pursue for their geriatric cancer pet.

Sensitivity Self-Assessment

After every appointment, assess your own performance as a veterinarian by asking yourself three simple questions: Did I serve the client? Did I serve the pet? Did I serve the human–animal bond? The human–animal bond is an entity unto itself, bigger than the pet alone or the client alone. A veterinarian may perform superbly as a medical practitioner to the pet and communicate accurately and clearly to the client, but without an understanding of The Bond, we are no more than mechanical engineers trying to fix a broken pet, or liaisons explaining to a client what is wrong with his or her pet. Our understanding of The Bond is the aesthetic that elevates our work into one of the most meaningful, passionate, and compassionate arenas of health care.

Defining the Human–Animal Bond

A working definition of this bond was proposed in a 1998 statement from the AVMA Committee on the Human–Animal Bond: "The human–animal bond is a mutually beneficial and dynamic relationship between people and other animals that is influenced by behaviors that are essential to the health and well-being of both. This includes, but is not limited to, emotional, psychological, and physical interactions of people, other animals, and the environment. The veterinarian's role in the human–animal bond is to maximize the potentials of this relationship between people and other animals." Dr. John S. Wright, past president of the American Association of Human–Animal Bond Veterinarians (AAH-ABV), proposes a simpler, more expansive definition: "The relationship between people, animals, and their environment. The AAH-ABV mission is to provide education, resources, and support that enhance the ability of veterinarians to create a positive and ethical relationship between people, animals, and their environment" (Wright 2005). The AAH-ABV is considering a name change to the Human Animal Bond Association (HABA), with which to embrace its paraprofessional members.

Because of The Bond, pet owners in the early 2000s began spending more money than ever before on their pets. They also spent more time on the Internet to become educated about their pets' medical conditions. This is good news for our profession because of its potential income. The bad news for those who entered veterinary medicine for monetary reasons is that the increase in pet owner spending is accompanied with more demanding standards. A few pet owners price shop but most want compassionate care when choosing veterinary medical providers. Clients no longer simply use the veterinary office nearest their home. They choose veterinarians and a veterinary staff based, in part, on their sensitivity and compassion. Pet lovers rely on their chosen pet(s) for spontaneous moments of playfulness, joy, and physical contact. Pets give people opportunities to give care and that enriches their lives with meaning, identity, and a closer connection with nature. Pet carers want their veterinarians to be cognizant and respectful of their special relationship. They want more than scholars; they want healers with intellectual charity who are not judgmental (Bustad 1996).

Keno's Case (If You Don't Communicate Well, Clients Will Go Elsewhere)

The Mannings were given a poor prognosis for Keno, an old M/N Beagle. He had epistaxis 1 week after his adoption. The initial computed tomography (CT) scan, rhinoscopy, and biopsy were negative for cancer. Two months later, Keno had a second episode of epistaxis. The new CT scan and biopsy confirmed nasal chondrosarcoma (CSA). The attending doctor immediately referred the Mannings to a radiation oncologist. During our phone consultation, they told me that they felt that the specialist was abrupt and looked bored and aloof during their consultation time. They said the doctor would not speak frankly with them or answer their questions to address their concerns. Mrs. Manning said, "We felt that we were talking to an attorney and not our veterinarian." When they asked if there were any more specific survival data that might favor Keno, they said that the doctor started doing math to show them what a median survival meant. Mrs. Manning said to me, "I'm an architect and my husband is an engineer. We both have MBA degrees. We did not need a math lesson!"

The radiation oncologist told the Mannings that Keno needed a third CT scan. Apparently, the second CT scan "was not good enough to determine if the cancer was in one side or in both sides of Keno's nasal cavity." She estimated the cost of treatment at $6,500.00. The Mannings asked what side effects Keno might have and the doctor told them she couldn't say because "it depends on the dog." She said that some get a bit of a burn and some develop blindness. Then the doctor gave some statistics and started to explain the averages in yet another math lesson. The Mannings asked the doctor, "If Keno were your dog, would you do it?" The doctor said, "That is a terribly unfair question – I get a discount. It was inappropriate of you to ask. How can you ask me that?"

Needless to say, the Mannings had a confidence crisis with this consult. When they asked for a record transfer, the office manager apologized. She said that the doctor may not have the best bedside manner but the techs and the treatment provided are excellent.

The Mannings told me that they were also looking for a Chinese medicine doctor to help Keno. They ultimately decided to drive $2^1/2$ hours in the opposite direction of the facility that provided the disappointing consult so Keno could have his radiation therapy elsewhere. Mrs. Manning said, "If the doctor treated us with boredom and indifference, we are afraid she would be like that with our dog too."

Ideally, the contemporary veterinarian looks at each person–pet relationship freshly and applies a caring focus on client concerns and the geriatric pet's well-being in the face of cancer. Celebrating the meaningfulness of The Bond between your clients and their geriatric pet(s) will be a constant and powerful practice refresher. The uniqueness of each client–pet relationship is inspiring and gives meaning and purpose to the hard work that veterinarians do on a daily basis. Take an interest! Enjoy the various facets in the relationships that create your practice. Treasuring The Bond will keep you afloat and help you avoid feelings of drowning, burnout, and compassion fatigue (see the section on compassion fatigue in Chapter 11).

Providing medical care for geriatric dogs and cats with cancer can be depressing and may contribute to compassion fatigue. It is especially disheartening if the pet was presented in an advanced stage of disease or if the client has money constraints that prohibit the best treatment. Often, the client can sense that the attending doctor has already written the pet off. The client sees through the doctor's professional veneer and finds a lack of sympathy. If you find that you are starting to care a bit less for your complex geriatric cancer patients, it may be time to take better care of yourself. Read the section on wellness and self-care by Dr. Kimberly Pope Robinson in this textbook.

A client can sense when his or her veterinarian is insensitive or does not have a clue about the human–animal bond or is withholding compassionate care. The client may feel underappreciated by a veterinarian who does not seem to value the client or the pet enough to offer supportive suggestions and medical care to help manage the geriatric pet's cancer. Pet owners can tell when their veterinarian prefers to euthanize their geriatric cancer pet rather than be bothered with the complexity of treating that pet's multiple problems. If the veterinarian steers the client toward euthanasia and the client does not want this, he or she will either find compassionate care for the pet elsewhere or will comply – only to endure intense guilt and regret for years to come.

The textbook case is the exception, mostly because clinical trials are run on ideal candidates. Textbooks are great. Where would we be without them? Oncology topics are covered with great detail in reference textbooks and in the veterinary literature. Each geriatric oncology case has a unique element of complexity if one looks for it. Many cases are atypical. Cancer care and diagnostics are on the verge of profound change and improvement. With the volume of material that a contemporary veterinarian must have in his or her head, it is a lifelong challenge just to keep all of the facts in place and up to date. However, this is not enough. Aside from having medical knowledge, veterinarians must also be able to think outside of the box. It is easy to fall into the trap of quoting textbook material, statistics, and so forth and be completely unable to provide individualized consultations or think outside of the box.

This may result in missed diagnoses and treatment delays and limit the quality and type of care that can be offered. Many patients have symptoms that would indicate a diagnosis that is true in 90% of cases. However, for the other 10%, do not automatically rule out the possibility of a diagnosis that is less common. Approximately 12% of the cases that look and feel like cancer are not cancer. Approximately 60% of 200 splenectomy patients at the University of Minnesota over 5 years had lesions that represented non-malignant lesions (mostly lymphoid hyperplasia) with hematoma formation instead of hemangiosarcoma (Modiano 2016). As much as we may suspect hemangiosarcoma, unless confirmed, it is ethical and optimistic to recommend splenectomy to control or eliminate the risk of hemorrhage and hope for a non-malignant diagnosis. Lead the client to as much information as he or she can handle. Let clients know what you are thinking and where you ideally would like to go with the workup of their geriatric pet's case in the best of circumstances.

Rodney's Case (One Enlarged Kidney May Lead to Another)

Rodney, a 14-year-old DSH M/N cat, developed an enlarged kidney. Fine needle aspiration (FNA) cytology was non-specific. The attending doctor recommended nephrectomy. The biopsy report diagnosed renal lymphoma. Rodney was given time to recover from surgery and then he was referred for an oncology consultation. Unfortunately, Rodney's remaining kidney enlarged during his 2-week recovery.

In situations like Rodney's, a geriatric oncologist would approach a mass in the abdominal cavity of an old cat differently and with more determination to get the diagnosis without nephrectomy. Most veterinary oncologists would strongly suspect lymphoma while ruling out differentials such as hydronephrosis, polycystic kidney disease, perirenal pseudocyst, or renal carcinoma. An oncologist would work hard to establish the diagnosis of renal lymphoma without the surgical intervention of nephrectomy in a geriatric feline oncology patient.

FNAs for large abdominal masses are often inconclusive due to cellular necrosis, cellular fragility, and heterogeneity within the mass. It is not unusual for me to examine up to 20 FNA slides from various sites of an abdominal mass. It takes patience to locate and identify the neoplastic cells that you are looking for. The extra effort is well worth it because it spares the geriatric patient the morbidity of surgery.

Before recommending nephrectomy for a patient like Rodney, it would be best to collect more FNA cells. We have been taught to use a 22-gauge needle with a non-aspiration technique. My preference is to use a $1^1/_2$-inch 27-gauge needle with gentle aspiration from multiple sites of the kidney.

The next best step would be to get several percutaneous Tru-cut needle core biopsy samples using ultrasonography. Take precautions to press the ultrasound probe over the needle track to control hemorrhage and observe the site with the ultrasound for at least 5 minutes to be certain that there is no sub-capsular bleeding. This approach is less invasive and a better next step considering Rodney's age and the prevalence for lymphoma (Caruso 2005). Rodney received unhelpful surgery that delayed his diagnosis and definitive treatment. Rodney was in poor condition at our first consultation and his family was so alarmed that they declined chemotherapy.

The 2016 Surgical Summit of the American College of Veterinary Surgeons hosted Dr. Erik Clary and myself for a full day of Ethics in Medico-Ethical Decision Making for End of Life Cancer Patients. We answered some tough questions: When is it too much surgery? How do we prevent overtreatment? When do we recommend hospice/Pawspice (Clary 2016a, 2016b, 2016c; Villalobos 2016a, 2016b, 2016c)?

Conversing with Clients

Compassionate conversation skills are a top priority for successful communication. How you say it is often more important than what you say. Clear explanations and written information will help you acquire your client's confidence and compliance for the complex home care accommodations often required in caring for geriatric oncology patients. Instruct carers to demonstrate enthusiasm or an upbeat playful attitude with treats when administering medications so the pet enjoys and looks forward to being medicated.

Maintain an Unconditionally Positive Attitude

The contemporary veterinarian must strive to show each client an unconditionally positive attitude. This is essential when addressing a geriatric cancer patient's specific issues and when answering questions about a disfiguring procedure such as amputation, mandibulectomy, or enucleation, or an upsetting condition (Small 1991). We must also strive to keep the client's "reality buttons" in focus with the expected prognosis. I like to draw a bell curve to demonstrate the expected prognosis and then point to the tail on the right that indicates long term survivors. I tell clients that we will do everything possible to place their geriatric cancer patient in the long survivor section. In addition to all of the other roles you will play as a veterinarian, you are also your client's barometer. What you say and how you say it can either help or hurt your client and your patient as well. Be aware of and sensitive to your client's state of mind and always seek balance in your communications.

Balance: Helping the Client's State of Mind

People get emotional when their geriatric pets are seriously ill. Cancer evokes fear, dread, and irrational behavior. Client education helps people understand which cancers are treatable. The family needs to be assured that many geriatric patients diagnosed with cancer can be cured, placed in remission, palliated, or maintained with an acceptable quality of life in Pawspice care. It is important to help clients stay rational and involved in the decision-making process. Help clients subtract reluctance about giving medications and convert to a positive intention speaking to their pet, "This will make you feel better." I often instruct clients to repeat this mantra when giving medications or when just relaxing with their pet. This is my favorite healing mantra: *Cell By Cell, You Will Be Well.*

Help Your Clients Keep Their Balance by Addressing Them on Their Level

People with all types of personalities own pets. Clients want and need your full attention. You need to keep a healthy two-way balance with the client. Make sure that you have your clients' full attention when you are speaking to them. Make sure you are concentrating on them while they are talking to you. Focus on them while you are listening to their geriatric pet's history, description, and duration of clinical signs. Some clients have the need to provide some personal information that impacts how they relate to their pet. Remember that because they live closely with their geriatric pet, they possess vital information that you, with all your education and experience, cannot possibly know. Be respectful and be a legendary listener eager to learn about their intimate knowledge of their pet. Be careful not to give your clients the impression that their intuitive feelings and knowledge are of no value to you.

If you find that your mind was not focused for charting information and you did not hear what the client said, simply ask the person to repeat it. The client knows that there is a lot on your mind. Asking a client to repeat the history or the duration of illness and the exact symptoms is a way of saying that you do not want to miss anything and that you want to chart it properly.

You may have to repeat your questions if the person seems evasive. For instance, it may take several questions to establish the rate of growth of a mass. When did you first notice it? What size was it at that time? When was it half the size that it is now? All of these questions need to be asked and answered to ascertain the history properly. Sometimes it is hard to get the client to commit to an answer, yet with patience and positive persistence, the information can be documented for the record.

Use good communication gestures such as looking directly at the client, sitting at his or her level, patting the patient, avoiding barriers such as the exam table. Use plain non-medical words to help your client understand the diagnosis and extent of cancer for the geriatric pet. If you need to use medical jargon, you should clearly define each term. Medical jargon is a sure way to lose a client's attention. The contemporary veterinarian counsels caregivers with appropriate hope balanced with realism, instead of the old "test and slaughter" philosophy (Butler et al. 1991). That old philosophy was prevalent 20–30 years ago, yet this bias still lingers with some clinicians. You understand many aspects of the medical situation regarding the pet better than the client. It is your obligation to share this information with the client any way you can; use handouts and web sites.

The first question you can ask a pet owner is, "What do you know so far about your pet's cancer?" It is surprising to find that many pet owners are inadequately and hastily informed about their pet's cancer problem.

There is a certain personality type who will chatter at you non-stop. Knowing when and how to politely excuse yourself from the rambling is essential. I have at times asked the chatterbox client to try very hard to slow down and listen to what I have to say because after all they are paying for my consultation. I do not want them to leave without the consult. I ask them to video or tape the session so they can review it later for clarity. Look for a break in the chatter and let the person know that you would like to talk with him or her more but that your main focus must remain with the patient. Tell the client that you have another patient waiting to be seen or a procedure that needs to be performed. Just excuse yourself politely when you can or ask a staff member to come into the room and help with the procedures or the discharge for the patient and the client.

Another personality type with high needs asks the same questions repeatedly in different ways. These clients are hoping you will tell them what they want to hear (Butler et al. 1991). They need to hear both the upside and the downside of what the cancer and its treatment options would entail, always with a kind and compassionate tone of voice.

There is a certain personality type who will NOT be interested in understanding the technical details of the geriatric cancer pet's medical situation. We should not force these clients off their balance with information overload. They do not want to listen to medical explanations. They only want to know how to care for the pet's medical condition properly. This type of client needs user-friendly information handouts the most, but will probably not read them. For clients like this, we often use long acting injectable medications for their pet and schedule the recheck exams to repeat the injections.

Mimzi's Case (Keep Clients Well Informed)

Mimzi, a 12-year-old F/S Pug, was due for a routine dental checkup. She had a few warts and some small bumps in her skin. A mass on her right shoulder bled after a visit to the groomer and it seemed to bother her. The warts and bumps were removed at the time of her dental checkup. Biopsy samples were not submitted. A few weeks later, Mimzi's right prescapular lymph node was enlarged. Antibiotics were given to fight the suspected infection. When the node did not reduce in size, FNA cytology slides were sent to the lab. The attending doctor telephoned the family and told them that Mimzi had a mast cell tumor.

Our consultation found that the family was poorly informed about mast cell cancer and the gravity of Mimzi's situation. It may have been a case of owner denial. However, the attending doctor's responsibility in geriatric oncology is to ensure that clients have a basic understanding of the extent of their pet's cancer and a general idea of the prognosis.

Dealing with Inappropriate Depression and Grief

When clients learn that their elderly pet has cancer, they are understandably depressed and frightened about what will happen. When delivering the diagnosis and prognosis of cancer, be aware that the client may become very depressed. Check to be sure that the client is hearing and understanding what you are saying. When delivering the prognosis, always explain that the survival data are generally derived from reference statistics about other animals with the same type of cancer.

Illustrate a bell curve and show the family that the majority of patients are in the middle part of the bell curve for survival time. Show them that there are always a small percentage of animals that have shorter and longer survivals at each end of the curve. Assure the clients that your oncology team will do everything possible to position their geriatric cancer patient in the longer survival group. If there is hope, an encouraging statement would be, "We can't change the given prognosis, but we can try to outlive it." Clients need to understand that your treatment at the clinic and their caregiving at home might help position their pet within the longer survival group of the bell curve.

Dealing with Anticipatory Grief

Pet loss is a special kind of grief. Much of it is anticipatory grief. It robs caregivers of energy and the ability to treasure and enjoy the precious time that they have left with their pet (Meyers 2000). It is important for veterinarians to identify this profound sorrow and try to improve this doubly sad situation. It often pops up at the time one receives the diagnosis of cancer and again with any bad news. Anticipatory grief is often not recognized by the attending veterinarian, even though most highly bonded pet owners will verbalize or act out their grief. Veterinarians and their staff members need to validate the carer's attachment for the pet and feelings of pending loss (Voith 1985). Sometimes the right words from the veterinarian can make the difference. It is also important to recommend pet-loss counseling. Group therapy sessions may be available through individual therapists who are qualified and interested in pet-loss counseling. Recommend an online chat room for anticipatory grief such as that conducted by the Association for Pet Loss and Bereavement.

At times like this, I might say, "You are experiencing life's richest emotions of love and loss. You will live through this and you will be okay. Your pet won't leave you until his job is done and you will know when his mission is completed. Do you feel the passion that Buddy gives you right now? Some people will never know the depth of your grief for Buddy. Their lives were not enriched in the way you have been enriched with Buddy."

Pet owners often tell me that they became more insightful and compassionate through pet loss. For Judy (see Buddy's case later in this chapter), I said, "You will be a much wiser person for the experience that Buddy gives you so that you will be prepared when a family member or close friend passes on. You can learn how to use these tools of insight and acceptance to help others who feel that they are in the same hopeless situation that you learned about so well with Buddy." Judy responded, "Buddy is my best friend. I wouldn't leave his side until it is over. Thank you for helping me. After Buddy is gone, I would like to help other people who are having trouble and feeling hopeless about losing a pet, like me." This statement was a good indicator that Judy was beginning to progress through the stages of grief. She was accepting that Buddy would go and she was thinking about helping others and creating new attachments.

To ensure further support for the client, we also inform the referring veterinarian of the situation. We ask the attending doctor to call the client and to alert his or her staff to provide as much comfort and support to the pet owner as possible during the pet's end of life care or "Pawspice" program. We also directly encourage the doctor to instruct the pet owner to seek counseling.

Disenfranchised Grief

A client's grief and sadness may be more intense by feelings of disenfranchisement. Few people truly understand the enormous emotional burden that pet illness and loss places on a person's morale. Many pet owners suffer from the insensitivity that others show regarding how they feel about their beloved pet's medical condition or impending death. This makes them feel deprived and disenfranchised because they cannot share their care-giving burden and their grief (Corbin 2004). Certainly, you and your staff members should not be among the people who do not understand how they feel. Do not let your associates and staff be aloof when carers are emotionally suffering. Do not let yourself or your staff ever join the veterinary insensitivity club!

Ask your clients if there is anyone they can count on for moral support. Let clients know that you and your staff understand what they are going through. Assure them that you are aware of their needs and that you and your team will help them to help their pet. Use creative optimism and present a positive, action-oriented attitude about solving each one of the geriatric pet's concurrent issues and complex medical problems. This gives clients more confidence that their geriatric cancer patient will be given every chance to survive as long as possible with a good quality of life.

Inappropriate Optimism: Keep Reality Buttons in Place

If, after a diagnosis of pet cancer, your client seems inappropriately optimistic, not understanding the seriousness of the pet's illness, communicate realism. You might say something like this: "You are paying me for my opinion and I want to make sure that you understand the gravity of Bullet's condition and prognosis. His time might be short. We need to make sure that you keep your reality buttons in place, so that if Bullet does well, you will know that he beat the odds. We can't change the poor prognosis that is dictated by the pathologist or the advanced stage of illness, but if you want us to treat him, there is a chance that we may be able to help Bullet outlive his prognosis."

Expect Shock and Dread

Many clinicians have told me that they are uncomfortable and do not know how to respond to clients who exhibit fear and grief. Some deal with this discomfort by just going on with the consult and ignoring the client's emotional display. They might point to the box of tissues, or offer a tissue, but they do not address or validate the client's sadness in a helpful way. Physicians also do a poor job preparing people for critical decisions. The vast majority of people in the US have never had an end of life discussion with a health care provider (2015). This omission of counsel, this lack of verbal acknowledgement, further disenfranchises that client's grief experience. It also alienates the client from your practice. Hire a grief counselor to come to a couple of staff meetings to provide skills and drills to provide emotional comfort to those who need it. Once you and your staff have the tools, the discomfort turns into a positive feeling of knowing you can acknowledge and offer empathy and help the client through the issues of pet illness, palliative therapy, and loss. Following are two true case scenarios with some verbal suggestions on how to address fear and grief on the phone or in the exam room.

Dori's Case (Wear Both Hats When Needed)

Maxine had a tissue in her trembling hand and was on the verge of tears when I entered the exam room. We discussed Dori's biopsy report, which diagnosed lingual squamous cell carcinoma (SCC). Oral examination was difficult, but the SCC invaded the entire base of Dori's tongue, making it stiff, ulcerated, and painful. I verified the poor prognosis that accompanies this type of cancer. Maxine looked at her 12-year-old F/S German Shepherd dog–mix and burst into tears. She could not suppress her intense feelings of loss, injustice, and regret. She said, "I love Dori. And I don't want her to suffer." Maxine had previously declined surgery and radiation therapy for Dori after learning that chemotherapy would have been only palliative.

Maxine reported, "Even though Dori lost 17 pounds and had trouble eating, she was still behaving close to normal and was cheerful in every other way." She asked me to do whatever I could for Dori to help her live a quality life until the end. When I introduced the concept of Pawspice and how to recognize and alleviate pain for Dori, Maxine burst into tears again. My other two exam rooms were full and there were people in the waiting room, but it was more important to focus on Maxine's distress for a few precious moments. I told Maxine that I was going to put on the pet loss counselor's hat for a few minutes. I knew that my other clients would understand completely.

I began by letting Maxine know that we would be there to help both her and Dori get through the next several months and that she was not alone in her grief. I said that pet loss often has the power to bring all of our personal losses to the surface and that grief makes one feel raw all over. I suggested that her tears were shed not only for Dori but also for other past losses – that these tears that come so freely may be called "tears of the ages."

Maxine then confided that she rescued Dori from the pound just after her brother had committed suicide. She said that her father had recently died and that she was holding his hand when he died. She said, "I just can't take another loss." Now we both recognized that Maxine's deep grief was truly for all of her losses. I suggested to Maxine that Dori might be helping her to deal with her repressed grief in a very special way. I told Maxine that Dori's cancer would give her time for reconciliation and that her passing may be a liberating gift to her. Maxine remained in distress.

When a client remains in distress, reach out and try to bring them to accept the situation. Even though I was behind schedule, it was important to help Maxine. It was time to share my personal beliefs with her by saying, "Each pet that shares our life comes to us with a special mission. Dori has a mission in your life and she won't leave you until it is accomplished."

This message is a very powerful tool that can bring deep meaning to the feelings that the caregiver is experiencing. It can also help to bring the grieving client to focus on to his or her personal life and the role that the old pal has played in the caregiver's life. Maxine told me that she was a smoker since childhood and that Dori would be her teacher to help her quit smoking.

When it seemed appropriate, I told Maxine that I needed to put my other hat back on, as Dori's doctor, and help to provide care and medical treatment to the best of my ability. We continued the office visit and made a treatment protocol for Dori that consisted of pain control, hand feeding, and immunonutrition. The daily protocol included monitoring Dori's weight, hydration, food intake, and scheduled rechecks to monitor the well-being of both pet and pet owner. Two days later, a follow-up phone call found Maxine feeling much better, as well as Dori, who lived well for another 4 months.

Over the years, this special message has helped uplift many of my upset clients: "The energy that you use to be anxious, depressed, and upset about Max's cancer is very powerful, and it has a negative impact on both you and Max. Instead, harness that energy and use it in a positive way. Then, you will be able to do more to help Max. Use your powerful energy to keep your appointments and learn more about the cancer and how to best care for Max. Your positive energy will help Max have a better chance and improve his quality of life."

Buddy's Case (Address Suicidal Tendencies)

Judy shared her life with Buddy, an 11-year-old M/N Golden Retriever who achieved a prolonged, stable remission with cutaneous lymphoma. When Buddy came out of remission and became resistant to treatment, Judy told me that she wanted to die if her sweet Buddy died.

Ignoring such a statement from a client would be very dangerous. When clients express this degree of depression, they are asking for your help. Never leave such an expression unanswered. If you are unable to help clients with their emotional responses to bad news, be sure to have a staff worker ready to step in. This is one of the other hats that we must wear as veterinarians. We are not therapists and should not delve too deeply into the client's emotions or thoughts, but we can be a friend and offer support and guidance to good counseling.

An appropriate, helpful response will validate the importance of the pet in the person's life, and express that you understand their feelings. For example: "I know how important Buddy is to you. Pets like Buddy come to us with a special mission on earth. Only you know what that mission is, because it is very personal. Your love and the joy that he gives you are the reasons for your deep sadness. Your sadness is a rich emotion, just as beautiful and rich as the love bond that you share with him."

It is helpful to ask distraught clients to tell you something special about The Bond that they share with their old pal. You can comfort clients with words like, "Buddy will always be with you, but in a different way. He will be in your sweet memories and always in your heart. Buddy will be like a jewel that you place in a special box and store safely away in your memory shelf. You can always open the memory box to see and hold the jewel whenever you want to. Our pets were not designed to live as long as we do. They come to us with an internal time clock, like an hourglass, that runs out long before ours. In fact, if you have one to three pets at a time, you will have up to 27 heartbreaks in your lifetime. Some of these heartbreaks, like how you're feeling about Buddy right now, will be harder on you than others." Many people remain stuck in their grief but are unable to express it. You might be able to help such a client by saying, "If you keep the grief inside, it will make a hard knot in your throat. If you release it and let it out and accept the inevitable, you will then be free to just be sad and go on with the business of living your life."

Consider Extenuating Circumstances

Veterinarians are constantly adjusting the puzzle of patient care based on time and money constraints of the client. Every person–pet combination has extenuating circumstances. Take these given factors, add into the equation the health issues and habits that are intrinsic to the geriatric cancer patient, and the result is the challenge of geriatric oncology. We need to know about all of these factors and their summation, in order to determine if there can be complete or partial compliance to a particular chemotherapy, radiation therapy, immunotherapy, or maintenance protocol.

Ask the client, "What is going on in your lives that may interfere or compete with the time commitment you need for your pet's treatment?" Some families have overwhelming interpersonal issues, or a concurrent crisis, or health issues that impact how they are able to care for their geriatric pet's comorbidities and the added burden of cancer care. Travel time and transportation issues for repetitive treatments may be difficult for people without cars or for those who are in and out of town due to work, parent care, or second homes. Money issues may exclude the preferred treatments and force the oncology team to treat the patient with a compromise protocol that has been adjusted to be more affordable. The pet's carers should not be judged or made to feel guilty. They should participate in the choices that are being made for the adjusted protocol. The oncology team must also inform these clients that the results may not be as successful when using the compromised protocol and that they must carefully monitor the patient for relapse or recurrence, which should prompt them to come in for a recheck.

Pawspice Care Philosophy

Pawspice is about veterinarians and their nursing staff helping clients to provide end of life palliative care at home for their terminally ill pets (TIPs). Family members need to fully understand that the word "palliation" actually means treatment for comfort, not cure. Often palliation is clearly the preferred mode of care for a geriatric oncology patient. Pawspice may include kinder gentler palliative cancer treatment such as metronomic chemotherapy, antiangiogenesis therapy, immunonutrition or integrative medications. Pawspice may include electroporation (electrochemotherapy) for difficult to remove tumors instead of standard wide excisional surgery. Palliative cancer treatment may be favored over standard curative treatment or euthanasia.

Emergency clinics should also present the option of hospice and the end of life vigil for TIPs with acute oncologic crisis such as hemoabdomen or cardiac tamponade. Our profession needs to move away from offering "either or" medicine by offering the Pawspice/hospice option. The client can sign a consent and release form that acknowledges the patient's dire condition and that they elect to go home with supportive medications that will comfort the pet during the hospice vigil. Providing the hospice vigil as an option relieves carers of being rushed or pushed to authorize their pet's death reluctantly and unwillingly with euthanasia.

The American Pet Association estimates that there are 170 million pets in the US (80 million dogs, 90 million cats) and that 16 million pets die each year. One million dogs will be diagnosed with cancer in the US per year (Nass and Gorby 2015). Cancer claims at least half of dogs and a third of cats over the age of 10. Organ failure erodes health in geriatric pets and ranks as the second most common cause of death. Most geriatric cancer patients are in physiologic decline with the aging process along with organ compromise and/or failure concurrently with their malignancies. As companion dogs and cats glide into their geriatric years, the human–animal bond that they share with their family gets stronger. As mentioned above, End of Life should be considered as a distinct stage of life due to specialized medical and psychosocial counseling skills needed.

We must face the fact that many geriatric cancer patients will not be treated due to owner reluctance, financial constraints, concurrent illness, or a logistical problem. We can and should still offer reluctant clients an up-to-date consultation or a referral so they can be fully informed of their options. Concern for the well-being and quality of life for the patient is first and foremost. Be sure to inform clients that there are kinder and more gentle ways to treat cancer if they want to consider slowing it down. However, there is a time to wholeheartedly admit to ourselves that despite our great medical advances, compassionate supportive care for TIPs and emotional support for their families is often the only and the very best medicine that we can provide at the end of the road for the human–animal bond.

If a geriatric pet is in the advanced or terminal stages of cancer at the time of diagnosis, various levels of palliative care, Pawspice, and pet hospice care should be recommended as highly effective priority options. The contemporary veterinarian offers palliation and Pawspice over the insensitive suggestion of euthanasia as per the old "test and slaughter" philosophy. The Pawspice option keeps TIPs and carers comfortably close to their familiar places and satisfies the need to nest for a private farewell. Pawspice offers pets and their families more time for hopefully slowing down the cancer and living through the decline process toward dying. Allowing more time for the end of life journey reduces the overwhelming and frightened feelings that death brings. It helps families see and accept death as a blessing (Fernandez 2016). Pawspice is often **the very best** care and support that veterinary medicine can offer TIPs while honoring the human–animal bond.

The most important ingredient to look for in yourself, your staff, and your clients is the willingness to provide comfort care for the geriatric cancer patient to assure peacefulness and quality of life. The purpose of Pawspice and hospice is to allow more time for the client to let go of his or her old pal with a longer, kinder, and intimate farewell. As long as the TIP is peaceful and pain-free, many tender private moments of quiet emotion and sweet conversation can be gratefully shared between the caregivers and their dying pets (see Chapter 10 on Pawspice).

Summary

No matter how the case turns out in the end, be assured that many carers with geriatric cancer pets want and need you to help them fight for their geriatric pet's life. The intensity of this cry for help places all veterinarians and their hospital staff on the emotional front line to help pet carers in the battle against cancer. It is always appropriate to acknowledge the reality of the geriatric oncology patient's prognosis and say, "We are working against the odds. Bella's time might be short." If you accept this challenge with compassion for your clients' feelings, your efforts will be appreciated and your practice will earn a positive reputation (Bustad 1996).

Assure clients that you will partner with them and offer the best guidance for decision making. Remember to follow Gawande's advice and ask carers, "What are your priorities, goals, fears and what tradeoffs are you willing to make to help your geriatric cancer pet as life approaches the end?" Then deliver the best care that you and your consultants can provide for the geriatric oncology patient, while honoring the human–animal bond. This means that you will be frank in your conversations and sincerely and compassionately discuss the patient's decline. When appropriate, you will acknowledge that seeking further medical therapy is futile and you will recommend transferring the failing patient into hospice for more intense palliative comfort care. You will encourage your clients to include friends and family in the hospice vigil. When possible, help the carers make aftercare arrangements and ensure that the patient will have a peaceful and painless passing either at your clinic or with home euthanasia services.

References

AVMA Committee on the Human–Animal Bond. 1998. *JAVMA* 212 (11):1675.

Borgatti, A., J.S. Koopmeiners, A.L. Winter, K. Steuber, D. Todhunter, J. Froelich, M. Henson, J.F. Modiano, and D. Vallera. 2015. Genetically engineered targeted toxin enhances survival in dogs with naturally-occurring incurable hemangiosarcoma. American Association for Cancer Research Annual Meeting Poster, UMN Animal Cancer Care and Research Program.

Bustad, L.K. 1996. *Compassion: Our last great hope – Selected speeches of Leo K. Bustad, DVM, PhD*, pp. 1–12. Renton, WA: Delta Society.

Butler, C.L., M.S. Lagoni, K.L. Dickinson, and S.J. Withrow. 1991. "Cancer." In *Animal illness and human emotion: Problems in veterinary medicine*, eds S.P. Cohen and C.E. Fudin, Vol. 3, No. 1, pp. 21–38. Philadelphia, PA: Lippincott.

Caruso, K.J. 2005. Feline enlarged kidney. *Clinician's Brief* (NAVC), September, pp. 41–42.

Clary, E. 2016a. A primer on veterinary ethics. *ACVS Surgical Summit Proceedings*, Seattle, WA.

Clary, E. 2016b. End-of-life medical ethics: Fundamental issues and principles (Part I). *ACVS Surgical Summit Proceedings*, Seattle, WA.

Clary, E. 2016c. End-of-life medical ethics: An thic of "Only Caring" (Part II). *ACVS Surgical Summit Proceedings*, Seattle, WA.

Corbin, J. 2004. A depth psychological analysis of the human–canine bond and its implications to the grief response: A phenomenological study. Personal Communication as an external reader, dissertation proposal. Pacifica Graduate Institute, Carpenteria, CA.

Fernandez, L. 2016. *Sacred gifts of a short life: Uncovering the wisdom of our pets end of life journeys.* Simi Valley, CA: Valstar Publishing.

Gawande, A., 2014. *Being mortal: Medicine and what matters in the end.* New York: Metropolitan Books, Henry Holt and Company.

Giuffrida, M.A. 2016. A systematic review of adverse event reporting in companion animal clinical trials evaluating cancer treatment. *JAVMA* 249 (9):1079–1087.

Hamlin, R.L. 1988. *Geriatric Medicine I, Veterinary Post Graduate Institute Course Proceedings*, ed. Robert R. Pensinger, pp. 140–202. Santa Cruz, CA.

Kitchell, B.E. 1988. Clinical oncology in the aging pet. *Geriatric Medicine I, Veterinary Post Graduate Institute Course Proceedings*, ed. Robert R. Pensinger, pp. 33–139, Santa Cruz, CA.

Meyers, B. 2000. "Anticipatory mourning and the human-animal bond: Clinical dimensions of anticipatory mourning." In *Theory and practice in working with the dying, their loved ones and caregivers*, pp. 537–564. Champaign, IL: Research Press.

Modiano, J.F. 2016. Personal Communication.

Nass, S.J., and H. Gorby. 2015. *The role of clinical studies for pets with naturally occurring tumors in translational cancer research: Workshop Summary*, 83 pp. NW, DC: National Academies Press (www.nap.edu21830).

Schoen, A.M. 1991. "Decision-making concerning pets with loss of autonomic function." In *Animal illness and human emotion: Problems in veterinary medicine*, eds S.P. Cohen and C.E. Fudin, Vol. 3, No. 1, pp. 61–72. Philadelphia, PA: Lippincott.

Scientific American, Science Agenda Editors, June 2015. A last right for dying patients: Health care providers do a poor job preparing people for critical decisions, p. 10.

Small, E.S. 1991. "Loathsome and disfiguring conditions." In *Animal illness and human emotion: Problems in veterinary medicine*, eds S.P. Cohen and C.E. Fudin, Vol. 3, No. 1, pp. 73–82. Philadelphia, PA: Lippincott.

Villalobos, A. 2016a. End of life medico-ethical decision making. *ACVS Surgical Summit Proceedings*, Seattle, WA.

Villalobos, A. 2016b. Preventing over treatment. *ACVS Surgical Summit Proceedings*, Seattle, WA.

Villalobos, A. 2016c. Veterinary hospice care: theory and practice. *ACVS Surgical Summit Proceedings*, Seattle, WA.

Voith, V.L. 1985. "Attachment of people to companion animals." In *Symposium on the Human–Companion Animal Bond*, Veterinary Clinics of North America, pp. 289–296. Philadelphia, PA: Saunders.

Wright, J.S., and the AAH-ABV Board Committee for Brochure Revision. 2005.

Suggested Reading

Abeloff, M.D., J.O. Armitage, J.E. Niederhuber, M.B. Kastan, and W.G. McKenna. 2004. *Clinical oncology*, 3rd edn. Philadelphia, PA: Churchill Livingstone.

American Association of Human-Animal Bond Veterinarians Newsletters and Human-Animal Bond Proceedings from AVMA, AAHA, NAVC (www.aahabv.org).

Balducci, L. (guest ed.). 1994. *Cancer Control: Journal of the Moffitt Cancer Center* 1 (2).

Balducci, L. 1994. Do we need geriatric oncology? *Cancer Control: Journal of the Moffitt Cancer Center* 1 (2):91–94.

Balducci, L., G.H. Lyman, W.B. Ershler, and M. Extermann (eds). 2004. *Comprehensive geriatric oncology*, 2nd edn. Oxon, UK: Taylor & Francis.

Creagan, E.T. 2001. *Mayo Clinic on healthy aging*. New York: Kensington.

De Jonge, F., and R. van den Bos. 2005. *The human–animal relationship: Forever and a day*. Assen, The Netherlands: Royal Van Gorcum.

DeVita, V.T., S. Hellman, S.A. Rosenberg (eds). 2001. *Cancer: Principles and practice of oncology*, 6th edn. Philadelphia, PA: Lippincott-Raven.

Team Advisor. 2005. Giving seniority to senior pets. *Clinician's Brief (NAVC)*, September, pp. 17–30.

Hunt, L. 2000. *Angel pawprints: Reflections on loving and losing a canine companion*. New York: Hyperion.

Villalobos, A.E. 1999. Pet hospice nurses the bond. *Veterinary Practice News*, September.

Villalobos, A.E. 2000. "Conceptualized end of life care: 'Pawspice' program for pets." In *AVMA Proceedings 2000*, pp.322–327. Schaumburg, IL: AVMA.

Villalobos, A.E. 2001. Comprehensive pain management vital to oncology patients. *Veterinary Practice News*, July.

Villalobos, A.E. 2002. Cancer pain: Understated shouldn't mean underestimated. *Veterinary Practice News*, July.

Villalobos, A.E. 2003. Cancer causes cachexia, an insidious weight loss. *Veterinary Practice News*, December.

Villalobos, A.E. 2004. The right words can make a difference. *Veterinary Practice News*, May.

Villalobos, A.E. 2004. Quality of life scale helps make final call. *Veterinary Practice News*, September.

Part Two

Chapter 3
The Warning Signs of Cancer in Geriatric Pets

The analysis of many a success or failure (in cancer management) often reveals the important role played by the physician or physicians who dealt with the case in its inception and their decisive influence on the eventual result. Where temporizing guesswork, amateurish approaches and defeatist attitudes may fail, intelligent understanding, prompt skillful treatment and a hopeful, compassionate attitude may succeed.

L.V. Ackerman, MD and J.A. del Regato, MD

Principles and Practice in Geriatric Oncology

The warning signs of cancer in geriatric dogs and cats may be subtle and masked by senescence, obesity, arthritis, cognitive dysfunction, dental disease, and so forth. Cancer is underestimated in geriatric dogs and cats because general signs of aging camouflage it. Cancer mimics signs of aging such as: "slowing down," lethargy, finicky appetite, loss of muscle mass (sarcopenia), weight gain, or enlargement of abdominal organs (organomegaly) that cause a distended abdomen. It is important to practice anticipatory medicine with geriatric dogs and cats. Be vigilant and look for cancer behind every warning sign no matter how subtle the sign may seem to be.

Early detection will provide geriatric cancer patients with the best chance of survival. Cancer diagnostics and care are on the verge of profound change and improvement due to advances in molecular research. Look for access to upcoming "liquid biopsy" tests that will screen dogs for cancer via a blood test and the CADETSM™ free catch urine test that will detect canine bladder cancer on free catch urine samples. The veterinarian's most important clinically relevant task is to recognize the premonitory warning signs of cancer during history taking and physical exam. Most types of cancer exhibit specific early (prodromal) warning signs. Following this, the geriatric patient begins to exhibit more location-specific or function-specific signs. As tumor size progresses further, the geriatric patient exhibits more obvious warning signs, such as evidence of a mass or a change or interruption of a routine function.

It is generally the pet owner (carer), the groomer, or the attending veterinarian who first detects a warning sign of cancer in an older pet. In my experience, there seems to be more owner reluctance, overprotection, and detection delay in geriatric pets. In many case histories, the pet caregiver and/or the attending veterinarian elected inaction. They took a conservative stance despite the presence of prodromal warning sign(s) because of the pet's advanced age. This inaction may be considered ageism or bias against old people and old pets. Ageism may limit the use of medical technology for geriatric

Canine and Feline Geriatric Oncology: Honoring the Human–Animal Bond, Second Edition. Alice Villalobos with Laurie Kaplan.
© 2018 John Wiley & Sons, Inc. Published 2018 by John Wiley & Sons, Inc.

pets, and may present an ethical dilemma for veterinarians who have the duty to act in the best interests of the patient.

Cancer in geriatric pets is often allowed to progress due to ignorance, owner denial, overprotection, reluctance, and various other circumstances and reasons resulting in detection delay. Clients are often unaware of the early signs of cancer in pets – client education is the best solution to this problem. The veterinarian can play an important role by educating clients one-to-one during office visits, with slide shows, videos, handouts, newsletters, web sites and downloads, and so forth. Incorporate client education during the waiting room time.

Some carers suspect that their geriatric pet may have cancer, but subconsciously or intentionally they delay taking the pet to their veterinarian. They may dread spending money (people without health insurance delay visits for over 6 weeks); they may be in denial. Some are afraid of finding a terminal problem. Others simply do not want to put their old pal through the inconvenience and stress that they fear cancer treatment will entail.

Detection delays are not all caused by uneducated or reluctant clients. In some cases, the client reported a problem based on existing warning signs, and the veterinarian failed to diagnose or delayed tests that would have revealed the diagnosis of cancer at an earlier stage. Such delay in detection can seal the fate of a companion animal that might have been treated successfully. For example, some owners report that they suspected that their old cat had cancer because of a chronic bleeding facial ulcer. The attending doctor did not diagnose the lesion(s) as facial squamous cell carcinoma (SCC), but instead prescribed an ineffective topical ointment.

Many cats with solar-induced SCC can be saved or spared nosectomy and pinnectomy if treated properly at the earliest stages using: cryotherapy, imiquimod cream (Aldara®) and other immuno-oncology products, electroporation, or laser therapy. Many advanced SCC lesions respond well to electroporation, radiation therapy, and potentially using intralesional injections of Yttrium 90 brachytherapy radiogel such as IsoPet™ (www.isopetsolutions.com). Attentive care will avoid complications and adverse events with geriatric cancer patients.

Warning Signs of Cancer in Dogs and Cats

It might be easier to think of the warning signs of cancer if we group them into three tangible symptom groups: palpable, physiologic, and behavioral. Please refer to the following group listings of the clinical warning signs of cancer and illness in pets.

Palpable Warning Signs

1. Enlarged lymph nodes (lymphadenopathy), abnormal swellings, or plaques that continue to grow in the skin.
2. Abnormal masses in the oral cavity, mammary glands, testicles, vaccine or injection sites, or enlarged abdominal organs (organomegaly).
3. Sores or ulcers that do not heal in 2 weeks, on the nose, ear tips, and face of white cats and ventrum of non-pigmented dog breeds.

Physiologic Warning Signs

4. Weight loss, cachexia.
5. Pale mucous membranes, icterus, jaundice, red or hyperemic areas on membranes.

6. Halitosis, more than one loose tooth at the same location.
7. Abdominal distention, organomegaly, fluid in the abdomen (ascites) or blood in the abdomen (hemoabdomen).
8. Red blotches in the skin (petechia, ecchymosis), bleeding or hemorrhage at any location, especially orifices such as nose, mouth, anus, urinary tract.

Behavioral Warning Signs

9. Anorexia, no interest in treats or delicious snacks.
10. Reduced energy or exercise intolerance, trouble breathing (dyspnea), coughing, gagging.
11. Trouble eating or swallowing (dysphagia), salivation, regurgitation, voice change, vomiting (emesis).
12. Chronic sneezing, unresponsive ocular discharge, unilateral nasal discharge.
13. Trouble urinating (dysuria, stranguria); blood in the urine (hematuria) that persists after initial therapy.
14. Diarrhea, straining to defecate (tenesmus), constipation, blood in the stools (hematochezia), change in shape of stools.
15. Lameness, painful movement, painful joints, hesitation to exercise.
16. Excessive urination and drinking (polyuria and polydipsia (PUPD): rule out chronic kidney disease (CKD), endocrinopathy, hypercalcemia, and hepatic disease.
17. Fainting or collapsing (syncope), muffled heartbeat, pericardial effusion, pleural effusion, fast breathing (tachypnea).
18. Weakness, stumbling, loss of balance (ataxia), loss of nerve function (paresis), behavior changes, pain, pain in the chest area (pleuralgia) when being picked up.

A revised list has been prepared in lay terminology of the warning signs of cancer and illness in pets for pet owners. This list (Table 3.2), along with an illustration for locating lymph nodes (Figure 3.19), is at the end of this chapter. Clinicians are invited to copy and distribute this list and illustration to clients and the companion animal community as educational material. Excellent free sources of information to recommend to pet owners can be found at: www.VeterinaryPartner.com, sponsored by Veterinary Information Network (VIN), and www.petcancercenter.org, which is an informative website that describes 35 types of cancer and leads viewers to the Veterinary Cancer Society (VCS) listings. See the 2016 *British Small Animal Veterinary Congress* article, "Pain assessment for your practice" by Dr. Sheilah Robertson, which can also be accessed on VIN.

Cancer mimics many other diseases, and unless cancer is diagnosed and treated, it is free to behave insidiously. Certain tumor types are well known for aggressiveness and ruthless behavior. However, almost every type of cancer (neoplasia) has a premonitory sign that can be identified in its preclinical stages. If definitive action is taken at the advent of the premonitory/prodromal signs, a resolution of disease, or at least a better outcome, is possible. New tests are being developed that will recognize circulating metastatic and cancer stem cells and will diagnose cancer in earlier stages.

The "let's wait and see" attitude of the veterinarian of the past must give way to a more contemporary "let's get a diagnosis" attitude. A veterinarian advising a client to "watch" a mass lesion is practicing illogical medicine. Most pet owners do not have the skills to know if a mass is behaving in a malignant manner. Any time that the fine needle aspirate cytology of a mass is not clearly benign to the clinician, it is always best to remove the mass and submit it for definitive diagnosis immediately. If the tumor is benign, that is good news. If the tissue *is* neoplastic, early detection will be invaluable in the ongoing management of that patient (Moore 2004).

Commonly Overlooked Prodromal Warning Signs of Cancer

Sadly, too many companion pets that experienced prodromal signs, which their caregivers were concerned about, progress into advanced stages of neoplasia before a diagnosis is made. Listen carefully to your clients. A red flag should go up when you hear a client casually or assertively report a specific or vague problem or a changed behavior in an older pet. It may be a sign that you discovered in this text or one you intuitively feel or scientifically know may indicate cancer.

Oral Cancers are Discovered Late

Geriatric pets (especially cats) with oral tumors are often diagnosed late in the course of their malignancy, despite the presence of early warning signs. Many carers do not pay attention to their pet's oral health. Signs that forewarn oral cancer are often noticed with mild curiosity and procrastination. Cats with bad breath or awkward chewing may be suspected as only having a minor dental issue. The family is not alarmed particularly when the pet remains alert and joyful and continues to eat. Think of an old cat with hyperthyroidism and an oral tumor driven by an increased appetite despite oral cancer pain. People detect oral tumors in dogs more readily because they pant and display an open mouth.

Prodromal Signs for Oral Cancer

Some of the early prodromal signs of oral cancer that pet owners often neglect to act upon are:

19. Pawing at the mouth, salivating, or leaving drops of blood in the water dish.
20. Holding or chewing food on one side of the mouth, dropping food, trouble picking it up.
21. Dysphagia or an awkward motion of the tongue while trying to chew.
22. A cat attempting to grasp food but dropping it.
23. A cat ignoring or walking away from food a moment after being very interested in eating it.
24. Halitosis: one person told me that her 15-year-old Beagle was frisky but had developed the worst halitosis. She told me that the dog was no longer allowed in the house.

Oral cancer can be difficult to diagnose in geriatric pets because some neoplastic lesions have no mass. This is especially true in senior cats with oral SCC. Lesions may appear only as lytic sites in the mandible or maxilla with loose infected teeth. Secondary infection automatically accompanies loose teeth. A typical scenario is the old cat with an infected oral SCC lesion. SCC clandestinely mimics dental disease and halitosis. The cat is taken to the veterinary hospital for a dental. The loose teeth are extracted, antibiotics are prescribed and the patient goes home. The cat returns in 30–90 days with obvious neoplasia at the old extraction site. The diagnosis could have been made at the time of the previous dental extraction had the attending clinician's index of suspicion been on high alert to rule out neoplasia. Dental radiographs might have identified abnormal lysis of bone at the lesion. At the previous dentistry, a deep socket tissue biopsy containing bone from the infected site could have been diagnostic.

Early detection of oral cancer and quick, aggressive action can save a pet's life. If the veterinary profession methodically educates the pet-owning public to link the subtle warning signs of oral cancer with a visit to a well-trained, suspicious veterinary clinician, more pets will be saved.

The Veterinary Team Can Educate Clients to Detect Oral Cancer

The veterinary team can be invaluable in teaching clients about oral cancer by doing the following:

25. Explain to clients that their pets will instinctively try to maintain a normal routine despite the pain and discomfort that oral cancer inflicts.
26. Show clients how to teach new pets to allow routine grooming and inspection of the entire mouth including visualizing the tonsils and under the tongue.
27. Demonstrate how to perform a mock oral inspection while pets are young (<13 weeks). It is never too late to ask clients to acclimate their geriatric pet to oral inspections so the pet is easier to examine on rechecks.
28. Instruct pet owners to brush their pet's teeth frequently and to schedule routine dental exams. If gingivitis, tartar, and halitosis are present, dental prophylaxis is essential.

Pet owners educated in this way will be more likely to detect oral neoplasia in its earliest stages.

Patches's Case (Blood in the Mouth 4 Months Before Diagnosis of Malignant Melanoma)

Janice Wilkinson allowed her dog, Patches, an F/S 8-year-old Springer–Retriever mix, to run back and forth along the fence, teasing and playing with the dog next door. Janice saw streaks of blood coming from Patches's mouth periodically. She thought that Patches cut herself chewing on the fence while taunting her canine neighbor. Janice did not see anything unusual when she inspected. Four months later, Janice noticed a fleshy red mass medial to Patches's upper left third premolar (LmaxP3). She took Patches to her local veterinarian immediately. A biopsy of the mass diagnosed spindle cell sarcoma but it could not rule out amelanotic melanoma. Our first consultation was at this point. Since the biological behavior of these two tumors is so different, a specific diagnosis was necessary. Janice authorized an immunohistochemical stain for differentiation. The tissue tested positive for the special tissue markers, MITF and S100. The presence of these protein markers on the spindle cells confirmed the diagnosis of oral malignant melanoma.

Knowing the aggressive nature of malignant melanoma helps us plan our treatment strategy to deal with metastatic disease as well as local control. Patches had a CT scan to determine bone involvement and define the borders of her lesion. She then had a caudal maxillectomy with 1 cm clean margins around the mass. This was followed by three sessions of chemotherapy with carboplatin and then she was entered into the Canine Melanoma Vaccine Study with the University of Wisconsin. This experimental vaccine was comprised of irradiated canine melanoma cells that were genetically engineered to produce human GM-CSF (an immune stimulant). Data obtained from this study from the Animal Cancer Treatment Program at the University of Wisconsin found benefit. ONCEPT™ is a xenogeneic (derived from a different species) vaccine for canine melanoma that targets the enzyme tyrosinase. Clinical trials that were under the direction of Dr. Phil Bergman, when he was at the Animal Medical Center in New York, showed benefit. ONCEPT™ gained United States Department of Agriculture (USDA) approval for use. There is now tremendous interest in immuno-oncology. This field offers precision or personalized medicine that uses the immune system to target the patient's own cancer cells based upon genomic information. One such approach uses vaccines made from the patient's own tumor cells, which are cultivated and modified to become recognized by the patient's innate immune system (CancerMoonshot2020.com).

Jake's Case (Ocular Discharge Was Jake's Early Warning Sign for SCC)

Lisa Neff said that Jake, her 12-year-old M/N DSH, had a "runny" right eye for months. There was no response with ophthalmic medications. Lisa occasionally saw Jake pawing at the left side of his mouth. Her attending veterinarian could not find any abnormalities on physical examination. A few weeks later, Lisa noticed that Jake was chewing food in the left side of his mouth. It took several months and a third trip to the veterinary hospital for Jake's problem to be recognized and diagnosed as oral cancer. Jake's attending doctor detected a softening of the hard palate on the right side due to an infiltrative lesion involving Jake's right maxilla. The biopsy diagnosed oral SCC.

Max's Case (Arthritis Treatment Masks Osteosarcoma)

Max Boman, a 10-year-old M/N Doberman Pinscher, exhibited periodic lameness due to osteoarthritis of his elbows and hips beginning when he was 7 years old. His attending doctor dispensed Rimadyl® to ease the painful symptoms. At each episode of lameness, Max seemed to do well for about 6 weeks, as long as he had his medication, but one such episode with left foreleg lameness did not respond. The Bomans noticed a firm swelling in the mid-caudal aspect of his left foreleg. Radiographs disclosed a lytic, demineralized lesion at the distal left ulna characteristic of osteosarcoma.

The opportunity for early diagnosis was missed because Max's symptoms were masked by concurrent arthritis and the usual treatment. Symptomatic treatment for arthritis provided enough palliation against cancer-induced bone pain. This scenario is more common today since dogs are receiving powerful non-steroidal anti-inflammatory drugs (NSAIDs) in multimodality protocols for arthritis pain. The prudent veterinarian must periodically recommend radiographs for lame senior and geriatric dogs – especially for large and giant breeds with a high prevalence for osteosarcoma (Figure 3.1). If the client declines radiography, it is best to note his or her refusal in the medical chart before prescribing a course of symptomatic relief for the patient.

Warning Signs of Skin Cancer in Cats

Apart from feline injection site sarcomas (FISSs), elderly cats are six times less likely to develop skin tumors than dogs. Benign tumors in cats may appear at any age and in any breed but are most likely to appear in geriatric Persian and Siamese cats. The median age for occurrence is 12 years. The most common benign tumors in geriatric cats may be present for many years without causing clinical concern. Benign skin tumors often appear as small, raised solitary masses covered with haired skin located on the head, back, trunk, or legs. They are superficial and generally do not cause alopecia, ulceration, pain, or invasion of surrounding tissue. These tumors may be solid, cystic, or pigmented and are generally cured with surgical excision. Basal cell tumors are the most common benign skin tumors of older cats.

Most malignant skin tumors in cats appear on the head, back, dorsum, legs, and mammary glands. They may be multiple, invasive, inflamed, ulcerated, coalescing, large, and erosive. They are locally invasive. Regional lymph node invasion and metastasis is uncommon except for mammary carcinoma, malignant melanoma, and at least 22.5% of long-term feline injection site sarcomas (FISS) cases (Hershey et al. 2000).

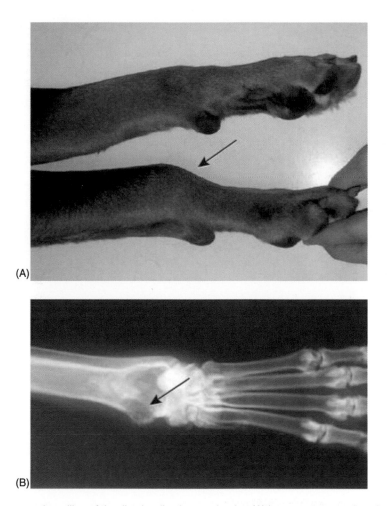

Figure 3.1. Lameness and swelling of the distal radius in a senior dog (A) is a common warning sign of bone cancer. This radiograph shows a lytic bone lesion, (B) typical of osteosarcoma.

FISS initially appears in the dermis and subcutis at typical vaccine or injection sites. The FISS Task Force recommends distal extremities for vaccination sites. Initially, a small inflammatory reaction nodule arises following vaccine. If the nodule fails to regress within 1–3 months or if it enlarges to 3cm in size, it should be biopsied (Figure 3.2). Initial wide surgical resection is required to control these invasive sarcomas.

Malignant squamous cell carcinoma (SCC), fibrosarcoma (FSA), mast cell tumor (MCT), and mammary carcinoma (MGAC) are the most common types of cancer afflicting geriatric cats. The feline sarcoma virus (FSV) causes multiple dermal masses in young cats infected with FeLV. It is rare and non-responsive to conventional treatment (Theilen, Madewell, and Gardner 1987).

Solar-Induced Skin Cancer in Cats: Non-Healing Lesions

SCC appears as chronic superficial crusting ulcers in the non-pigmented facial area of cats. Lesions most commonly appear on the ear tips, nose, lips, and temporal skin. Here are some typical quotes from cat owners: "I didn't know that it would be cancer"; "I thought he had dirt on his nose";

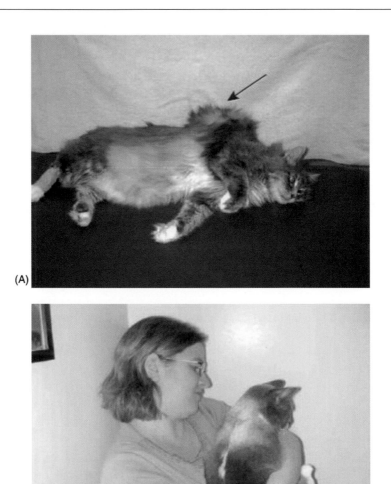

(A)

(B)

Figure 3.2. FISS arises as an inflammatory nodule, which transitions into malignancy and enlarges at vaccine or injection sites. Tumors can become very large (A). Abby shows her radiation therapy site where the hair grew in white as we celebrated her fifth anniversary of survival from FISS, with her carer (B).

"I thought he scratched his nose"; "He always rubs his nose on the screen door"; "I thought he got his ear scratched in a fight"; "I thought it was a stye in her eyelid" (Figure 3.3).

Initial lesions appear as inflamed sunburned skin with crusting sores. If the sores persist for over 2 weeks, carcinoma in situ is the most likely answer. A presumptive working diagnosis for actinic lesions or SCC would be warranted whether or not the owner permits a biopsy for verification. The superficial ulcerative lesions of carcinoma in situ are easily treated with cryotherapy or laser therapy and may respond to topical use of imiquimod (Aldara^{TM}) cream, immuno-oncology products. Moderately invasive lesions may be controlled by surgical excision, cryotherapy, laser ablation, or electrochemotherapy (ECT). Advanced lesions require radiation therapy, isotope therapy, or electroporation (EP) (see the section on ECT/EP at the end of Chapter 6). Instruct pet owners to keep white cats inside between 10:00 a.m. and 4:00 p.m. to avoid sun exposure.

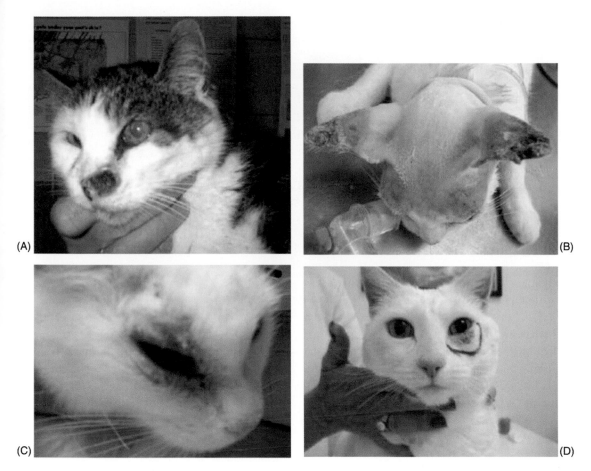

Figure 3.3.   Solar-induced nasal planum SCC in a cat (A). Solar-induced SCC on the pinnae and the temporal areas of a 20-year-old white cat (B). SCC lesions appearing on upper (C) and lower (D) eyelids of white cats exposed to the sun.

Warning Signs of Solar-Induced Squamous Cell Carcinoma (SCC)

Dogs with non-pigmented ventrum skin are at risk for SCC and from solar exposure. Breeds most commonly affected with solar-induced SCC in my practice are Pit Bulls, White Boxers, Dalmatians (Figure 3.4A), and Harlequin Great Danes. Typical warning signs of SCC on sun-exposed skin include prodromal lesions that first appear as inflamed patchy sunburn (Figure 3.4B). Early SCC lesions appear as patchy red blemishes, which may ulcerate. Advanced lesions become proliferative fleshy masses, which may hemorrhage. American Pit Bull siblings Bella and Stella developed a full array of SCC lesions (Figure 3.5). They are shown before and after therapy.

Warning Signs of Cutaneous Hemangiosarcoma

Actinic cutaneous hemangiosarcoma is a solar-induced vascular skin cancer that occurs in the non-pigmented ventral skin of dogs that like to sunbathe. Greyhounds, Italian Greyhounds, Whippets, American Pit Bulls, American Staffordshire Terriers, Basset Hounds, Beagles, Dalmatians, White Boxers, English Springer Spaniels, and Salukis are among the breeds more commonly affected. Early

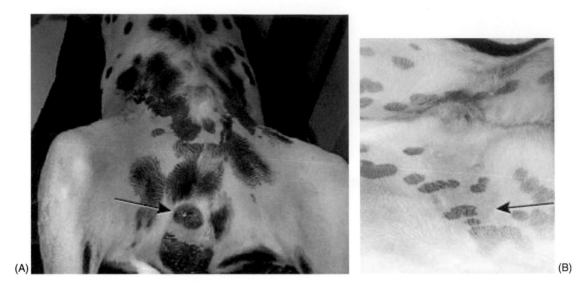

(A)

(B)

Figure 3.4. SCC in a Dalmatian's unpigmented ventrum skin due to solar exposure. The lesions metastasized to the inguinal lymph nodes (A). Patient with chronic sunburn: a prodromal sign (B).

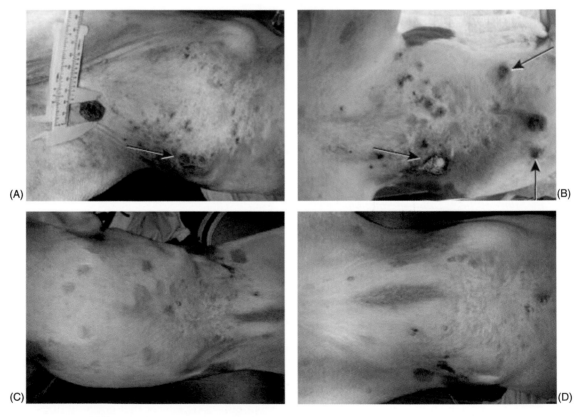

(A)

(B)

(C)

(D)

Figure 3.5. Both Pit Bull siblings, Bella (A) and Stella (B), have solar-induced SCC, which responded to a combination of surgery, cryosurgery (C, D), and oral maintenance with Agaricus immunonutrition.

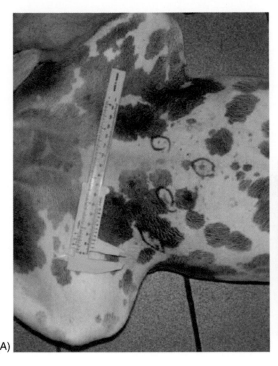
(A)

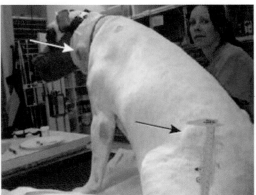
(B)

Figure 3.6.   Actinic dermal hemangiosarcoma lesions during a cryotherapy session for Penny Burchfield (A), an 11-year-old Pit Bull. Penny needs periodic cryotherapy for new lesions as they emerge over a 3-year period. Cutaneous non-actinic hemangiosarcoma is due to multisystemic hemangiosarcoma in Buddy Lebuarn, a 9-year-old American Pit Bull (B).

lesions appear as flat red spots, red blisters, or bluish blood-filled dermal cysts. Some tumors may appear as raised cystic lesions that easily hemorrhage. These lesions should be treated because they may metastasize.

Non-actinic cutaneous hemangiosarcoma is rare. It is a cutaneous manifestation from multicentric hemangiosarcoma (Figure 3.6B). Breeds reported with greater prevalence are Bernese Mountain Dogs, Boxers, German Shepherd Dogs, and Golden Retrievers (Goldschmidt and Hendrick 2002).

Penny's Case (She Had a Rash That Would Not Go Away)

Penny Burchfield, an 8-year-old F/S Pit Bull mix, was plagued with skin allergies. She developed little red spots on the skin of her underside. Her family thought the red spots were "just another rash," but the spots did not go away with topical or systemic treatment for allergies. Penny was referred to a dermatologist, who diagnosed cutaneous hemangiosarcoma (cHSA) by punch biopsy. It is a cancer of the superficial capillaries in delicate skin and generally does not exhibit the aggressive biological behavior of visceral hemangiosarcoma. Penny was given Accutane®, an expensive retinoid, for a year and a half. The cHSA lesions did not regress. She developed a small, fleshy mass on her right flank that was removed during a routine dental examination. Her attending veterinarian submitted the mass for histopathology and found that the mass was an incompletely removed grade II MCT.

We met Penny for consultation regarding the MCT. She had over 50 cHSA lesions (Figure 3.6A). Since Accutane™ was not helpful, we recommended cryotherapy for the numerous cHSA lesions. More than three years passed since that first consultation. Penny developed new cHSA lesions every few months and had periodic cryotherapy as needed. New MCTs appeared yearly and were widely excised. Eventually, Penny passed away after she developed acute hemoabdomen from a ruptured hemangiosarcoma of her spleen. There is good reason to address cHSA lesions early in their clinical course as some may metastasize to the viscera.

Cutaneous Lymphoma: Often Misdiagnosed as Dermatitis

Cutaneous lymphoma (CL) has many manifestations that may run over a variable length of time. It may first appear as flaky and/or inflamed, hyperemic skin with or without pruritis. One client commented that his pet's skin looked as if it was producing ashes. In many cases of CL, the owner and the attending doctor notice flaky skin, dandruff, dermatitis, folliculitis, macules, plaques, and pododermatitis for several months, or longer, before skin biopsies are taken. Lesions may be crusted, ulcerated, alopecic, pigmented, and pruritic and may wax and wane. CL is rare in cats.

Most cases of CL are histologically diagnosed in older dogs as cutaneous T-cell epitheliotrophic lymphoma. It is also known by its old misnomer, *mycosis fungoides* (MF), because the lesions mimic fungal disease. Non-epitheliotrophic cutaneous lymphoma lesions may be B- or T-cell. Painful, inflamed lesions often appear in the oral cavity, eyelids, and body orifices. CL may respond to initial chemotherapy for short remissions but most patients die within a year of diagnosis (Figures 3.7 and 3.8). With the advent of immunotherapeutics, we may be able to improve survival times.

Jack's Case (CL Can Easily Be Misdiagnosed as Dermatitis)

Jack Watson, a 10-year-old M/N Golden Retriever, developed non-pruritic, flaky, scaly skin. His attending doctor treated the differential list that included flea allergy dermatitis, atopic dermatitis, pyoderma, and food allergies. Over a period of 6 months, Jack's skin appeared inflamed and would dry, causing large pieces of dried skin to peel and flake. Later, Jack developed macules and plaques of thickened skin. Several punch biopsy specimens were sent for histopathology. He was diagnosed with cutaneous T-cell lymphoma.

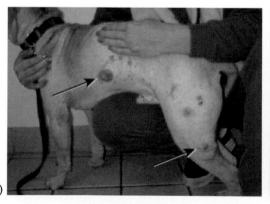
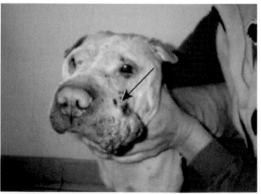

(A) (B)

Figure 3.7.   Shar-Pei with cutaneous lymphoma. Most cases are diagnosed as T-cell epitheliotrophic lymphoma.

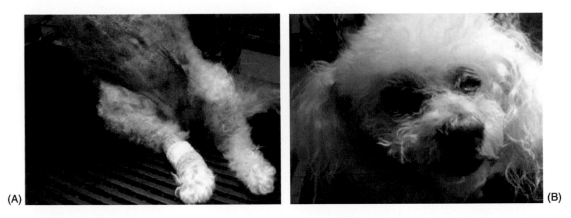

Figure 3.8. Cutaneous lymphoma appeared as inflamed hyperemic dry skin, which mimicked allergic dermatitis, for several months before diagnosis in this 16-year-old Poodle (A). Notice the late-stage lesions in her eyelids (B). Mitzie also had painful oral lesions.

Mast Cell Tumors (MCT)

One in five skin tumors, which appear as innocent fatty tumors or fleshy wide-based warts, may actually be MCT. Boxer and Bulldog breeds are at greater risk although any breed may be affected. Mast cells are normally present in all tissues of the body and function in allergic reactions and local control of vascular tone. There are greater numbers of mast cells in airways and around body openings. Some MCTs appear rapidly on the face, feet, or axilla resembling insect bites. Do not cling to this diagnosis if the swelling lasts over 2 days. MCTs may also arise in the feline spleen or along the intestinal tract or in the liver. On occasion, some MCTs acquire the behavior of infiltrating lymphomas. In these cases, mast cells are found in the bone marrow and in the peripheral blood as mast cell leukemia.

Lucy's Case (The Family Thought She Had Hairballs)

Lucy, a 12-year-old F/S DSH, started vomiting once or twice daily for several weeks. The family initially felt Lucy's problem was hairballs. The vomiting episodes were unresponsive to initial treatment. When her vomiting episodes became more frequent and more dramatic, she was referred for consultation. Endoscopic exam found a fleshy red lesion involving the pylorus, which was diagnosed as MCT. She responded well to surgical excision and chemotherapy for at least 6 months until lost to follow-up.

Biological Behavior of Mast Cell Tumors

Mast cell tumors behave variably depending on their grade and location. Lesions in mucocutaneous junctions, groin, axilla, and mammary chain are more aggressive in my experience, although one report found no difference (Sfiligoi et al. 2005). Some tumors appear and regress and reappear. Rapid growth rate (doubling time), geriatric age greater than 8 years, metastatic disease at the time of diagnosis, and relapse are factors that negatively affect prognosis.

Cytograding mast cell tumors based on the Kiupel method is very helpful to determine if a particular tumor is likely to be aggressive. The presence of multinucleated cells, and a mitotic index >4/10 high power fields indicates high grade disease (Scarpa et al. 2014). The MCT Panel stains for KIT, Ki-67,

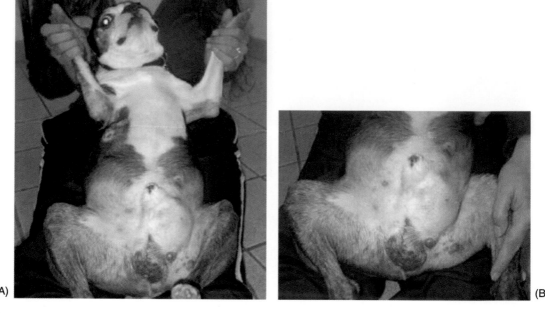

Figure 3.9. Buddy had a pedunculated mass on his left caudal thigh for 3 years. It was removed without a biopsy. The lesion was metastatic to Buddy's inguinal node and the mammary lymphatic vessels.

PCNA, Agnors, and IDT mutation analysis. Tissue can also be sent to Innogenics for the Enlight™ assay to differentiate and suggest treatment options. This may be useful in predicting behavior and response to selected and targeted therapy.

Buddy's Case (An Innocent-Looking Skin Mass Can Kill)

Buddy, a 10-year-old M/N Boston Terrier, had a pedunculated mass on his left caudal thigh for 3 years. At first, the mass looked like an innocent skin tag. It changed suddenly one day and looked more like a mushroom. The mass was removed during a routine dental procedure without a biopsy. Within a month, Buddy's thigh and his left popliteal lymph node became swollen. FNA cytology revealed malignant mast cells. The lesion was metastatic to Buddy's inguinal node and the mammary lymphatic vessels (Figure 3.9).

All brachycephalic dogs are prone to MCTs. Therefore, it is best to perform an FNA on even the most innocent-looking indolent skin lesions in a brachycephalic dog prior to removal. In this way, a wider surgical excision and biopsy for grading, staging, and treatment can be planned.

Hanny's Case (MCT Present for 3 Years, Then Lymphoma)

Hanny Jackson, a 9-year-old F/S Golden Retriever, had a recent history of hypothyroidism, urinary tract infection (UTI), and a grade I MCT. Thyroid supplementation helped Hanny shed 16 pounds over 4 months. She developed several new dermal and subcutaneous masses. The attending doctor recommended removal and biopsy. If the biopsy indicated MCT, then a second deeper excision may be needed. He also warned that more lumps might develop.

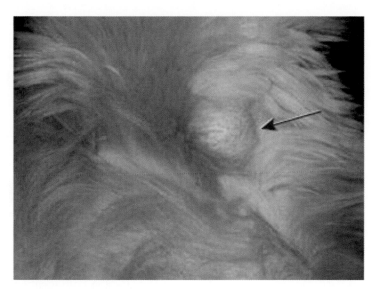

Figure 3.10. This innocent-looking mast cell tumor was present for 3 years in the right axilla of Hanny, an older Golden Retriever.

It was at this point that Mr. Jackson was referred to our service for consultation. Hanny had six skin tumors. A mass in her right axilla was $1.2 \times 1.2 \times 0.5 \text{cm}^3$. It was a pearl-colored, hairless dermal tumor of 3 years duration (Figure 3.10). Mr. Jackson said that he had asked his veterinarian about the mass but was told that it was not a problem.

Three of the six skin tumors revealed sheets of mast cells on FNA cytology, including the right axillary mass. The MCTs were removed widely and diagnosed as grade I-II MCTs on histopathology. Hanny received oral chlorambucil and prednisone and weekly vinblastine IV chemotherapy for 8 weeks followed by a tapering schedule. Six months later, Hanny exhibited generalized lymphadenopathy. FNA cytology was consistent with lymphoma. Immunohistochemical stains were positive for CD79a, which classified it as a B-cell lymphoma.

This scenario illustrates the vulnerability of geriatric cancer patients to second primary cancers, especially for Golden Retrievers and Boxers. It would be expected that Hanny's lymphoma would be more resistant to treatment due to previous use of steroids for her MCT. Fortunately, she achieved remission with induction chemotherapy.

Rapidly Growing Masses in the Skin

Mast cell tumors may appear suddenly. They may appear as angry, fleshy, inflamed masses that have no hair (epilate). Some MCTs have a glassy appearance on denuded skin. Some have a very rapid growth rate. Some may appear as a bee sting and cause a large swelling.

Max's Case (MCT Misdiagnosed as a Bee Sting, Then a Spider Bite)

Max Anselmo, a 10-year-old M/N Aussie, suddenly developed a swelling on the right side of his nose that was treated as a bee sting. The swelling shrank marginally with antihistamines and steroids but returned. Mike took Max back to the vet, who then suspected a spider bite. Four weeks went by on symptomatic treatment while Max's muzzle remained swollen. Mike noticed that a lymph node in Max's neck was enlarged. The attending veterinarian took FNA samples that diagnosed both the muzzle and node swelling to be mast cell cancer. He responded to radiation and chemotherapy for several months; however, he developed systemic involvement. Diagnosis a month earlier might have changed the outcome for Max.

Some MCTs appear and then disappear and may go undiagnosed because of this transient feature.

Katie's Case (An Educated Owner Was Suspicious of MCT)

John Haddon read one of my local newspaper columns about MCT. It said that some MCTs could appear and then disappear due to histamine release, causing a local inflammatory response. John's 3-year-old F/S Rhodesian Ridgeback, Katie, had a marble-sized mass in the skin behind her ear that disappeared. A few days later, John noticed that another mass appeared on the opposite side of Katie's neck. Because of what he read, John brought Katie to our clinic for an examination.

FNA cytology of each site found sheets of mast cells present at both locations. A third MCT was found on her proximal hind thigh. We surgically excised a section of skin that contained both the palpable mass and the regressed mass. We also removed the mass on her thigh with wide margins. The tumors were grade II MCT on histopathology. Katie developed a new crop of MCTs about every 3 years and lived to age 11.

Warning Signs of Mammary Cancer in Dogs

Many people feel guilty that they didn't recognize the early warning signs of mammary cancer in their dog. Here are some typical quotes: "I thought it was a cyst"; "The tumors didn't bother her"; "My vet said to keep an eye on it"; "One thing led to another and we didn't get back to the pet hospital when they grew"; "We wanted her to have a litter first but we never got around to it"; "My husband wants to keep her natural"; "We didn't know that if you spay a female dog or cat before she goes into heat, it protects her from breast cancer" (Figure 3.11).

Since the 1970s, our profession has accepted that one out of four intact female dogs over 4 years of age is at risk for developing one or more breast tumors. However, recent data on specific breeds (Labrador and Golden Retrievers) has found a lower risk (Hart 2016). Malignant mammary carcinomas are diagnosed in 50% of mammary tumors and half of these carcinomas metastasize to draining lymph nodes and lungs via a plexus of lymphatic vessels within 1 year. Ovarian hormones, progesterone and estrogen, cause sensitization and promotion in mammary tissues, resulting in point mutations in the genes that initiate tumor growth causing field cancerization. Ovariohysterectomy (OVH) surgery prior to 6 months of age is preventative while OVH surgery prior to $2\frac{1}{2}$ years of age has a sparing effect. The best age for OVH in large, athletic dogs has been examined by evaluation of the long-term effects of gonadal removal of male and females of various breeds. It may be best to wait until after 12 months to allow growth plate closure to offset joint disorders. Female Golden Retrievers that remain intact may benefit with a reduced rate of lymphoma, hemangiosarcoma, mast cell tumor, and did not seem to be at great risk for mammary cancer (Hart 2014).

Ginger's Case (Biopsy All Mammary Tumors at Initial Surgery)

Ginger Meeks, a female 10-year-old Australian Shepherd, went to work every day at various construction sites and herded sheep on the family's ranch. She had one litter and was never

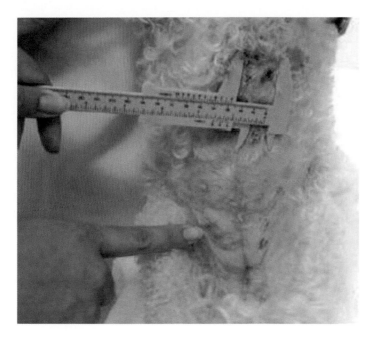

Figure 3.11. Breast tumors in an intact female geriatric Poodle.

spayed. Ginger developed two mammary tumors that were probably not noticed for some time due to her thick coat. When the family noticed the tumors, the masses felt like walnuts. Ginger's veterinarian performed a lumpectomy but submitted no biopsy at that time.

Shortly after, several tumors recurred at the site. A second surgery was performed; this time, a mastectomy and biopsy verified mammary adenocarcinoma. The biopsy did not detail the margins because only a small sample of tumor tissue was submitted for diagnosis (see Chapter 5 on biopsy techniques and pathology and Chapter 6 on surgical margins).

Within a month, Ginger developed angry red, weeping, raised dermal rashes emanating up to 6cm in all directions from the incision site. At that point Ginger's family came to our service for consultation (Figure 3.12A). She was in severe pain from the lesions to the point where she had trouble walking. Mammary cancer invasive into the cutaneous lymphatics is known as

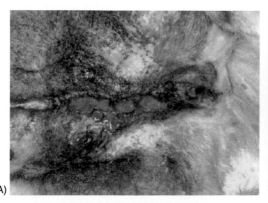
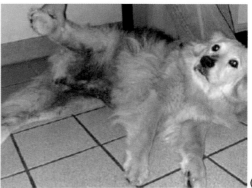

(A)   (B)

Figure 3.12. Breast cancer in the cutaneous lymphatics is known as inflammatory mammary adenocarcinoma or inflammatory carcinoma. It exhibits a very aggressive behavior and is universally fatal. The lesion infiltrated the suture line (A). Notice the swollen right rear leg in this patient (B).

inflammatory mammary adenocarcinoma or inflammatory carcinoma. It has a very aggressive biologic behavior. The family declined chemotherapy due to the poor prognosis. We provided palliative anti-inflammatory therapy and pain medication and entered her into Pawspice care. It may not be fair to speculate, but Ginger may have had a different course if the first surgery had been a mastectomy with a biopsy. However, the mechanisms that cause inflammatory carcinoma are not fully understood (Figure 3.12B).

Breast Tumors in Cats: Malignant Mammary Carcinoma

Most cats that remained intact while young are prone to breast cancer when they are 10–12 years old, but tumors may appear at any age. Mammary tumors are the third most common tumors in cats and over 80% are malignant and behave aggressively. Siamese cats are at twice the risk as other cat breeds. Most carers who notice these tumors delay visiting their veterinarian for several months or until they notice a discharge from involved nipples or a second mass. By that time, there may be ulcers, infiltration of lymphatics, or swelling and edema. Radical mastectomy is superior to lumpectomy to minimize recurrence. Tumors over 3cm have a poor prognosis due to early metastasis.

Cancer of the Nasal Passages

Nasal passage cancer develops insidiously in older pets. It composes up to 2.4% of reported canine tumors and is more common in long-nosed (dolichocephalic) dogs and rare in cats. The most common tissue types found in canine nasal passage cancer are nasal respiratory carcinoma, SCC, fibrosarcoma, chondrosarcoma, and lymphoma. Lymphoma and respiratory adenocarcinoma are the most common tissue types found in feline nasal tumors. Treatment is frustrating because 68% of dogs with nasal cancer do poorly with the best of treatment. There is encouragement from a study that employed follow-up CT scan and surgical exenteration of residual disease following radiation therapy, which more than doubled median survival times (Adams et al. 2005).

The early warning signs of nasal cancer in dogs or cats are unilateral nasal and/or ocular discharge, epistaxis, stridor, loss of smell, facial or palatine deformity, loose teeth, and, sometimes, pawing at the face. Late-stage signs would exhibit a deformity along the dorsal aspect of the maxillary bones or over the paranasal and frontal sinuses. Some pets present a raised or pitting facial deformity. The deformity may involve the maxilla. Some pets exhibit a firm or soft focal, raised mass protruding below, around, or between the eyes. Some cases may have a softening and bowing out of the hard palate due to demineralization of the palatine bone. In every case of facial deformity, there is bone lysis and tumor invasion at that site. There may be a tremendous amount of mucus and phlegm clogged in the passages and sinuses. The stridor, discharge, sneezing, and epistaxis and blood spraying cause great distress for the family.

Most cases of nasal cancer exhibit sporadic signs, which show progression over a period of about 3 months before they are actually diagnosed. Initially the clinical signs fit the assumption that the pet has one of a various number of afflictions of the nasal passages. Occasionally, a dog may sneeze out tissue that can be sent for histopathology.

Most clinicians would rightly suspect that the geriatric patient has rhinitis or allergies or an inhaled foreign body. Initial rhinoscopy may find no lesions while cultures find the usual pathogens. The diagnosis of rhinitis may suffice for a time. The presence of oral–nasal fistula or pain from infected or extracted teeth may complicate matters and mask the diagnosis.

Rufus's Case (One Episode of Epistaxis Can Forewarn Cancer)

Rufus, a 10-year-old M/N Black Lab belonging to Trudy Gleason, had a single episode of epistaxis. He started snoring over the following 4 months. After a second episode of epistaxis, his attending veterinarian performed rhinoscopy and biopsy, which yielded the diagnosis of nasal passage chondrosarcoma. Rufus was referred for radiation therapy. Trudy was told that nothing else could be done for Rufus and that his chances for survival past another 3–6 months would be all that she should expect. Trudy did not want radiation for Rufus and came in for a second opinion. Treatment with 6 cycles of carboplatin every 21 days then with increasing intervals along with immunonutrition helped Rufus survive another 3 years with a great quality of life. Rufus accompanied Trudy on 30 Ten Kilometer walks during his 3 year Pawspice before recurrence.

Blue's Case (Episodic Epistaxis Forewarns Nasal Cancer)

Blue Monahan, F/S, an 11-year-old Aussie, had an episode of nasal bleeding. A CT scan and rhinoscopy with biopsy were negative. Three months later, Blue had a second episode of nasal bleeding. This time around, the CT scan and biopsy confirmed nasal chondrosarcoma. Blue was given essentially the same poor prognosis that Rufus (just discussed) had been given. The family asked me for a second opinion, which led me to recommend radiation therapy, carboplatin, and immunonutrition.

Suede's Case (Clients Don't Report Some Warning Signs)

Suede, a 9-year-old male Chocolate Labrador Retriever belonging to Susie Saddle, had a senior wellness "tumor watch" exam including chest and abdominal X-rays. The exam showed no signs of tumor activity. Two months later, Suede sneezed out a chunk of tissue. Susie took the mass to her local pet hospital to submit for pathology. Suede was diagnosed with SCC. It was at this point that Susie admitted that Suede had been sneezing for 5 months. She did not mention the sneezing or occasional epistaxis during Suede's wellness exam because she thought the sneezing was from allergies or inhaled weeds or dust. She admitted to not reading our brochure that describes the warning signs of cancer. Do not assume that your clients will take the time to read handouts or newsletters.

Instruct your room assistants to review the checklist of warning signs for cancer and illness during senior wellness exams and geriatric checkups (see Table 3.2 at the end of the chapter).

Warning Signs of Abdominal Masses

Geriatric dogs and cats are very deceiving as they develop indolent abdominal tumors. They may appear to be slowing down or look as if they are gaining weight. Some pets show subtle reluctance to get up, a change in behavior, or lethargy. Others develop nausea, vomiting, weakness, straining, obstructions, diarrhea, hematochezia, lethargy, hemoabdomen, and so forth. Unfortunately, most abdominal masses are detected late in geriatric pets.

Warning Signs of GI Lymphoma in Cats

Although there has been a drop in FeLV-related lymphomas in cats, there is a rise in non-viral intestinal lymphoma with and without pre-existing inflammatory bowel disease (Louwerens, London, and

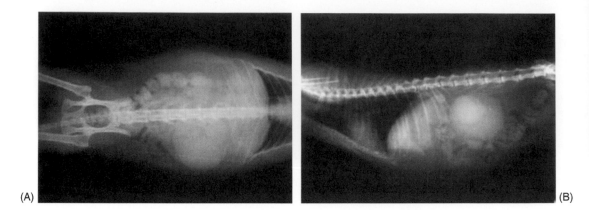

(A)   (B)

Figure 3.13.   Radiographs showing renomegaly.

Pederson 2005; Cotter 2005). Soft stools, diarrhea, and chronic weight loss in older cats are important warning signs to rule out GI lymphoma. These skinny old cats often have normal values in their blood work and normal X-rays on their workup. Intestines may feel ropey on palpation. Many of these cats do not have palpable masses in the abdomen. If there is no response to dietary management, further diagnostic tests are indicated.

Endoscopy and biopsy of inflamed and suspicious (cobble stone) looking lesions may establish the diagnosis of intestinal lymphoma. At times, the only way to get a definitive diagnosis is with exploratory surgery and full thickness tissue samples taken from several areas of the intestinal tract. For cats with abdominal masses, FNA cytology or Tru-cut needle core tissue samples may establish the diagnosis without subjecting the geriatric oncology patient to the stress of exploratory surgery (Figure 3.13).

Warning Signs of Hepatic Tumors

Geriatric pets are more prone to develop hepatic neoplasia as they age. The warning signs are non-specific during the early stages but may include polydipsia, abdominal distension, nausea, anorexia, elevated liver enzymes, icterus, vomiting, pain, and lethargy. Obesity, hypothyroidism, and Cushing's disease are concurrent conditions that may camouflage the warning signs of hepatic tumors in geriatric pets.

Mitzie's Case (Elevated Liver Enzymes Are a Clue)

Mitzie, a 13-year-old F/S Beagle belonging to Roberta Karsch, had a history of colitis with acute episodes three to four times a year. Mitzie gradually developed an enlarged abdomen and drank more water as she aged. Her doctor considered Cushing's disease and ran all the tests. The liver enzymes were up but she was negative for Cushing's. Radiographs indicated a large hepatic mass or hepatomegaly. Abdominal ultrasound detected a 15cm mass in the central caudal liver displacing her gallbladder caudal and to the left of midline. Roberta elected exploratory laparotomy. The surgeon performed a right liver lobectomy and gallbladder excision. The diagnosis was biliary adenocarcinoma. We treated Mitzie with chemotherapy for 4 months. She developed multifocal recurrence in her liver with elevations of her hepatic enzymes, ascites, and abdominal distension (Figure 3.14).

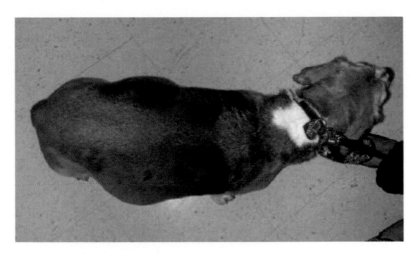

Figure 3.14. Mitzie Karsch, a 13-year-old F/S Beagle, had a right liver lobectomy and gallbladder excision for a 15cm hepatic mass. The diagnosis was biliary adenocarcinoma. Her early warning signs were masked by concurrent: colitis, overweight body condition score, and Cushing's disease. Mitzie's ascites recurred.

Alfie's Case (My Own Dog's Liver Cancer Was Insidious)

Alfie, my own $11^{1}/_{2}$-year-old Australian Shepherd, showed some hesitation to go on his morning walk without his rimadyl. In retrospect, it was out of character for Alfie to stay on the floor during a car ride. He usually jumped on the seat to look out the window with Alaska, our Great Pyrenees. Alfie was alert, active, and still interested in food when my associate, Dr. Kathleen Carson, commented on him, saying Alfie looks "a little geriatric." I examined him carefully and palpated a large, firm mass in his anterior abdomen. I could feel his ribs and realized that Alfie had mild muscle wasting from cancer cachexia. From that moment forward, Alfie knew that I knew. He acted like the sick dog he truly was, dutifully enduring his workup with radiographs, ultrasound, and FNAs, which indicated a bizarre sarcoma. Exploratory celiotomy found metastatic lesions throughout the entire hepatic parenchyma, mesenteric nodes, gallbladder, and serosa. We had said our goodbyes to Alfie before he went under anesthesia. When the surgeon told us the malignancy was inoperable, we sent him scampering carefree over the rainbow bridge. The histologic diagnosis was a highly malignant undifferentiated carcinoma of unknown origin.

Warning Signs of Splenic Tumors

German Shepherd Dogs, Golden Retrievers, Portuguese Water Dogs and other large-breed dogs are prone to develop splenic tumors. Geriatric dogs show very few warning signs during the early indolent stages of splenic hemangiosarcoma. It is a very aggressive vascular cancer, which is thought to arise from CD34-positive stem cells (hemangioblasts) from bone marrow origin (Modiano and Helfand 2005). Pale mucous membranes, slowing down, hesitation to exercise, or distended abdomen may be signs of splenic hemangiosarcoma, but most dogs are diagnosed only after acute abdominal hemorrhage of a splenic mass. It is good to note that of 200 dogs that had splenectomy at the University of Minnesota, 60% were not hemangiosarcoma (Modiano 2016a).

It makes sense to screen all susceptible breeds over the age of 5. Proactive screening would include survey abdominal X-rays and/or ultrasound examinations every 6 months to check for splenic hemangiosarcoma (HSA). We may be able to extend the survival times in cases that are detected before splenic rupture. Very few dogs with splenic tumors are lucky enough to be diagnosed early. That situation may change with new tests to detect circulating hemangioblasts by sorting with flow cytometry. Soon you will be able to send 3 ml of anticoagulated blood to a laboratory for detection of HSA in dogs at risk. Soon we may be using a new endothelial vaccine (in clinical trials) that may help dogs survive this dreaded cancer. In addition to early detection, we may soon be able to *prevent* HSA by using a specific low dose bacterial toxin that targets specific EGF and UPA receptors on HSA's progenitor cancer stem cells. This new generation of preventative therapy is called chemoprophylaxis for HSA (Modiano 2016b).

Chloe's Case (Screen High-Risk Breeds; Surgery Is Best Before Splenic Rupture)

Chloe Foreman, a 12-year-old German Shepherd Dog, accompanied her pal, Max, for his final farewell after a 1-year battle with nasal chondrosarcoma. Mr. Foreman admits that he focused all his attention on Max's radiation therapy, recurrence, and overdue bills. He did not take Chloe for an exam when her coat turned dull, she lost weight, and started itching. Right after Max was euthanized, Mr. Foreman asked the attending doctor to examine Chloe. He said, "The doctor's face turned white when she palpated Chloe's abdomen." The doctor discovered a large mass in the area of the spleen. That day, Chloe had blood work, radiographs, ultrasound, and exploratory surgery. She was referred to our service for consultation and follow-up care. Mr. Foreman could not afford costly chemotherapy for HSA. He settled for vincristine, Cytoxan, piroxicam, doxycycline, and immunonutrition. Chloe gained back 15 pounds and her shiny coat. She survived over 16 months postsplenectomy.

Marty's Case (Not All Bleeding Spleens Are a Death Sentence)

Marty Lloyd, a 19-year-old, 90-pound M/N Collie belonging to Gary Lloyd, presented with acute onset of weakness and pale mucous membranes. Abdominal radiographs and a four-quadrant abdominal tap indicated that this crisis was due to a bleeding tumor in his spleen. Ultrasound-guided FNA of a $6 \times 6cm^2$ cavitated splenic mass failed to confirm hemangiosarcoma on cytology. The mass was confined to Marty's spleen. Radiographs showing three views of the thorax were clear and his organ function panel was within normal limits. He had anemia (PCV 20%). We felt that Marty, despite his advanced age, would survive exploratory laparotomy and splenectomy because his performance assessment and body condition prior to this episode was excellent for a dog of 19 years. We told Gary that 80% of bleeding, cavitated splenic tumors are malignant hemangiosarcomas or cancer of some type but that 20% are benign hematomas. If the bleeding was controlled with splenectomy and if Marty survived the postoperative period, there was an 80% chance that Marty would only have another 3–4 months to live.

Gary responded with an amazing look of relief and said, "Why wouldn't I want to do this? You are telling me that if you operate that he has a good chance to live 3–4 months and a 20% chance of living longer than that! Why would I not want to give him a chance?" Gary turned my grim statistics into his golden window of opportunity. Old Marty made it through the surgical procedure. He lived 3 more years, with the help of acupuncture, chiropractic, and immunonutrition to the ripe old age of 22.

Chronic Hematuria Heralds Bladder or Prostate Cancer

Transitional cell carcinoma (TCC) of the bladder causes disturbance of urine flow and hematuria and initially mimics a urinary tract infection (|UTI). TCC represents 1–2 of all canine cancer and is very rare in cats. Prostate cancer may also cause hematuria and mimic UTI as it often evades early diagnosis. Prostate cancer represents about 1% of all canine cancers and is extremely rare in cats. Antibiotics often create an apparent improvement, masking symptoms, which can delay detection and diagnosis of these insidious cancers. Persistent hematuria should urge pursuit of the diagnosis with a rectal exam, a reliable urine assay, bladder and prostate ultrasound, and/or cystoscopy.

The CADET *BRAF* Mutation Detection Assay is now available for early detection of TCC in urine. Since the BRAF mutation is present on 85% of all canine TCC cells, the mutant gene can be detected in as few as 10 cells in a urine sample. The good news is that cancer can be detected up to 4 months or longer before it becomes evident. The test will be available to dog owners and veterinarians. It does not yield false positives and is not affected by the presence of blood, bacteria, or inflammation (www.SentinelBiomedical.com).

A tumor antigen test (V-BTA Test, Bion Diagnostic Sciences, Redmond, WA) may help diagnose TCC when used with cytology as a screening test. Unfortunately, hematuria causes false positives. Since hematuria is the chief symptom in TCC, the test alone is limited. Most labs will run the test but its application in hematuria cases may need to be interpreted alongside cytology, ultrasound, or double contrast radiography, which visualizes lesions.

Surgery is seldom helpful in TCC because of widespread seeding, unless the lesion is confined to the apex of the bladder. Surgery is rarely the first choice in prostate cancer due to the extent of disease at diagnosis and complications. Stereotactic radiation may be the best option to palliate selected cases.

Sacsha's Case (Persistent Hematuria Signals Bladder Cancer)

Sacsha Podowlski, a 17-year-old Samoyed–Shepherd mix, was treated for three episodes of UTI and hematuria over an 18-month period. He was on soloxine for hypothyroidism and carprofen (Rimadyl®) for chronic arthritis. Abdominal ultrasound revealed a large mass along the left wall of the bladder. A urethral catheter was used to aspirate cells from the wall lesion for cytology. Sacsha was diagnosed with TCC. He responded to chemotherapy with mitoxantrone for a short period, with an improved quality of life. Sacsha had a beautiful wake before his home euthanasia with his family and friends from happy dog park days.

Winter's Case (Bladder Stones and UTI May Mask Bladder Cancer)

Winter Tobo, a 15-year-old M/N Cocker Spaniel who had been successfully cured of MCT 5 years previously, presented with a history of UTIs and chronic hematuria. The condition was initially responsive to antibiotics, but recently the hematuria persisted. Two large bladder stones were identified on plain radiography, which explained the hematuria. At cystotomy, the bladder mucosa appeared fleshy and abnormal. Tissue was submitted for biopsy, which diagnosed TCC. Winter's cystotomy incision dehisced and he was taken to an emergency clinic for care. Budget constraints forced the family to opt for euthanasia.

Warning Signs of Colon Tumors

Colorectal neoplasia is associated with maldigestion, weight loss, bloody stools (hematochezia), tenesmus, diarrhea, abnormally shaped feces, and obstruction. Many geriatric patients are at advanced stages of disease when tumors become large enough to cause symptoms. One of my geriatric oncology patients exhibited sporadic hematochezia over 5 years before the family consented for a workup.

Lucky's Case (Tenesmus and Change in Stool Shape Warned of Cancer)

Joan Scheid noticed that her 14-year-old M/N Scottish Terrier mix, Lucky, was straining and that his stools were flattened or leaf shaped. A rectal exam was normal, but a barium enema found a solitary mass in the colon. Joan opted for exploratory laparotomy. The mass was removed with wide margins followed by anastomosis. The mass was diagnosed on histopathology as a leiomyosarcoma. The mass could have been intestinal adenocarcinoma or MCT but Lucky was indeed a lucky dog because this sarcoma is associated with long survival following excision. Lucky lived to be 17 years of age.

Warning Signs of Anal Sac Carcinoma

Anal sac tumors may become quite large before a dog exhibits symptoms due to the innate elasticity of the anal sphincter. Some tumors protrude and may be noticed at an early stage. Most grow alongside the distal rectum and may expand to 5–8cm in large dogs before being noticed. Straining to defecate (tenesmus), bleeding, malodorous anal discharge, abnormal bowel movements, or stool drifting off to one side during elimination are all warning signs of anal or perianal tumors. Some dogs are not diagnosed until they have trouble defecating due to metastases and enlargement of the sublumbar/iliac nodes from the primary anal sac mass. These lymph nodes may expand enormously, placing firm pressure on the colon and causing tenesmus, change in the shape of the patient's stool, and ultimately obstruction and distant pulmonary metastasis.

Dealing with Geriatric Caregivers with Geriatric Pets

Veterinarians need to be especially careful when dealing with elderly pet owners and their geriatric oncology pets. They may have trouble remembering instructions and keeping things in order. Elderly people are also burdened with their own doctor visits and concurrent conditions such as arthritis, heart disease, diabetes, and hearing and vision deficits. We cannot expect them to wrestle with their pet to give pills or be responsible for difficult home care procedures and wound care.

Lady, Jax, Prince, and Boy's Case (Screen All Geriatric Pets in the Same Household)

The Conners, an elderly couple, shared their lives with three cats and a dog that were all geriatrics. Lady, their beloved 13-year-old F/S DSH, developed a third recurrence of FVAS and was referred to our service. One year into Lady's treatment, Jax, their M/N 12-year-old DLH, started salivating. He was in too much pain to allow an oral exam. Under sedation, we found that a huge fleshy mass had completely obstructed his pharynx, making intubation impossible. We were amazed that Jax's problem had gone unnoticed in the Conner household for so long. Mr. Conner said that Jax had quit eating dry food a couple of months before. Somehow Jax could swallow soft food without dysphagia, gagging, or pawing at his mouth.

A few months later, the Conners noted a large firm mass in the right axilla of their 12-year-old M/N Shepherd-Malamute, Prince. The mass was $8 \times 8 \times 8cm^3$ and diagnosed as sweat gland adenocarcinoma. Prince was a big, energetic dog and difficult for the elderly couple to manage for brushing, bathing, or walking. Mr. Conner did not see or feel the mass until it was obvious due to Prince's thick undercoat and hefty appearance.

At age 16, Lady (a 3-year FVAS survivor) started losing weight. Her appetite remained excellent. On physical exam, we palpated a small thyroid nodule and small tumors in her caudal left mammary glands measuring $1.5 \times 1 \times 1cm^3$. Hyperthyroidism and mammary adenocarcinoma were diagnosed and treated. Six months later, Lady developed diarrhea and weight loss. GI lymphoma was diagnosed and treated. Lady succumbed to renal failure at age 17. A year later, Lady's son, Boy, developed loose stools and weight loss. He was diagnosed with GI lymphoma at age 17 and treated.

This scenario is common in households where people and pets are aging together. Mr. Conner was burdened with doctor visits and hospitalizations for Mrs. Conner's diabetes and heart condition. Veterinarians need to be proactive with elderly clients who have elderly pets. We can establish routine visits to carefully examine and screen the family's geriatric pets. Hopefully, we will identify problems, including cancer, at early stages.

Acute Warning Signs

Cancer creates acute symptoms due to its insidious indolent nature. Cancer can bypass prodromal signs and build momentum within the host. Some caregivers reported that the cancer figuratively burst out like the creature in the movie *Alien*. Acute signs are more than warning signs; they are often so obvious that they are direct indicators. Acute signs put attending doctors on high alert to strongly suspect cancer in their geriatric patients. Older patients admitted for acute collapse, seizures, dyspnea, obstruction, pathological fractures, blood dyscrasias, septic fevers, and low blood glucose should be worked up to rule out neoplasia.

Collapse or Seizures: May Be a Ruptured Abdominal Mass or Brain Tumor

A dog with a splenic or hepatic mass might be playing, then suddenly lie down and be unable to move. A dog with an insulinoma may have a seizure or collapse. A cat with spinal lymphoma may become paralyzed. A dog with a brain tumor or a cat a meningioma may have seizures. A dog with a bleeding hemangiosarcoma of the right atrium may collapse due to cardiac tamponade and pericardial effusion. A geriatric oncology patient with coagulopathy may collapse suddenly.

Jinx's Case (It Can Happen at Your Clinic)

Jose Alfaro, who has worked diligently and faithfully for 43 years at our clinic, lifted Jinx, a 13-year-old M/N Old English Sheepdog, to place him in the bath tub. Jose called out "code blue" because Jinx collapsed in the tub. Abdominal centesis and ultrasound led to the immediate clinical diagnosis of ruptured splenic hemangiosarcoma with metastatic foci in the liver. The family declined further care due to Jinx's advanced age and poor prognosis.

Dyspnea: May Indicate Thoracic Masses or Effusions

Anterior mediastinal masses (AMMs), especially in cats, are very insidious because they grow without much attention until they reach a critical mass. They cause pleural effusion and may cause esophageal obstruction. A cat with AMM may exhibit acute respiratory distress, tachypnea, and vomiting. A cat with anterior mediastinal lymphoma may have acute collapse after exercise. Geriatric oncology patients with occult disseminated disease may develop respiratory distress syndrome or acute systemic inflammatory response syndrome (SIRS).

Shelby's Case (She Died Suddenly without Complaint)

Shelby, an intact 8-year-old Rottweiler, had a decreased appetite and mild lethargy. The only abnormality on her database was thrombocytopenia. Abdominal ultrasound found metastatic cancer in her liver. On her first visit, Shelby jumped out of the car, walked into our office, collapsed, and died on the spot, releasing copious amounts of fluid from her lungs. We presume she had SIRS. Shelby's family was in shock because she did not act like she was dying.

Pathological Fracture: May Be Osteosarcoma

Many working breed dogs with osteosarcoma (OSA) are able to hide their pain. The first warning sign that a pet caregiver may have to herald osteosarcoma may be an acute pathological fracture. One in five OSA Greyhounds will have a spontaneous pathological fracture with no previous warning signs.

Stars's Case (We Kept Waiting for It to Happen)

Julie and Kevin Jennings loved Stars, their $12^1/_2$- year-old M/N Greyhound. Julie and I were best friends, and we marveled that Stars had not yet developed OSA in his geriatric years. One Sunday morning, when Julie was out of town, Kevin called me in a panic. Stars had slipped in the kitchen and was extremely painful in his right hind leg. X-rays diagnosed a pathological fracture at the proximal right femur. We did not tell Julie. Instead, I picked her up at the LAX airport, and personally gave Julie the sad news. She cried all the way home. Julie and Kevin slept with Stars downstairs that night and said their goodbyes. When they were ready, I came over to the house and helped Stars peacefully transition over the Rainbow Bridge.

Ozzy's Case (Greyhounds with Osteosarcoma May Not Know It)

Ozzy Marquod, a 9-year-old M/N Greyhound, had a pathological fracture as the first warning sign of bone cancer for his family. Ozzy was jumping out of the car when he went suddenly lame. Radiographs identified the characteristic lesions for osteosarcoma of the left distal radius. Ozzy had an amputation and received carboplatin chemotherapy and immunonutrition. The advent of immunotherapy given in combination with carboplatin chemotherapy may prolong overall survival times in newly diagnosed bone cancer patients.

Noodles's Case (Indoor Cats Can Have Pathological Fractures)

Noodles Marcus, a $17^1/_2$-year-old indoor Siamese cat, was found acutely limping on his left hind leg. Noodles had been diagnosed with advanced stage GI lymphoma 3 years previously. Noodles was considered one of our miracle cats because his cachexia was extreme, yet he regained his weight on chemotherapy. All the while he had CRF. Mr. Marcus leaves the country often, so Noodles received maintenance chemotherapy sporadically. Radiographs identified a left tibial fracture with displacement and demineralization of the bone. The fracture was repaired with a plate and a biopsy was taken to rule out lymphoma. The histopathology report diagnosed osteosarcoma at the fracture site. Noodles recovered from surgery but his loose stools and cachexia returned due to recurrence of his GI lymphoma, which seemed to be exacerbated from the stress of surgery. We started Noodles back on chemotherapy but he did not do well and was lost to follow-up.

Acute Pain or Paresis: May Be from Spinal Cord Tumors

Acute onset of severe pain or paresis may be the first warning sign of a spinal cord tumor. Vertebral body masses or any primary or metastatic tumor that invades the spinal canal or impinges on the spinal cord may cause acute onset of pain and/or paresis. This type of compressive pain is very difficult to control with analgesics. Imaging is the best way to diagnose these lesions.

Behavior Changes: May Be from Brain Tumors

Many brain tumors are not malignant but because they compete for space in the cranial vault, by their very nature, they exert pressure on the brain and kill the host. Many geriatric oncology patients with brain tumors are not diagnosed until a precipitating acute warning sign appears such as: seizures, behavior changes, circling, ataxia, stumbling, head pressing, blindness, paresis, etc.

Amanda's Case (Meningiomas in Cats Grow Slowly)

Amanda, an F/S 17-year-old DSH, started howling around the house more frequently and during the day over a 6-month period. The symptoms seemed to abate with antianxiety medications. She became more aloof, which was attributed to the medication. Then one day she started circling to the left. Magnetic resonance imaging (MRI) found a large mass consistent with a meningioma in the left posterior fossa/cerebellopontine angle. The mass explained Amanda's behavior changes.

Misty's Case (Something Was Wrong for 6 Months)

Misty D'Amico, a 13-year-old F/S West Highland White Terrier, was in and out of the hospital for 6 months with general complaints about weak rear legs, chronic UTIs, hypothyroidism, ear infections, chronic gagging, lethargy, occasional loss of balance, and a dwindling appetite. One night Misty had a massive seizure and was rushed to the emergency room. An MRI found a large inoperable mass in her parasagital frontal lobes that had invaded through the ethmoid plate (Figure 3.15).

Paraneoplastic Syndromes

Paraneoplastic syndromes (PNSs) are plentiful in geriatric cancer patients. Older animals may bypass the prodromal warning signs of cancer and exhibit a PNS, which is a secondary cancer, as their first warning sign. A good working definition for PNS is: an aberration of physiology, function, or structure that is mediated by the production or the release of chemicals, hormones, or hormone-like molecules or cytokines, which exert an effect that is distant from and unrelated to the size or mass of a primary

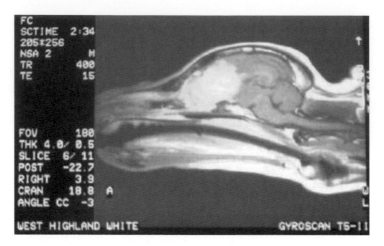

Figure 3.15. Misty, a 13-year-old F/S West Highland White Terrier, had vague prodromal warning signs for 6 months prior to diagnosis. MRI showed a large inoperable mass in the parasagittal frontal lobes invading through the ethmoid plate.

tumor. Older pets are commonly rushed to emergency rooms due to acute onset of severe PNS symptoms, which evoke the emergency room clinician (criticalist) or attending doctors to pursue the diagnosis of cancer as the primary problem.

PNSs have some of the longest names in medical terminology with prefixes of "hypo" and "hyper" followed by "inemias" (e.g., hyperheparinemia, hyperinsulinemia, hypergammaglobulinemia). The syndromes affect multiple sites and systems and have variable morbidity. These aberrant conditions torment the geriatric cancer patient with adverse metabolic changes and hormonal imbalances. Geriatric patients are often subdued and less active, which can divert the discovery of a metabolic imbalance until the patient is in advanced crisis.

A host of cytokines and endocrine substances have been discovered in the past 4 decades in the study of cellular metabolism (metabolomics). These "new players" are produced or overexpressed by neoplastic cell clones originating from organs and tissues. Many of these cellular products were unheard of when half of our profession attended veterinary school. A cadre of interleukins, interferons, prostaglandins, enzymes, and co-factors regulate intracellular and extracellular functions and cell surface signaling. Any one of these proteins may be overproduced (overexpressed) by neoplastic transformation of their progenitor cells. As researchers gain more understanding of the intricate chemistry of cellular metabolism and cancer, we may be able to exploit their underlying mechanisms as therapeutic targets (Hahn 2005).

Any malignancy that originates in or affects the bone marrow and its hematopoietic stem cells may induce a PNS. The most common hematologic effects from malignancy are anemia of chronic disease followed by blood loss anemia, microangiopathic anemia (common in hemangiosarcoma), and immune-mediated hemolytic anemia. Thrombocytopenia and coagulation disorders are also common. Hyperestrogenism from Sertoli cell tumors, interstitial (Leydig) cell tumors of the testes of older dogs, and ovarian tumors may induce hypoplastic anemia, leucopenia, and thrombocytopenia. Degranulating mast cell tumors release heparin (hyperheparinemia) and may induce petechiation, ecchymosis, and hemorrhage due to PNS coagulopathies. FeLV and FIV retroviral infections exert effects in the bone marrow tissue of cats, resulting in immunosuppression, anemia, leukopenia, pancytopenia, leukemias, and lymphomas that can produce any number of PNSs.

The dramatic effects seen with PNSs often create life-threatening complications for the already compromised geriatric oncology patient. Renal failure and heart failure can be sequelae from severe malignant hypercalcemia. However, if the geriatric oncology patient has pre-existing CRF and/or heart disease, the patient is impacted more heavily by the PNS and the window of opportunity to respond is diminished. Insulinomas cause hypoglycemia, inducing seizures, weakness, and coma. PNS-related epistaxis may occur in a geriatric dog due to hyperviscosity syndrome resulting from immunoglobulin production from malignant plasma cells in multiple myeloma. Hemangiosarcoma induces fatigue and acute collapse due to chronic anemia, acute blood loss anemia, immune mediated anemia, and coagulopathies. Gastrointestinal ulceration is commonly found in mast cell cancer patients due to hyperhistaminemia or due to hypergastrinemia in patients with gastrinoma. Any one of these PNSs is an urgent care challenge that requires intense supportive care with 24 hour per day management.

Cancer cachexia, anemia, fever, and hypoproteinemia are commonly encountered in geriatric oncology patients. Hypercalcemia, GI ulceration, protein-losing enteropathy (GI lymphoma in cats), and hypoglycemia are commonly seen syndromes. Glomerulonephritis and neurologic problems, hyperestrogenism, hypertrophic osteopathy, and hypergammaglobulinemia are also frequently encountered. Many problems that parallel the symptoms of PNS are actually iatrogenic, due to perioperative complications or to adverse effects related to chemotherapy or radiation therapy. It is up to the attending clinician to establish the cause of the paraneoplastic condition.

Endocrine PNS

Most endocrinopathies in geriatric pets are oncologic in nature. Feline hyperthyroidism and hyperadrenocorticism or Cushing's disease, by definition, fit the PNS category. Thyroid tumors cause distant effects on the function and condition of the heart and kidneys in feline hyperthyroidism. Either primary cause (pituitary tumor or adrenal tumor) in Cushing's disease is essentially neoplastic in nature. Feline hyperthyroidism and hyperadrenocorticism may be among the most common PNSs seen in geriatric pets.

Endocrine-Like PNS

In addition to hypercalcemia of malignancy (HM), veterinarians may encounter other endocrine-like PNSs. Any malignancy that originates from an endocrine organ or tissue that upregulates the production of a product of an endocrine organ may induce a PNS. Pancreatic tumors produce a variety of biologically active hormones that adversely affect the geriatric oncology patient.

Insulinomas are pancreatic beta-islet cell tumors that secrete insulin, causing elevated levels, which cause hypoglycemia and are manifested by the patient as weakness, ataxia, seizures, and coma. PNS hypoglycemia may also be caused by disturbances of other metabolic pathways by non-islet cell tumor functions or products such as insulin-like growth factors.

Gastrinomas are non-islet cell pancreatic tumors that secrete gastrin, which causes gastroduodenal ulcers, blood loss, vomiting, and pain. This PNS is known as the Zollinger-Ellison syndrome in human medicine. Increased epinephrine and norepinephrine from pheochromocytoma (adrenal gland neoplasia) causes PNS hypertension, restlessness, and related disorders.

It is up to the diagnostic acumen of the clinician and good laboratory support to feather out the various causes of any one of the panoply of PNSs that can potentially affect aging companion animals.

Hematologic PNS

PNSs are commonly manifested as hematologic abnormalities, such as anemia, monoclonal gammopathies, thrombocytopenia, thrombocytosis, platelet dysfunction, hypoproteinemia, coagulopathies, and disseminated intravascular coagulation (DIC). These PNSs are most often associated with hemangiosarcoma in older dogs. Overproduction of red blood cells (erythrocytosis) and neutrophils (leukemoid reaction or neutrophilic leukocytosis) and eosinophils can be due to excess secretion of stimulatory glycoproteins and cytokines from tumor cell clones.

Dermal PNS

The skin is a target organ that may reflect distant effects from primary tumors. Some cutaneous PNSs have been described in animals such as alopecia, cutaneous flushing, necrolytic migratory erythema, nodular dermatofibrosis and ischemic necrosis of the hind digits, pemphigus vulgaris, and pruritis. We should also include calcinosis cutis and feminization and virilization syndrome in this category. There are certainly other cutaneous manifestations of neoplasia that are yet to be reported.

Some PNSs are manifested as abnormalities in the skin, such as nodular dermatofibrosis on the legs of Shepherd breed dogs with renal cystadenocarcinoma, vasodilation, and cutaneous flushing from adrenal tumors or mast cell degranulation and release of vasoactive substances such as histamine and heparin. Pancreatic alpha cell clones can secrete glucagon and cause erosive blisters (necrolytic migratory erythema). Older cats may develop ventral alopecia and painful footpad disease from biliary and metastatic pancreatic carcinomas in the liver.

Simply put, PNSs are disorders that accompany or precede the diagnosis of certain malignancies. Encountering one of these varied disorders may be the pet owner's first warning sign and your initial clue to work up the geriatric patient for cancer. The most dramatic PNS is HM. It is generally associated with T-cell lymphoma and various adenocarcinomas, most notably anal sac apocrine adenocarcinoma. Older dogs may develop other endocrine-like PNSs such as hyperadrenocorticism from pituitary adenomas, adrenal tumors, or, rarely, primary lung tumors. Older dogs may develop hypoglycemia, which is most commonly caused by insulinoma. Other common PNSs are anorexia, cachexia, protein-losing enteropathy, fever, and pain.

Of the many PNSs, several merit descriptions and more attention to help familiarize you with the most important features of these baffling cancer-associated syndromes.

Anorexia and Hepatic Lipidosis

Cancer-related anorexia and hepatic lipidosis are common problems in feline geriatric oncology patients. The condition may persist on a long term basis and become the overriding cause of death. When owners encounter a change in eating behavior, we should consider it a red flag for anorexia. Anorectic cats may approach the dish, stare at the food, and then back off, appearing to be nauseated. Some gag. Some cats will make a grinding sound with their mouth as if they have temporomandibular joint disease. I associate this grinding sound with a poor long term prognosis. In my experience, it appears in cats with weight loss, poor hydration, and one of the viral infections, FeLV, feline infectious peritonitis (FIP), or FIV.

Thoughts on Feline Anorexia

Scholars have long wondered about the odd, aloof psyche of the anorectic feline. One viable theory can be found in the April 15, 1999, *JAVMA*, where Dr. Frank McMillan comprehensively reviews the vast data about how stress causes neuropeptides ("negative endorphins") to form in the body, which negatively affects emotions and health. Cats are very "oral"-based animals. They seem to enjoy using their tongues to clean themselves and they socially enjoy licking others. It is easy to conclude that gingivitis, stomatitis, or any illness (especially oral and GI neoplasia) would cause pain and stress in cats and a "negative nueropeptide" flood resulting in loss of appetite. It is obvious that other factors such as mood, texture, smell, or change of food also alter the mental states that influence a cat's appetite. Capromorelin (Entyce™) has shown efficacy for stimulation of appetite in clinical studies in cats. It will be a welcome Rx to improve appetite in cats.

Treatment for Anorectic Cats: The Feeding Tube

An essential supportive treatment for geriatric cats with cancer-related anorexia and cats with hepatic lipodosis-related anorexia is esophageal feeding tube placement. Old malnourished cats with chronic kidney disease (CKD) need feeding tube placement when they are unable to consume enough calories to maintain a positive energy balance. It is best to recommend placing a feeding tube in any geriatric cat with a history of unresponsive anorexia and cachexia. When planning cancer treatments or procedures that are expected to initiate anorexia or add stress to the already anorectic geriatric cat, an esophageal or nasogastric feeding tube should be considered as standard supportive care.

Missy's Case (Offset Anticipated Anorexia)

Missy, a geriatric feline, refused to eat for 2 weeks following mastectomy for mammary adeno-carcinoma. Missy needed a second chain mastectomy for breast cancer management. I recommended that a feeding tube be placed as a prophylactic measure. This precaution was not only important to the success of the surgery but was also a factor in the family's decision to have the second surgery done.

Oral medications such as capromorelin, mirtazapine at one-quarter of a 15mg tablet q 48 hours, Xanex® at 1.5mg per day, and cyproheptadine at 2mg twice daily, and prednisone or prednisolone can stimulate the appetite. Entyce®, capromorlin oral solution, is expected to be approved for use in cats in 2018. Megestrol acetate 10mg IM may help. An IV injection of diazepam (1.5mg) diluted to 1 ml with dextrose solution may arouse a cat's appetite for 30 minutes, but it is troublesome to repeat frequently. There are ways to coax a cat to eat. Petting the cat, putting food on the paws or on the nose, and warming food to room temperature to release aroma may help. Because cats love the ritual of eating, dramatizing the preparation and sounds (the can opener) of serving the food often sparks the cat's interest.

Cats do not particularly love the way mice taste, but they do love to chase moving things and play. Maria Peterson of Santa Monica, CA, found that tossing food (chase) or tying it to a string (play) will often prompt an anorectic cat to start eating again. Offering different flavors of food, especially fresh shrimp and salmon, may spark an anorectic geriatric cat's appetite.

Assess hydration in front of the cat's family and show them how to monitor it by stretching and then releasing the skin to see if it springs back. Many anorectic cats are sent home with bags of fluids and vitamins for subcutaneous injection by their carers.

Before sending the client home with a geriatric cat that needs medicating and home care, always make it a point to clearly demonstrate the proper method of giving pills, liquids, vitamins, capsules, and especially administering SQ fluids. It is easy for the veterinary staff to administer SQ fluids and force feedings, but often impossible for the caregiver to muster up the courage to use a needle or to force-feed their sweet, independent-minded, stubborn feline. With detailed demonstration and coaching, most clients feel that they have made a real "breakthrough" when they master the technique and gain the skills needed to properly support their geriatric cat at home.

Teach carers several ways to force (hand) feed their geriatric cat. Opening a cat's mouth can be difficult, but with skillful instruction, most pet owners are willing and able to hand feed if necessary. Patrick and Timothy Strong of Los Angeles used hand feedings for their $16^{1}/_{2}$-year-old M/N cat, Montgomery, following splenectomy for mast cell infiltration. Montgomery enjoyed an excellent quality of life until age 21. Gene Behrman of Manhattan Beach, CA, kept Biggs, his 16-year-old M/N cat with CKD, on daily SQ fluids until Biggs reached the ripe old age of 22.

Some carers are willing to hand-feed their cat but the cat will not accept it. This causes great stress to the family and stresses the human–animal bond if the cat avoids them. This situation obligates the attending doctor to solve the problem. If a cat is losing weight rapidly, we strongly and enthusiastically suggest feeding tube placement as the best solution to this problem. The placement of a feeding tube became widely accepted as the life-saving step for resolving hepatic lipidosis. Encourage feeding tube placement as routine supportive care for all stubborn cases of feline anorexia, especially for cats with oral cancer. It should not make a difference if the reason a cat will not eat is terminal or temporary. Providing good nutritional support is imperative on a daily basis.

Esophagostomy feeding tubes are the most commonly utilized method for tube feeding anorectic cats. Nasal feeding tubes are utilized on a temporary basis but are too cumbersome and easily removed by the patient. We used to place gastric feeding peg tubes via endoscopy at surgery. Since the more practical technique for placement of an esophageal feeding tube was described, we use it almost exclusively (Ogilvie and Moore 2001).

Once the esophageal feeding tube is in place, the nightmare of force-feeding an unwilling cat is over. Recommend a healthy liquid diet designed to meet the feline patient's specific nutritional needs. It can be fed along with pulverized medications through the tube. Pet owners truly appreciate the opportunity to provide proper nutrition to their geriatric cats without the angst that force-feeding entails. In fact, caregivers may become dependent on the feeding tube. They may feel fearful and frustrated if the feeding tube accidentally comes out. In this case, simply comfort the family and replace the tube if the patient still needs it. Once the feeding tube is removed, the caregivers have to resume the work of directly administering medications over the objections of their cat.

Cats with Oral Cancer Require Feeding Tubes

Cats have variable early warning signs for oral cancer, such as ocular discharge, pawing at the mouth, loose teeth, and halitosis. However, they are often not diagnosed until the family notices a swelling either in the mandible or maxilla. Because cats are independent and do not open their mouth to pant as dogs do, their oral tumors are usually discovered in advanced stages. Cats with lingual tumors seem more demoralized than cats with tumors located in the dental arcades and the hard palate. The prognosis for long term survival in geriatric cats with oral tumors is generally poor, especially with lingual squamous cell carcinoma (SCC).

The first positive article about mandibulectomy in cats came from our oncology practice (Hutson et al. 1992). It reported on a series of seven cats that had mandibulectomy followed by radiation therapy for SCC of the mandible. This small series of cats had prolonged tumor-free intervals, and this report is referred to as an encouraging reference article. Our cats did well because they all had feeding tubes placed at the time of their mandibulectomy. They did not lose weight because we kept them in a positive nutritional status despite the predictable loss of appetite during their course of

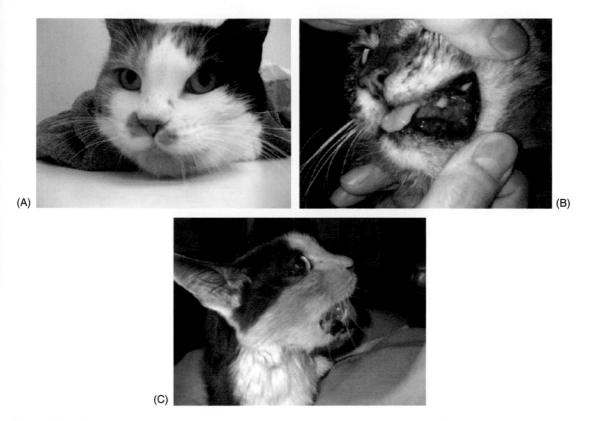

Figure 3.16. Oral tumors are generally discovered late in cats. Shandi Payner had an ocular discharge, increased salivation (A), and dental extractions prior to the diagnosis of SCC of her right maxilla. Oral SCC in the left mandible (B) and sublingual area (C) in an older cat.

therapy. The esophageal feeding tubes remained in place well after completion of radiation therapy and chemotherapy. Today, we would consider using electroporation or Yittrium-90 brachytherapy as excellent front line options for cytoreducing oral tumors in cats. Read the electrochemotherapy section in Chapter 6.

Shandi's Case (Ocular Discharge and Pawing at Her Mouth Were Her Warning Signs)

Shandi Payner, a 14-year-old DSH calico cat, had early warning signs of a "runny eye" and occasional pawing at her mouth on the right side. She quit eating dry food. When she had overt dysphagia, the family took her to their veterinarian for an exam. A firm swelling of her right maxilla was discovered (Figure 3.16). The family elected to place a feeding tube when Shandi could no longer eat but declined conventional therapy due to the poor prognosis.

Scrappy's Case (Sudden Enlargement of the Mandible Can Signal SCC)

Scrappy Irvine, a 12-year-old M/N DSH, suddenly developed a firm swelling on the rostral mandible. The family was familiar with our warning signs of cancer brochure because their family dog, Ebony, a 10-year-old Blue Heeler cross, was successfully treated for splenic hemangiosarcoma during the previous 18 months. They called immediately requesting tests and treatment for Scrappy. Biopsy of the mass verified SCC. They elected mandibulectomy, feeding tube placement, and follow-up radiation therapy to the surgical site and neck nodes. Scrappy had 3 follow-up chemotherapy treatments with carboplatin. Scrappy had no recurrence of oral SCC during a 5-year follow-up.

Sarcopenia versus Cancer Cachexia, an Insidious PNS

Prior to the clinical detection of cancer, many geriatric animals may exhibit a general loss of weight and muscle mass (sarcopenia) with or without the loss of fat. Sarcopenia is now recognized as an insidious, multifactorial geriatric syndrome generally associated with underlying chronic illness that contributes to frailty. The World Small Animal Veterinary Association (WSAVA) has excellent charts to assess sarcopenia in dogs and cats using muscle condition scores described as: normal, mild, moderate, to severe.

> http://www.wsava.org/sites/default/files/Muscle%20condition%20score%20chartCats.pdf
> http://www.wsava.org/sites/default/files/Muscle%20condition%20score%20chart%202013.pdf

Companion animals with cancer may develop catabolic wasting of muscle mass and tissue (cachexia) because they are in a hypermetabolic state, which causes involuntary weight loss. Cancer cachexia is an insidious process that contributes to poor outcomes. Cachexia may occur while the pet maintains a good appetite, attitude, and activity level. For a time, the geriatric oncology patient may be able to fool the best and most highly bonded caregivers. Weight loss starts to become obvious when the pet has lost 6–10% of their normal weight. Due to dogs and cats having fur, many pet owners do not recognize cachexia and are surprised to discover that their old pal dropped so much weight. Some people explain away their elder pet's weight loss with the rationale that this is just part of the aging process. In reality, their pet is wasting away before their eyes (Figure 3.17A).

In some cases, cancer cachexia is the only visible warning sign of illness or neoplasia. The mechanism for this profound involuntary weight loss is still not fully understood. Some scientists feel that the mechanism of cancer cachexia is put into action due to abnormalities in carbohydrate, protein and lipid metabolism, and cytokine dysregulation (Figure 3.17B).

Metabolic Abnormalities in Cancer Cachexia

Cancer cells metabolize glucose differently than normal cells. The end product of the abnormal cell's anaerobic glycolysis is lactic acid. It requires energy from the body to convert the lactate back into glucose. In addition to this metabolic disturbance in carbohydrate metabolism, cancer patients have abnormal glucose formation, disposal, oxidation, and turnover. Cancer patients have been shown to have elevated insulin levels and exhibit more insulin resistance than normal. If the geriatric oncology patient is overweight or has diabetes or Cushing's disease, insulin resistance may be compounded.

Cancer patients have lower levels of amino acids and high-density lipoproteins (HDL) and high levels of low-density triglycerides, resulting in disturbances of protein and lipid metabolism. Some cancer cells cannot access fat as an energy source. This situation has opened the door to the concept of starving the cancer and feeding the patient as a nutritional approach to managing the cancer patient.

Along with the metabolic abnormalities of cancer cachexia, the cancer patient experiences immune system suppression and extreme physiologic stress. After several months of weight loss, the

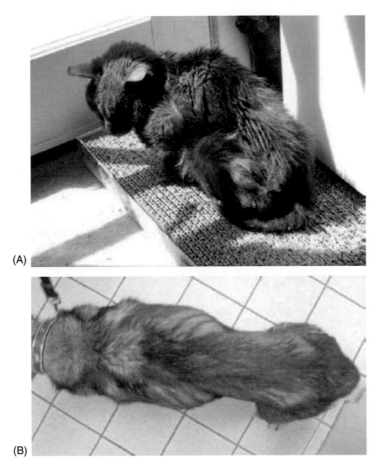

(A)

(B)

Figure 3.17.   Cancer cachexia: weight loss becomes obvious when 6–10% of the pet's normal weight is lost. Some people feel their elder pet's weight loss is part of the aging process.

debilitated pet may start to exhibit signs such as decreased exercise tolerance, GI disturbances, or lethargy. This behavior is what most often prompts a visit to the veterinarian. Decline in the condition of pets with cancer cachexia may leave the animal in such a state of debilitation and dehydration that attempts to help them surgically or medically may be fraught with complications.

The oncologist and the referring doctor must determine if the pet is capable of surviving suggested standard procedures and protocols that are generally used to diagnose and treat the cancer. Unfortunately, despite the removal of the primary tumor or the achievement of remission in lymphoma via chemotherapy, the metabolic abnormalities of cancer cachexia may persist. It is unsafe to deliver cancer therapy to debilitated geriatric oncology patients. We must first restore them to a metabolically balanced state of hydration and nutrition. Encourage the pet owner to rehabilitate his or her pet at home whenever possible with quality nutrition and supplements so the pet will be more able to tolerate the treatment modalities selected to battle the cancer.

When cancer cachexia is identified, many caregivers are shocked that their companion pet has lost so much weight. They feel cheated that the cancer was so insidious. This very situation happened in my own household. My $11\frac{1}{2}$-year-old Australian Shepherd, Alfie, developed cancer cachexia without me noticing it. His case was described earlier.

Weight Loss: An Insidious Warning Sign of Cancer

Soft stools, diarrhea, and chronic weight loss in older cats are important warning signs to rule out GI lymphoma. Cachectic cats often have normal values in their blood work and normal radiographs for their preliminary workup. The intestines may feel ropey on palpation. Many cases do not have masses in the abdomen. If there is no response to dietary management, further diagnostic tests are indicated. Endoscopy with biopsy of inflamed and suspicious (cobble stone) looking gut lesions may establish the diagnosis of intestinal lymphoma. At times, the only way to get a definitive diagnosis is with exploratory surgery with full thickness tissue samples taken from several areas of the intestinal tract. For cats with abdominal masses, FNA cytology or a Tru-cut tissue sample may establish the diagnosis without subjecting the patient to the stress of surgery.

How Cancer Causes Anemia

As cancer cells gain momentum in the body they acquire the physical ability and the cellular mechanisms that cause various types of anemias. This makes anemia one of the most common paraneoplastic syndromes encountered in practice. Up to one in four pets with cancer may have an associated anemia. Since geriatric dogs and cats frequently have concurrent illnesses, such as hypothyroidism, CRF, or chronic active hepatitis (CAH), they may not have the regenerative abilities needed to deal with their anemia. Anemia is more common and may be profound in dogs with hemangiosarcoma and Sertoli cell tumor due to estrogen suppression of the bone marrow. Anemia is found in cats infected with FeLV and FIV. It may accompany the diagnosis of lymphoma, especially if they have advanced renal lymphoma. Any animal with myeloproliferative disease will also have anemia due to myelopthesic crowding of the bone marrow. Anemia may appear with any type of cancer. The types of anemia most commonly encountered with oncology patients are described as follows:

1. Anemia of chronic disease (ACD) exhibits normochromic, normocytic red cells.
2. Blood loss anemia (BLA) exhibits hypochromic, microcytic red blood cells.
3. Microangiopathic hemolytic anemia (MAHA) exhibits schistocytosis (shearing of red blood cells, or RBCs) and hemolysis often due to disseminated intravascular coagulation (DIC).
4. Immune mediated hemolytic anemia (IMHA) exhibits spherocytosis, hemolysis, and regeneration of RBCs with elevated reticulocytes. The tumor releases tumor-associated antigens that prompt the immune system to react to and destroy its own RBCs. Consequently, the victimized RBCs are fragile and undergo hemolysis.
   The mechanisms that result in anemia may be intertwined with one another to complicate matters for the geriatric oncology patient and the clinician. Dogs with hemangiosarcoma often experience BLA due to acute rupture of a splenic mass and hemoabdomen. Yet the dog may have been "slowing down" for several weeks while the tumor caused MAHA and low-grade DIC. Circulating RBCs and platelets get fragmented as they bump into strands of fibrin that clog the tiny abnormal blood vessels and microvasculature that compose the matrix of the tumor. Fibrin strands also form in small capillary vessels when animals develop DIC, further pushing the intravascular injury and destruction of red cells.
5. Myelopthesic anemia (MA) results when the bone marrow is invaded with cancer cells. The normal precursor cells for erythropoiesis are crowded out with pressure from the neoplastic cells.

This type of anemia is often associated with the leukemias and it may be complicated with ACD. Myelopthesic anemia, as a paraneoplastic anemia, may also be caused by other yet-to-be-described cytokines. There may be other functions and other inhibitors of growth factors produced by malignant cells that have the power to dysregulate the function of normal bone marrow cells.

6. Bone marrow hypoplasia (BMH) is found in dogs with Sertoli cell tumor due to the hypersecretion of estrogen, which is suppressive to RBC formation in the bone marrow. This condition is likely to occur in senior cryptorchid dogs (most commonly reported in German Shepherd dogs) that have not been surgically explored for removal of their retained testicle(s). Prevention for this type of BMH in any case would be early neutering.

7. Hypersplenism causes anemia with an exaggerated hemolytic function that clears RBCs from the circulation.

8. Erythophagocytosis can also cause anemia. It occurs due to an aberration of phagocytic macrophages found in malignant and systemic histiocytosis of Bernese Mountain dogs and malignant fibrous histiocytoma of the spleen.

9. Iatrogenic anemia may result from chemotherapeutic suppression of blood precursor cells in the bone marrow. Aging is associated with a reduced stem cell reserve, which makes the geriatric oncology patient more susceptible to chemotherapy-related anemia. The anemia is slowly progressive with long-term chemotherapy and may cause the hematocrit to be as low as 20 as opposed to a normal low of 37. Chemotherapy-induced anemia is an expected side effect in treating people because higher doses are used. The dose range and frequency of veterinary chemotherapy protocols is generally lower than that used for humans and therefore not injurious to the animal's bone marrow. The anemia caused by veterinary chemotherapy does not become a clinically significant issue. The offending drug should be suspended, reduced, or given less frequently if the anemia becomes a problem. Erythropoietin may help boost the hematocrit in cases where we cannot safely discontinue chemotherapy (such as resistant lymphomas).

Treatment for Paraneoplastic Anemias

Geriatric pets often have chronic borderline anemia due to stem cell depletion, lack of regenerative responses, myelofibrosis, diminished reserve, and physiologic stress.

Treatment of the geriatric oncology patient for any of the paraneoplastic anemias described above should be aimed at correcting the anemia while targeting the primary tumor with surgical intervention or chemotherapeutic control. Transfusions or the use of Biopure® or HemoPure™ (an oxygen carrying solution) could be used as a rescue measure in patients with life-threatening blood loss and myelopthesic and hypoplastic anemias. Its effect lasted only 18–19 hours before transfusion was needed (Hale 2005). There were issues with adverse events and the company filed for bankruptcy in 2009.

Erythropoietin (Epogen®, epoetin-alfa, Procrit®, Darbopoetin®) is a glycoprotein growth hormone secreted by the kidney, which acts on stem cells of the bone marrow to stimulate RBC production. Recombinant DNA technology allows erythropoietin to be commercially available for use in the treatment of anemia. It is of great value in cases that are responsive. Antibody formation is a problem in both dogs and cats. New erythropoietin products made specifically for dogs or cats or both may become available. Ideally, it would be great to have a megakaryocyte-stimulating factor but, as of this writing, there is no product on the market.

It is wise to advise carers to feed small amounts of highly digestible food at 1–2 hour intervals to their severely anemic pets to keep their blood flow from diverting to meet the demands for digestion of a large meal.

Noche's Case (Anemia Reduces Tolerance to Pre-existing Airway Disease)

Noche Holbrach, a 14-year-old F/S Lab mix, was being treated for resistant small cell lymphoma. She developed chronic anemia, presumably from chemotherapy. Noche had concurrent chronic obstructive airway disease that caused hypoxic episodes when she was excited. The anemia lowered her threshold of endurance during these respiratory distress episodes. We used epogen to stabilize Noche's hematocrit. The anemia resolved when we increased the interval between treatments during her remissions. It recurred when she needed chemotherapy dose escalation to treat her lymphoma as she developed resistance.

Frisco's Case (Limb Sarcomas Can Induce PNS)

Frisco Antonelli, a 12-year-old male Yellow Lab, was limping for 10 days by the time Ms. Antonelli felt that he was in pain. She suspected a muscle pull. Frisco's doctor found a soft tissue swelling in the left thigh. Radiographs found no bone involvement. Frisco was sent home on etogesic 300mg as needed with the plan to rule out trauma, lipoma, or neoplasia. Two weeks later, Frisco started whining and limping again. A biopsy of the mass was scheduled for several days later.

On the day of anesthesia, an in-house PCV was 34% and a panel was sent to an outside lab. Chest radiographs showed a possible metastatic lesion in the left caudal lung lobe. Five to six tissue samples were taken. The tissue appeared to be blood clots but were surgically taken and submitted for histopathology. The following day, the panel reported low hemoglobin of 10.8 g/dl and a low hematocrit of 32% with nucleated RBCs of 9% along with four comments: polychromasia 2, macrocytosis 1, hypochromasia 1, and anisocytosis 2. The pathology report was inconclusive.

Ten days after the procedure, Frisco was referred to a surgical specialty clinic for another surgical biopsy. During the preanesthetic workup, chest radiographs demonstrated progressive metastatic disease. Frisco was referred to an oncologist who suggested a repeat biopsy procedure, palliative radiation therapy, or euthanasia. He was given a prescription for Tramadol® 50mg BID for pain and Tussigon® 5mg 1–2 tablets BID or TID as needed for coughing. The family was referred to our service for emotional support for themselves and Pawspice care for Frisco.

We made the presumptive diagnosis that we were working with an aggressive soft tissue sarcoma such as hemangiosarcoma. This would explain the coagulation disorder, the metastases, and the anemia. We gave the family information on hemangiosarcoma and explained the biological behavior of this relentless cancer and entered Frisco into Pawspice care. A week later, Frisco was doing much better clinically, although he remained anemic. Three weeks later, his hematocrit dropped to 18% and his platelet count was 80,000. We explained that the anemia and thrombocytopenia were from internal blood loss, a myelopthesic effect of the cancer and/or immune mediated pathways. The family declined a blood transfusion or Biopure. We advised strict rest for Frisco. He did very well for 2 more days. He ate a big breakfast on the third day and slowed down during the day and declined his dinner. Late that evening Frisco became dyspneic and weaker. That is when the family called me for advice. We decided to let him pass away in his loving home. Ms. Antonelli brought me yellow roses that bloomed their hearts out on my deck for a long time, reminding me of Frisco.

Hypercalcemia of Malignancy (HM)

Hypercalcemia of malignancy (HM) is a very distinctive and one of the most urgent paraneoplastic syndromes. Unfortunately, geriatric oncology patients with concurrent diseases, such as Cushing's disease, CRF, or hepatic disease may already be drinking large amounts of water (polydipsic) and urinating large amounts (polyuria). Paraneoplastic syndromes are aberrations of function or structure associated with cancer that are not related to the actual mass itself. Dogs and, less often, cats may develop classic HM associated most commonly with lymphoma, and then a host of other tumors, most notably apocrine gland anal sac adenocarcinoma, multiple myeloma, thymoma, thyroid carcinoma, bone tumors, squamous cell carcinoma, mammary gland carcinoma, and, of course, primary parathyroid tumors.

Certain clones of cancer cells produce a parathormone (PTH) like hormone PTH-rp (related peptide). It parallels PTH secreted by the normal parathyroid gland with related gene sequences identical to real PTH. PTH-rp pulls calcium from the bones and causes electrolyte and metabolic havoc and can precipitate renal failure in the geriatric cancer patient.

Warning Signs of Hypercalcemia of Malignancy (HM)

HM is a paraneoplastic syndrome that is associated with some cases of lymphoma, anal sac carcinomas, and miscellaneous other tumors. The early clinical signs are polydipsia and polyuria (PUPD) with an inability to concentrate urine. As the dog gets sicker, they develop lethargy, vomiting, dehydration, bradycardia, hypertension, weakness, tremors, constipation, depression, and, in severe cases, stupor, coma, and seizures. Whenever the calcium level is near or greater than 18mg/dl, the case must be considered a medical emergency as the kidneys undergo life-threatening vasoconstriction. With such reduced blood flow through the kidneys, the glomerular filtration rate (GFR) drops and cellular degeneration and calcification set in.

Harley's Case (If a Lymphoma Dog Is Sick, Check the Calcium)

Dr. Harlan called to brief me about the Jones family and Harley, their M/N 8-year-old Boxer, with generalized lymphadenopathy. A fine needle aspirate confirmed the diagnosis as lymphoma. The Jones family were his favorite clients and would be calling to speak to me before making an appointment. When Mr. Jones called, he had the usual questions about prognosis with treatment. I asked him about Harley and sensed that Harley was not feeling well. He had a poor appetite and PUPD. He was not on any steroids.

I instructed the family to go immediately back to Dr. Harlan's office and have a serum calcium level check and chest radiographs. Sure enough, Harley had HM, causing slight elevations of his renal values. He did not have an anterior mediastinal mass or symptoms of myasthenia gravis. Harley spent a few days in the hospital on fluids, diuretics, and steroids to resolve his HM. He was feeling much better by the time we started definitive chemotherapy. Most Boxers have T-cell lymphomas, which are more resistant to treatment and long-term survival (Lurie et al. 2004; Modiano and Helfand 2005). Harley's first complete remission lasted over 24 months!

Workup and Treatment of Hypercalcemia of Malignancy (HM)

HM patients may be so sick that emergency fluid therapy (0.9% saline diuresis) must first be given for stabilization *before* the cancer can be treated. It is tempting to use steroids immediately because steroids reduce HM by inhibiting prostaglandins, osteoclastic activity, and calcium uptake. To establish a diagnosis and determine the underlying cause, it is important to do a rectal exam, harvest samples of enlarged lymph nodes, and take X-rays of chest and abdomen to rule out a thymic or abdominal mass *before* the administration of steroids. If no evidence of cancer is found on this initial assessment, it is wise to do a bone marrow aspiration and FNA of the liver and spleen. Use a $1^1/_2$-inch 27-gauge needle for FNA. If the cytology is negative, proceed with abdominal ultrasound in pursuit of a definitive diagnosis and then proceed with corticosteroids.

Steroids will obscure the diagnosis of lymphoma. Steroids have a direct cytotoxic effect on lymphoblasts, causing the cell surface membrane to become more fragile. The cells undergo lysis and appear as non-diagnostic cellular debris on the FNA cytology slides. If the lymphoblasts are in cytotoxic lysis, they may not be diagnostic on cytology or on histopathology slides. It is possible to run immunocytochemistry or immunohistochemical stains on the intercellular debris present on FNA cytology samples and non-diagnostic tissue samples. For example, the presence of positive staining for CD79a and negative staining for CD3 protein markers in the cell debris would suggest a B-cell immunophenotype of the lymphoma.

The best plan of action is to gather all FNA slides and Tru-cut biopsy samples during the initial hours that the pet is in the hospital on IV fluid therapy. Use saline diuresis to rehydrate the patient and increase the GFR. Once the patient is rehydrated, it is safe to follow with furosemide at 1–4mg/kg at 8–24 hour intervals to directly inhibit further calcium absorption. Use prednisone orally at 1mg/kg once or twice daily. Bisphosphonates are helpful in lowering HM. Pamidronate at 1mg/kg IV infusion over 30–60 minutes every 3–6 weeks is helpful. Alendronate (Fosamax®) at 10mg/dog/day. Always give oral bisphosphonates with a water chaser so the tablet gets into the stomach.

Treat the primary tumor with chemotherapy or surgery as quickly as possible while maintaining diuresis and monitoring renal and cardiac function.

Induction chemotherapy protocols for lymphoma and more detailed treatment for refractory HM are covered in many texts. Hypercalcemic lymphoma patients have more trouble maintaining prolonged remissions and survival, especially if they also exhibited an anterior mediastinal mass or signs of muscular weakness (myasthenia gravis). Most of the hypercalcemic lymphomas are of the T-cell phenotype. Unfortunately, T-cell lymphomas are generally more resistant to chemotherapy treatment than the B-cell phenotype lymphomas. This holds true in both dogs and cats. Using mitoxantrone versus Adriamycin in the CHOP protocol and lomustine during maintenance and Tanovea® for rescue may benefit T-cell lymphoma patients.

JR's Case (Perianal Anal Tumors Go Unobserved for a Long Time)

JR Radke, a 13-year-old F/S German Shepherd dog mix, was referred with a history of bilateral pannus, urinary incontinence, and a large right-sided perianal gland carcinoma. Looking back, her warning signs dealt with the primary tumor with an 8-week history of licking her anal area. The referring hospital treated JR for an impacted anal gland without much improvement. The large mass was discovered on a recheck and considered inoperable. An incisional biopsy was performed for a definitive diagnosis. The pathology report described the mass to be a well-differentiated perianal gland carcinoma. Mr. Radke was referred to our service for definitive treatment.

After a thorough consultation, with full disclosure of the potential side effects including anal sphincter incontinence, Mr. Radke elected to proceed with definitive treatment. JR's presurgical workup radiographs and blood work revealed HM. Her reported calcium level was 14.4 and her corrected calcium was 13.3mg/dl. JR responded well to preoperative aggressive saline diuresis followed by excisional biopsy with intralesional chemotherapy and intracavitary (intraoperative) radiation therapy (directed into the tumor bed). The margins were clean and the HM resolved. Five months later, JR presented with a $3 \times 3cm^2$ firm mass at 4 o'clock on the right side of her anal sphincter. Mr. Radke thought that this was a recurrence but she did not have HM with this mass. I felt the mass was a de novo tumor, pointing out the lack of HM and its location on the opposite side of the sphincter. The new mass was excised using our intraoperative protocol. Histopathology revealed a poorly differentiated rhabdomyosarcoma. There was no recurrence of HM during JR's 20-month survival.

Harley Jones's Case (When a Lymphoma Dog Feels Sick, Check the Calcium)

Harley Jones, a 5-year-old male Boxer, was referred for multicentric lymphoma. During our pre-visit conversation, Mr. Jones mentioned that Harley had a poor appetite. I asked about his water intake and discovered that Harley had PUPD. This was an indicator that Harley may have an anterior mediastinal mass with HM or sepsis. Since stage III lymphoma cases should be feeling well, I advised Mr. Jones to take Harley directly to his attending doctor for an exam, chest X-rays, and to check the calcium level. Harley had a serum calcium level of 14.7 and a corrected calcium level of 13.1mg/dl and slight elevations of his BUN and serum creatinine. The chest X-rays were negative for AMM. Harley was given the appropriate treatment with fluids and diuretics and was able to avoid renal damage.

Harley Stall's Case (HM May Result with Bone Metastases)

Harley Stall, a 9-year-old Yellow Lab, was referred following incomplete removal of a large apocrine gland adenocarcinoma of the anal sac. Harley responded well for 3 months until he developed PUPD. His corrected serum calcium was 14.68mg/dl. A large firm mass was palpated on rectal exam. Lateral abdominal radiographs demonstrated enlarged sublumbar/iliac nodes. Calcium levels were not taken prior to his first surgery. Harley received intense saline diuresis, steroids, and furosemide to reduce his serum calcium.

At exploratory laparotomy, the mass was declared inoperable by the attending board-certified surgeon performing the surgery, as the mass had the density of bone. Harley recovered and was discharged with instructions for the family to give one liter of saline SQ BID, oral etidronate (at 5mg/kg/day with a water chaser), and gastroprotectants. We presumed Harley's hypercalcemia was due to bone metastases releasing osteoclast-activating factor or tumor-associated prostaglandins because his primary tumor did not manifest clinical signs of HM.

We entered Harley into Pawspice care and continued medical management of the HM. Our strategic plan was to offer supportive comfort care with SQ fluids, chemotherapy, steroids, and other measures (diet modification with low calcium content). With teamwork and great home care, we kept Harley's calcium level down for 3 months. Without the SQ fluids, his serum calcium level would rise to 14.3mg/dl. With time, the tenesmus increased and the family became exhausted with Harley's medical management and the chore of administering the SQ fluids to such a big dog over a prolonged time. The Stalls were pleased that Harley had a good quality of life and that he was able to give them a long farewell.

Pain Is a Warning Sign and a Paraneoplastic Syndrome

As a warning sign, cancer pain is all too often overlooked in the geriatric oncology patient. Pain is considered a paraneoplastic syndrome. It is estimated that up to 20% of the 65 million dogs in the United States may suffer from osteoarthritis pain and less than half receive veterinary care. Pain neglect may become an important welfare and ethical issue (Robertson 2016). Since pre-existing pain is commonly present in older animals with other concurrent geriatric conditions, cancer pain is often accepted as part of the problem and misinterpreted. Chronic pain in sedentary geriatric dogs and cats is generally undertreated when compared to pain in more active younger animals. Geriatric pets may have a lower threshold to pain and many seem to accommodate to their chronic pain. Older animals may be more stoical than younger, more active, excitable animals. Most geriatric dogs and cats have periodontal disease and arthritis. Pet caregivers feel that their old pets have adjusted well to living with chronic low-level pain.

The warning signs of cancer pain in geriatric oncology patients are associated with reduced energy, exercise intolerance, trouble breathing, coughing, gagging, dysphagia, regurgitation, vomiting food or bile, tenesmus, constipation, lameness, stiffness, reluctance to move, hesitation to exercise, painful extremities, breathlessness, increased panting, anxiety, disorientation, dizziness, paralysis, behavior changes, teeth grinding, vocalizations, agitation, crying, and so forth (French et al. 2000).

Chronic pain in the geriatric oncology patient may wax and wane with variations in the weather and activities and concurrent conditions (Figure 3.18). Pet owners interpret this waxing and waning as good days or bad days for their old pal without thinking about the underpinnings of cancer pain. These circumstances explain why cancer pain may be passed over in older pets when the pain is actually a warning sign of cancer.

When cancer pain is superimposed on the comorbidities of the geriatric patient, it may be initially misinterpreted, greatly underestimated, passively accepted, or dismissed by the family and the attending doctor. See Chapter 7 for more details regarding the recognition of pain and its management in geriatric cancer patients.

Older cats probably suffer more untreated pain than dogs due to their aloof, quiet nature. The warning signs of pain in cats appear as subtle behavior changes such as decreased self-grooming; increased sleeping; avoidance of food, water, and petting; withdrawal from normal interactions; change in sleeping places; litter box indiscretions; postural changes; hissing or growling when touched; purring; salivation; dysphagia; and so forth (Smith 2005). An excellent online source for clients on cancer pain written in 5 languages is: http://www.petcancercenter.org/Supportive_Care_Pain_management.html.

Client Education

Use Table 3.2 ("Warning Signs of Cancer and Illness in Pets"), along with Figure 3.19 for locating lymph nodes, in a monthly newsletter or in a client education handout for clients in your waiting room or exam rooms. This list is regrouped and reworded for the public from the routinely used list of cancer warning signs for the veterinarian (Table 3.1).

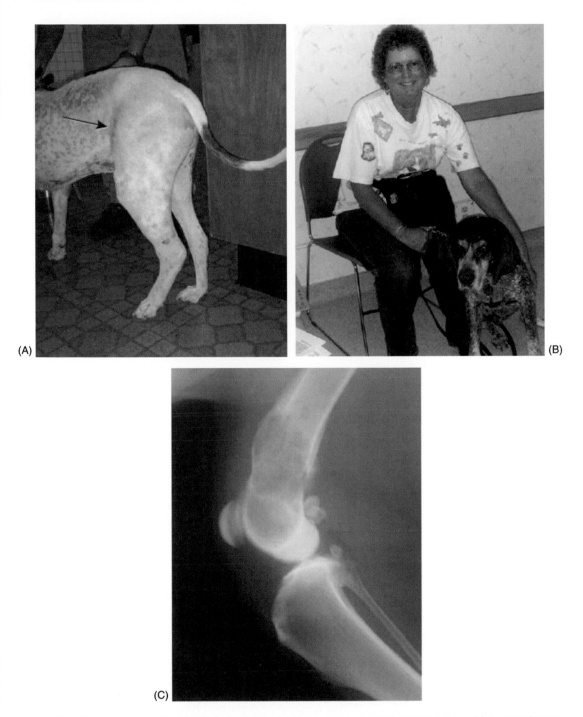

Figure 3.18. This 12-year-old Pit Bull (A) had advanced osetosarcoma of the left proximal tibia, which caused severe swelling and pain. Maggie, a 13-year-old German Shorthaired Pointer (B), with radiographs consistent with osteosarcoma in her right distal femur (C). Following amputation, Maggie had a wonderful quality of life for 5 months.

Table 3.1. Problems That Early Warning Signs May Signal

Warning Signs of Illness or Cancer	What or Where the Problem May Be	Type of Cancer to Rule Out
Sores that do not heal	Skin, face, abdomen	Skin cancer, squamous cell
Abnormal swellings on any part of the body surface that continue to grow	Infections or tumors of skin, lymph glands, mouth, nipples, testicles, anus	Skin cancer, lymphoma Breast, testicular cancer Oral, anal cancer
Weight loss, loss of appetite, loss of energy, pale gums	Illness, fever, cancer, abdominal mass	Visceral (internal) cancer Hemangiosarcoma
Bad breath, loose teeth, offensive odor, chronic sneezing, or runny nose/eyes	Dental disease, infection, nasal passage infection, tonsillitis	Oral cancer, nasal cancer, tonsilar cancer
Difficulty eating or swallowing, salivation, vomiting, regurgitation	Dental disease, foreign body ingestion, inflammation, ulcers	Oral, esophageal cancer, stomach cancer, intestinal cancer
Difficulty breathing, urinating, or defecating, prolonged elimination effort, change in shape of stools	Asthma, bronchitis, pneumonia, bladder, prostate, colon problems, constipation	Lung cancer, bladder cancer, prostate cancer, intestinal cancer, anal sac cancer
Trouble walking, or rising, hesitation to exercise, distended abdomen, reluctance to jump	Arthritis, hip dysplasia, orthopedic problems, misalignment, bloat, overeating	Bone cancer, joint capsule cancer, abdominal mass
Persistent lameness or stiffness, holding up a leg	Injury, fracture, arthritis	Bone cancer, nail bed cancer
Bleeding or discharge from any body opening, bloody nose, diarrhea, blood in the urine or feces	Bleeding disorders, uterine infection (pyometra), infections, inflammations, colitis, inflammatory bowel	Oral, nasal, urinary, rectal, auricular (ear), eye cancer, intestinal cancer, uterine cancer, multiple myeloma
Increased water intake or urine output, change in color of membranes to pale or yellow jaundice	Kidney disease Liver disease, anemia Diabetes Hormonal imbalance	Liver cancer Pituitary tumor Neuroendocrine tumor Abdominal mass
Behavior changes, fainting Change in routine	Behavior problem	Benign brain tumor (meningioma)
Head pressing, seizures	Epilepsy	Brain cancer
Unequal size of pupils	Meningitis, liver disease	Liver cancer
Pain	Try to localize the pain	Bone, spinal cord tumor, oral tumor, abdominal mass Ulcerated skin tumor

Use a cell phone or digital camera to take pictures of patients with enlarged lymph nodes, breast tumors, oral tumors, and skin tumors before and after surgery. It is always best to place calipers on the tumors to show the measurement. Put together a picture album, digital photo collection, or a PowerPoint slide show. Develop a personalized talk to have with clients when their pet is having a senior wellness exam, about the various tumor types and the warning signs of cancer. Show your slides and be sure to educate clients to look for masses at vaccination and injection sites. You may also want to give them the AVMA brochures on the warning signs of cancer.

Table 3.2.   Warning Signs of Cancer and Illness in Pets
Clinicians have permission to copy this table for distribution to pet caregivers.

The warning signs of cancer are easy to confuse with the warning signs of other illnesses. Cancer mimics other diseases. Use this checklist to recognize cancer's warning signs. Know what those signs indicate. If you see any of these physical changes in your pet, inform your veterinarian immediately and schedule a checkup.

Changes you can feel:
  1. Abnormal swellings that continue to grow in the skin, especially enlarged lymph nodes.
  2. Abnormal lumps in the mouth, mammary glands, testicles, vaccine sites, abdomen.
  3. Sores or ulcers that do not heal in 2 weeks on the nose, ear tips, and face, particularly of white cats and in the white underside skin of dogs, particularly Italian Greyhounds, Whippets, and Bulldog breeds.

Physiological changes you can see:
  4. Weight loss (use a baby scale to weigh cats and small dogs once every 2–4 weeks).
  5. Pale gums and mucous membranes, yellow (jaundice) membranes, bruising.
  6. Bad breath (halitosis) or more than one loose tooth at the same location.
  7. Distended abdomen, fluid in the abdomen, blood in the abdomen.
  8. Small red spots or red discoloration of the skin due to leaky capillaries, bleeding at any location, especially body openings.

Behavioral changes:
  9. Appetite loss.
 10. Difficulty eating, excessive salivation, spitting up (regurgitation), vomiting food or bile.
 11. Chronic sneezing, discharge from the eyes, unilateral nasal discharge, noisy breathing.
 12. Difficulty urinating, blood in the urine that persists after therapy.
 13. Excessive urine output, increased water drinking (kidney, liver problems, diabetes, etc.).
 14. Loose stools (diarrhea), straining to defecate, constipation, blood or mucus in the stool.
 15. Reduced energy or exercise intolerance, trouble breathing, coughing, gagging.
 16. Lameness, painful movement, painful joints, hesitation to exercise.
 17. Weakness, disorientation, dizziness, paralysis, pain.
 18. Fainting, muffled heart beat, breathlessness, increased panting, anxiety.

Where are my pet's lymph nodes?

There are five major external lymph nodes on either side of a dog or cat.

From Bullet's nose to his tail:
   1 Submandibular
   2 Prescapular
   3 Axillary
   4 Inguinal
   5 Popliteal

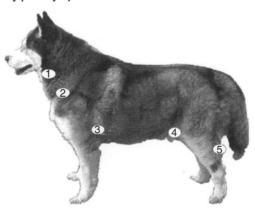

Figure 3.19.   Lymph node location from *Help Your Dog Fight Cancer*, by Laurie Kaplan with Dr. Alice Villalobos (2016). Printed with permission from JanGen Press.

The contemporary veterinarian also finds opportunities to reach out to the local community of pet owners with topics that favor health and longevity for the family pet. Over the years, I have enjoyed speaking to dog clubs; agility clubs; pet store clientele; Rotary, Kiwanis, and Lion's Clubs; women's clubs; garden clubs; and schoolrooms to familiarize people with the early warning signs of cancer and illness in their companion pets. I also educate people about cancer in humans. People are amazed to hear that cats living with smokers are at higher risk for oral and GI neoplasia. They need to know what to look for at vaccine and injection sites. They appreciate learning that lawn chemicals can cause bladder cancer and lymphoma in dogs. Talks with a comparative aspect geared toward the audience, young or old, may help save a life.

An interesting slide show, presented by you at a Rotary or Kiwanis Club meeting, promotes community awareness for pet health. It shows that you are a caring veterinarian and it is a very good practice builder.

References

Ackerman, L.V., and J.A. del Regato. 1978. American Joint Committee on Staging and End-Results Reporting, Manual for Staging of Cancer. Quoted in *Clinical oncology: A multidisciplinary approach for physicians and students*, 7th edn, ed. P. Rubin, p. 667. Philadelphia, PA: Saunders.

Adams, W.M., D.E. Bjorling, J.F. McAnulty, et al. 2005. Outcome of accelerated radiotherapy alone or accelerated radiotherapy followed by exenteration of the nasal cavity in dogs with intransal neoplasia: 53 cases (1990–2002). *JAVMA* 227 (6):936–941.

Cotter, S.M. 2005. What ever happened to feline leukemia virus? *Proceedings of the Sierra Veterinary Medical Association*, February, pp. 113–116.

French, E., et al. 2000. Assessment of pain in laboratory animals. *National AALAS Meeting*. Available at www.colostate.edu/depts/lar/Pain_Assessment.doc.

Giving seniority to senior pets. 2005. Team Advisor, *Clinician's Brief (NAVC)*, September, pp. 17–30.

Goldschmidt, M.H., and M.J. Hendrick. 2002. "Tumors of the skin and soft tissues." In *Tumors in domestic animals*, 4th edn, ed. D.J. Meuten, pp. 45–117. Ames, IA: Iowa State Press.

Hahn, K.H. 2005. A cellular revolution. *Veterinary Practice News* September.

Hale, A.S. 2005. Practical canine blood transfusion. *Clinician's Brief (NAVC)*, September.

Hart, B.L., L.A. Hart, A.P. Thigpen, and N.H. Willits. 2014. Long-term health effects of neutering dogs: Comparison of Labrador Retrievers with Golden Retrievers. *PlosOne*, doi:10.1371/journal.pone.0102241.

Hart, B.L., L.A. Hart, A.P. Thigpen, and N.H. Willits. 2016. Neutering of German Shepherd Dogs: Associated joint disorders, cancers and urinary incontinence. *Veterinary Medical Science* 2:191–199, dpo:10.1002/vms3.34.

Hershey, A.E., K.U. Sorenmo, M.J. Hendrick, et al. 2000. Prognosis for vaccine associated sarcoma after excision. *JAVMA* 216:58–61.

Hutson, C.A., C.C. Willauer, E.J. Walder, et al. 1992. Treatment of mandibular squamous cell carcinoma in cats by use of mandibulectomy and radiotherapy: Seven cases (1987–1989). *JAVMA* 202:777–781.

Kaplan, L. 2016. *Help your dog fight cancer: Empowerment for dog owners*. Briarcliff, NY: JanGen Press, LLC.

Louwerens, M., C.A. London, and N.C. Pederson. 2005. Feline lymphoma in the post-feline leukemia virus era. *JVIM* 19 (3):329–335.

Lurie, D.M., M.D. Lucroy, S.M. Griffey, E. Simonson, and B.R. Madewell. 2004. T-cell derived malignant lymphoma in the boxer breed. *Veterinary and Comparative Oncology* 2 (3):171–175.

Modiano, J.F., and S.C. Helfand. 2005. Innovations in the diagnosis of canine hemangiosarcoma. Personal Communication, *VCS NL* 29 (1):4–5.

Modiano, J.F. 2016a. Personal Communication.

Modiano, J.F. 2016b. Innovations in cancer treatment and prevention *World Veterinary Cancer Congress*, Foz do Iguassu, Brazil.

Moore, A.S. 2004. Biopsy of suspected injection-induced sarcoma in cats. *Clinician's Brief (NAVC)* June:13–19.

Ogilvie, G.K., and A.S. Moore. 2001. "Nutritional support." In *Feline oncology: A comprehensive guide to compassionate care*, pp. 113–125. Trenton, NJ: Veterinary Learning Systems.

Robertson, S. 2016. Pain assessment for your practice. *British Small Animal Veterinary Congress* (BSAVC) (http://www.vin.com/doc/?lld=7227442).

Scarpa, F., S. Sabattini, and G. Bettini. 2014. Cytological grading of canine cutaneous mast cell tumors. *Veterinary and Comparative Oncology* 14 (3):245–251.

Sfiligoi, G., K.M. Rassnick, J.M. Scarlett, N.C. Northrup, and T.L. Geiger. 2005. Outcome of dogs with mast cell tumors in the inguinal or perineal region versus other cutaneous locations: 124 cases (1990–2001). *JAVMA* 226:1368–1374.

Smith, L.J. 2005. Practical analgesia in cats. *Veterinary Medicine* August:602–609.

Theilen, G.H., B.R. Madewell, and M.B. Gardner. 1987. "Hematopoietic neoplasms, sarcomas and related neoplasms." In *Veterinary cancer medicine*, eds G.H. Theilen and B.R. Madewell, pp. 345–381. Philadelphia, PA: Lea & Febiger.

Suggested Reading

Abeloff, M.D., J.O. Armitage, J.E. Niederhuber, M.B. Kastan, and W.G. McKenna. 2004. *Clinical oncology*, 3rd edn. Philadelphia, PA: Churchill Livingstone.

Balducci, L. (guest ed.). 1994. *Cancer Control: Journal of the Moffitt Cancer Center* 1 (2).

Balducci, L., G.H. Lyman, W.B. Ershler, and M. Extermann (eds). 2004. *Comprehensive geriatric oncology*, 2nd edn. Oxon, UK: Taylor & Francis.

DeVita, V.T., S. Hellman, S.A. Rosenberg (eds). 2001. *Cancer: Principles and practice of oncology*, 6th edn. Philadelphia, PA: Lippincott-Raven.

Dobson, J., and D. Lascelles. 2003. *BSAVA manual of canine and feline oncology*, 2nd edn. Quedgeley, Gloucestershire, England: British Small Animal Veterinary Association.

Hoffman, R., E.J. Benz Jr., S.J. Shattil, B. Furie, H.J. Cohen, L.E. Silberstein, and P. McGlave (eds). 2005. *Hematology basic principles and practice*, 4th edn. Philadelphia, PA: Elsevier.

Meuten, D.J. 2002. *Tumors in domestic animals*, 4th ed., Ames, IA: Iowa State Press.

Morrison, W.B. 2002. *Cancer in dogs and cats: Medical and surgical management*, 2nd edn. Jackson, WY: Teton New Media.

Moulton, J.E. (ed.). 1990. *Tumors in domestic animals*, 3rd edn. Berkeley, CA: University of California Press.

Ogilvie, G.K., and A.S. Moore. 1995. *Managing the veterinary cancer patient*. Trenton, NJ: Veterinary Learning Systems.

Ogilvie, G.K., and A.S. Moore. 2001. *Feline oncology*. Trenton, NJ: Veterinary Learning Systems.

Theilen, G.H., and B.R. Madewell. 1987. *Veterinary cancer medicine*. Philadelphia, PA: Lea & Febiger.

Withrow, S.J., and E.G. MacEwen (eds). 2001. *Small animal clinical oncology*, 3rd edn. Philadelphia, PA: Saunders.

Chapter 4
Basic Types of Cancer and Their Biological Behavior

When you have chosen your part, abide by it, and do not weakly try to reconcile yourself with the world…If you would serve your brother because it is fit for you to serve him, do not take back your words when you find that prudent people do not commend you.

Ralph Waldo Emerson

Introduction

Cancer is the all-encompassing name given to over two hundred various types of abnormal cell production (neoplasia) and related syndromes. A good working definition, proposed in *Tumors in Domestic Animals,* is: "A Neoplasm is a mass of tissue generated by cells capable of division which have acquired either permanent expressible heritable change or stable epigenetic change so that the cells no longer respond appropriately to one or more normal tissue-organizing stimuli, chemical or physical, intracellular or extracellular, in the organism in which it occurs" (Cullen, Page, and Misdorp 2002).

Cancer cells exhibit various behaviors. Cancer's complex behavior has been eloquently described as exhibiting traits belonging to birds, rabbits, or turtles, in an article titled, *OVERKILL*, by Atul Gawande, MD. Some tumors behave like birds that fly from the source, or rabbits that hop from one lymph node to the next, or turtles that stay put and do not travel far (Gawande 2014). This is a good concept to keep in mind.

Neoplastic cell types are categorized either as mesenchymal or epidermal. A binomial system categorizes all forms of neoplasia according to benign or malignant behavior and their mesenchymal or epithelial cell type of origin. Mesenchymal refers to connective tissue, muscle, blood, and all endothelial cells, including mesothelium, synovium, and meninges. Epidermal refers to squamous cells of the skin, all glands, all cells lining tubular tracts and cells of neuroectodermal origin, including melanocytes (Cullen, Page, and Misdorp 2002).

Practicing veterinarians can more readily address oncology on a clinical basis by placing tumors within five major group divisions. By understanding cancer cell types within the construct of these major group divisions, the diagnosis, management, supportive care, and chemoprevention for geriatric patients may be more approachable. The clinician may also address cancer according to its location in the body, such as head and neck tumors versus abdominal tumors. This approach often employs specific shared treatments.

Canine and Feline Geriatric Oncology: Honoring the Human–Animal Bond, Second Edition. Alice Villalobos with Laurie Kaplan.
© 2018 John Wiley & Sons, Inc. Published 2018 by John Wiley & Sons, Inc.

Some malignant tumors grow so rapidly that they are difficult for the pathologist to classify. They may be reported as undifferentiated. Think of these as renegade cells that grow so fast that they have no time to pick up the morphological characteristics of their cell of origin. We can consider these cells to be "dedifferentiated." When pathologists cannot identify the cell of origin, they may describe the tumor as "anaplastic carcinoma or undifferentiated sarcoma." New diagnostic tests using molecular and genetic profiling (see Chapter 5) will add to our ability to classify anaplastic cells and indicate therapeutic options. Ask your pathologist if these differentiation tests are available.

The attending doctor needs to have a basic understanding of the origin of a particular tumor and its biological behavior, because the geriatric cancer patient's welfare is at stake. The Dog Aging Project is directed by Dr. Dan Promislow, who is also the founding Director of the Canine Longevity Consortium, generating information on environmental and genetic factors that affect the aging process and how aging impacts cancer in geriatric dogs (www.dogagingproject.com). For clinical purposes, we can consider grouping cancer into the following five major categories:

1. Carcinomas: cancer that arises from skin cells, mucous membranes, cells from glands and internal organs, or cells that form the lining of body cavities. Cancer arising from glandular tissue is often referred to as adenocarcinoma (AC).
2. Sarcomas: cancer arising from connective tissues such as bone, muscle, and fibrous connective tissue and from various types of cells that reside in the body, such as mast cells, melanocytes, plasma cells, and dendritic cells.
3. Blood cancer: cancer arising from hematopoietic tissues and lymph nodes or other lymphatic tissue, causing leukemias and lymphomas, respectively. Hemangiosarcoma may be included in this category.
4. Nervous system cancer: cancer arising within the brain, in the spinal cord, or in nerve cells.
5. Miscellaneous and uncertain cell types: histiocytic tumors, difficult-to-classify malignancies, and tumors of uncertain origin.

Carcinomas

Carcinomas arise from epidermal cells in the skin, from cells that form the lining of cavities, or from cells forming the inner surface of an organ. Many carcinomas, especially mammary tumors, testicular tumors, and perianal and sweat gland tumors, appear on the surface of the body and are initially noticed by the pet owner, whereas carcinomas that arise in the viscera remain insidious and occult until the pet becomes symptomatic.

Squamous cell carcinoma (SCC) arises in non-pigmented facial skin of older white cats and in the ventrum of light-skinned dogs due to chronic solar irradiation. Non-actinic SCC may arise anywhere in the oral cavity affecting the tongue, tonsils, and esophagus. Non-actinic SCC may also arise in the nasal sinuses, respiratory tract, and nail beds of both dogs and cats. Some reports have associated SCC of the tonsils in dogs with environmental pollution. Cats exposed to environmental tobacco smoke for five or more years are at an increased risk of developing oral SCC and GI lymphoma (Snyder, Bertone, and Moore 2001).

Carcinomas may arise from nasal respiratory epithelium at any location in the nasal passages and may involve the sinuses, extend between the eyes, involve ethmoid plate, and invade into the calvarium and brain. They cause turbinate destruction, unilateral nasal discharge, epistaxis, and facial deformity.

Carcinomas arising in the thorax in older dogs and cats include aortic body (heart-based) tumors, esophageal carcinoma, and respiratory and bronchogenic carcinoma. Primary lung tumors are rare in old cats but SCC is the most common cell type. In the feline, malignant cells may metastasize to the digits as a final event. Primary lung tumors generally appear as a solitary round mass in the caudal lung lobes in both dogs and cats.

Adenocarcinomas

The term "adenocarcinoma" (AC) applies more specifically to tumors that arise in glandular tissues of the skin and viscera and form glands within the neoplasm. Adenomas are benign tumors of glandular cells. Over time, some adenomas may transition into malignant tumors. The skin and mucous membranes commonly give rise to carcinomas in dogs and cats as they age. AC may arise in the ciliary body of the eye and occasionally in the glands of the eyelids. Dogs are prone to develop sebaceous, mammary, anal sac, perianal, salivary, and sweat gland tumors. Cats are prone to develop squamous cell carcinomas, basal cell tumors, and mammary tumors. Perianal tumors in male dogs and mammary tumors in female dogs and cats are sex-hormone related.

Mammary tumors are encountered in 25% of most breeds of older intact female dogs and in most breeds of older female dogs that had OVH after $2^1/_2$ years of age. Recent studies find low rates of mammary tumors in intact female Golden and Labrador Retrievers and German Shepherds (Hart et al. 2014, 2016). Half of canine mammary tumors are malignant and 50% of this group die within 1 year. Mammary tumors are less common in cats; however, more than 90% are malignant AC with a high rate of fatality if greater than 3 cm in size. Cats that had OVH late in life are more prone to develop mammary AC.

ACs may originate from glands in the abdomen, such as liver, colon, intestine, stomach, kidney, bladder, pancreas, prostate, and the adrenal glands. Widespread dissemination of cancer in the abdomen and throughout the body is given the term "carcinomatosis," but this term may also include other tissue types.

ACs may also originate from any gland in the neuroendocrine or reproductive system, such as the thyroid glands, pancreas, adrenal glands, pituitary gland, choroid plexus, ovaries, uterus, testicles, and prostate. This type of tumor often causes paraneoplastic syndromes related to their particular cell products. Sertoli cell, interstitial (Leydig) cell, and seminoma of the testicle may produce estrogen, causing feminizing syndrome and hypoplastic or aplastic anemia.

Anal sac AC or apocrine gland AC of the anal sac originate in the pouch-like glands located on each side of the anus and the most common carcinoma (25%) associated with malignant hypercalcemia. It is rare in cats. Spaniel breeds and German Shepherds are more commonly affected, showing signs of tenesmus, change in stool size, blood in the stool, and polydipsia. Note that canine lymphoma is the most common cause of malignant hypercalcemia, but a number of other malignancies may also cause this potentially life-threatening paraneoplastic syndrome.

Most mesotheliomas are classified as ACs although they have mesenchymal elements. They are rarely found in geriatric dogs and cats. Mesotheliomas arise from the serosal lining of the thorax, pericardium, and peritoneum, causing malignant effusions. In humans, mesotheliomas are associated with mining and working with asbestos.

Behavior of Carcinomas and Adenocarcinomas

Most ACs have an aggressive biological behavior with a persistent tendency for local and distant metastasis. Local recurrence following surgery is common. Local and regional lymph node invasion is common, followed by widespread dissemination. Most ACs expand to a detectable size by accumulation of cells and outward exponential growth. Various proliferative mechanisms drive tumor growth, especially angiogenesis. Mechanisms that promote cell membrane dissolution cause direct extension of neoplastic cells into local tissues, lymphatic vessels, and capillaries, setting the stage for cancer cells to enter the vascular and lymphatic system via diapedesis and achieve dissemination. Some cancer cells engaged in metastasis may bypass local sentinel lymph nodes.

Metastatic lesions are generally not detected in veterinary medicine until they can be palpated, seen, or imaged with X-rays, ultrasound, and scans. Lesions generally appear as nodular cell clones in the lungs, liver, spleen, abdomen, brain, or eyes and may further (but less commonly) metastasize to bone, skin, or toes.

Symptoms of metastatic disease may be sub-acute or chronic. Affected pets may develop coughing, gagging, exercise intolerance, dyspnea, ascites, or abdominal distention. Primary tumors of the lung and metastatic lesions may cause hypertrophic osteopathy (HO), a painful swelling of the legs due to periosteal new bone growth along the long bones of the limbs. Pulmonary metastases often demonstrate a "cannon ball" appearance or a patchy interstitial pattern on radiographs of the lung fields. Pulmonary and/or abdominal effusion is a common sequel of end stage metastatic carcinomas and adenocarcinomas.

Sarcomas

Sarcomas are malignancies that include all mesenchymal connective tissues, all endothelial cells, muscle tissue, bone, bone marrow, blood, mast cells, melanocytes, and miscellaneous cells. Sarcomas have a variable clinical appearance and have been subdivided into their palpable texture as soft tissue sarcomas vs. sarcomas of bone (firm) and blood (hematopoietic), which includes the leukemias and lymphomas. Various mesenchymal cell types give rise to distinctive neoplasms such as mast cell tumors, malignant melanoma, plasma cell tumors, and histiocytic (dendritic) cell tumors. These are also soft tissue sarcomas by definition. Sarcomas are so variable that they are often regarded as clinically distinct and comprise four of the five major cancer groupings as discussed in this book.

Soft Tissue Sarcomas

STSs arise in the connective tissues of the body, such as the skin, muscle, blood vessels, and fibrous tissue. Most STSs form a mass that is palpable on the surface of the body. However, some STSs that may originate from pluripotent stem cells of the bone marrow, such as transformed hemangioblasts, that insidiously lead to hemangiosarcoma, may arise as tumors anywhere in the body (Modiano and Helfand 2005). Look for the new "liquid biopsy" that may be able to detect circulating cancer cells prior to clinical manifestation (Modiano 2016).

Sarcomas of Bone

Osteosarcoma is the most commonly found bone tumor in dogs and cats. The other sarcomas of bone are chondrosarcoma, synovial cell sarcoma, and malignancies arising from any other bone constituent. Large and giant breed dogs are more prone to osteosarcoma at growth plates than are medium and small breed dogs. Bone tumors are relatively rare and less aggressive in cats, affecting them in their senior to geriatric years.

Bone may be secondarily infiltrated by metastatic carcinomas and other sarcomas. However, dogs and cats do not experience the high rate of bone invasion from metastatic cancer that is seen in humans. There may be a protective mechanism that spares bone from metastatic disease in dogs and cats, or perhaps they simply do not survive long enough for this to occur. As animal cancer patients survive longer, we may see more late metastases to the bones. Metastases to bone are recognized in canine osteosarcoma patients previously treated with chemotherapy. It seems that chemotherapy may have protected patients from lung metastasis but left them vulnerable to bone metastasis.

Osteosarcoma exhibits an aggressive biologic behavior in dogs. Radiographs show lysis and destruction of normal bone architecture and cortex at the primary site. Elevation of the periosteum to form Codman's triangle is considered pathognomonic for osteosarcoma. Tumor growth, inflammation, and expansion cause invasion through the cortex into surrounding tissues. Lytic lesions and stretching of the periosteum cause intense pain, which may be worse at night.

Dogs may develop pathological fractures at the tumor site due to stress on the weakened bone. Micrometastasis to the lungs occurs early in the course of disease, resulting in pulmonary lesions that compromise respiratory function within 4 to 6 months in most untreated cases. Cats rarely develop pathological fractures and metastasis to the lungs is slow to develop. Therefore, amputation may be curative in cats.

Feline Injection Site Sarcoma

Some cats have a genetic tendency toward developing soft tissue sarcoma (STS) at vaccine and injection sites. Chronic inflammation at the injection site creates inflammatory tissue, which promotes and initiates malignant sarcoma cells via mechanisms including genetic alterations of the tumor suppressor gene, *p53*. The situation was illuminated in 1991 by a letter to the editor in *JAVMA* by Dr. Mattie Hendrick, a pathologist at the University of Pennsylvania. She noted an increase in the number of cats with interscapular fibrosarcomas and theorized that aluminum hydroxide adjuvant, observed as a blue staining substance at vaccine sites, may play a role in creating the inflammatory response leading to malignant soft tissue sarcomas (Hendrick and Goldschmidt 1991).

This tumorigenic phenomenon was originally given the name "feline vaccine-associated sarcoma" (FVAS). It has since been renamed feline injection site sarcoma (FISS). It has a bimodal appearance with the second peak affecting senior and geriatric cats. If a cat develops a mass at a vaccination site that persists over 3 months, it should be highly suspected as FISS and treated as such (Moore 2004). The Vaccine Associated Feline Sarcoma Task Force (VAFSTF) was organized to unify the profession's efforts at understanding the carcinogenesis, pathogenesis, therapy, and prevention of FISS. The VAFSTF reached a consensus to review protocols and rationale for vaccination of cats.

FISS behaves aggressively and has a high rate of recurrence and fatality. The neoplasm has tentacles that infiltrate deeply below the mass and along facial planes, resulting in incomplete surgical resections. In addition, macrophages that engulf the aluminum hydroxide adjuvant may travel and create new foci of inflammation that may transition into new malignant sarcomas.

Unfortunately, the recurrence rate is greater than 90% within 6–12 months following routine surgery. When a board certified surgeon performs excision, the tumor-free interval is greater because wider and deeper margins are attained. When surgery is followed by radiation therapy, the rate of recurrence is reduced to 50% within 1 year. Approximately 25% of long term survivors develop metastases to the lungs. FISS can be prevented via a personalized lifestyle vaccine program that minimizes overvaccination, and by using fewer injections. Using non-adjuvanted vaccines for cats may eliminate tumor formation (Macy 2005).

Biological Behavior of Sarcomas

The biological behavior of STS is variable. Some tumors tend to remain in the local site of origin, while others metastasize. Tumors that remain localized still have the potential to kill because they recur after surgery and often become quite large and debilitating over time.

Geriatric pets are good candidates for treatment of STS if the patient is considered to be in good health and condition at the time of diagnosis. If the patient has concurrent illness, the overall survival time may be limited. Geriatric patients are more easily stressed from multiple surgeries or from the rigors of radiation therapy, chemotherapy, recurrence, and tumor burden.

The STSs that tend to remain localized fall into a large group that may be treated with a similar strategy. Aggressive surgery is generally required. If STS is approached casually without a good strategic plan prior to surgery, inadequate removal and recurrence is likely. The morphologic shape of STS may be imagined as an octopus with tentacles extending laterally into facial planes and deeply into structures below the mass.

A well-thought-out plan for total removal of STS is required. Unfortunately, many STSs are incompletely or inadequately removed. Well-intended clinicians who lack the surgical oncology skills for enblock definitive surgery may attempt to "debulk" a mass that could be completely excised by a board certified or qualified surgeon. It is important for the client to understand that if residual cancer cells remain in the body after the initial surgery, the cancer has *not* been removed. It has only been debulked, despite the good intention of the attending doctor and the healthy appearance of the surgery site.

Tumor removal can be a very humbling process, due to the high rate of failure in specific tumor types, especially STS. The surgeon's goal in surgical oncology is to gain complete removal of the mass with adequate margins of 2 to 3 cm beyond the extensions of the mass. Many surgeons feel and state with confidence that they "got it all." An excision may appear complete even when the microscopic examination finds narrow margins or dirty margins (see Figures 1.1 and 5.7). However, all remaining cancer cells are immortal. They are committed to grow into a recurrent tumor and metastasize, to accomplish their fatal agenda.

An incomplete first surgery may cause an interruption in the normal tissue planes. Additionally, growth factors involved in the wound healing process at the surgery site may allow residual cancer cells to behave more aggressively. Some sarcomas, such as hemangiopericytoma, seem to select a more aggressive cell line to grow back after successive surgeries and may transition toward fibrosarcomas.

Blood (Hematopoietic) Cancer

Malignancies of hematopoietic cells and lymphoid tissue are commonly referred to as blood cancer and include the leukemias, meyloproliferative disorders, and lymphomas. The leukemias are further classified according to the cell of origin, such as lymphoblastic, chronic lymphocytic, myelogenous, acute myelogenous, granulocytic, multiple myeloma (plasma cell), erythroleukemia, and so forth. Lymphomas are commonly diagnosed in dogs and cats and claim high mortality. There is a retroviral etiology in cats related to FeLV and FIV infection, but as yet no viral etiology has been found in dogs. The August 2016 issue of *Veterinary and Comparative Oncology* was devoted to canine and feline non-Hodgkin lymphoma. It gathered key publications regarding classification systems to further identify types and assign prognostic information based on immunological markers, gene expression profiling, and molecular and protein profiling.

Blood Cancer in Dogs

Lymphomas in dogs are described as large cell, blastic, cleaved cell, small cell, T-cell, B-cell, mantle cell, or cutaneous T-cell lymphoma (which includes mycosis fungoides). For prognostic and therapeutic information, clinicians are encouraged to pursue immunophenotyping to differentiate T-cell versus B-cell lymphoma. Canine T-cell lymphoma is less responsive than B-cell lymphoma. Boxers were found to have more T-cell lymphomas than most other breeds (Lurie et al. 2004), while geriatric dogs over 14 years of age were found to have more B-cell lymphomas (Modiano and Helfand 2005). This knowledge enables the attending clinician to more confidently determine an individual patient's prognosis and predict patient response to combination chemotherapy. Geriatric lymphoma patients benefit from induction chemotherapy as soon as an FNA diagnosis of lymphoma is established. Delaying treatment while waiting for histopathology and immunophenotyping results may allow the disease to advance and compromise the chances of treatment success.

Ted Valli and members of the American College of Veterinary Pathologists determined the value and ease of application of the WHO's system with a large study. This classification of canine nodal and extranodal lymphoma was published in the *WHO International Histological Classification of Tumours of Domestic Animals* in 2002. Each category and subtype in this system constitutes a well-described and documented disease entity, rather than a general cell type or morphology. Immunophenotype, disease topography, and signalment were evaluated by 17 pathologists and compared for accuracy and consistency. An effort was made to create acceptance of a single international nomenclature and criteria of recognition and classification for hematopoietic neoplasms in dogs (Valli 2005).

The study enrolled 300 cases from North America and Europe from oncology practices, pathology services, private practices, and colleges of veterinary medicine. In each case, the clinic and the animal carer signed an agreement permitting the use of tissues for research purposes. The client financed examinations, staging, nodal excision, and diagnostic procedures (including pathology and immunohistochemistry) to determine phenotype. Patients were treated by their local oncologist/clinician within the philosophy and financial means of the pet's owners.

The overall accuracy of the 17 pathologists was 83% to 87%. When tested for reproducibility, agreement between first diagnosis and the second diagnosis ranged between 40% and 87% (Valli et al. 2011).

Blood Cancer in Cats

Retroviral infection with FeLV and FIV increases the risk for affected cats to develop lymphoma, leukemia, meyloproliferative disorders, and immunosuppression. Historically, over one-third of all feline cancer deaths were FeLV related (Cotter, Hardy, and Essex 1975). In addition, deaths occur from anemia and infections due to viral injury of the immune system. The current prevalence of FeLV in healthy US pet cats is less than 1%, down from 5% during the 1970s and 1980s. This decrease is mostly due to test and isolation/removal programs.

The type of lymphoma diagnosed in cats has changed over the past 30 years. In the past, 50% of cats with hematopoietic malignancy had acute leukemia and 50%had lymphoma. The mediastinal form of lymphoma was most common and appeared in young cats. Cats with lymphoma tested 70% positive for FeLV or were positive with virus isolation.

Today, we see more FeLV-negative lymphomas, 70% of which are the alimentary form of the disease (Cotter, Hardy, and Essex 2005). Variations in the viral subtypes and other causes for lymphoma, such as exposure to environmental carcinogens and tobacco smoke, may explain this. Chronic exposure to cigarette smoke has been associated with the occurrence of lymphoma of the gastrointestinal tract in cats (Snyder, Bertone, and Moore 2001). Since 24% of adult people smoke cigarettes, and many of them own cats, there is an enormous population of cats at risk from chronic exposure to second and third hand tobacco smoke carcinogenesis as they age.

Many cats have a history of inflammatory bowel disease and weight loss prior to the diagnosis of GI lymphoma. Older cats with poorly differentiated GI lymphoma do poorly if they are debilitated at the time of diagnosis. It is difficult to monitor these patients because signs of progressive disease often mimic chemotherapy toxicity. The T- or B-cell phenotype is fairly evenly distributed in feline lymphoma. Phenotyping is not prognostically significant in cats. Predictive factors remain elusive. An initial complete response to therapy was found to be the only significant factor affecting survival for a series of 38 lymphoma cats. The average age was 11 years and 47% achieved complete remission with a median survival of 654 days (Milner et al. 2005). A recent prospective clinical trial in 26 cats also found that response can only be assessed during and not before treatment, emphasizing the need for molecular and genetic markers that allow for prognostication before treatment is begun (Limmer et al. 2016).

The attending clinician should avoid stressful diagnostic surgery in sick cats in preference to non-invasive diagnostic techniques such as FNA or Tru-cut biopsy. Many of these older cats have concurrent conditions such as cancer cachexia, chronic renal failure, heart disease, hyperthyroidism, diabetes, and so forth. Treatment and supportive care for these cats requires skill, patience, and initiative. It is imperative to address each one of the geriatric patient's comorbidites and balance effective chemotherapy in the face of other concurrent illnesses.

CNS Tumors

Tumors that arise in the brain, brainstem, and spinal cord are extremely difficult to manage in the veterinary patient. In part, this is due to typically late diagnosis. Many dog and cat patients tolerate the initial growth of CNS tumors without overt symptoms. The undiagnosed tumor progresses until compression by the calvarium or the spinal canal causes the animal to exhibit the signs of CNS neoplasia, such as behavior changes, seizures, circling head tilt, ataxia, blindness, or paresis.

A workup and complete neurologic examination may localize the lesion. For confirmation, imaging with MRI, CT, or PET scan can visualize the lesion. If a mass is localized, situated peripherally, and accessible by surgery, then the patient may benefit. Radiation therapy may be very helpful to control some brain tumors and spinal tumors.

PP's Recurrent Meningioma

One of my 19-year-old, geriatric feline patients named PP entered Pawspice as a 5-year survivor, following two surgeries for a large meningioma that caused blindness and circling. When PP's symptoms of blindness, circling, and imbalance recurred for the second time, her family did not want a third surgery. PP responded to our palliative oral brain tumor protocol using: Oil of Evening Primrose capsules 458 mg BID, prednisone 5 mg BID and metronomic lomustine at 3–3.5 mg/m^2/day. PP regained her vision and ability to jump and enjoyed a good quality of life during her Pawspice, which lasted for an unexpected 8 months.

Choroid plexus tumors are classified as carcinomas although they arise in the brain stem. They are not amenable to surgery and they are resistant to radiation therapy. Tumors that arise from nerve cells, including neurofibroma, neurofibrosarcoma, and nerve sheath tumor (schwannoma), are best treated as locally invasive sarcomas with wide surgical excision followed by external beam radiation therapy when feasible.

Miscellaneous Tumors and Tumors of Unknown Origin

Histiocytes are cells that have tiny extensions or dendrites on the cell surface (dendritic cells) such as macrophages, monocytes, and Langerhans cells. When transformed into their neoplastic counterparts, they multiply rapidly and infiltrate viscera. The cells often accelerate their signaling to phagocytize red cells and sometimes other white cells and other "self-cells," causing illness. Histiocytic tumors create a confusing set of syndromes.

Tumor cell markers are used to differentiate the cell of origin because these lesions can be confused with anaplastic carcinomas or diffuse large cell lymphoma. The most advanced collection of tumor cell markers for dendritic cells has been developed in the laboratory of Dr. Peter Moore in the Department of Pathology at the University of California, Davis. Unfortunately, as of this writing, the knowledge for tumor makers has served for diagnostic purposes only. When immunohistochemical (IH) stains become more readily available, we may be able to run a detailed analysis to identify the cell type more clearly and plan for more strategic therapy.

Bernese Mountain Dogs (BMDs) are genetically predisposed to malignant histiocytosis (MH). Other susceptible breeds are Rottweilers, Golden, Labrador, and Flat-Coated Retrievers, and Doberman Pinschers. MH is rare in cats. The malignant cells in MH originate from the pet's own immune system. There is controversy as to the cell type. MH may originate from a mutated clone of tissue macrophages but there is also a theory that BMDs genetically lack the ability to suppress tumor cell proliferation.

Another type of histiocytic tumor behaves as a somewhat localized but aggressive soft tissue sarcoma. Malignant fibrous histiocytoma (MFH) appears in middle aged and older dogs and cats. The tumors appear most often in Golden Retrievers and Rottweilers. These tumors may appear on the limbs and skin or in the spleen as a solitary growth but in this case they also have a multiorgan variant. MFH may also arise at injection and vaccine sites in cats. These localized tumors need to be aggressively excised. With follow-up radiation therapy or chemotherapy, some patients may have a variable tumor-free interval that may extend from a few months to years.

The tumors discussed in the following section are the most common histiocytic tumors encountered in general practice. Patients with these tumors need a thorough workup with histology and staging to distinguish cutaneous from systemic histiocytosis and MH.

Histiocytic Tumors

1. Malignant histiocytosis (MH) is the most aggressive histiocytic syndrome. MH most commonly affects the lymph nodes, viscera, eyes, CNS, and skin of older male BMDs and Rottweilers but can appear in Golden Retrievers, Miniature Schnauzers, Tibetan Terriers, and cats. The cells of origin are malignant tissue macrophages that show erythrophagocytosis and simultaneously infiltrate multiple organs and skin. MH is rapidly fatal. Some tumors may be misdiagnosed as granulomatous inflammation. Any clinician examining a sick BMD with CNS or ocular signs should be very suspicious and request special IH stains on cytology or tissue samples to rule out MH.
2. Systemic histiocytosis (SH) arises in the skin of younger BMDs and spreads to lymph nodes and viscera. The cells do not look malignant on cytology but show erythrophagocytosis. The disease

runs its course over a longer period of time than MH but eventually causes the patient's death. Leflunomide (an orphan drug) at 4 mg/kg PO SID has been proposed as somewhat helpful in both MH and SH but it causes GI toxicity when used with prednisone. Azathioprine and cyclosporine may also be of help.

3. Cutaneous histiocytosis (CH) is a multifocal proliferative variant of solitary cutaneous histiocytoma that remains restricted to the skin. This condition affects the nose, nasal mucosa, muzzle, and dorsum skin of BMDs, Briards, Collie breeds, and Golden Retrievers. The cells of origin for CH are dermal dendritic cells (positive for lysozyme marker on IH stains), whereas dermal Langerhans cells give rise to solitary histiocytomas found in young dogs. Lesions wax and wane over time but do not involve lymph nodes or viscera. Most pathologists do not classify these tumors as malignant but they do proliferate due to lack of tumor suppressor gene function. Some tumors may regress spontaneously. The tumors generally respond to steroids, surgery, or cryotherapy. L-asparaginase and azathioprine may also be used to achieve remissions.

4. Malignant fibrous histiocytoma (MFH), formally known as giant cell tumor, behaves like a very aggressive soft tissue sarcoma in both dogs and cats. The cell of origin is often undetermined but may come from pleomorphic fibroblast-like cells that exhibit cartwheel patterns or an inflammatory variant with bizarre histiocyte-like cells that arise in the spleen. These tumors contain spindle and round cells. Because they can be confused with carcinomas, fibrosarcomas, or osteosarcomas, special stains are in order. The behavior of MFH is variable but most often fatal. The solitary cutaneous/subcutaneous masses can be excised with some success. The multicentric form of MFH is very resistant to conventional attempts at treatment.

Miscellaneous Tumors

1. Plasma cell tumors have many names, including plasmacytoma, reticulum cell sarcoma, Merkel cell tumor of neuroendocrine origin, atypical histiocytoma, and cutaneous plasma cell tumor. They can also be misdiagnosed as MH. They are rare in cats. What pulls all these misnomers together is testing for the presence of immunoglobulin (IgG or lambda light chains) in the cytoplasm of the cells with immunofluorecense or immunoperoxidase stains. Plasma cell tumors appear as fleshy solitary or multiple cutaneous or oral neoplasms. They typically have a benign behavior (despite their wild cellular pleomorphism) when completely removed and they respond to radiation and chemotherapy. They do not cause monoclonal gammopathy and do not metastasize to bone. If you see widespread lesions, they are more likely to be metastatic from a primary multiple myeloma in the bone marrow. Both multiple myeloma and IgM macroglobulinemia are responsive to chemotherapy with chlorambucil and prednisone.

2. Pulmonary lymphomatoid granulomatosis (PLG) is rare. It appears as large masses in the lungs of dogs. The cell of origin is a pleomorphic population of atypical lymphoid infiltrates around and invading vessels. The majority of cases respond to chemotherapy protocols used for lymphoma and patients have similar median survival times as lymphoma dogs.

Rocky's Case (Systemic Histiocytosis Is Mean)

Rocky Racinto, a 10-year-old M/N Boxer, developed multiple, raised erythematous dermal lesions on his face, eyelids, and dorsum along with interdigital hyperemia and pruritis. The pathologist could not distinguish the cell type as cutaneous versus systemic histiocytosis.

Rocky's clinical appearance warranted a poor prognosis. Mr. Racinto, who worked night shifts as an orderly in a hospital, wanted to save Rocky but he had a limited budget. We recommended IH stains CD3 and CD79a to confirm systemic histiocytosis, but he was satisfied with my clinical impression and elected to spend his money on therapy. Rocky had a short regression of his tumors following induction with vincristine, L-asparaginase, and prednisone. His facial and cutaneous lesions cleared up.

Following the first treatment of Adriamycin, Rocky experienced nausea and vomiting. Two weeks later, he had an acute onset of severe upper airway dyspnea for 24 hours. On exam, he had pharyngeal edema and a firm swelling in the neck with parasympathetic paralysis. Radiographs identified a mass that deviated his trachea at the larynx and megaesophagus. We presumed that Rocky had progressive disease. His cutaneous lesions remained reduced with some crusting, despite the internal devastation caused by the malignancy and its fatal agenda.

Bingo's Case (Have Optimism – Cancer Can Be Cured!)

Bingo, a 9-year-old male Bernese Mountain Dog, was adopted by the Snyder family after retiring from the show ring. Bingo developed a rapidly growing $8 \times 5 \times 5$ cm³ subcutaneous mass in the area of the fourth mammary gland. The biopsy report was MFH. No other lesions were found on a complete workup. The Snyders had a strong bond with Bingo and knew that his line had longevity until 10 to 12 years of age. The family had some financial constraints and asked me to recommend the most valuable and cost-effective procedure that could be done. They elected our multimodality protocol with wide, deep surgical excision, intralesional chemotherapy, and intraoperative radiation therapy for curative intent. They declined postoperative external beam radiation and chemotherapy due to the costs. Bingo lived cancer free for 3 more years, until age 12, when he developed fulminant MH.

Letty's Case (Plasma Cell Tumors Are Not All Bad)

Letty Klint, a 10-year-old F/S King Charles Spaniel mix, developed a 1 cm mass in the gum tissue of her right caudal maxilla. Plain radiographs showed some bone loss. The mass was excised by her local veterinarian with narrow margins. During our consultation, the family told me that they had spoken to several other doctors: a holistic doctor, a family friend, and two veterinarians from their local practice. They also needed specific quotes for procedures and told me that they had financial constraints. I recommended either maxillectomy or radiation therapy for this generally localized oral tumor. The Klints declined invasive surgery. We referred them for a radiation therapy consultation. A CT scan was recommended to assess for bone invasion before the radiation therapy or surgical maxillectomy.

The scan showed no abnormalities and the Klints declined treatment for Letty. Their reasoning was, "Since there was nothing about the CT scan that was abnormal, we are having doubts about the diagnosis from the pathologist. Since there was no evidence of local recurrence, we decided that there was no evidence that would make us put Letty through either option at this time." The Klints made a follow-up plan with their local doctor to have oral X-rays every 3 months. They said that they would not consider a follow-up CT scan at the cost of $750.00. On a follow-up call four months later, Letty remained tumor free.

Fluffy's Case (She Outlived the Prognosis)

Fluffy Lockart, a 10-year-old F/S DSH, belonged to Liz Lockart, who lived and worked at Jones Veterinary Hospital in Santa Monica. Fluffy developed a $5 \times 5 \times 6$ cm^3 solitary histiocytic lymphoma on her right hind leg. The pathologist gave a poor prognosis of 90% mortality within 6 months. Liz declined amputation and elected debulking surgery with intraoperative radiation therapy (RTx) followed by 12 fractions of external beam RTx to the field and chemotherapy. Fluffy was in remission for 10 months, at which time she developed popliteal and inguinal lymph node enlargement. The recurrence was resistant to treatment and within 30 days she developed fulminant disease involving the spleen, liver, and lungs. Liz was satisfied and proud that Fluffy had outlived her prognosis.

Approaching Cancer According to Location

Another way to manage the complexity of oncology cases encountered in geriatric patients would be to approach them by location (Figure 4.1). You may find this clinical approach more appealing as the tumors, by virtue of their location, have many management features in common. Once the tumor is localized, it can be approached as a carcinoma or a sarcoma at that particular site. Clinicians can factor in the geriatric patient's comorbidities, body condition, and performance assessment as they view tumors from a location perspective. Weighing all these factors helps the clinician with decision making for management of the most common malignancies in geriatric oncology patients.

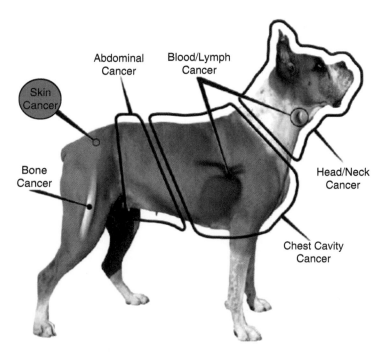

Figure 4.1.   Cancer can be named by its location. Approaching cancer according to its location helps to manage the complexity of oncology treatments.

Malignant Skin and Subcutaneous Tumors

Carcinomas: squamous cell, sebaceous, mammary, testicular, anal sac, perianal, salivary, sweat gland, basal cell, nail bed SCC, etc.

Sarcomas: mast cell tumors, fibrosarcoma, liposarcoma, neurofibrosarcoma (nerve sheath tumor), myxofibrosarcoma, hemangiopericytoma, cutaneous actinic hemangiosarcoma, cutaneous non-actinic hemangiosarcoma, malignant melanoma, nail bed melanoma, rhabdomyosarcoma, leiomyosarcoma, transmissible venereal tumor (TVT), cutaneous plasmacytomas, etc.

Malignant Head and Neck Tumors

Carcinomas: oral SCC and thyroid, salivary, ceruminous gland (otic), and ciliary body (ocular) carcinomas, etc.

Sarcomas: oral and facial fibrosarcoma, mast cell tumor, oral and facial malignant melanoma, etc.

Oral tumors: SCC, fibrosarcoma, malignant melanoma, osteosarcoma, acanthomatous epulis, etc.

Nasal tumors: nasal planum SCC, nasal respiratory carcinoma, chondrosarcoma, etc.

Brain tumors: glial tumors (more common in older, brachycephalic dogs), ependymoma, choroid plexus tumors, meningiomas (more common in old cats), etc.

Malignant Chest Cavity Tumors

Secondary: metastatic pulmonary disease may be from either mesenchymal or epidermal origin malignancy.

Carcinoma: bronchogenic carcinoma, squamous cell carcinoma, esophageal carcinoma, heart base (aortic body), cardiac tumors, mesothelioma, etc.

Sarcoma: thymoma, thymic (mediastinal) lymphoma, hemangiosarcoma of myocardium, malignant histiocytosis, and lymphomatoid granulomatosis.

Malignant Abdominal Cavity Tumors

Carcinomas: gastrointestinal, splenic, hepatic, pancreatic, adrenal (pheochromocytoma), renal, bladder (transitional cell carcinoma), prostatic, gonadal cancer (ovarian, uterine, and retained testicular tumors), mesothelioma, carcinomatosis, etc.

Sarcomas: hemangiosarcoma, lymphoma, leiomyosarcoma, mast cell tumor, malignant histiocytosis, extramedullary plasmacytomas, miscellaneous, etc.

Bone Cancer

Osteosarcoma, chondrosarcoma, fibrosarcoma, giant cell, synovial cell sarcoma, secondary metastases, etc.

Blood Cancer

Lymphomas, leukemias, multiple myeloma, myeloproliferative disorders, hemangiosarcoma, etc.

Summary

Cancer becomes more prevalent and complex in companion animals as they age due to reduced immunosurveillance and the comorbidities associated with aging. Clinicians may categorize neoplasia according to its benign or malignant behavior and according to its mesenchymal or epithelial origin to help in decision making for geriatric pets. Grouping cancer into the five major categories such as carcinoma, sarcoma, blood cancer, nervous system cancer, and miscellaneous cell types helps to understand its biological behavior. Tumors may also be clinically approached by location (Figure 4.1). Many tumors share similar management features due to their location. This basic information along with new genetic and molecular diagnostic tests may allow the attending doctor to make early recommendations for pet owners to consider during the difficult process of decision making. Clients need to know all available treatment options, including clinical trials and the option of palliative cancer care with the Pawspice concept, and when to seek comfort care with hospice for geriatric pets with cancer.

References

Cotter, S.M., W.D. Hardy, and M. Essex. 1975. Association of feline leukemia virus with lymphosarcoma and other disorders in the cat. *JAVMA* 166:449–454.

Cullen, J.M., R. Page, and W. Misdorp. 2002. "An overview of cancer pathogenesis, diagnosis, and management." In *Tumors in domestic animals*, 4th edn, ed. D.J. Meuten, pp. 3–43. Ames, IA: Iowa State Press.

Gawande, A. 2014. OVERKILL: An avalanche of unnecessary medical care is harming patients physically and financially. *Annals of Health Care, The New Yorker Magazine*, October 15th.

Hart, B.L., L.A. Hart, A.P. Thigpen, and N.H. Willits. 2014. Long-term health effects of neutering dogs: Comparison of Labrador Retrievers with Golden Retrievers. *PlosOne*. doi:10.1371/journal.pone.0102241.

Hart, B.L., L.A. Hart, A.P. Thigpen, and N.H. Willits. 2016. Neutering of German Shepherd Dogs: Associated joint disorders, cancers and urinary incontinence. *Veterinary Medicine and Science* 2:191–199. doi:10.1002/vms3.34.

Hendrick, M.J., and M.H. Goldschmidt. 1991. Do injection site reactions induce fibrosarcomas in cats? *JAVMA* 199:968.

Limmer, S., N. Eberle, V. Nerschbach, I. Nolte, and D. Betz. 2016. Treatment of feline lymphoma using a 12-week, maintenance-free combination chemotherapy protocol in 26 cats. *Veterinary and Comparative Oncology* 14 (S1):21–10. doi: 10.1111/vco.12082.

Lurie, D.M., M.D. Lucroy, S.M. Griffey, E. Simmonson, and B.R. Madewell. 2004. T-cell derived lymphoma in the boxer breed. *Veterinary and Comparative Oncology* 2 (3):171–175.

Macy, D.W. 2005. The big, the bad, the ugly: Fibrosarcomas. *AVMA Convention Notes, Merial Symposium*, pp. 47–53.

Milner, R.J., J. Peyton, K. Cooke, L.J. Fox, et al. 2005. Response rates and survival times for cats with lymphoma treated with the University of Wisconsin–Madison chemotherapy protocol: 38 cases (1996–2003). *JAVMA* 227 (7):1118–1122.

Modiano, J.F. 2016. Where the future lies: Innovations in cancer treatment and prevention. *3rd World Veterinary Cancer Congress Proceedings*.

Modiano, J.F., and S.C. Helfand. 2005. Innovations in the diagnosis of hemangiosarcoma. Personal Communication, *VCS NL* 29 (1):4–5.

Moore, A.S. 2004. Biopsy of suspected injection-induced sarcoma in cats. *NAVC Clinician's Brief*, June, pp. 13–19.

Snyder, L.A., E.R. Bertone, and A.S. Moore. 2001. Environmental tobacco smoke exposure and *p53* expression in feline lymphoma. *Veterinary Cancer Society Proceedings*, p. 5.

Valli, V.E., 2005. Canine lymphoma: International review and evaluation. Personal Communication, *VCS NL* 29 (1).

Valli, V.E., et al. 2011. Classification of canine malignant lymphoma according to the World Health Organization criteria. *Veterinary Pathology*, 48 (1):198–211. doi: 10.1177/0300985810379428.

Veterinary and Comparative Oncology, 2016. *Lymphoma*, Vol. 14, Supplement 1, August, Argyle & Pecceu (eds).

Suggested Reading

Meuten, D.J. (ed.). 2000. *Tumors in domestic animals*, 4th edn. Ames, IA: Iowa State Press.

Villalobos, A.E. (ed.). 2010. "Tumors of the skin and soft tissues." In *The Merck Veterinary Manual*, 10th edn, ed. C.M. Kahn, pp. 764–789. Whitehouse Station, NJ: Merck & Co.

Chapter 5

Generating the Diagnosis and Prognosis of Cancer in Geriatric Pets

If you were this patient, are these the diagnostics and treatments that you would like to have your doctor choose?

Carl A. Osborne, DVM, ACVIM

Principles and Perspective for Diagnosis in Geriatric Cancer Patients

It is essential to establish a working and definitive diagnosis to properly manage cancer in geriatric patients. However, by their very nature, geriatric oncology patients pose more diagnostic dilemmas due to age-related changes and comorbidities, which compete for medical attention and reduce the patient's tolerance to stress (see Table 2.2). We must also document the geriatric patient's clinical condition and functional performance (see Chapter 8). Each geriatric patient is unique and should be evaluated with the concept that age itself is not a disease but a physiologic condition in which cancer is more commonly found. Cancer is currently a more treatable disease in dogs and cats, but the first doctor consulted often determines the fate of the geriatric pet with cancer. This emphasizes the importance of education in geriatric oncology so that we can meet our clients' expectations for expertise and professional help when cancer strikes their aging pets.

If a biopsy or diagnostic procedure places the geriatric patient at risk or if the procedure is as stressful as the treatment, you are completely justified in getting the biopsy along the way. There are many instances where having the definitive diagnosis of a suspected cancer would not alter your immediate recommendation or the pet owner's decision for palliative or curative clinical control. Exemptions from the academic pursuit of a definitive diagnosis *before* a definitive procedure would be justified, especially for geriatric oncology patients, when making recommendations for cancer types where we have a high rate of diagnostic confidence based upon imaging. These procedures would include: splenectomy for suspected hemangiosarcoma; amputations for suspected osteosarcoma; lobectomy for a solitary lung mass; mandibulectomy for a suspected fibrosarcoma, melanoma, or squamous cell carcinoma (SCC); and craniotomy for a suspected benign brain tumor.

Generating the diagnosis of cancer places a negative burden on the geriatric oncology patient if it requires sedation or anesthesia. Cancer and related paraneoplastic syndromes interact with the geriatric patient's concurrent illnesses and onboard medications. We can alert our clients that in the future we may only need a "liquid biopsy" via a blood test for diagnosis. All these considerations have a direct impact on the methods we choose to establish the diagnosis and staging of cancer. Your clients

Canine and Feline Geriatric Oncology: Honoring the Human–Animal Bond, Second Edition. Alice Villalobos with Laurie Kaplan.
© 2018 John Wiley & Sons, Inc. Published 2018 by John Wiley & Sons, Inc.

will appreciate your efforts to provide a rapid cost-effective diagnosis or presumptive diagnosis of cancer that will assist them in decision making for their geriatric pets.

Diagnostic Tools and Techniques Used for Diagnosis and Staging Cancer

Basic tools and techniques essential for diagnosis of cancer in geriatric patients include:

1. Calipers and cartoon body maps to measure and document location of tumors in the chart.
2. Point of service laboratory tests (including complete blood count (CBC), chemistries, and electrolytes).
3. FNA cytology with direct microscopic examinations and laboratory confirmation.
4. New methylene blue stain for cytology and impression smears.
5. Punch biopsy and Tru-cut (Travenol Labs Inc., Deerfield, IL) needle core biopsy instruments, scalpel blade/handle, needle holder, suture scissors, suture, skin glue, staples.
6. Imaging machines: diagnostic X-ray and ultrasound (if possible).
7. Local anesthetic, safe sedation, and anesthesia protocols for minor and major diagnostic procedures.
8. A 10% formalin solution in a capped bottle, lab request form with history, and cartoon body map.

Utilization of sophisticated diagnostic tools and techniques involving ultrasound, endoscopy, computed tomography (CT), magnetic resonance imaging (MRI), and positron emission tomography (PET) scanning or nuclear medicine requires collaboration with colleagues in specialty services. New technology imaging provides three-dimensional color visualization of tumors for staging and treatment planning. The most important goal for the practitioner to keep in mind is to gather as much information as possible with the least amount of stress to the geriatric cancer patient. Actively involve your clients in the diagnostic quest every step of the way so they feel satisfied that you are keeping them informed. This partnership enables the family to make good choices. When thorough and continuous involvement through good communication with the caregiver fails to occur, misunderstandings and dissatisfaction issues regarding cost of care and ultimate outcome of therapy are much more likely to happen.

Fine Needle Aspiration Cytology: A Very Handy but Underutilized Tool

In-house FNA cytology examination is a very inexpensive and rewarding diagnostic tool that is a consistent favorable practice builder. FNA helps to characterize skin tumors, lymph nodes, thoracic and abdominal masses, and effusions. It is definitely worth your while to gain confidence and some expertise in performing in-house cytology. My preference is to look at FNA cytology slides under the microscope immediately to get an idea of what type of tumor we are dealing with. Clinicians who read their cytology slides in-house offer a tremendous point of service value that translates into an immediate medical and therapeutic advantage for their geriatric oncology patients.

FNA cells fall into these general categories: lipid, sebum, inflammation, infection, normal benign, hyperplastic, or abnormal cells. Abnormal cells appear bizarre and may exhibit one or more characteristics of malignancy. Characteristics that are easy to detect on cytologic examination that would suggest malignancy are macrocytosis, anisocytosis (variable cell sizes), pleomorphism (variable cell forms), anisokaryosis (variable nuclear sizes), and karyomegaly (large nuclei). In addition, the cells may manifest a high nuclear-to-cytoplasmic ratio, variable staining intensity of cytoplasm, variable sizes and shapes of nucleoli, and increased or abnormal mitotic figures (Meyer 2001; Cowell 2003).

It is easy and clinically very important to distinguish mast cell tumors (MCTs) from lipomas, wide-based warts, and masses that arise in the dermis and SQ tissues of geriatric pets. Cytograding of mast cell aspirates (based on number of mitoses, multinucleated cells, bizarre nuclei, and karyomegaly) can provide helpful insights for on the spot clinical decision making (Scarpa et al. 2014). After screening for the blue granules in MCTs and black granules in melanomas, your job is to recognize the bizarre spindle cells of sarcomas and secretory vacuoles or epithelial appearance of carcinoma cells. Never postpone FNA of enlarged lymph nodes in geriatric oncology patients. They have a much higher cancer risk than younger animals. Lymph node cytology is quick, easy, and rewarding. What is most important with in-house cytology is that you can generally start a plan of action using it as a point of service information source while laboratory confirmation is pending (Cowell 2003).

It is essential for clinicians working with geriatric cancer patients to use a reliable reference laboratory staffed with veterinary pathologists or clinical pathologists to read their cytology samples. There is a 15% variation between interpretations for cancer in human pathology versus veterinary pathology. We have enough variations with pathologists in our own profession without asking for more variables. Identify which pathologist specializes in reading cytology slides and direct your slide specimens and questions to that individual. Turnaround time for samples submitted to your diagnostic laboratory should be within 24–48 hours to expedite patient management. Clients should not have to wait more than a few working days for results.

Lady's Case (Client Satisfaction Is Very Important)

Lady White, a 10-year-old Great Dane belonging to Dr. Angel White, a physician and researcher working at UCLA, developed a large swelling at the right distal radius. Dr. White, who breeds and rescues Great Danes, noticed the mass a week before presentation. I listened carefully to her issues and sensed her distress. She wanted to confirm her own presumptive clinical diagnosis of bone cancer without subjecting Lady's already painful leg to the recommended core biopsies. She had declined thoracic and limb X-rays due to reluctance to submit Lady to sedation or anesthesia.

After a supportive consultation, our staff was able to lift Lady on to the X-ray table and take an AP view of her right distal radius. The lesion appeared radiographically consistent with osteosarcoma. Using a local anesthetic injection of lidocaine and using the X-ray to identify the most lytic area of the lesion, I performed FNA with a 20-gauge needle. The cytology sample was stained with new methylene blue and immediately examined. It revealed osteoclasts and wild sarcomatous cells.

I invited Dr. White to view the cells at the microscope. She took a long look at the cells and then turned toward me with tears filling her eyes and said, "This was all that I needed to help me make my decision. Thank you for helping me to spare Lady from stress and pain." Dr. White has continued to use our oncology service for over 20 years.

If you suspect cancer upon viewing X-rays and FNA cytology, inform the pet owner of your suspicion and provide a short list of differential diagnoses to rule out. Pet owners appreciate a correct diagnosis when it is arrived at quickly, before their anxieties reach high levels. A prompt diagnosis also allows the clinician to advise clients regarding the next best step in the workup, staging, and subsequent discussion of the most suitable therapeutic options. The attending doctor should be the geriatric cancer patient's advocate in decision making. Your clinical judgment, common sense, compassion, and courage can help aging pets derive maximum benefit from diagnostic procedures with minimum morbidity.

Large Aspiration Needle Chop for Firm Tumors

There is a predictable glitch when it comes to FNAs of firm tumors. Be suspicious of firm masses because they are often sarcomas. Because these tumors do not exfoliate well and tend to yield non-diagnostic results, it is important to invest your time and energy into obtaining worthwhile cellular samples from firm masses. Do not submit acellular samples from firm masses to the lab for cytology. This common failure to harvest cells from firm masses for cytology only wastes your time and your clients' time and money.

Harvesting cellular samples from firm masses is essential for an accurate diagnosis. To address this predictable problem, ratchet up your FNA technique by using a relatively large bore needle as an augur. Thrust an 18-gauge needle attached to a 6 or 12 cc syringe into the center of the tumor, and then briskly angle the needle off to one side before aspirating. This will enable you to capture a tiny core of cells for aspiration cytology. Repeat this procedure in two other directions using the same entry point until enough cells are harvested for cytology, always keeping the needle within the mass. This technique allows the end of the 18-gauge needle to chop off tiny cores of cells for retrieval and cytology. I call this version of fine needle aspiration "large aspiration needle chop" (LANC). The next step is to place a few drops of new methylene blue stain or diff quick stain and view the cells immediately. The LANC technique yields tissue for optimum diagnostic success. You will find that you get a higher rate of positive confirmations using LANC cytology on firm masses.

Many cases of feline vaccine-associated sarcomas (FVASs) and canine soft tissue sarcomas (STS) experience delayed diagnosis due to the submission of acellular samples using routine FNA techniques.

Keno's Case (Don't Allow the Opportunity for Diagnosis to Slip Away)

Keri noticed a firm interscapular mass on her elderly cat, Keno. Her local veterinarian performed routine FNA, which was non-diagnostic. Keri, who was in the process of moving, drove cross-country with Keno under the incorrect assumption that the mass was benign or not of grave danger.

Three months later, the mass was much larger with extensions that delved toward the dorsal spinous processes. Keri's new doctor referred Keno to our service for consultation. We used the LANC technique and within a few minutes, confirmed that Keno had feline injection site sarcoma (FISS). If the LANC technique had been used for Keno's original FNA, it probably would have been diagnostic. Without a proper diagnosis, Keri felt that she lacked the information that she needed to treat Keno's mass quickly and appropriately. A review of the original records revealed that her doctor advised surgical biopsy if the mass did not regress. Keri felt that her doctor should have put her on high alert to rule out cancer without the intimidation of general anesthesia.

LANC would predictably increase the opportunities to establish initial diagnoses in numerous geriatric pets presenting with firm tissue masses. Estimates reveal that there could be as many as 22,000 cats developing vaccine-associated sarcomas every year in the United States, with no change in prevalence worldwide since 1993 (Ford 2004; Kass et al. 1993; Gobar and Kass 2002). Geriatric cats are prone due to the cumulative effect of vaccines over time. The LANC technique provides caregivers one more diagnostic option that may spare the pet from sedation or anesthesia.

FNA should be included in the routine physical exam for any geriatric patient with a mass since 33% of all tumors in dogs and 25% of all tumors in cats arise in the skin (Vail and Withrow 2001; Cowell 2003). My curiosity wants an instant answer and new methylene blue staining makes it easy to immediately view FNA slides under the microscope before submitting the rinsed slides to a clinical pathologist for confirmations as needed. Inform clients that your initial in-house cytology exam is a quality control procedure to locate significant cells. If the first set of FNA slides is not worthy for submission to the laboratory, it is convenient to approach the patient for more cells.

Use a body cartoon map to document the size, location, and FNA diagnosis of skin masses for the medical chart (Figure 5.1A). Be sure to review the basic cytology slides in this section. This collection will help you to differentiate cells so that you can identify mast cells, leukemia, lymphoma, sarcoma, malignant melanoma, and carcinoma cells. You can offer basic cytology as a point of service test for your clients (Figures 5.1B through 5.6).

Characteristics of Cancer in Cytology

Neoplastic cells are often surrounded by inflammatory cells, cells undergoing apoptosis, areas of hypoxia, cell debris, and necrosis. This explains the complex and heterogeneous nature of tumors and why FNA samples cannot be relied upon to rule out cancer entirely. The consortium of variable cells and areas inside malignant tumors causes an inherent error factor of 15% for cytology. The characteristics of malignant cells are similar to the cytograding of mast cells mentioned above. Look for: clusters and nests of cells, bizarre and irregular cells, multinucleated cells, multiple nucleoli in the nucleus of cells, variable nuclear-to-cytoplasmic ratio, and spindle-shaped cells. Foamy contents in cells is characteristic of glandular carcinomas (adenocarcinomas). Numerous large lymphoblasts indicate lymphoma (see Figures 5.1 to 5.6). On some occasions and with certain tumor types, such as feline abdominal masses, persistence is very important and rewarding. I often look at 15 to 20 slides before finding enough intact cells that are representative for diagnostic cytology. If you see 10 or more intact lymphoblasts on a cytology slide from a senior cat with an abdominal mass, you have a working diagnosis of lymphoma. Finding diagnostic cells is very rewarding, especially when it enables you to spare an elderly pet the rigors of exploratory laparotomy. When the cytology findings correlate with the clinical appearance of a mass, it negates the need and expense of sending the slides to the laboratory for further assessment unless you need to document the diagnosis with professional laboratory confirmation. This saves both hospital and client added expense of using a professional laboratory to report the obvious.

Nikki's Case (Don't Assume Mast Cell Recurrence until Proven)

Nikki Alvarez, a 12-year-old F/S Shar-Pei, presented with a firm, distended abdomen. Two and a half years previously, we had treated Nikki for MCT of the hard palate with external beam radiation therapy. Nikki was cancer free and on our cure list for MCT. Nikki presented to her local vet with a history of vomiting and reduced appetite. Her doctor palpated a huge abdominal mass on the left side of her abdomen, which he believed was an enlarged spleen. He found that Nikki also had greatly elevated liver enzymes. The referring doctor worried that the splenomegaly might be due to metastatic mast cell cancer.

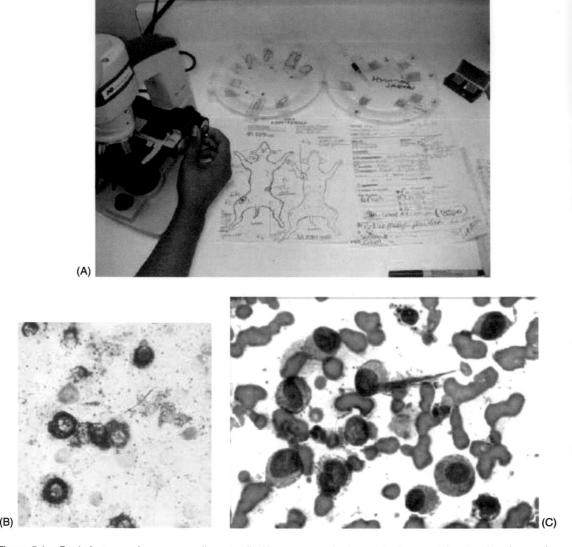

Figure 5.1. Basic features of common malignant cells. Use a cartoon body map to document the size, location, and FNA diagnosis of skin masses for the medical chart (A). Mast cells stained with new methylene blue (B) and with Romanowsky staining (C). Notice the cytoplasmic granules that may be released into the extracellular fluid. (B) Contributed by Deborah C. Bernreuter, DVM, MS, Veterinary Clinical Pathologist, IDEXX Labs. (C) Photographed specimens from the author's clinic by Dr. Lon Rich, DVM, ACVCP, Antech Labs.

Ms. Alvarez requested an evaluation for surgery. We performed abdominal ultrasound and FNA of the mass to rule out metastatic MCT. During the ultrasound study, we found moderate ascites and a normal spleen, which was displaced and compressed by a large hepatic mass. The left liver lobe was enormously enlarged and numerous hyper and hypoechoic lesions were imaged in the right liver lobes as well.

We used ultrasound for guided FNAs of the mass. The mass was firm and did not exfoliate cells for our initial cytology study, which did not contain mast cells. We performed another series of FNAs using $1\frac{1}{2}$-inch long 22-gauge needles. By using our special version of FNA

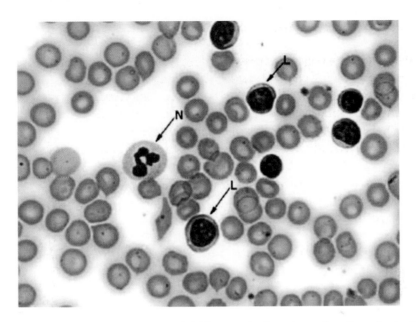

Figure 5.2. Leukemia: lymphoblasts (L), neutrophil (N). Photographed specimens from the author's clinic by Dr. Lon Rich, DVM, ACVCP, Antech Labs.

using the LANC technique, we were able to aspirate representative cells for cytology. The cells were stained with new methylene blue and a cover slip was placed over them. The harvested cells had the appearance of hepatocytes and demonstrated several characteristics of malignancy. We also identified some cells that were spindle shaped. Ms. Alvarez wanted surgery for Nikki, if it would afford her a reasonable chance for 3 to 4 months of quality life afterwards.

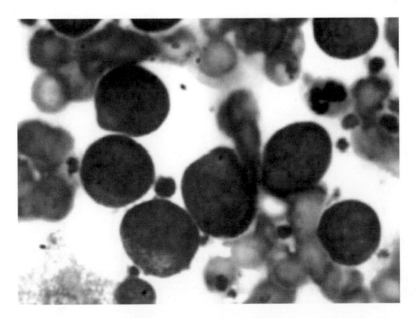

Figure 5.3. Lymphoblasts from an enlarged lymph node. Malignant lymphoma cells are large (blue staining) cells with large nuclei and nucleoli. Contributed by Deborah C. Bernreuter, DVM, MS, Veterinary Clinical Pathologist, IDEXX Labs.

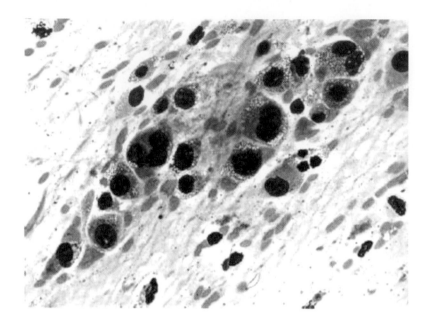

Figure 5.4.   Sarcoma from FVAS: notice the bizarre spindle-shaped cells. Photographed specimens from the author's clinic by Dr. Lon Rich, DVM, ACVCP, Antech Labs.

Based on the findings, we advised Ms. Alvarez to enter Nikki into our end of life care Pawspice program. We offered antiemetics and pain control medications and recommended feeding Nikki a liquid diet compatible with liver failure such as Hill's L/D canned food. We also placed Nikki on several supplements that were supportive of liver function. Nikki lived another 47 days in the comfort of her home in Pawspice care.

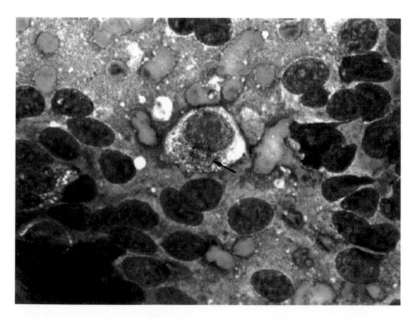

Figure 5.5.   Malignant melanoma, showing cytoplasmic black granules. Photographed specimens from the author's clinic by Dr. Lon Rich, DVM, ACVCP, Antech Labs.

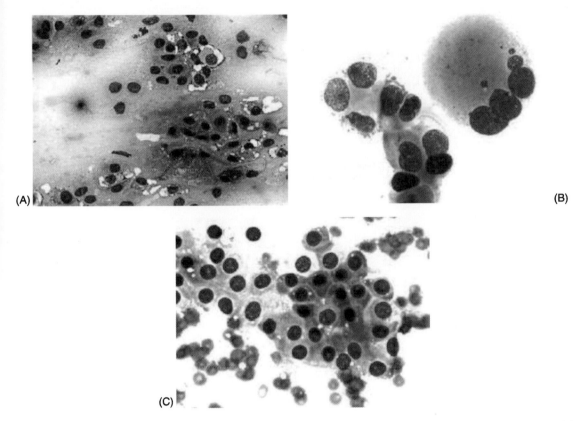

Figure 5.6.   Carcinoma (A). Carcinoma showing secretory material (B). Thyroid carcinoma with pink secretory material representing colloid (C). (A) Photographed specimens from the author's clinic by Dr. Lon Rich, DVM, ACVCP, Antech Labs. (B) and (C) Contributed by Deborah C. Bernreuter, DVM, MS, Veterinary Clinical Pathologist, IDEXX Labs.

Punch and Tru-cut Core Biopsy Needle Techniques

Every veterinarian should have quick access to small gauge punch biopsy instruments and Tru-cut needles. The instruments should be handy in the exam rooms, treatment rooms, and in the ultrasound room. Diagnostic biopsies can be taken from most skin tumors of well-behaved geriatric pets simply with the use of local anesthesia and skin glue to control bleeding (Ogilvie and Moore 1995).

Nervous or stressed patients need relaxation and analgesia for many diagnostic procedures. We prefer to use a short-acting intramuscular sedation such as dexmedetomidine (Dexdomitor®) in clinically healthy older patients using the IM dose table in the package insert. It can be reversed with atipamezole (Antisedan®). The low dose combination of Dexdomitor® with butorphanol at 0.4mg/kg delivers smooth sedation with analgesia, allowing most minor procedures. It has the advantage of reversal with Antisedan® and smooth recovery. Dexdomitor and butorphanol are compatible in solution with one another and can be drawn into a 1ml tuberculin (TB) syringe. The combo may also be administered intravenously using the IV dose table provided in the package insert via a butterfly catheter in place. This combination is safe for physiologically healthy patients with normal cardiac function. We seldom need the high dose sedation. Use the Plumb's Veterinary Drugs text or AP as a reliable source for more detailed guidelines.

For nervous geriatric and/or frail patients and for patients with cardiac disease, the best choice for IM or IV sedation would be a short acting opioid such as fentanyl in combination with a short acting benzodiazepine such as midazolam or IV propofol (Diprivan^{TM}). It is very important not to stress the nervous geriatric cancer patients. Always use a mild sedative if the patient gets anxious when being held by staff or allow the procedures to be done in the presence of the pet owner if possible. Monitoring the geriatric cancer patient is essential.

Skin glue is very handy to seal small punctures and incisions if needed. Staples, clips, or sutures are also appropriate for skin apposition following punch biopsy. We often administer an injectable antibiotic at the time of the biopsy procedure if the tumor is infected or if the patient has concurrent UTI, dental disease, pyoderma, or any other antibiotic responsive condition that may affect the postbiopsy period.

Incisional versus Excisional Surgical Biopsy for Diagnosis

If general anesthesia is required to harvest tissue for biopsy in a geriatric patient, a preliminary database including mucosal clotting time is essential prior to the procedure. It should include a thorough physical exam, a profile to determine organ function, a urinalysis, chest and abdominal X-rays, and abdominal ultrasound if indicated. Sterile surgical technique is employed to prepare the site. When using a punch, Tru-cut biopsy needle, or a scalpel, make sure that the incision penetrates into the tumor without traumatizing the tissue. Take deep samples at several sites in larger masses. Blot blood from the sample and place it on cardboard or wood tongue depressor with an orientation mark. Provide the pathologist with a cartoon drawing or digital picture that describes the lesion (Kunkle and Akucewich 2005).

Inflammation, necrosis, and tumor heterogeneity may obscure the diagnosis; therefore, it is best to take several samples along different tracts. Tissue samples taken at the periphery of the mass often have more viable cells and yield more information regarding invasiveness. The needle track used to harvest the biopsy must be recorded or marked on a map or directly on the skin with ink or sutures. If and when the tumor is excised, irradiated, or treated with electroporation, the biopsy track(s) must also be included in the excision, in the radiation therapy field, or the ablation field respectively. For bone marrow aspirations and biopsy of lytic bone lesions, be sure biopsy needle placement is accurate and that you collect cells from several sites so that a representative sample may be harvested (Friedrichs and Young 2005; Withrow 2001).

It is quite easy to insert a Tru-cut needle instrument into a lymph node or tumor for diagnostic histopathology and tumor grade. Tru-cut biopsy is especially useful before attempting surgical excision of any mass scheduled for surgery. An unknown excised mass has the potential to be a malignant tumor such as a MCT or a soft tissue sarcoma. Most well-behaved geriatric patients only require a topical or locally injected anesthetic for Tru-cut biopsy, as it is a minor procedure. Taking a punch biopsy even with the smallest gauge instrument requires an injection of local anesthetic and mild sedation.

Some doctors prefer the rapid induction and rapid recovery achieved using inhalant sevoflurane as a "sedative" technique. Geriatric cats can be conveniently given IV propofol or inhalant anesthetics in an anesthetic chamber and maintained with mask delivery. During sedation, look for other minor procedures that can be done to enhance the geriatric oncology patient's quality of life, such as trimming overgrown nails, dental and ear cleaning, coat care, and so forth. This added care is especially important for older cats with oral tumors. These patients drool on their legs and paws, so their coats are generally unkempt and require constant cleaning.

Gunter's Case (The First Surgery Can Be More Effective with FNA)

Gunter Fillmore, an 8-year-old, 98-pound M/N Weimaraner, developed a mass that appeared suddenly in the medial aspect of his right elbow. We treated him for a soft tissue sarcoma in the footpad of his left front leg the previous year. Gunter's attending doctor removed the mass immediately and submitted it for histopathology. Ms. Fillmore called me in despair after learning that the mass was a grade I–II MCT excised with narrow margins. She felt that Gunter had lost his battle against cancer. I explained that the two tumors were unrelated and recommended a consultation to review the biopsy report and discuss options for dealing with the new tumor. The report described it as well differentiated with a low mitotic index. The margins were complete but inadequate for MCT. Gunter was referred to a board certified surgeon for excisional biopsy of the entire tumor bed. In my opinion, the second surgery could have been avoided for Gunter if his attending doctor performed FNA prior to surgery or used the rule of thumb principle of acquiring margins at least the size of the mass.

Some clinicians prefer to remove a suspicious mass quickly and get it over with. They often feel confident that their margins are seemingly complete at the first attempt. They submit the tissue to the pathologist and feel satisfied that they are serving their clients well by this approach. Their intent may be to avoid problems associated with biopsy of potentially "excitable" tumors or to avoid problems following the incisional biopsy procedure itself. However, this approach may not be the best procedure for the patient. Attending doctors must think clearly and analytically about gathering more information on tumors prior to excisional surgery. At the very least, the clinician should determine if the mass is an MCT to plan for adequate 2–3cm margins. If the surgeon knows preoperatively that a mass is a sarcoma or carcinoma, the patient is more likely to benefit with a wider, deeper excision and a true cut or wedge biopsy of the local and regional lymph nodes for staging purposes.

When excising a mass without the precaution of FNA cytology, it is best to acquire wide, deep margins around the mass that are at least the same size as the mass itself. This extra measure at surgery may achieve adequate margins around the tumor and save the patient a second surgery if the mass is subsequently found to be a malignancy.

Histopathology Terms: Adequate versus Complete Margins

The terms "complete margins" and "adequate margins" are often used by pathologists. They may seem interchangeable, but the distinction is of great significance to the patient's survival. When veterinarians read the word "complete" in the report, they want to believe that they "got it all" and that the surgery was complete enough for the case. In reality, "complete" indicates only that the tumor was removed in its entirety and does not indicate that the margins around the tumor are adequate for decreased recurrence or increased survival time.

The achievement of "adequate margins" occurs when the margins around the completely removed mass are wide enough to expect a lowered recurrence rate and an increased tumor-free interval. Complete margins are not as good as adequate margins, although the literal interpretations of these words

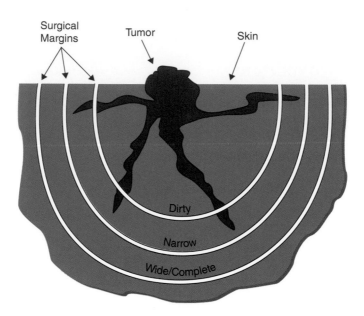

Figure 5.7. The octopus-shaped malignancy showing dirty, narrow, and adequate surgical margins.

in pathology reports have been misleading clinicians for many years. Be very clear about the clinical significance of terminology and the definition of the words that your pathologist uses (Figure 5.7).

Intraoperative Cytology

A quick and inexpensive way to determine clean margins during surgery can be achieved by using intraoperative cytology. This is an underutilized diagnostic procedure that can make a big difference in the efficacy of surgical excisions. Intraoperative cytology has the potential to dramatically decrease recurrence rates and increase the tumor-free interval as well as patient survival times. We use intraoperative cytology most often when dealing with known MCTs, SCC, and soft tissue sarcomas.

When an undiagnosed mass is removed, use intraoperative cytology to determine the nature of the mass. Before placing the mass in the specimen jar for histopathology, make impression smears from a cut surface of the mass and look for mast cells or sarcoma cells. This information gives the surgeon the opportunity to excise the mass more aggressively, and perhaps to spare the patient a second surgery.

To examine margins, make impression smears of the anterior, posterior, lateral, medial, and deep margins. Place the marked slides on a paper plate and examine them immediately under the microscope. If malignant cells are found on one or two of the slides, the surgeon knows where to cut more deeply to gain clean margins before closure. This requires cooperation between the surgeon and the person reading the slides and patience on the surgeon's part to wait for a go ahead before closure. It also extends anesthesia time for the patient, but with practiced teamwork between the surgeon and the reader, this time can be kept to a minimum.

I tell pet owners that this technique is the closest thing to Moh's surgery that we can offer our cancer patients. Moh's surgery involves the luxury of having frozen sections analyzed by a pathologist during surgery with immediate feedback to the surgeon to guide the adequacy of the excision. Intraoperative cytology is a practical and rewarding procedure that adds direct value to the veterinary surgical oncology effort and success. We use this technique as margin studies for known tumors and it is a valuable adjunct in routine mass excisions as well.

Sunshine's Case (Intraoperative Cytology Saves Lives)

Sunshine Johnson, an 8-year-old Afghan Hound with SCC of the rostral maxilla, was on the surgery table. Repeated intraoperative cytology slides found tumor cells streaming upward from the mass. Cancer cells were identified along the intended dorsal incision and invaded into the base of her nasal frenulum. I guided our surgeon to expand the excision dorsally. He provided me with several margin samples containing cancer cells. After several more cuts, the samples became free of malignant cells. I called Ms. Johnson during surgery to explain that there would be an unanticipated cosmetic defect because we had to take some of Sunshine's frenulum to gain clean margins. Sunshine developed osteosarcoma at 11 years of age and lived three-legged to the ripe old age of 12. She remained cancer free at her rostral maxilla.

A Word About Unhelpful Diagnostic Abdominal Surgery

FNA is overlooked far too often as a reliable diagnostic tool in the assessment of abdominal masses, especially in the senior and geriatric feline. Veterinarians often recommend exploratory surgery without suggesting FNA or ultrasound to better characterize the pet's abdominal mass. All too often, the caregiver is referred exclusively for surgical consultation after initial palpation or imaging of an abdominal mass.

The same push for exploratory laparotomy may also come from the surgeon following ultrasonography that anatomically visualizes but does not diagnose the patient's mass. The surgeon should not be more focused on the priority of removing an abdominal mass over the discovery of what the mass is. Geriatric cats are better served when the surgeon first rules out lymphoma, the most common cause of abdominal masses in cats. For non-obstructed patients, medical management is better than surgery.

Being rushed into abdominal surgery for mass removal is a problem for cats everywhere, especially for debilitated cats. Many elderly cats with GI or abdominal lymphoma can be definitively diagnosed with diligent sampling via percutaneous FNA cytology or true cut needle biopsy of their abdominal masses without the systemic stress of exploratory surgery. In fact, abdominal surgery is often counterproductive and may be a major setback for the geriatric patient.

Tessa's Case (Splenectomy Is Not Always Needed)

Tessa was an F/S DSH brown senior cat around 14 to 16 years old. Tessa was lethargic around the house. Her attending doctor initially referred Tessa to an internist for abdominal ultrasound evaluation. She had palpated small kidneys and felt that Tessa needed a more thorough workup. The ultrasound study found a 2.5cm, highly echogenic mass in the tail of the spleen. FNA was not performed at that time.

At discharge, the internist recommended splenectomy as the treatment of choice with no further diagnostic tests. Bonney, Tessa's carer, asked if there was a test that could be done to figure out if the mass needed to be removed. The internist told her that it was better to just remove it. Bonney declined the surgery, fearing that Tessa was too old. She shared this fear with the attending doctor, who then referred her to our service for FNA of the splenic mass and a second opinion.

We located the mass in the spleen on ultrasound and obtained an FNA from the mass using a 27-gauge needle for FNA We were able to aspirate several slide samples for cytology. We diagnosed the mass as lymphocytic hyperplasia on FNA. Our professional laboratory confirmed the diagnosis. This condition in the spleen, mesenteric lymph nodes, or intestines may be a precursor to lymphoma. We discussed options with Bonney and she elected to place Tessa on conservative chemotherapy to see if there was a response. This option would address the problem and avoid the angst and the debilitation of surgery. Tessa started to feel better from the moment that her treatment with oral prednisone and chlorambucil began. The mass reduced in size and, after 8 weeks of oral chemotherapy, Bonney elected to discontinue treatment because Tessa was feeling much better and resisted being medicated.

The trauma of cancer surgery, recovery, and hospitalization may stress a geriatric feline lymphoma patient into a downward spiral. Following exploratory surgery for the diagnosis of lymphoma, the surgeon and/or attending doctor often informs the owner that definitive chemotherapy must be postponed because it delays wound healing. This precaution is justified for recovery of geriatric patients with intestinal anastomosis. It is sound advice to delay definitive chemotherapy for these patients, but a 10–14 day delay may allow the patient's cancer to advance and reduce the chances for survival. The patient may recover in the hospital under doctor's care but lack specific care needed to deal with the rampant lymphoma.

When asked to consult in such scenarios, I tell pet owners that oncologists think differently. The cancer does not arrest itself and wait on the sidelines while the patient is healing. Over the years, this has been my experience when dealing with abdominal (GI, renal, hepatic splenic) lymphoma in the feline. Oncologists work hard to finesse a diagnosis from a feline patient's heterogeneous abdominal tumors with diligent FNA cytology or Tru-cut needle biopsy and impression smears. Acquiring a relatively non-invasive diagnosis allows the safe and immediate use of induction chemotherapy and avoids subjecting geriatric cats to unhelpful or deleterious surgery.

Sweet's Case (Cytology Can Preclude Surgery)

Sweet, a 14-year-old F/S DSH, was in the arms of her high-strung, nervous carer, who paced the room repeating, "She is the love of my life." The timing was horrible. She was getting married in a week, merging two families together, moving to a new home, and leaving for a 3-week honeymoon. Sweet was vomiting and had anorexia for 1 week. Her attending veterinarian palpated an abdominal mass and scheduled Sweet for ultrasound. The visiting radiologist, who performed the study, found a 1cm thickened bowel loop extending 6cm but did not do FNA for cytologic diagnosis.

A consultation with the staff surgeon was scheduled at the time of pickup. The surgeon advised immediate exploratory surgery with the intention of removing the affected bowel. Sweet's owner was overwhelmed and declined surgery. She wanted to take Sweet home for a few days to think about it and get a second opinion. During our consultation, we explained that the most common type of cancer in the feline abdomen was lymphoma and that we might be able to diagnose the tumor via FNA and treat it medically.

We located the mass with ultrasound and performed ultrasound-guided FNA. The cytology slides were clearly diagnostic for lymphoma. We advised chemotherapy to see if it might reduce the mass without surgical intervention. We were given permission to administer chemotherapy, antiemetics, and an esophageal feeding tube.

Since the family would be on honeymoon for 3 weeks, we used L-asparaginase for induction and Adriamycin for its 3-week activity against lymphoma. The family was relieved that we were able to make a diagnosis and start definitive treatment without surgery. Sweet's family was tormented with the emotional and financial burden of continuing chemotherapy and supportive care. After a few days, the new family realized that they had no time for the rigors of feeding and medicating and could not budget for the estimated costs. The family was able to arrive at this difficult realization based upon the FNA diagnosis and initiation of therapy without surgery.

Wally's Case (Look for Pitting Defects)

Wally, a 12-year-old Old English Sheepdog, developed a right-sided nasal discharge. Wally's referring veterinarian was unable to find a foreign body or any lesions worthy of biopsy during routine rhinoscopy using an otoscope. At presentation, there was no facial deformity, but on careful palpation of Wally's muzzle, a pitting defect was found, located along the proximal right side of his dorsal muzzle. FNA through this 1cm lesion identified numerous malignant SCC cells on cytological examination.

Point-of-Service Panels and Cytology of Fresh Blood Smears

Being curious and accurate about the immediate health status of the geriatric oncology patient allows instant decision making that may be life-saving. Point-of-service laboratory evaluations for cancer patients reduce the guesswork and the omission of potentially life-saving stat care and supportive services. The need is most evident when dealing with oncology patients that have profound leukopenia, hypercalcemia, renal damage, or sepsis. A certain percent of geriatric oncology patients will present in preclinical and/or precritical functional compromise. Identifying these complicating conditions on a stat basis clearly saves lives. The benefits to the patient are obvious and enhance the rewards found in successful case management.

World-famous Dr. Oscar Schalm was my hematology instructor at the University of California, Davis. He stressed the importance of looking directly at a patient's blood. If you practice oncology, you will lose animals unless you are prepared to look at fresh blood smears. In certain instances, you need to know what the patient's blood cells look like on a stat basis in order to identify or verify morphologic abnormalities such as leukemia (Figure 5.2), leukopenia, thrombocytopenia, autoagglutination, poikilocytosis, reticulocytosis, nucleated red blood cells, and so forth. Only if you know what your patient's blood looks like will you know when to disagree with the machines.

Look at fresh blood smears alongside automated CBC results. At each recheck visit for cancer patients, especially for chemotherapy patients, we need to directly evaluate some of the abnormalities reported by automated CBC units. When the white blood cell count is high, we must verify that we are dealing with leukocytosis versus leukemia. If there is a low white blood cell count or a low platelet count, look at a fresh blood smear to verify the findings. Sometimes there are plenty of platelets, but they are clumped and will not read accurately on the automated units. If the white blood cell (WBC) is extremely low, the machine will not register any results and you must look at the smear directly to assess the presence or absence of white cells.

Leukopenia should be determined on a stat basis at your clinic for urgent care decision making. The sample can be sent to a professional laboratory for an exact count, but if you depend on an outside lab for this value, the patient may be in crisis before the lab results are in. If the clinic's lab equipment is unreliable or breaks down, you will need to look directly at the cells to expedite a decision. If in doubt, hold off on chemotherapy and provide supportive care until you get the results back from the lab.

It is convenient to use point-of-service (in-house) CBC equipment and chemistry machines to immediately assess the patient's hematology and organ function status. This information is required for on-the-spot decision making and dose adjustment before writing up orders for a patient's chemotherapy. Some of our referral clinicians do not have point-of-service laboratory equipment and they are unprepared or reluctant to examine fresh blood smears. They ask their clients to bring the pet in for blood work 1 or 2 days in advance of the chemotherapy date. This is acceptable but certainly places one more time-consuming burden on the client.

We often get a call from an attending clinician when a cancer patient presents with signs of chemotherapy toxicity or an adverse reaction. I always ask the doctor to take a CBC and examine a fresh blood smear. I ask the clinician to prepare the slides properly with special attention to the feathered edges and to assess white blood cells and platelets to see if they are present in normal or high numbers or absent. As a rule of thumb, if there are less than one to four white blood cells per high power field, we are dealing with leukopenia. If the patient is not febrile and has between two and four white blood cells per high power field, supportive care with outpatient antibiotics and symptomatic care may be all that is needed.

This clinical assessment is easily accomplished with an outpatient visit. The pet may be discharged with instructions for the pet owner to monitor the temperature twice daily, SQ fluids, oral antibiotics, and so forth. If there are less than or only zero to two white blood cells per high power field and the patient is febrile or sick, then immediate hospitalization is needed for IV fluids, antibiotics, and neupogen along with intense supportive care (see the section on adverse effects of cancer therapy in geriatric pets in Chapter 6). Immediate and direct assessment of the fresh blood smear, electrolytes, and blood chemistries is essential in providing the best care for the ongoing needs of geriatric cancer patients, especially those receiving chemotherapy. Adverse events are not unusual and reporting in clinical studies using chemotherapy has become more reliable since 2011 when the Veterinary Cooperative Oncology Group (VCOG) adopted the Common Terminology Criteria for Adverse Events (CTCAE) (Giuffrida 2016).

Clinical Pathology and the Geriatric Cancer Patient

Elder pets are referred to our oncology service with a smorgasbord of concurrent conditions and diagnostic dilemmas. Geriatric cancer patients may have halitosis, polyarthritis, and/or endocarditis related to their advanced dental disease. Older dogs often have mild to severe arthritis, chronic heart disease, hypothyroidism, Cushing's disease, diabetes, or other ailments. Always ask the family if the pet is on any over-the-counter drugs, such as aspirin or a cannabinoid preparation from a local dispensary or an online supplier for arthritis pain, etc.

Geriatric cats may also have concurrent hyperthyroidism, heart murmurs, inflammatory bowel disease (IBD), feline triad disease, chronic kidney disease (CKD), obesity, diabetes, dehydration, and cachexia, to name some of their more common problems. For geriatric cancer patients, chemistry profiles should be rechecked if the most recent panel was done more than a month ago.

The new profile may restate the previous general organ function abnormalities such as elevated hepatic enzymes, alkaline phosphatase, renal disease, or endocrinopathy. The urine analysis may reveal a sub-clinical urinary tract infection or show low specific gravity or bilirubinuria or microalbuminuria. If the BUN and creatinine are elevated preoperatively, then the patient's values must be monitored postoperatively. These pretreatment values must also be reevaluated before starting chemotherapy and during the course of chemotherapy to make the proper dosage adjustments.

When treating senior and geriatric pets with cancer, concurrent organ compromise must be carefully diagnosed and kept in mind during the diagnostic workup. These patients will require dose reduction of at least 25% and up to 50%, depending on the degree of organ compromise. Precautions for pets with CKD may necessitate admitting the patient into the hospital the day before procedures such as surgery or drug administrations that are expected to compromise renal function. The CKD patient can be given IV fluids during the 12–24 hours before treatment or before surgery. After the procedure, the patient may require 24-hour follow-up on IV fluids for 1 or 2 days in recovery. You may need to adjust the CKD patient's diet and make recommendations for daily SQ fluids as home care maintenance.

If CKD patients are to receive chemotherapy, elevated renal values signal the need for a dose reduction, especially for those drugs that are excreted by the kidneys (cyclophosphamide, vincristine, carboplatin, etc.). For dogs with CKD or compromised glomerular filtration rate (GFR), cisplatin should *not* be used because it is extremely nephrotoxic and would invite disaster. Cats should *never* be given cisplatin because it is extremely toxic to felines, causing respiratory failure. We only use very small doses of diluted cisplatin (1–6mg diluted 1:1 with sterile water) for intralesional injection prior to electroporation (EP)/electrochemotherapy (ECT).

Geriatric animals with compromised renal and/or hepatic function do not eliminate chemotherapy drugs properly. They may become toxic and exhibit adverse events and signs of overdose with vomiting, diarrhea, anorexia, fever, immunosuppression, and leukopenia. Some pets may develop sepsis or pancreatitis, which may be fatal if the problem is not identified early and treated vigorously. The trouble with treating debilitated cancer patients is that it can be difficult to determine if it is the patient's illness or the treatment that is causing a specific problem. It is best to presume that the chemotherapy is the culprit. Prepare your client to handle grade 1–3 adverse events by sending home a "Cancer Care Package" that includes: a thermometer, antibiotics, antiemetics, and antidiarrheal medications. Each medication must be clearly labeled for their purpose.

Elderly pets, especially those with compromised or marginal organ function, require reduction of the initial chemotherapy dose by 25–30%. When using doxorubicin/Adriamycin in geriatric large and giant breed dogs or in dogs with heart disease, I generally use a split dose schedule instead of using the maximum tolerated dose (MTD). This split technique involves administering a proper therapeutic dose of drug but divided over a longer time span of several days to 1 week. The split dose schedule has become my preferred method for administering Adriamycin to geriatric large and giant dogs. We administer 20mg/m^2 on the initial treatment day and then another 20mg/m^2 6–8 days later, working it into the protocol.

The split dose method addresses the thinking that large breed dogs are underdosed with the meter squared (m^2) scale. It also addresses the need to use precautions to limit the cardio and GI toxicity of Adriamycin. If the patient is able to handle the initial dose of drug without significant adverse events, and CBC and blood chemistries remain normal, dose escalation toward the MTD at the following cycle would then be considered for that patient.

When clinicians commit to the philosophy of close observation of the CBC and organ function, at all stages of the workup and during all stages of treatment, the patient benefits and the clients will be pleased. If you can, on a preliminary basis, evaluate the cells of any mass in question, assess a fresh blood smear, and react quickly to adapt therapy to the geriatric patient's organ function and needs, then you are practicing responsive medicine. It is exhilarating to know that you can provide great service for the geriatric cancer patient and to feel on top of your chosen profession.

Imaging Detectable Tumors

A mass must be at least 0.5–1 cm before it can be visualized by most anatomic imaging techniques used in veterinary practices today. Newer functional imaging techniques may detect smaller nodules at 3–5 mm. A small mass contains up to a billion cells by the time it is detectable. The inherent problem with traditional anatomic imaging of tumors is that we are looking for a mass. Unfortunately, by the time enough cancer cells have accumulated to form a detectable mass, it may have already experienced up to 25 doubling times and released its athletic cells to metastasize under the radar of the geriatric oncology patient's immunosurveillance system.

The use of anatomic imaging in the management of cancer patients is essential, but it cannot definitively diagnose a mass as a malignancy. The differentials may be inflammation or infection. This domain belongs to pathology. The value of visualizing a few malignant cells in the microscope remains the final word in the diagnosis of cancer. Imaging is used to locate, to stage, to guide for FNA and biopsy, for follow-up assessments, to monitor for recurrence, and for guiding the delivery of therapeutic or ablative agents.

Imaging Tumors with Radiography

Imaging with radiographs is the cornerstone of anatomic imaging services in most veterinary practices. The field of diagnostic radiology offers excellent textbooks for positioning, exposing, and reading. The points I would like to stress are quality and quantity. For senior and geriatric pets, radiographs should be suggested more often, especially as part of their routine senior wellness exams.

All coughing, limping, vomiting, and straining in elderly pets and pets with abdominal distension, have a justifiable need for radiographs. The thorax is not fully evaluated for tumors unless three views are assessed (right and left lateral views as well as the ventrodorsal (VD) view). Thoracic tumors that are not visible in usual two-view routine films may be found in the left lateral exposure. If you are restricted from taking three views of the thorax because of an owner's financial constraints, inform your client that the study will be limited. Tell your client that this limited approach is a "scout" study.

If your facility is inconvenient for radiology or if your staff members have objections to the restraining techniques for using the equipment, it is essential to make the necessary changes so that radiography is a welcome procedure. Establish safe protocols for mild sedation for geriatric patients. The proper size X-ray cassettes should be on hand and they should be cleaned routinely. The proper film for the job should be available, such as non-screen mammography film for high-detail open mouth radiographs of the nasal passages, maxilla, and mandible. Good technique is essential to get high-resolution films of the skull and nasal passages, especially if dental film and dental radiography are not set up in your practice. All X-ray films should be marked properly for easy identification of the dates to compare recheck radiographs as you follow the patient's progress.

Digital radiography offers tremendous advantages and versatility. The equipment is expensive but it makes sense for high-volume practices to make the investment. If your practice takes a lot of radiographs, the overall savings on staff time, film, processors, and maintenance fees for processors may offset the initial capital investment in the long run.

Imaging Tumors with Ultrasound

My personal favorite diagnostic imaging instrument is the ultrasound machine. During the 1970s at UCLA Medical School, I helped Hal Snow, DVM, teach radiology students to use real-time fluoroscopic imaging for placing catheters in dogs that we ran from the femoral artery into the heart or from the carotid artery into a brain tumor.

My first ultrasound unit was purchased in 1982. We upgrade ultrasound machines every few years. There is nothing more enjoyable for me than to invite our clients and the patient into our ultrasound procedure room, or to bring the unit into the exam room. We instruct clients to verbally comfort their pet and to encourage the pet to stay in position in the v-cut boat while they witness the ultrasound study. It is easy to determine if a mass is solid, cystic, or cavitated. We use ultrasound imaging for anatomical detection of tumors, for staging, for guiding FNA and Tru-cut needles, for centesis, for guiding the delivery of intralesional therapy, and for monitoring tumors during follow-up.

One of the most frequent uses of ultrasound in my practice is to evaluate patients on a per-region basis and for routine periodic follow-up assessments. We check on the size of a bladder tumor to see if it has reduced after chemotherapy and we image the patient's kidneys to see whether or not hydronephrosis has developed. We may evaluate the progress of metastatic hepatic lesions and primary masses to evaluate their response to therapy. In cats with abdominal or anterior mediastinal masses, we use the ultrasound to guide us for centesis of effusions, to guide FNA, and to monitor progress.

It is very easy to teach a technical staff to collect urine from a small bladder using the ultrasound for guidance. Ultrasound also offers the ease of identifying structures in patients with ascites when X-rays provide poor resolution. You can assess PUPD in intact female patients for pyometra and you can check that a Golden Retriever with weakness and muffled heart sounds to immediately rule out pericardial effusion from right atrial hemangiosarcoma. There is nothing like having an ultrasound machine at your beck and call to excite and enhance your practice.

The terminology used to describe structures during ultrasound evaluation employs lengthy words such as hypoechogenic and hyperechogenic, cavitations, granularity, transitional zones, artifacts, and nodularity. For this reason, I suggest using a special ultrasound report form with all of the appropriate words so that the description of each organ may be checked off to expedite reporting and record keeping. We take digital pictures of the images for storage. Ultrasound-guided FNAs and true cut biopsies of tumors in the abdomen are routinely used for diagnosis and staging. Peripherally located thoracic masses may also lend themselves for ultrasound-guided FNA when accessible. Occasionally, thoracic masses are situated peripherally enough so that it is considered safe to proceed with ultrasound-guided Tru-cut biopsy.

Ali's Case (An Old Akita Struggled Before Thoracotomy)

Ali Dehener, a 12-year-old F/S Akita, had a long history of gagging episodes. She started with a mild cough that progressed for 2–3 months. Referral chest X-rays showed complete consolidation of the left lung lobe. In my opinion, Ali's pulmonary condition posed an anesthetic risk for diagnostic procedures. During consultation, we advised ultrasound-guided percutaneous FNA without sedation or anesthesia. We infiltrated a local anesthetic into the intercostal site selected for percutaneous FNA and inserted a $1^1/_2$-inch 27-gauge needle through the involved lung lobe into the mass and aspirated gently. Our FNA cytology samples contained mucinous debris and an occasional cluster of round pleomorphic cells. The cells possessed several malignant characteristics consistent with carcinoma. Our working diagnosis was primary bronchogenic adenocarcinoma and our clinical pathologist confirmed it. Chest X-rays showed no hilar adenopathy. Based on this information and normal blood values, I was ready to send Ali to surgery right away but our surgeon insisted on a CT scan prior to thoracotomy. Ali suffered a major setback following the anesthesia and positioning protocol for the CT. Mucus and debris spilled into her airways, causing fever of 106 degrees and pneumonia. She was hospitalized for 7 days on IV antibiotics. The CT confirmed that her cancer was localized in one lung lobe. Ali underwent lobectomy and survived an additional year with excellent quality of life until recurrence.

Note: A standing tracheal wash procedure may also be helpful in cases like this. When there is a history of coughing or if x-rays identify lesions close to the major bronchi, tracheal washing may yield material for culture and sensitivity tests and for cytology.

Screening Senior and Geriatric Patients with Imaging

It is easy and convenient to screen the abdomen and heart with ultrasound. My ideal would be to hold semi-annual ultrasound wellness exams to check the spleens and hearts of senior and geriatric Portuguese Water Dogs, Boxers, Chesapeake, Labrador and Golden Retrievers, and German Shepherd Dogs to rule out hemangiosarcoma. Until routine blood samples can detect cancer in pets, imaging exams are not overly cautious because as many as 2.5 million dogs are estimated to die of hemangiosarcoma in the United States each year (Lamerato-Kozicki et al. 2006). Proactive breed-screening makes sense since one in five Golden Retrievers is diagnosed with hemangiosarcoma at the average age range of 7–9 years old, and one in seven to eight get lymphoma at the average age range of 6–8 years old (Modiano 2016). The Golden Retriever Club National Survey found that 67% of males and 57% of females die of cancer and that the largest males are more prone (Glickman, Glickman, and Thorpe 2000). The Morris Animal Fund is conducting the "Golden Retriever Lifetime Study" to gather prospective data in the US.

Since 50% of dogs and 30% of cats over 10 years of age die of cancer, it makes sense to consider using available methods of inexpensive imaging for screening with X-rays and ultrasound as part of a complete wellness exam. Several laboratories are racing to develop reliable and reasonably priced laboratory and/or blood "liquid biopsy" tests that can screen for sarcoma, carcinoma, and lymphoma by identifying tumor genetic biomarkers in dogs and cats. Some of the first generations tests had variable reliability if they cross-reacted with inflammation. These newer tests will greatly assist our opportunity for earlier diagnosis of cancer and may serve to monitor treatment success or recurrence. Until these tests become routinely available, we must rely on the physical exam and current methods of anatomical imaging for proactive screening of our highly valued geriatric patients.

Imaging Tumors with CT, MRI, and PET

Computed tomography (CT) and magnetic resonance imaging (MRI) and positron emission tomography (PET) are very helpful non-invasive technologies that can be used in the workup and staging of the geriatric cancer patient. CT, MRI, and PET enable us to make better treatment decisions because we know more about the anatomic extent of the patient's tumor.

CT scans the body using ionizing radiation in the form of X-rays. Sir Godfrey Hounsfield, who made the first CT scan machine in the 1970s, developed practical CT. He shared the 1979 Nobel Prize in medicine with physicist Allan Cormack, who wrote the first theoretical papers on the CT scan system.

Today, newer generation CT scanners require only minutes to yield excellent studies for bone, soft tissue, and vasculature with the use of enhancement agents that allow better contrast. Contrasted CT is very helpful for selecting operable tumors, such as prostate tumors, in humans. CT is used to visualize whether neoplasia is confined within the prostatic capsule or if it involves the urethra. This technology can be used for dogs to determine if an early stage prostatic tumor is operable (Henderson 2004, 2005). In veterinary medicine, CT is currently the preferred method for anatomic imaging of tracheobronchial lymph nodes in patients with primary lung tumors prior to surgery. The prognosis for survival postlobectomy exceeds 1 year for dogs with negative node studies versus only 6 months for dogs with infiltrated or enlarged tracheobronchial nodes. CT imaging is also very helpful in evaluating the chest for the diagnosis of metastatic disease.

Ulla's Case (Always Offer Clients All the Options)

Ursula was passionate in her quest to do the right thing for her beloved Ulla, a 9-year-old F/S Rottweiler. She came to us for consultation following a rib resection for Ulla's osteosarcoma (OSA). A bone scan performed prior to the rib resection was negative for metastatic disease. Ulla's chemotherapy treatments went well. She received six treatments of carboplatin in rotation with two cycles of Adriamycin. Eight months later, Ulla started having petite mal seizure-like episodes. We were very suspicious of metastatic disease but unable to document it with routine three-view chest X-rays. FNA by our LANC technique, described previously in this chapter, found no significant cells. Ursula expressed anxiety about spending so much family money on Ulla. We discussed the value of further imaging. If the results of the study were not going to change Ulla's treatment, then it would be a pointless expense. I learned more about the power of the human–animal bond and the inquiring mind of Ursula when, a few weeks later, she opted to have a CT scan of Ulla's lungs. The CT scan revealed that Ulla had seven or eight small metastatic lesions of variable size, distributed in multiple lung lobes. These small metastatic lesions were not detected in her most recent radiographs.

Ursula came in for a heart-to-heart consultation about her options. She felt that she just had to know what was causing Ulla's seizure-like episodes and now that she knew, she could deal with the grief. Ulla was not a good candidate for metastatectomy. She could try to enter a study using inhalation therapy with liposome-encapsulated interleukin-2 conducted by Dr. Chand Khanna in Minnesota. We called Dr. Khanna only to discover that the study was over.

We learned from Ursula and Ulla not to allow an owner's verbalizations about expenses to preclude discussion of the best procedures, including initial diagnostics and follow-up studies, even when the anticipated results may not change the treatment. Always inform clients of all the options. Ulla's seizure-like episodes may have been due to decreased oxygen flow or metastases to the brain. Ursula did not pursue an MRI of Ulla's brain to rule this out. She needed the information from the thoracic CT study to make her decision to stop further treatment and place Ulla in Pawspice and ultimately hospice care.

There will be more carers, like Ursula, who will want to use advanced imaging for follow-up and monitoring of their geriatric oncology patient's progress. We should suggest it more often, especially since the newer machines require less time. If the patient is calm, only mild sedation may be needed, and in some cases, no sedation.

MRI delivers pulsed radiofrequency waves into the patient. Signals from the radiofrequency waves are picked up by a special magnetic coil and then processed by a computer for anatomic imaging. Paul Lauterbur first generated MRI images in the 1970s. During the 1980s, MRI machines were installed in most major health care facilities because it was regarded as superior for imaging brain, spinal cord, and musculoskeletal regions. In the early 1980s, our UCLA Animal Tumor Resource Facility lost its orthovoltage machine space to install the new MRI. Contrast agents such as gadolinium enhance the visualization of tumors by detecting variations in vascular permeability.

CT, MRI, and PET studies are divided into image slices, spaced along the patient's body like slices from a loaf of bread. These slices can be sectioned in several planes: transverse, longitudinal, and dorsal. PET technology can detect clusters of cells based upon their metabolism of radiolabeled glucose given IV prior to the scan. This functional imaging technology may detect metastatic tumor cells before they can be visualized by MRI or CT. MRI technology can localize tumors that are not detectable by X-ray or ultrasonography. MRI has excellent sensitivity for the imaging and evaluation of tumors in soft tissues, especially the liver, spleen, and adrenal glands.

Contrast agents may be administered IV to enhance and distinguish tumors in soft tissues. All veterinary patients must be heavily sedated or anesthetized and placed in a stationary position on a table that moves the body within the strong magnetic field for scanning. It is understandable why many owners of geriatric cancer pets are reluctant to subject their pet to anesthesia for the purpose of CT or MRI imaging, which restricts the clinician's ability to provide a definitive diagnosis. However, if there is an imaging facility within referral distance with a newer, faster imaging unit, the patient may be safely scanned in 7 minutes with little to no sedation.

Positron Emission Tomography

Positron emission tomography (PET) is a functional imaging technique that uses radionuclide tracers that target glycolysis. Increased glucose metabolism is a distinguishing metabolic and functional characteristic of all malignant cells. Therefore, glycolysis is the most practical functional target used in PET scanning today because smaller metastatic lesions can be detected. This has an impact on the early staging and restaging of tumors, and avoids false positive diagnoses due to its reliance on targeting the cancer cells' glycolysis function. It is rapidly replacing the use of strictly anatomical imaging prior to high-risk exploratory and therapeutic procedures in human medicine. PET scanning is available at some veterinary colleges and it will become more available for veterinary patients in the future.

Hybrid Imaging Technology

Improvements in non-invasive imaging technology will have great value for our geriatric cancer patients. Hybrid machines that fuse PET with CT or MRI can deliver more accurate images and detect smaller tumors in difficult locations such as the mediastinum and pulmonary parenchyma. This exciting combination of functional and anatomical imaging enables us to detect and locate very early metastatic disease.

This unprecedented detection of early metastatic disease has created the problem of stage migration. For example, patients with one or two 1–9 mm pulmonary metastases and patients with gross disease (multiple 1–5cm nodules) will be stratified in the same stage. This is an important consideration in understanding the discrepancy between how cancer patients have been staged in the past and how they are now staged. The modern-day oncology workup will classify more cancer patients as being in a more advanced stage than in the past. These more comprehensively scanned cases migrated from a lower to a higher stage. We would expect these cases to have better survival times than their historical peer stage cases. Tumors detected by hybrid technology have much less volume than anatomically staged tumors. Therefore, interpreting survival data will be challenging because the PET/CT/MRI fusion scanned patients will appear to have more prolonged survivals than the anatomically scanned same stage patients.

Evaluation of therapeutic agents such as targeted therapies will be very difficult to interpret unless new sub-staging is established to address the issue of stage migration discrepancy. Taking this problem into account is an obvious necessity. The gridlock of scientific bureaucracy and marketing pressures (which may override ethical considerations) of some drug companies may allow some drugs to appear more efficacious than they actually would be with further scrutiny. When hybrid imaging technology becomes available to our veterinary patients, they will endure fewer futile thoracotomies and laparotomies. Veterinary patients will also benefit from more accurate field analysis for image guided radiation therapy (IGRT), stereotactic radiosurgery (SRS), and follow-up assessments.

Nuclear Imaging with Radioisotopes

The terms "radiopharmaceutical," "radiochemical," and "radioisotope" are used interchangeably in nuclear imaging. Radiopharmaceuticals can assess the function of cells and provide images of organ system function. Radiopharmaceutical compounds are composed of a gamma radiation-emitting substance and a specific drug that functionally seeks or is taken up by a structure or organ. The emissions are picked up by a gamma camera as black dots on an image screen. Nuclear imaging can reveal occult disease, such as "hot spots" in bone. It can demonstrate the amount of uptake by the liver in patients with hepatic shunts and/or liver failure.

Nuclear imaging and radiopharmaceutical medicine are commonly used in veterinary medicine both diagnostically and therapeutically for the thyroid gland. Technetium-99 radioisotope is used for radionuclide or scintigraphy bone scans, while Samarium-153 isotope is used to treat some bone tumors and bone metastases.

The most commonly used radioisotope for imaging the thyroid glands in geriatric cats is technetium-99 pertechnetate. This compound is readily taken up by the thyroid glands. It is short acting and inexpensive. Technetium-99 pertechnetate is used for pretreatment assessment of the size and location of hyperthyroid glands and can detect aberrant, ectopic tissue or nodules. Iodine-131 (I-131), a potent beta and gamma emitter, is used for treatment where indicated. It has a long half-life of 8 days and is used most commonly to ablate hyperthyroid adenomas in older cats. Yttrium-90 is a beta emitting radioisotope that is administered as an intralesional therapy for hepatic tumors in people. Y-90 has a promising future for intralesional use in accessible tumors of companion animals (www.IsoPetSolutions.com).

Bone Scans and Function Scans

Technetium-99 (Tc99) is commonly combined with methylene diphosphonate and used to detect metastatic "hot spots" in skeletal bone. As we search for metastatic disease in the workup for osteosarcoma patients and as we monitor our geriatric cancer patients for metastases, there is an increasing role for radioisotope bone scans. To assess lymph nodes, liver, and spleen, Tc99 is combined with sulfur colloid. When this compound is introduced to the body, it is taken up by phagocytosis into the monocyte–macrophage system and yields readable function scans.

Generally, patients are referred to facilities that have the permits and expertise in this specialized area of nuclear medicine. The information that is gained from the uptake studies is used for individualized patient treatment planning. For a more in-depth review of nuclear medicine, see Widmer's Chapter 16 in W.B. Morrison's book *Cancer in Dogs and Cats: Medical and Surgical Management* (2002) and basic nuclear medicine texts.

Screening Strategy for Active Surveillance

Screening geriatric veterinary patients for cancer makes sense, since they are at very high risk for developing cancer the older they get. There are ongoing national campaigns promoting biennial physical exams for geriatric pets by the AVMA, AAHA, the Animal Cancer Foundation, the CataLyst Council, and the Morris Animal Foundation.

It is estimated that six million cats will be diagnosed with cancer in the US per year as found by the CataLyst Council™. The Morris Animal Foundation states that 12 million dogs and cats will be diagnosed with cancer in the US every year. Dogs are more prone to cancer than cats. It is estimated that 8,000–10,000 will be diagnosed with bone cancer, 80,000 with bladder cancer, over 300,000 with lymphoma, and up to 2.5 million with hemangiosarcoma yearly in the US. It is unknown how many dogs will develop mast cell cancer, soft tissue sarcomas, oral tumors, and so forth.

In addition to a comprehensive panel, the geriatric checkup should include CBC and urine analysis, as well as chest and abdominal X-rays. For large and giant breed dogs at risk for hemangiosarcoma (especially Golden and Chesapeake Bay Retrievers, German Shepherds, Portuguese Water Dogs, and Rottweilers), I recommend a quick ultrasound of the abdomen that checks the spleen and liver every six months. When the "liquid biopsy," which can detect circulating cancer cells, becomes routinely available, it should replace the need for using ultrasound imaging as the screening tool. The CADETSM™ free catch urine test for bladder cancer will also be useful in comprehensive cancer screening, especially in older Scottish Terriers at 20 times higher risk.

The controversy against whole body screening for humans uses two basic arguments: lead bias and length bias. It is theorized that if slow-growing tumors are detected earlier, they may be more amenable to treatment and cure. Lead bias counters this theory because if there is no effect from treatment, a cancer retains its natural behavior and kills the patient in a given time period no matter when the diagnosis is made. Although the patient lives longer from the date of diagnosis, early detection and early treatment have made no difference in overall survival time. It is estimated that one-third of human health care costs result from overscreening, overdiagnosis, and overtreatment of non-threatening tumors. Atul Gawande, MD, author of *Being Mortal*, discussed this situation in 2014 in *The New Yorker* in his insightful article titled *OVERKILL*.

Length bias gives us a good example when looking at canine hemangiosarcoma, which occurs in one of five Golden Retrievers in the US. Most affected patients survive less than 4 months postdiagnosis. The argument against whole body screening contends that it would be less likely that a "hot" tumor (such as hemangiosarcoma) would be detected by a screening procedure at 6–8 month intervals. If the diagnosis is made 1–2 months earlier, and the patient lives 5 or 6 months from diagnosis, it would appear that early detection has made a difference, where in actuality, it did not (Balducci

2004). Early detection via blood tests ("liquid biopsy") that detect neoantigens specific for transformed hemangioblasts will become available to general practitioners for easy screening of susceptible dogs (Modiano 2016).

The only comfort here is that postoperative survival for dogs with non-ruptured splenic hemangiosarcoma is longer than for ruptured cases. We need more survival information on dogs diagnosed early at a preclinical stage using the new detection blood tests or screening abdominal and cardiac ultrasound in order to know if treated patients are receiving a survival benefit.

Staging Cancer

At the very least, the diagnosis and workup of the geriatric cancer patient should provide the clinician and the pet owner with a preliminary clinical stage of the pet's cancer. Staging uses all of the clinical data collected from a patient, including blood work, urine analysis, radiographs, ultrasound, cytology of locoregional nodes, spleen, liver and bone marrow, biopsy, immunophenotyping, CT, MRI, bone marrow aspirates, core biopsy, bone scan, and so forth. In addition, staging acknowledges if the patient is symptomatic and/or has paraneoplastic disease.

Full knowledge about the impact of staging on each type of cancer enables the clinician to provide accurate information and advice to help the pet owner with decision making. I have comforted clients who were under the impression that stage III lymphoma was a very bad indicator for their seemingly healthy dogs. In most other types of cancer, advanced stage III carries a much more negative prognosis than it does for lymphoma. Clients who are misinformed and jump to conclusions tend to make irreversible decisions that they may later regret and that may endanger their pet's chances for treatment and survival.

Most solid tumors are staged using the straightforward tumor, node, metastasis (TNM) system (Table 5.1). Accurate staging helps everyone involved in the case to speak the same language and allows the clinician to give a more accurate prognosis. Low stage patients generally live longer and have better survival rates than high stage patients. Staging assists in treatment planning and is also used in follow-up evaluations to see if therapy has downstaged the tumor. Staging is also used in clinical research to distinguish cases from one another for meaningful interpretation of survival data. Newer, more sensitive, and specific diagnostic hybrid imaging technology will classify current patients into a later stage of disease than previously. This results in stage migration will cause survival data of lower stage patients to appear improved, as discussed above.

The World Health Organization (WHO) TNM staging system has been adapted for animals. The TNM system is commonly used for evaluating primary solid tumors, other than lymphoma, in dogs and cats for pre- and posttreatment evaluations. "T" refers to the size of the primary tumor: adding numbers after the letters indicates degrees of growth or extent of the disease, a sort of shorthand notation. T0 is no tumor (this code can be used postop as pT0), T1 is used for carcinoma in situ (superficial) tumors <3cm, T2 is 3–5cm, T3 is >5cm, and T4 is very large. "N" refers to the local lymph node involvement: N0 is normal, N1 is local involvement and moveable, N2 is regional involvement and moveable, and N3 is fixed node involvement. "M" refers to metastases: some oncologists use MX to indicate undetermined status for metastases, M0 indicates no metastases, and M1 indicates metastases beyond regional nodes (Morrison 2002).

When general staging systems are applied to cats and toy breeds, we meet with some frustration. We find poor analogy, especially in oral, head, and neck tumors, due to the minimal size of the head in canine toy breeds and in the feline. A 1cm mass in a cat's mouth is comparable to a 3cm mass in

Table 5.1.   TNM Table

Using TNM for Primary Tumor (T) Staging

Skin	T1	T2	T3	T4
Skin	<3cm	3–5cm	>5cm	
Skin	Minor involvement		Major involvement	
Fascia, muscle, and thoracic wall	With or without fascia or muscle		Thoracic or abdominal wall fixation	

T*	Description of Primary Tumor
Tis	Preinvasive carcinoma (carcinoma in situ)
T1	Tumor, 2cm maximal diameter, superficial or exophytic
T2	Tumor 2–5cm maximal diameter or with minimal invasion irrespective of size
T3	Tumor >5cm or with invasion of the subcutis irrespective of size
T4	Invasion of other structures, e.g., fascia, muscle, cartilage or bone

*T is subclassified: (a) with (b) without bone involvement.

N Group	Regional Lymph Nodes
N0	Regional lymph nodes not palpable
N1	Movable ipslateral nodes
	N1a Nodes not considered to contain growth*
	N1b Nodes considered to contain growth*
N2	Movable contralateral or bilateral nodes
	N2a Nodes not considered to contain growth*
	N2b Nodes considered to contain growth*
N3	Fixed nodes

M Group	Distant Metastasis
M0	No evidence of distant metastases
**M1	Distant metastases present – specify sites

* (–) = histologically negative, (+) = histologically positive.
** Distant nodes to be included.

Source: Morrison, W.B. 2002. "Using TNM for primary tumor (T) staging." In *Cancer in dogs and cats: Medical and surgical management*, 2nd edn. Jackson, WY: Teton New Media.

the mouth of a human or large dog. Most WHO staging schemes are applicable to medium, large, and giant breed dogs. The most important principle is to document the appearance, size, and extent of a neoplastic disorder and to make clinical staging an integral part of your initial workup. More details will be added to the staging process as further diagnostic information is gathered.

Canine Lymphoma Staging System

Canine lymphoma accounts for 20–25% of all canine malignancies and it occurs 2–5 times more frequently in dogs than in people. The WHO lymphoma staging system commonly used for dogs and cats was set up in 1980. The scheme applies well for dogs, because 84% present with multicentric lymphadenomegaly. It has less application for cats. Cats are generally categorized into the anatomic forms of lymphoma such as alimentary, mediastinal, multicentric, extranodal (renal, hepatic, spinal, etc.). Feline lymphomas are also grouped histologically into low, intermediate, or high grade depending on mitotic index, T- or B-cell type, and involvement.

Table 5.2. World Health Organization (WHO) Clinical Staging System for Lymphosarcoma in Domestic Animals

Anatomic Site
A. Generalized
B. Alimentary
C. Thymic
D. Skin
E. Leukemia (true) (a)
F. Others (including solitary, renal)
Stage* (to include anatomic site: A, B, C, D, E, or F)
I. Involvement limited to a single node or lymphoid tissue in a single organ (b)
II. Involvement of many lymph nodes in a regional area (tonsils)
III. Generalized lymph node involvement, liver and/or spleen involvement (stage III)
IV. Manifestation in the blood and involvement of bone marrow and/or other organ

*Each stage (I, II, III, IV) is subclassified: (a) without symptoms, (b) with symptoms.
(a) Only blood and bone marrow involved.
(b) Excluding bone marrow.
Source: Vail, D.M., E.G. MacEwen, and K.M. Young. 2001. "Hematopoietic tumors, canine lymphoma and lymphoid leukemias." In *Small animal clinical oncology,* 3rd edn, eds S.J. Withrow and E.G. MacEwen, pp. 558–590, Table 28-4. Philadelphia, PA: Saunders.

The WHO scheme stages dogs with lymphoma according to nodal involvement. Dogs are staged I, II, III, or IV and are further sub-classified as (a) clinically well, asymptomatic or (b) sick, followed by the letter designations: h = hepatic, s = splenic, and b = bone marrow, indicating organ involvement (Table 5.2). Well patients with generalized multicentric lymphadenomegaly may generally be considered to be in clinical stage IIIa. Patients that are sick have organomegaly, enlarged sternal, hilar, and iliac nodes, anemia, or pulmonary involvement and should be considered to be in clinically advanced stages.

Phenotyping Lymphoma and Leukemia for Prognosis and Treatment

The microscopic appearance and molecular composition of lymphoma cells is an important aspect for diagnosis, classification, and prognosis. T- or B-cell phenotyping of canine lymphomas is helpful as a confirmation tool and as a valuable guide for prognosis, treatment adjustment, and future lymphoma vaccine selection. Immunophenotyping of tissue or cytology slides can be performed at most veterinary laboratories by using antibodies against lymphocyte cell markers. The cluster determinant CD3 marker is used for T lymphocyte distinction and the CD79a marker is used for B lymphocyte identification. B-cells make antibodies and T-cells differentiate into Natural Killer (NK) cells, helper T-cells, etc., which kill virally infected cells, pathogens, and cancer cells. Flow cytometry and PARR (PCR for antigen receptor rearrangements) are tests that detect specific CD proteins on the lymphocyte cell surface. This technology is excellent to confirm lymphoma or leukemia in ambiguous cases with suggestive cytology (Avery 2014). In general, one out of three lymphoma dogs will have the more resistant T-cell subtype. An observational study of archived lymphoma tissue found that 82% of 50 Boxers, 50% of 22 Golden Retrievers, and 19% of 37 Rottweilers had T-cell lymphomas (Lurie, Lucroy, and Griffey 2004). Another study of 1,263 dogs with lymphoma representing 87 breeds had similar findings (Modiano et al. 2005).

T-cell subtype lymphomas in dogs are more likely to exhibit hypercalcemia, mediastinal mass, myasthenia gravis, shorter first remission times and shorter survival times than B-cell patients. We educate our clients about the importance of phenotyping, how the information helps us decide which drugs to use, and how it affects their dog's overall prognosis. We often counsel clients with the thought; *"B is better and T is terrible."* Subtype and histologic information on feline lymphomas does not yield prognostic information as to response rates (Limmer et al. 2016).

Precise clinical staging of an individual lymphoma patient is not considered reliable without X-rays and a core bone marrow biopsy. Bone marrow cytology is evaluated to rule out leukemic involvement. Hawkins, Morrison, and DeNicola (1993) found that 33% of 47 dogs with lymphoma had pulmonary parenchymal evidence of involvement on X-ray evaluation and could be further cytologically evaluated with bronchoalveolar lavage.

Clients who are highly bonded to their lymphoma pets will probably elect the best combination chemotherapy no matter what clinical stage or phenotype is determined. For this reason and for financial considerations, many veterinarians do not pursue thorough diagnostic testing and bone marrow cytology for precise staging. This is especially true in cats, as lymphoma represents a diverse group of lesions and further diagnostic information has not been helpful to predict response rates and may not change how feline lymphoma patients are initially treated.

A Proposed International Prognostic Index for Canine Lymphoma

There are over 50 different types of lymphoma in human medicine with unique risk factors, epidemiologic features, prognosis, and outcome. Dr. V.E. Valli, who spent most of his career as a pathologist focused on canine and feline lymphoma at the University of Illinois, asked veterinarians and oncologists to participate in a global study to update the staging of canine lymphomas to relate to outcome. This collaborative study published 992 cases that correlated different subtypes with response to therapy (Valli et al. 2013). Others have contributed information from Europe (Ponce 2015).

Veterinary and Comparative Oncology devoted a special supplemental issue on Lymphoma in August, 2016. It is an excellent update of the pathophysiology, diagnosis, classification, and potential new therapies for canine and feline lymphomas.

Tumor Markers for Diagnosis of Cancer and Targeted Therapy

The study of proteins (proteomics) has opened the molecular Pandora's box that is the cancer cell's milieu. Scientists have only identified a small fraction of the millions of proteins and regulatory DNA switches that control genes in the body. Certain proteins act as growth factors, enzymes, and signals and may be overexpressed on the surface and in the cytoplasm of cancer cells and help mark various tissue types. The proteins are unique to each type of cell and these analyses yield a "bar code" that reveals cell and tissue identity.

Checkpoint inhibitors block docking sites that reduce the T-cells' ability to recognize and kill cancer cells. The most studied checkpoint inhibitor is programed death ligand-1 (PD-L1). It is a gene that plays a key role in protecting cancer cells from T-cell mediated destruction. Signals can hijack DNA repair pathways that shorten telomeres. Tests to identify specific proteins, or markers, are used to differentiate tumors on a molecular basis, opening up new areas of research and potential targets for drug therapy. As a group, tumor markers can identify a host of molecules that can be indicators of tumor cell type, function, growth factors, tumor presence, response, or recurrence. Each of these proteins, signals, and switches have names and acronyms that add great complexity to the alphabet soup milieu, which is immuno-oncology today.

There will be more useable and specific tumor markers and tests developed to identify, characterize, and target malignant tumors in the future. Some markers are used to detect tumor activity or recurrence. Other markers will be used to tell us if a tumor contains sites that would be susceptible to targeted therapies, such as antiapoptosis, antiangiogenesis, and kinase, telomerase, or metalloproteinase inhibitors. These special marker tests may be run on cytology slides, serum, biopsy, or fresh tissue samples.

Tumor marker tests may employ immunohistochemical stain techniques, polymerase chain reaction (PCR) technology, spectrophotometry, gel electrophoresis, or some other intricate technology for identification of selected proteins or for gene mapping. For example, tumor markers may identify the presence of tumor suppressor genes such as the well-characterized *p53* gene found in canine osteosarcoma. Tumor markers may be used to follow tumors as they transition from their dormant stage into their more threatening proliferative stage as with Ki-67, the nuclear antigen found in proliferating mast cell sarcomas and proliferating mammary adenocarcinomas. The constitutive activation gene, *C-kit* (CD117), is a proto-oncogene that can be used both as a screening tool and as a target for treatment. *C-kit* undergoes mutations in several cancers and can be detected by PCR. *C-kit* serves as a useful target for small molecules and gene therapy, to control recurrent or inoperable mast cell cancer in dogs.

In the field of proteomics, tumors are not identified by morphology, grading, or staging. Instead, tumors are characterized as being positive or negative for expression of a certain set of protein receptors on analysis. One important set of growth factor protein receptors to be familiar with belongs to the angiopoietin family of receptors: vascular endothelial growth factor receptor (VEGFR), platelet-derived growth factor receptor (PDGFR), fibroblastic growth factor receptor (FGFR), and Tie1/2. Information about the presence or absence of expression of these protein receptors links investigators to the type of signaling pathways that a particular cancer type uses. The angiopoietin family of receptors signals for endothelial cell migration, proliferation, and coordination for the process of angiogenesis that is vital for cancer cell proliferation and survival (Abeloff et al. 2004).

A diagnostic flow cytometry test may become available that will detect the ontogeny of hemangiosarcoma by the expression of cell-surface determinants of circulating transformed hemangioblastic stem cells in dogs. This may confirm the diagnosis and assist in monitoring minimal residual disease after surgical removal. The test will be most useful as a screening test if it can reliably detect HSA in its early stages and if there is targeted therapy available for patients testing positive (Lamerato-Koziki et al. 2006). More tumor expression patterns and specific marker families will be identified for future diagnostic screening and testing in cancer patients. This will give researchers targets with which they will be able to develop specific drugs, ligand-targeted bacterial toxins, and/or vaccines specifically for that individual. This approach will enable the delivery of precision or personalized medicine for veterinary patients. This approach may be kinder and more gentle on geriatric cancer patients than the current standard of care surgery, chemotherapy, and radiation therapy protocols.

Gene Microarray Results Can Guide Therapeutic Options

Veterinarians have access to and can use the technique of tissue microarrays. This sophisticated technique surveys a special slide for diagnosis of immunoreactivity and genetic makeup of certain cancers. How can we use the information? Identifying the molecular players in cancer cell pathways opens targets for development of drugs and vaccines to attack the cancer at vulnerable sites.

If we learn from a diagnostic microarray test whether or not an OSA patient's tumors express COX-2 activity, then we know that an NSAID would be a helpful therapy. Unfortunately, only a low percentage of primary OSAs do express COX-2. Microarray assessments of OSA pulmonary metastases have found an upregulated expression of COX-2. Therefore, COX-2 inhibitors may be more helpful in the metastatic phase of OSA versus the primary phase.

NSAIDs such as piroxicam, meloxicam, carprofen, deracoxib, and thalidomide (a glutamic acid derivative) have cyclooxygenase-2 (COX-2) inhibition activity and antiangiogenesis activity. It is also understood that COX-2 inhibition confers some antitumor effects in bladder cancer, squamous cell carcinoma (SCC), and other cancers that overexpress COX-2. However, what is the role of NSAIDs in OSA management?

COX-2 inhibitors can be used in all OSA cases from day 1, whether or not the pet owner elected amputation. The primary purpose of selecting a COX-2 inhibitor for the management of OSA is that it offers pain control. The secondary purpose is that there is a 10% chance that the drug may inhibit the primary tumor. Nitrogen-containing bisphosphonates that exert antiresorptive effects are also used for these two purposes. A kinder and gentler approach in palliative cancer medicine for geriatric cancer patients is to select drugs with a dual purpose. These drugs reduce pain in unamputated patients while providing additional therapeutic advantage against metastatic disease in both amputated and unamputated patients. The use of zoledronate and meloxicam reduced oral bone loss and tumor growth in an orthotopic mouse model of bone-invasive feline oral SCC. This well-tolerated combinatorial approach may palliate older cats afflicted with oral SCC (Martin et al. 2015).

Complimentary or Alternative Methods Used in the Diagnosis of Cancer

Complementary and alternative medicine involves diagnostic tests that assess blood, urine, feces, and tissues, as in conventional medicine, but it also includes the assessment of hair samples, muscle resistance testing, biofeedback, pulse palpation, tongue examination, iris reading, and more. Some of these tests are controversial and disputed, but they generally reveal the diagnosis of toxicity and immunosuppression. The fundamental toxicity comes from heavy metals and environmental carcinogens. Immunosuppression comes from the malignancy and stress reactions due to allergies to specific foods, antibiotics, drugs, chemotherapy, steroids, and so forth. The patient is tested further and generally withdrawn from the offending agent and placed on a detoxification program and a rebalancing program to regain a stronger energy field. Cancer patients are often put on special diets and supplements as well.

If a client wants to pursue alternative diagnostics and therapy for their geriatric cancer pet, it is an opportunity to counsel them. Recommend that they simultaneously take advantage of modern technology along with the complimentary medicine. Recommend that they create an integrative program that dovetails the most effective treatments from each branch of medicine so that their geriatric cancer pet receives the maximum benefit. Since conventional Western medicine modalities do not offer comprehensive treatment solutions for all patients and all tumors, many pet owners seek complementary and alternative therapies to integrate into their geriatric cancer pet's treatment plan.

Veterinarians will increasingly be challenged to remain open-minded and somewhat knowledgeable about alternative approaches. Regardless of personal biases against alternative therapies, the contemporary veterinarian refers clients seeking alternative care to local practitioners who provide alternative care. The nurturing and palliative aspect of alternative medicine, such as massage, acupuncture, and nutritional counseling, serves the geriatric cancer patient in a very positive way.

Summary

Geriatric patients present many diagnostic challenges when they develop cancer. Geriatric patients present in all stages of cancer, from early to advanced, superimposed on all stages of organ system compromise, which compete for the patient's morbidity and mortality (Fouchi et al. 2016). Many of these patients have been previously referred to specialists for cataract removal, orthopedic surgery, dental care, and internal medical issues. They come into the clinic with various degrees of information and history from one or several attending veterinarians. When the actual diagnosis and stage of disease has not been established, the challenge is to pinpoint the diagnosis and extent of the problem by staging the patient against the backdrop of its physical and health status.

For definitive diagnosis, it is necessary to biopsy all suspicious tissue and then use anatomic and/or functional imaging to accurately stage the patient. The process of decision making should be a partnership between the patient's carers and the veterinarian. Offer the owner information, with handouts and a list of online sources, and help them access all available options for their pet's therapy. Help them with medicoethical end of life decision making. Then support and treat the patient within the owner's parameters. Be mindful that newer, more sensitive, and specific diagnostic technology will become available, such as faster 3D imaging and the endothelial precursor cell (EPC) test for hemangiosarcoma. This new technology will detect cancer at its earlier stages, but will also cast more cases in more advanced stages of disease, resulting in stage migration issues. Therefore, it may be difficult to provide answers to those inquiring about the prognosis for their geriatric cancer pet with comorbidities because a survival prediction based on previous evidence-based medicine using ideal patients may be difficult to interpret.

Thorough, compassionate communication is essential when delivering the diagnosis and prognosis of cancer. Keep in mind that most carers love their geriatric pets and do not want their pet to die. Compassionate, high-touch communication with sincerity and concern for the care and management of the geriatric cancer patient is as important as our high-tech machines, tests, drugs, and surgical skills.

Note: If you are interested in learning about ongoing studies conducted by the Veterinary Cooperative Oncology Group, see the Veterinary Cancer Society web site at www.vetcancersociety.org. The AVMA Animal Health Studies Database (AAHSD) has recently become the clearing house for all current clinical trials. Go to https://ebusiness.avma.org/aahsd/more_info/search_for_studies.aspx.

Scooter's Case (Some Skinny Cats Can Respond)

Scooter Abrams, a $12\frac{1}{2}$-year-old F/S DSH, was referred for management of nasal planum SCC. On physical exam, Scooter was emaciated, dehydrated, and had an elevated heart rate. She was hyperactive, very excitable, and impossible to handle without sedation. Scooter also had that wide-eyed, surprised look found in hyperthyroid cats. Her body weight was only 4.75 pounds from her normal 8 pounds. Scooter's referring veterinarian had recently diagnosed her with hyperthyroidism: T-4 (RIA) = 11.63 (normal = 0.8–4.0µg/dl) and Free T-4 (RIA) = 8.36 (normal = 0.5–2.5). Mr. Abrams used fish-flavored compounded methimazole (tapazole) at 5mg BID. The biopsy of two nasal planum lesions reported carcinoma in situ. Although Scooter's lesions would be responsive to cryotherapy, she had cachexia, was clinically hyperthyroid, fractious, and a very poor candidate for sedation. Mr. Abrams was apprised of the risk.

We used IM Domitor sedation, took a blood sample, and treated Scooter's SCC lesions with liquid nitrogen cryotherapy. Mr. Abrams was instructed to give SQ fluids at home, along with a calorie-dense diet, and to continue methimazole at 5mg twice daily. On recheck, Scooter's T-4 by radioimmunoassay (RIA) climbed from 11.63 to 13.72µg/dl on the compounded tapazole. Mr. Abrams was asked to discontinue the compounded tapazole and give Scooter the tablet form. One week later, her T-4 (RIA) rose to 15.06µg/dl. The normal T-4 (RIA) range for our laboratory was 0.8–4.0µg/dl.

We referred Scooter to Dr. John Amman, a radiologist, for nuclear imaging of her thyroid glands and a GFR scan to evaluate her renal function. Our intention was to see if iodine 131 treatment would normalize her T-4 level. Tc99m DTPA was used for the GFR study. The GFR value for her left kidney was 2.88ml/min/kg and the right was 2.1ml/min/kg (normal >2.5ml/min/kg). Her renal function was considered within normal limits. After 1 hour, Scooter was given Tc99 pertechnetate to image her thyroid glands. Scooter's right thyroid gland was enlarged and her left gland had increased uptake.

Iodine 131 was given but Scooter's T-4 levels remained elevated following two treatments. Her thyroid glands were imaged again on the gamma camera and there was no change over 2 months. Ultrasound exam revealed a large circumscribed mass with an intact capsule. Lack of response of the right thyroid to treatment is consistent with thyroid carcinoma (Amman 2002). Scooter had thyroidectomy and follow-up monitoring of her calcium levels.

Thyroidectomized patients may experience life-threatening hypocalcemia, due to accompanying inadvertent parathyroidectomy. Scooter required calcium gluconate only once during her 2-day postthyroidectomy hospitalization period. Scooter's T-4 normalized following surgery and she gained weight. Her nasal SCC lesions resolved with cryotherapy.

One year later, Scooter presented with new SCC lesions on her opposite nostril. The lesions were treated with cryotherapy. Her T-4 remained normal and her nose remained cancer free for 3 more years. At age 16, Scooter presented weighing $4\frac{1}{2}$ pounds and vomiting. She had slightly pale mucus membranes, fleas, an elevated heart rate of 160, and her T-4 was elevated to 11 (Figure 5.8). Scooter was placed on 2.5mg propranolol (Inderal®) BID, oral methimazole (Tapazole®), and a calorie-dense diet. This time, her T-4 value dropped quickly. Her renal function remained unaffected but she did not gain weight. Chest X-rays found a mass in the caudal lung field, which we presumed was either metastatic thyroid carcinoma or primary

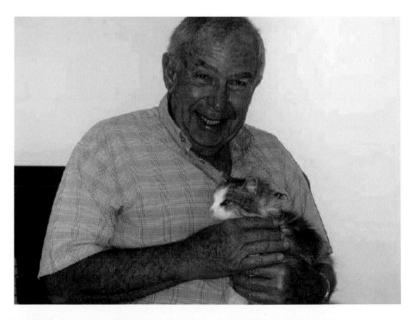

Figure 5.8.   Mr. Abrams and 18-year-old Scooter: treated for nasal planum SCC, cachexia, sarcopenia, malignant thyroid carcinoma, and hyperthyroidism. One year later Scooter developed either presumptive primary pulmonary carcinoma or metastatic thyroid carcinoma and entered the hospice phase of our Pawspice program.

pulmonary carcinoma. Further diagnosis did not matter as she was too frail for cancer therapy. Metronomic therapy might have been an option as it is associated with minimal adverse events. Scooter entered the hospice phase of our Pawspice care program, fluctuating between 4 and $5^1/_2$ pounds. Surprisingly, she gained $^1/_2$ pound in 2 weeks after injections with T-Cyte®, a thymic signaling protein that stimulates helper CD4 T-cell function and numbers, interleukin 2 (IL-2) production, and erythropoiesis (Beardsley et al. 2005).

References

Abeloff, M.D., J.O. Armitage, J.E. Niederhuber, M.B. Kastan, and W.G. McKenna. 2004. *Clinical Oncology*, 3rd edn. Philadelphia, PA: Churchill Livingstone.

Amman, J.F. 2002. Personal Communication, July 3, 2002.

Avery, A. 2014 Testing for lymphoma and leukemia in dogs and cats. *Veterinary Cancer Society Proceedings*, pp. 179–188.

Balducci L. (ed.). 2004. "Part 4: The influence of aging on prevention, diagnosis and treatment of cancer." In *Comprehensive geriatric oncology*, 2nd edn, eds L. Balducci, G.H. Lyman, W.B. Ershler, and M. Extermann, pp. 207–309. Oxon, UK: Taylor & Francis.

Beardsley, T.R., T-Cyte® Therapeutics, and C.A. Bansall. 2005. The role of lymphocyte T-cell immunomodulator (LTCI) in amplification of helper CD-4 cell response, IL-2 production, and hematopoiesis. Personal Communication, September.

Cowell, R.L. 2003. Cytology Part II. *Veterinary Clinics of North America* 3 (1):47–67.

Friedrichs, K.R., and K.M. Young. 2005. How to collect diagnostic bone marrow samples. *Veterinary Medicine* August:578–588.

Ford, R. 2004. New research into vaccine-associated feline sarcomas. As quoted by the *141st AVMA Annual Convention News*, July 28, pp. 1, 15.

Fouchi, T., S. Bains, M.C. Lee, et al. 2016. Impact of increasing age on cause-specific mortality and morbidity in patients with Stage I non-small-cell lung cancer: A competing risks analysis. *Journal of Clinical Oncology* 162 (234):150–177.

Giuffrida, M.A. 2016. A systematic review of adverse event reporting in companion animal clinical trials evaluating cancer treatment. *JAVMA* 249 (9):1079–1087.

Glickman, L., N. Glickman, and R. Thorpe. 2000. *The Golden Retriever Club of America national health survey*, August 15 (http://www.grca.org/healthsurvey.pdf).

Gobar, G.M., and P.H. Kass. 2002. World wide web-based survey of vaccination practices, postvaccinal reactions, and vaccine site associated sarcomas in cats. *JAVMA* 220:1477–1482.

Hawkins, E.C., W.B. Morrison, D.D. DeNicola, et al. 1993. Cytologic analysis of bronchoalveolar lavage fluid from 47 dogs with multicentric malignant lymphoma. *JAVMA* 203:1418–1425.

Henderson, R.A. 2004. Prostatectomy: Is it time for a revisit? *VCS NL* 28 (3).

Henderson, R.A. 2005. Personal Communication, *VCS NL*, Spring.

Kass, P.H., et al. 1993. Epidemiologic evidence for a causal relation between vaccination and fibrosarcoma tumorigenesis in cats. *JAVMA* 203:396–405.

Kunkle, G.A., and L. Akucewich. 2005. Obtaining a skin biopsy for histopathologic evaluation. *NAVC Clinician's Brief* August:15–18.

Lamerato-Koziki, A.R., K.M. Helm, C.M. Jubala, G.C. Cutter, and J.F. Modiano. 2006. Canine hemangiosarcoma originates from hematopoietic precursors with potential for endothelial differentiation. *Experimental Hematology* 34 (7):870–878.

Limmer, S., N. Eberle, V. Nerschback, I. Nolte, and D. Betz. 2016. Treatment of feline lymphoma using a 12-week, maintenance-free combination chemotherapy protocol in 26 cats. *Veterinary and Comparative Oncology* 14 (S1):21–30. doi: 10.1111/vco.12082.

Lurie, D.M., M.D. Lucroy, and S.M. Griffey. 2004. T-cell-derived malignant lymphoma in the Boxer breed. *Veterinary and Comparative Oncology* 2 (3):171–175.

Martin, C.K., W.P. Dirkson, M.M. Carlton, et al. 2015. Combined zolendonic acid and meloxicam reduced bone loss and tumor growth in an orthotopic mouse model of bone-invasive oral squamous cell carcinoma. *Veterinary and Comparative Oncology* 13 (3):203–217. doi: 10.1111/vco.12037.

Meyer, D.J. 2001. "The essentials of diagnostic cytology in clinical oncology." In *Small animal clinical oncology*, 3rd edn, eds S.J. Withrow and E.G. MacEwen, pp. 54–63. Philadelphia, PA: Saunders.

Modiano, J.F. 2016. Where the future lies: Innovations in cancer treatment and prevention. *World Veterinary Cancer Congress*, Foz de Iguassu, Brazil.

Modiano, J.F., M. Breen, R.C. Burnett, et al. 2005. Distinct B-cell and T-cell lymphoproliferative disease prevalence among dog breeds indicates heritable risk. *Cancer Research* 65 (13):5654 (www.aacrjournals.org).

Morrison, W.B. 2002. "Principles of cancer diagnosis." In *Cancer in dogs and cats: Medical and surgical management*, 2nd edn, pp. 57–177. Jackson, WY: Teton New Media.

Ogilvie, G.K., and A.S. Moore. 1995. "Section 1: Biopsy, managing the veterinary cancer patient. In *Managing the veterinary cancer patient*, eds G. Ogilvie and A. Moore, pp. 1–47. Trenton, NJ: Veterinary Learning Systems.

Ponce, F. 2015. Update on the treatment and prognosis of canine lymphoma. *European Society of Veterinary Oncology Proceedings*.

Scarpa, F., S. Sabattini, and G. Bettini. 2014. Cytological grading of canine cutaneous mast cell tumors. *Veterinary and Comparative Oncology* 14 (3):245–251.

Vail, D.M., and S.J. Withrow. 2001. "Tumors of the skin and subcutaneous tissues." In *Small animal clinical oncology*, 3rd edn, eds S.J. Withrow and E.G. MacEwen, pp. 233–260. Philadelphia, PA: Saunders.

Valli, V.E., Kass, P.H., San Myint, M., Scott, F., 2013. Canine lymphomas: association of classification type, disease stage, tumor subtype, mitotic rate, and treatment with survival, Veterinary Pathology, Vol. 50, Issue 5, p738-748.

Veterinary and Comparative Oncology, 2016. *Lymphoma*, Vol. 14, Supplement 1, August, eds Argyle, Thamm, and Pecceu.

Widmer, W.R. 2002. "Alternative imaging for the diagnosis of cancer." In *Cancer in dogs and cats: Medical and surgical management*, ed. W.B. Morrison, pp. 177–204. Jackson, WY: Teton New Media.

Withrow, S.J. 2001. "Biopsy principles." In *Small animal clinical oncology*, 3rd edn, eds S.J. Withrow and E.G. MacEwen, pp. 63–70. Philadelphia, PA: Saunders.

Part Three

Chapter 6
Treating Cancer in Geriatric Pets

We must uphold the traditional value of sharing and caring by avoiding the contemporary code of making and taking, with indifference to the needs of others.

Dr. Carl A. Osborne, DVM, PhD, ACVIM (AVMA News 2005)

Chapter 6 has the following sections: Principles and Philosophic Perspective for Treating Geriatric Cancer Patients; The Role of Surgery in Cancer Management and "When Is It Too Much Surgery"; Chemotherapy in the Management of Geriatric Cancer; Adverse Effects of Cancer Therapy in Geriatric Pets; The Role of Radiation Therapy in Cancer Management; Immunotherapy, Cancer Vaccines, and Gene Therapy; Antiangiogenesis Therapy with Metronomic Chemotherapy; Chemoprevention and Immunonutrition for Cancer Patients; Integrative and Alternative Medicine; and Electrochemotherapy (ECT)/Electroporation (EP). Each topic is immense, but will be distilled into essential aspects for treating the most common cancers in geriatric dogs and cats along with supporting our patients and their families at the end of life.

Principles and Philosophic Perspective for Treating Geriatric Cancer Patients

Veterinary medicine is one of the few professions that hold the keys to a person's heart. We have a wonderful opportunity to enter the eye of an emotional storm and provide a healing atmosphere for both the geriatric cancer patient and their family. The goals of this section are to muster your enthusiasm, increase your knowledge, and hone your skills for treating cancer in geriatric patients. It takes a positive attitude and clinical courage to treat any pet's cancer definitively. Yet more skill and thoughtfulness are required to successfully treat and care for geriatric cancer patients. Just as importantly, it takes wisdom and courage to realize that a certain patient has passed the window of benefit from known conventional therapies at hand.

Because cancer can be insidious in older pets and resilient, it often wins the battle despite the noble effort that veterinarians and pet owners put forth. However, the rewards of treating and caring for geriatric cancer patients are well worth the effort. When geriatric pets are past the window of definitive therapeutic benefit, palliative Pawspice care, which embraces kinder and gentler cancer medicine and transitions to hospice at the end of life, comes to the forefront. We can develop this aspect of practice into an expected and respected end of life care program for older patients with advanced cancer. One client, Roberta, wrote a thank you note that said it well: "If Mitzi could have lived on love, she would have lived forever."

This chapter discusses using a multimodality approach for treatment of general types of cancer, such as adenocarcinomas and sarcomas. An overview of the most common treatment protocols for

Canine and Feline Geriatric Oncology: Honoring the Human–Animal Bond, Second Edition. Alice Villalobos with Laurie Kaplan.
© 2018 John Wiley & Sons, Inc. Published 2018 by John Wiley & Sons, Inc.

the most common types of cancer is provided. As new information explodes on us every day, we must expect to change and improve our protocols constantly. New technology, drugs, and vaccines will target different molecular mechanisms of malignancy and may produce more options for our geriatric oncology patients. The CancerMoonShot2020 is dedicated to developing immunotherapy and other technologies that may, in the future, be able to diagnose, prevent, and target primary and metastatic disease. The goal of the CancerMoonShot2020 program is to transform cancer into a chronic disease, rather than a terminal disease. We must be aware of and be willing to incorporate innovative drugs, biotechnology, supportive therapies, and effective supplements into our existing protocols.

Furthermore, we must be willing to adapt mainstream therapies to individual client and patient needs, even if that means we enter some uncharted territory with some innovative yet logical adaptations of known therapies. With the advent of precision or personalized cancer therapy, based upon the patient's molecular targets, we will soon have that opportunity. The most important objective must always be to provide the greatest benefit for the patient while respecting the emotional, financial, and physical capabilities of the patient's family. This ultimate consideration will provide the best quality of medicine for the individual geriatric cancer patient and client situation.

In addition, there are no two oncologists who treat their geriatric cancer patients the very same way or with the same bedside manner. This explains why your clients will get different opinions and impressions from different consultants. For this book, I was asked to share my personal perspectives and approach to geriatric oncology and tell you the way I treat my patients. This is not a "how to" but rather "a way to" approach cancer management in geriatric patients. As a disclaimer, please always verify drug doses and schedules for your patients.

There is no secret or mystery about what I have been doing for the past 40 plus years. This book is a vehicle through which I can share with decades of experience admixing geriatric oncology, Pawspice, hospice, and the human–animal bond. I hope that this book will help you minister a greater number of geriatric cancer patients into a longer and higher quality of life. If these pages provide insight and have a positive impact on practitioners to develop and practice the art of geriatric veterinary oncology, then the input and production of this textbook as a tool to advance the care given to geriatric cancer pets will have accomplished its goal.

Contemporary oncology research reaches into the molecular frontier of genomics, proteomics, and immuno-oncology. The acronyms and codes for the language of proteomics will force readers of oncology literature to swim (or sink) in a cumbersome pool of alphabet soup. There are hundreds of acronyms and sequence numbers that represent receptors, ligands, signaling and cross-link proteins, pathway promoters, and inhibitors. These proteins play specific roles in cell metabolism, proliferation, migration, programmed cell death or suicide (apoptosis), etc. Proteomics gives scientists the keys to unlock, target, inhibit, and rearrange the signals of cellular mechanisms that promote carcinogenesis, angiogenesis, metastasis, apoptosis, etc. This era has rediscovered One Medicine and is at the crest of development of new types of targeted therapies that will help to curb cancer for patients of all species and all ages.

Researchers will develop reliable diagnostic tests called "liquid biopsies" that will detect cancer in its earliest stages by its circulating markers. Early detection allows us to apply new cancer prevention therapies to at-risk patients, to more effectively offset cancer's fatal agenda. Targeted therapies bind to specific proteins on the surface of tumor cells and inhibit activity that is vital for tumor cell division, immortality, and metastasis. There is excitement with the development of inhibitors of the programed death ligand (PD-L1), which plays a key role in protecting cancer cells from T-cell mediated destruction and immunosurveillance. There will be many advances in conventional protocols for veterinary cancer prevention, detection, and treatment because of artificial intelligence, such as IBM

Watson. This artificial intelligence helps researchers with its ability to quickly review the vast world literature, to improve diagnostic accuracy, and to suggest therapeutic applications for personalized cancer management. IBM Watson can digest the enormous minutiae in the molecular alphabet soup more quickly than humanly possible. Once the complex folds and spirals of the genomic and proteomic recipe for neoplasia is divulged, scientists can unfold and target its pathways with powerful and precise technology to prevent and control cancer (Vail 2006a; Modiano 2016).

Veterinarians contact me daily to fill in the lines left out of their oncology textbooks. They feel intimidated and uncertain about geriatric oncology, yet are motivated to learn more because their clients are asking for more expertise and help. The first and most useful principle of geriatric oncology is to practice with compassionate understanding while comprehending the whole patient. Since so many of my patients have done exceptionally well under my philosophy of care, this information needs to be shared beyond the confines and the limited reach of my private oncology practices. This chapter offers a fresh, compassionate, and practical addition to the excellent literature already available in veterinary oncology.

Each geriatric cancer patient is unique and must be individualized by the stage of disease, concurrent conditions, comorbid illnesses, and the pet owner's economic situation, logistics, personal philosophy, and time commitment. The attending doctor must coordinate decision making and treatment choices. Most difficult surgical oncology cases and all radiation therapy cases are referred to specialists. Surgical oncology and radiation oncology require more complex planning for geriatric oncology patients. Consultations for the administration of chemotherapy protocols used in medical oncology can be achieved more readily.

Clinicians have recently become more interested in using chemotherapy in practice. Chemotherapy protocols are plentiful, but they must often be modified and adjusted by the attending doctor as needed based on factors such as: body score condition, hydration status, performance, organ function, and so forth. Variations in chemotherapy drug sequencing and doses are common because the recommended treatment plans must be adapted to the responses and needs of each individual geriatric cancer patient. Customizing protocols is not always easy to do while staying within the boundaries of the pet owner's wishes and financial resources. Clients will appreciate the integration of these principles into your style of practice. Such flexibility shows pet caregivers that the well-being of their geriatric pet is important to you and that you respect their personal issues.

Consult with an oncologist at your reference laboratory for the latest chemotherapy options to assist your client in decision making. Make an attempt to check with at least two or three current sources to verify that the protocols described in this chapter are still the current and favored way to treat the particular neoplasia that affects your patient. The best local source to check would be your state's veterinary college, or any veterinary college with an oncology service. The Veterinary Cancer Society (VCS), founded in 1976, has an online directory that will help you locate a VCS Member nearest to you: www.vetcancersociety.org/pet-owners/find-an-oncologist/.

Oncology information abounds on the Internet. Some professors regularly provide blogs and notes online, as illustrated by Dr. Neal Mauldin's current blog at www.petcureoncology.com, which supports stereotactic radiotherapy (SRS). Drs. Tony Moore and Angela Frimberger have an online private oncology consultation service for veterinarians at www.vetoncologyconsults.com, providing access to Body Surface Area Charts. Free human oncology medical information is available at www.Medscape.com. The National Library of Medicine hosts www.pubmed.gov, with access to MEDLINE, its flagship database.

The Veterinary Information Network (VIN) offers members ("Vinners") interactive online courses, consultations, and information at your fingertips to verify the latest treatment protocols with specialists in chat rooms at www.VIN.com. You and your clients can also download and copy user-friendly client information at www.VeterinaryPartner.com, a free online service from VIN. VetFolio.com is an online educational resource that combines information from the North American Veterinary Community (NAVC, VMX) and The American Animal Hospital Association (AAHA). Members of Vetstream, at www.vetstream.com, have access to Vetlexicon, their online species specific libraries: Canis, Felis, Lapis and Equis. Data are from the *BSAVA Manual of Canine and Feline Oncology* text with updates by Dobson and Lascelles (2003). By searching for the latest online information, you will be aware of the most up-to-date cancer treatments for your geriatric patients. Consider using telemedicine to consult with experts about your cases. Create an online safe friendship circle with like-minded colleagues with whom you can discuss your cases. Keep an open mind and always seek and learn new information. You may need to unlearn and bury old ideas that have become outdated. Use the Internet to keep up with new drugs and recommendations to add to existing protocols that may extend remission and survival times for geriatric cancer patients. Expert oncology management advice and unit-dose treatment supplies are provided for specific patients for members of www.oncurapartners.com.

Many pet owners are members of pet cancer support groups on the Internet. They share their experiences and feelings regarding their pet's cancer. Some groups focus on a particular cancer type in dogs or cats. Pet owners discuss treatments, adverse events, and the care their pet is receiving. They also discuss their pet's diet and they search for diets that may discourage cancer cells. They offer one another support and a safe haven for people to express their feelings without the common "It's just a dog!" or "It's just a cat!" response.

Because chemotherapy is thought to be immunosuppressive, many Internet users are convinced that it will harm their older pet. Veterinarians need to be able to discuss the issues and the myths that concern clients. We can assure clients that cancer itself is immunosuppressive. A study of 21 dogs on chemotherapy found that they responded to vaccination as well as normal dogs. Combination chemotherapy caused these dogs more immunosuppression than single-agent therapy. However, some tumor vaccines are given concurrently with certain chemotherapy agents such as Cytoxan® to enhance the vaccine's antitumor activity (Walter et al. 2006).

Many Internet group members become extensively educated about protocols and medical oncology. When an owner speaks knowledgeably about cancer treatment, rather than being offended or annoyed, always applaud their quest and dedication to their pet's well-being.

When a cherished cancer pet passes away, their online support group members are very helpful in providing validation and heartfelt compassion within a safe peer group. Pet lovers often create touching email tributes in honor of their deceased pet to share with the group. I often ask my clients to write a eulogy about their pet and to email it to me. We may post it on our web site if the family agrees.

Be forewarned that Internet support group members chat candidly about their veterinarians! They post comments about bedside manner and they share their assessment of their veterinarian's motivation level and competence in treating their pet. Occasionally, someone might complain online at Yelp or RipOff. It is hard not to be upset if this happens but it is best not to take it personally. Stack up all your thank you cards and read them to show yourself that you are valued and loved for what you do to help animals and that one bad Yelp is not the end of the world. Simply by keeping an unconditionally positive attitude toward every client and focusing on the human–animal bond, while serving the geriatric cancer patient, you will remain in the good graces of the Internet support group network.

Ask questions about the pet and enjoy discovering unique features in the history of each geriatric pet that you treat. Cancer therapy almost always needs to be individualized to satisfy clients' special situations and considerations. One of the best ways to approach a geriatric oncology case is to assure pet carers that you will take the time to tailor a protocol for their geriatric pet's particular needs and stay within their financial ability, without ever making them feel guilty about financial constraints.

Overview of the Four Musketeers of Cancer Therapy

The "Three Musketeers" used in conventional cancer treatment are surgery, chemotherapy, and radiation therapy. The coarse terms used for these techniques are cut, poison, and burn. Most clinicians make the decision to perform surgery on a cancer patient with the blessings of their clients. However, it is often in the geriatric pet's best interest to consult a medical oncologist at the initial stages of treatment, before engaging a surgeon. Medical oncologists think differently from surgeons, internists, or radiation therapists when it comes to treating geriatric cancer patients. Medical oncologists might bring in immunotherapy as the "Fourth Musketeer" to fight the cancer.

Oncologists generally attempt to obtain a diagnosis and staging information in an efficient, patient-sparing way. This is especially beneficial for the geriatric cancer patient that may be compromised with the effects of aging and other concurrent illnesses. Oncologists understand the behavior and growth rate of various cancers and will generally move more quickly toward definitive therapy following diagnostic procedures. Proper imaging and staging may conclude that interventions such as surgery would be unhelpful or useless for some geriatric cancer patients (Hahn 2006). The first surgery is the opportune time to harvest cancer cells for autologous cancer vaccine production that may prevent or delay progression, recurrence, or metastasis. An example of a multi-indication dendritic cell cancer vaccine would be IFx-VET.com.

Rather than putting off therapy for the sacred 2-week healing period following surgery, medical and surgical oncologists often consider using neoadjuvant chemotherapy, palliative radiation therapy, sterotactic radiosurgery, immunotherapy, or a combination of treatments before, during, or shortly after cancer surgery. This may prevent the patient's cancer from robustly skipping to a higher stage. Postponing treatment until after the postoperative healing period may allow the malignant cells time to recruit and recur. If the patient is not scheduled for chemotherapy until 2 weeks after surgery, the residual tumor has a window of opportunity to undergo further cell divisions.

Most autologous vaccines take 3-4 weeks for production and may be used alongside conventional or metronomic chemotherapy or instead of chemotherapy. Using immunotherapy as the "Fourth Muskateer" is an excellent, kinder, and more gentle treatment option for geriatric cancer patients.

Unhelpful Surgery

I have witnessed the rapid postoperative onslaught and/or recurrence of excised high-grade abdominal lymphomas. Some tumors return to presurgical dimensions within 10–20 days post-op. One 17-year-old cat with an enlarged kidney underwent a nephrectomy because an FNA was non-diagnostic. The histology report diagnosed renal lymphoma. This old cat was presented to our service for management 2 weeks postnephrectomy. His remaining kidney was huge and the BUN and creatinine were elevated compared to presurgery levels. This scenario is undesirable for pet owners who readily consent in good faith to their doctor's recommendation for major surgery. It was unfortunate for this geriatric cat that many practitioners are reluctant to pursue ultrasound-guided percutaneous renal biopsy in the clinical evaluation of their patients. A Tru-cut needle biopsy of the enlarged kidney may have yielded a precise histologic diagnosis without the stress of nephrectomy (Vaden et al. 2005). Due to adherence to an unnecessary chemotherapy delay following unnecessary surgery and its conventional postsurgical "waiting period," this old cat's renal lymphoma was allowed to robustly move onward with its fatal agenda.

Weezie's Case (Exploratory Surgery May Delay Needed Therapy)

Weezie, a 12-year-old M/N DSH, started to decline and was taken to his local veterinarian for an exam. The doctor palpated an abdominal mass. Despite the fact that Weezie was eating and passing stool, the doctor recommended immediate exploratory surgery. The family requested more diagnostics. They were referred to a surgical specialist, who performed an abdominal ultrasound to visualize the mass. The surgeon strongly recommended exploratory surgery to remove the mass and biopsy, even though Weezie was eating and passing stool. The owners felt that they were given no other choice and surgery seemed to them to be the best course of action at that time. At surgery, a 6.8cm mass was removed from the mesenteric nodes and intestine. The diagnosis was lymphoma, present in the kidneys, intestines, and mesenteric nodes. The recommendation was to start chemotherapy after recovery. Recovery was uneventful and sutures were removed 2 weeks postop.

One week later, Weezie started to decline again. That is when I received a desperate call and we fitted Weezie into our schedule on the following day. A large abdominal mass was palpated along with an enlarged kidney with elevations of the BUN and creatinine.

An oncologist would have approached this case differently. A palpable mass in the abdomen of an FeLV negative geriatric cat can be presumed to be lymphoma until proven otherwise. Cells can be characterized via persistent, diligent, percutaneous FNA cytology or Tru-cut biopsy. This non-surgical evaluation technique can diagnose lymphoma and avoid unhelpful surgery in cases like Weezie's. With infiltrative, low volume intestinal lymphoma, endoscopy may be successful for diagnosis; however, surgery is often required to harvest full thickness samples of intestine for definitive diagnosis.

In Weezie's case, surgery and the subsequent postponement of chemotherapy were not helpful. Chemotherapy for high grade abdominal lymphoma in cats and dogs is helpful when administered postoperatively within hours or within the first few days following surgery. In the postoperative setting, it is best to omit prednisone for the first 7–10 days. We adjust the protocol to sequence the induction drugs over several days rather than administering them simultaneously in order to use the best window of therapeutic opportunity for the patient's sake. The anticipating clinician often feels caught in a medical dilemma. Most choose to wait until after healing of the surgical wounds rather than administer perioperative chemotherapy in time to halt the relentless spread of the lymphoma. What would you do if this was your cat?

Neoadjuvant and Perioperative Therapy

Neoadjuvant (prior to surgery) and/or perioperative chemotherapy (including intralesional or intracavitary administration during surgery) are valuable combination therapy tools that are underutilized in oncology practice. See the section on "Electrochemotherapy (ECT)/Electroporation (EP)," a technology used more often in South America and Europe that exquisitely combines this approach during surgery.

Tumors need to undergo only seven or eight doublings after clinical detection to be fatal. Some cancers such as hemangiosarcoma and osteosarcoma synchronize with bone marrow derived progenitor host cells. These host cells are home to tumor-specific premetastatic sites and form cellular clusters that encourage metastasis and angiogenesis (Kaplan et al. 2005). Therefore, by the time we see cancer in our patients, time is running out.

When a lymphoma patient has recovered fully from anesthesia and is on IV fluids, I may administer an induction chemotherapy drug in divided doses over 24 hours. High grade lymphoma has a relentless agenda of its own and does not wait idly for 2 weeks while the patient recovers from surgery. Therefore, we need to finesse the art of medicine in these cases as a matter of life and death.

We need to take courage and do what we can to safely control the neoplastic dynamics of the individual cancer patient. This may go against generalized textbook recommendations that depict healing times as sacrosanct. Viewing the surgery day as day 0, I give a 50% dose of vincristine on day 1. If the patient is doing well, the other 50% of vincristine may be given on day 2. L-asparaginase at 400mg/m^2 on either day 1 or 2 is an excellent perioperative chemotherapy choice for lymphoma patients, depending on the case. We hold off the use of prednisone until day 6 or 7 postop.

If a cancer patient is a candidate for radiation therapy (RTx), it is best to schedule a consult with a radiation oncologist before surgery and before ordering expensive diagnostic tests. Early referral may save the client money and spare the pet from unnecessary or redundant testing. The preliminary imaging used for the radiation therapy workup and dosimetry, for example, may favor CT over MRI. The radiation oncologist can set up the geriatric pet with diagnostic and therapeutic step-savers from the start. For instance, instead of ordering an MRI for a suspected brain tumor, the medical oncologist would order a CT scan if the owner is considering RTx. CT is more readily used to interface with a computerized radiation and dosimetry treatment plan. RTx can be safely started within a few days after surgery. In many cases, palliative radiation therapy or setereotactic radiosurgery (SRS) can be delivered in high fractions over a short time, using 1–3 treatments. If available and affordable, SRS may offer tumor shrinkage and control advantages for the geriatric cancer patient that may preclude the need for surgery (www.petcureoncology.com).

The attending surgeon may be asked to mark the tumor field with clips so that the radiation oncologist has proper orientation. The oncologist may request intralesional or intracavitary chemotherapy administration into the tumor bed following excision. In many cases, RTx is started as soon as possible after surgery, bypassing the 2-week delay recommended by many surgeons. At times, RTx is delivered prior to surgical removal. To ensure fewer oversights and more efficient and beneficial care for the geriatric cancer patient, the team approach is best. This team approach requires that the attending doctor and the specialists who are working up the patient are in good collaborative communication with the oncologist in charge of the case.

Novel Approaches

Novel approaches for treating cancer in animals are on the horizon. These new therapies may include: check point inhibitors in combination with harvesting cancer cells for culture and vaccine production; gene therapy using vaccines delivered via electroporation; targeted therapy using small molecules against certain cellular components; immunotherapy for specific tumor types; intratumor injections using jet guns or electrochemotherapy or radioisotopes, such as Yttrium 90, and the use of antiangiogenesis compounds. From the vast research and collaborative work being done in the field and with the help of CancerMoonShot2020, it seems apparent that these new treatments will be added to the arsenal of currently used anticancer techniques in the near future.

Novel therapies are designed to attack basic mechanisms of tumorigenesis and metastasis by a variety of cancers. It may be that after we cut, zap, burn, freeze, and poison the primary tumor, we will be able to arrest cancer's recurrence using novel medications. Ideally, we may soon be able to employ preventative strategies by using canine cancer vaccine "cocktails" that prevent OSA, LSA, and HSA (Modiano 2016). There will be smart, small, and stealthy molecules and monoclonal antibodies that target cancer's complex alphabet soup of multiple pathway signals and mechanisms, such as PD-L1, tyrosine kinase receptors, telomere-regulated apoptosis, angiogenesis, and micrometastasis.

Smart Molecules

Tyrosine kinase is the enzyme target for "smart" and small molecule drugs. Gleevec® (Imatinib, Mesylate) is an example of one of the first successfully used small molecule drugs. It inhibits a kinase in the abnormal Philadelphia chromosome found in chronic myelogenous leukemia (CML) patients. Gleevec blocks the receptor tyrosine kinase (RTK) kit at its adenosine triphosphate (ATP)-binding site. Another small molecule drug, Erbitux®, blocks the ability of cancer cells to absorb growth factors. Avastin® is a small molecule drug that thwarts angiogenesis. Other small molecule inhibitors of kinases that are potentially useful against cancer are Tarceva®, Iressa®, Cetuximab®, Astra®, Erptinob®, and Bevacizumab®. Be prepared to encounter and make good use of many other new products as they are released for clinical use.

Masitinib (Masivet®) is an RTK inhibitor developed by AB Science. Toceranib (Palladia®, SU11654) is a small molecule drug developed by Pfizer®, specifically as a veterinary product. They are intracellular competitive inhibitors of ATP at the RTK domain and inhibit *c-Kit* phosphorylation. Toceranib and masitinib cause tumor regression and inhibition of cell growth by inducing cell cycle arrest and apoptosis. These drugs have efficacy against various tumors. Dogs with mast cell tumors treated with toceranib had response rates ranging up to 55% (London 2004). The long-term efficacy, adverse events, oral dose scheduling, availability, and maintenance costs will affect how veterinarians incorporate these and other new smart drugs into the contemporary management of geriatric cancer patients.

Understanding proteomic technology is an esoteric endeavor. It requires an in-depth taste for the alphabet soup used to name the milieu of cellular proteins. Suffice it to say that breakthroughs in the aforementioned technologies may soon make them available and affordable for practical applications in veterinary oncology.

Your clients will soon be reading, in lifestyle magazines and on the Internet, about clinical trials using small molecule drugs as they are developed and marketed for targeted cancer therapy. They will know that this new class of drugs has broad efficacy against cancer, especially against mast cell tumors. If new drugs have tolerable adverse events and are affordable, people will want them to be used for their older pets with cancer. Therefore, an understanding of the tools of molecular biology, the concept of dysregulated cell signaling by cancer cells, and targeted therapy by small molecules should be incorporated into the contemporary veterinarian's approach toward the treatment of cancer in the geriatric patient.

Multimodality, Combinatorial Therapy

Multidisciplinary, multimodality, or combinatorial therapy for the treatment of cancer means that more than one method is used to treat a malignancy (Dobson, Cohen, and Gould 2004). Generally, this refers to using combinations of conventional surgery, radiation, and chemotherapy, but soon it will include immunotherapy or immuno-oncology. Proper sequencing of the various treatments may enhance the efficacy of multimodality therapy. For instance, some oncologists theorize that preoperative radiation therapy or stereotactic radiosurgery is more helpful than postoperative radiation therapy for large, aggressive sarcomas. Others, including myself, feel that intraoperative therapy is particularly effective. The advantages proposed for preoperative radiation therapy would be improved tumor control at surgery by shrinking the mass and destroying its tentacles and satellites. The advantages for intraoperative radiation therapy would be that the tumor bed is sterilized beyond the incision planes. In addition, chemotherapy may be added before surgery (neoadjuvant) or during surgery (intralesional/intracavitary). Revolutionary for surgical oncologists will be the use of fluorescence-based photodynamic imaging techniques that enhance the visualization of malignant tumor cells during surgery. This technology will improve the surgeon's ability to achieve adequate clean margins and identify involved sentinel lymph nodes (Lowik 2016).

Many caregivers want an aggressive surgical technique to address a malignant tumor on their geriatric pet but they do not want to subject their pet to repetitive follow-up treatments. The use of multimodality intraoperative techniques serves the wishes of these families well.

What is Integrative Therapy?

Integrative medicine is healing-oriented medicine that is informed by evidence and considers the whole patient. It emphasizes the relationship between doctor and patient or client and makes use of all appropriate healthcare therapies, both conventional and alternative/complimentary to achieve optimal health.

There is a recent trend for conventional practitioners to acknowledge the benefits and use of nutritional supplements and some "alternative" or complimentary medicine. Conventional practices embrace the nutrition and supplement field by marketing commercial diets that feature nutraceuticals, antioxidants, and evidence-based supplements. Specialized diets are formulated to treat chronic degenerative conditions associated with aging, such as arthritis, cognitive syndrome, hepatic, cardiac, and renal disease, cancer, and so forth. This concept opens a rational door into the field of chemoprevention, nutrigenomics, immunonutrition, and some aspects of complementary and alternative medicine.

Integrative therapy involves the simultaneous use of conventional therapy, including multimodality combinatorial therapy, along with some techniques of complimentary therapy that may enhance the overall treatment outcome. Complementary and alternative medicine (CAM) may include chemoprevention, immunonutrition using evidence-based supplements, acupuncture, chiropractic, massage therapy, herbal medicine, and so on. Many veterinarians use, suggest, or condone selected holistic remedies or preparations to treat specific chronic unresponsive conditions in their geriatric cancer patients.

Overall, the most important therapeutic ingredient to offer in geriatric oncology is supportive care for both the patients and their people.

The Role of Surgery in Cancer Management and "When Is It Too Much Surgery"

If we did the things we are capable of doing, we would literally astound ourselves.

Thomas Edison

Surgery is considered the most aggressive, hands-on approach for solid tumors. However, since the mechanisms of metastases often elude even the most aggressive radical surgeries, a multimodality, multidisciplinary combinatorial approach is now being used to improve patient survival. We must forever be aware of how the 100-year tenure of Halstead's radical breast resection beliefs ended with a paradigm shift. Despite conflict and emotional opposition, Dr. Bernard Fischer demonstrated no benefit with Halstead's radical mastectomy approach. He demonstrated that simple mastectomy and excision of involved lymph nodes, followed with or without regional radiation therapy, yielded similar survival times without the morbidity of aggressive surgery. Data were provided from multicenter clinical trials. Fischer's clinical trials developed and emphasized the importance of evidence-based medicine in the 1980s.

The same ethical issues are alive today with some MD pancreatic surgeons who stubbornly insist on up-front surgery instead of accepting the evidence that surgery following cytoreductive chemotherapy yields more cancer-free margins and longer survival times for patients with pancreatic carcinoma. The American Academy of Veterinary Surgeons asked me to answer the question: "*When is it too much surgery?*" for a potential keynote topic at their 2016 Surgical Summit. This concept turned into a day track titled, *Ethics in Surgical Decision Making*, with Dr. Erik Clary, ACVS. The bioethical issues discussed and opinions stated in this text are mine, based upon many years of experience. Review the three articles: *End of Life Medico-Ethical Decision Making in Veterinary Oncology*, *Preventing Over-Treatment*, and *Veterinary Hospice Care: Theory and Practice*, in the 2016 ACVS Proceedings.

Surgery is the mainstay treatment used for management of localized invasive tumors. The very first surgery performed on a mass is the single procedure that may give the geriatric cancer patient the best chance of survival. Therefore, the principles of surgical oncology are an important set of rules to apply diligently at the very first surgery. The preoperative workup, the surgical plan, the perioperative support, and client advice are just as important as the anesthesia and the surgical procedure when dealing with geriatric cancer patients.

Surgery is widely used in cancer management as a diagnostic tool to biopsy and to stage cancer. Surgery is also used frequently to debulk tumors (cytoreduction), to palliate life-threatening conditions (as with splenectomy for ruptured splenic hemangiosarcoma), and to reduce pain (as with amputation for osteosarcoma (OSA)). Surgery is used in cancer patients to bypass lesions, to remove obstructions, to relieve pressure exerted by a tumor, to establish drainage, to clear airways, and to place vascular access catheters and stents. Biliary stenting is a less invasive alternative to biliary rerouting to palliate dogs with extrahepatic biliary obstruction caused by pancreatic adenocarcinoma or bile duct carcinoma (Mayhew et al. 2006).

Surgical reconstruction and graft techniques are used to repair defects created by large mass excisions, tumor necrosis, and postradiation necrosis. Surgery is used to debride necrotic tumor tissue and wounds and repair extravasation defects. Cytoreductive surgery may correct abnormalities such as malignant hypercalcemia generating from anal sac carcinoma and other PTHrp-producing tumors. Surgery may correct disease syndromes from other hormone-producing tumors such as insulinomas, gastrinomas, Sertoli cell tumors, seminomas, and adrenal tumors in dogs. Surgical lobectomy is helpful for dogs with solitary primary pulmonary masses, while metastatectomy may help in selected cases. Hepatocellular carcinomas localized to a single liver lobe also benefit from lobectomy.

Surgery may prevent cancer. Spay and neuter programs reduce breast cancer incidence for many dog breeds except for Labrador and Golden Retrievers (Hart et al. 2014). Surgery to remove both mammary chains in feline breast cancer is considered the best preventative approach to extend survival when performed in early stage disease, prior to micrometastasis from the primary tumor.

Surgery is life-saving when used to remove obstructions, control splenic hemorrhage, excise masses, and keep lumens patent and functional. Surgery is also used in the management of cancer to place feeding tubes, vascular access ports, stents, and stomas, and to palliate painful lesions. Surgery is the best pain control for OSA. The alleviation of pain is one of the primary goals accomplished with amputation of an OSA limb.

Surgical oncologists will use fluorescence-based photodynamic imaging techniques that enhance the visualization of malignant tumor cells during surgery. This image-guided cancer surgery technology will improve the surgeon's ability to achieve adequate clean margins and identify involved sentinel lymph nodes (Lowik 2016).

Special Considerations for Surgery

Any and all surgical procedures performed on a geriatric cancer patient should be directed at improving the patient's well-being. In addition, the client's concept of well-being for his or her pet should be discussed and respected. When improper planning leaves the patient with no benefit from the procedure, surgery was clearly the wrong approach. It is easy to say "wrong approach" after the fact, but the veterinary surgeon must weigh the facts beforehand and operate when the risk–benefit ratio favors the geriatric oncology patient. Careful attention to perioperative supportive care of the geriatric patient creates a smooth recovery and minimal hospitalization period.

Surgery should never be recommended perfunctorily and prematurely. Surgery generally contributes added stress to the compromised geriatric patient and may cause more unintended harm than good. These cases should be managed with finesse to spare the patient the stress of surgery whenever possible. I am all for surgery when it is realistically expected to be helpful to the geriatric cancer patient.

Surgery should never be recommended as a single modality for debulking non-localized tumors. When used without follow-up modalities for overall tumor control, debulking surgery for metastatic tumors may be essentially unhelpful in winning prolonged longevity for the patient. Debulking surgery is especially stressful in frail geriatric and debilitated patients. In fact, surgery alone may actually hasten the patient's death. This effect was shown to be true for nasal passage cancer patients undergoing rhinotomy alone, but if they had radiation followed by rhinotomy for residual disease found on follow-up CT, they had longer survival times. Unfortunately, the best surgery and the best radiation therapy are still limited in their ability to cure cancer that is metastatic. Surgery and radiation therapy can be curative only for those patients that have completely localized tumors.

Every geriatric patient about to have surgery for a solid tumor would benefit from comprehensive preoperative diagnostics and thoughtful presurgical planning. Attention to the principles of surgical oncology and the aggressive pursuit of clean wide margins may successfully remove the entire mass. I like to use intraoperative cytology to assist the surgeon in pursuit of clean margins. With intraoperative cytology, for instance, a well-planned and successful maxillectomy or mandibulectomy in a dog may result in a cure for acanthomatous epulis and freedom from recurrence of local disease from fibrosarcoma or squamous cell carcinoma. The two latter cases often benefit with follow-up radiation therapy to increase the tumor-free interval.

For oral malignant melanoma, we can achieve excellent local control with surgical mandibulectomy or maxillectomy. Electroporation/electrochemotherapy and stereotactic radiation therapy are also great options to control difficult to excise oral tumors. However, we must expect metastasis at 10 months postsurgery. It is important to educate clients about the biological behavior and prognosis of malignant melanoma to help with decision making for follow-up therapy. Malignant melanoma patients need further therapy to address metastasis. Options include: harvesting cancer tissue for autologous dendritic cell vaccine production, using transdermal Oncept® Canine Melanoma Vaccine or another melanoma vaccine, and/or using carboplatin chemotherapy.

Amputations of limbs for locally aggressive sarcomas in dogs and cats may be curative for most cases where the tumor is distal enough for wide clean margins. If a large sarcoma is located in the proximal part of the limb and surgical margins are inadequate, recurrence is likely. This case would benefit from postoperative radiation therapy. This case may also benefit from debulking followed by intraoperative or postoperative electroporation/electrochemotherapy, with the intention to save the limb. If amputation is performed for a primary bone malignancy in the dog, further systemic therapy with carboplatin chemotherapy, metronomic chemotherapy, chemoprevention, and vaccine therapy is indicated to prolong or prevent metastases.

Scintigraphy uses radiomimetic chemicals to identify "hot spots" in bone. It is used prior to surgery, for staging, and to monitor progression of the disease on follow-up. If chest X-rays and the bone scan are negative, surgery has the potential to cure the patient. The best X-rays, CT, MRI, and scintigraphy cannot identify a single malignant cell, or even cell clusters. Always educate clients regarding our frustration with the potential for metastasis. Fusion or hybrid scanners that combine positron emission tomography (PET) with CT or MRI are more sensitive in their ability to detect small metastatic lesions than conventional imaging techniques.

With improved preoperative evaluation and staging of the mass using new and improved imaging techniques, more success is expected from surgery because the cases will be better selected. This is especially true with peripherally located brain tumors.

When a surgeon approaches the patient with the full intention to perform complete excisional biopsy of a sarcoma or carcinoma, the patient will have improved survival. The amputation of a limb for osteosarcoma generally does not prolong a dog's life span without follow-up carboplatin chemotherapy and the potential benefit of immunotherapy. Combinatorial innovative modalities, such as inhaled liposome encapsulated IL-2, IV immunomodulators, specific antitumor vaccine, Samarium 153 (bone-targeting radiopharmaceutical Quadramet®), metastatectomy, and small molecule therapy, may address metastasis and enhance survival times for OSA patients when used in addition to chemotherapy and vaccine therapy.

A General Rule of Thumb for Oncologic Surgery

There is a general rule of thumb that most general practice surgeons would do well to incorporate into their surgical plan when approaching an unknown mass. The strategic plan would be to remove a diameter of tissue laterally and ventrally around the primary tumor that is at least half of (optimally equal to) the size of the primary mass itself. If this plan were universally adopted, more pets could be spared second surgeries and recurrences, and more lives could be saved. For all mast cell tumors, the ideal margins are at least 2–3cm laterally and ventrally. For tumors that lay across bone, ligament, nerves, and other vital structures, at least one fascial plane should be removed below the mass. Otherwise, the surgery will be incomplete.

Most general practice surgery is unhelpful for cats with feline injection site sarcoma (FISS). Board certified surgeons and those surgeons who plan aggressively to achieve wider and deeper margins do create longer tumor-free intervals and potential cures for FISS cases. Surgery performed by the local practitioner for this vicious malignancy is best used strictly as an incisional diagnostic tool prior to referral of the case to a specialist for definitive surgery. I consider general surgery to be the wrong approach for FISS. This iatrogenic malignancy needs extreme measures with wide and deep margins at the very first excisional procedure to do the cat justice. Anything short of an early aggressive and definitive approach to the excision of a sarcoma is unjustified in today's knowledgeable atmosphere. The use of Merial's ALVAC®, a recombinant canarypox virus expressing the feline interleukin-2 (*IL-2*) gene, administered locally prior to excision or into the tumor bed after excision, has been shown to reduce recurrence of FISS and other tumor types.

Excisional biopsy of a large anal sac tumor that involves over half of the anal sphincter may cause fecal incontinence. The use of laser or radiation therapy may be better options to cytoreduce these cases. Excision of the caudal rectal area to remove tumors may cause permanent fecal incontinence. Electroporation/electrochemotherapy may also be very helpful in controlling anal sac tumors.

Multifocal mast cell cancer may be helped by surgery if the tumors are well differentiated, limited in number, and expected to be localized to no more than three areas. Surgery is unhelpful in widespread multifocal mast cell cancer. It is better to address all multifocal lesions with a systemic therapy than to attempt surgical removal.

Abdominal Surgery

The outcome for exploratory laparotomy has fewer surprises and is more successful if there has been appropriate presurgical evaluation. Abdominal X-rays are informative, but abdominal ultrasound and imaging with CT or MRI can reveal more information and make a big difference in decision making.

Cytoreductive surgery is very helpful in patients with hormone-producing tumors such as gastrinomas, insulinomas, adrenal tumors, and metastatic anal sac tumors associated with hypercalcemia in dogs. Dogs with massive hepatocellular carcinomas localized to the left liver lobe benefit more with lobectomy versus conservative medical management (Liptak et al. 2004). Many geriatric patients with liver tumors are poor surgical candidates due to high tumor burden, tumor location, involvement of vasculature, poor hepatic function, or a combination of these issues.Many locoregional ablation techniques have been developed for treatment of primary and secondary hepatic tumors in compromised patients such as: cryotherapy, chemoembolization, radioembolization using Y-90, laser ablation, electroporation, radiofrequency ablation, and microwave ablation (Yang et al. 2017).

Hemangiosarcoma Surgery

Emergency surgery to remove a bleeding splenic mass that is suspected to be hemangiosarcoma is very dramatic and can be immediately lifesaving. Hemangiosarcoma surgery does not spare the majority of geriatric oncology patients from the ravages of metastatic disease and death within 3 months. It is important for clients to be made aware of the prognosis prior to electing surgery. We can be more optimistic in recommending splenectomy because 60% of splenic lesions may be benign, as documented in the last 200 cases followed at the University of Minnesota (Personal Communication, Modiano 2016).

If the family declines surgery yet is reluctant to euthanize their pet, it is appropriate to allow the patient to be released with a consent form so the family has the opportunity to go home for the hospice vigil. There is no harm in offering some hope as some patients may stabilize because with rest and supportive care, the blood may be resorbed. Some dogs with hemoabdomen will stabilize within a few days with strict rest, a belly wrap, Yunnan Baiyao at 48mg/kg BID, and supportive care. Families appreciate the opportunity to have a more private and extended farewell with their pet during these days of quiet rest. I have received heartfelt thank you letters from pet owners who were able to enjoy precious time at home during the hospice vigil with their dog following acute hemoabdomen.

Breakthrough research from the labs of Drs. Modiano and Breen may completely change the outlook of surgery for patients with non-cutaneous hemangiosarcoma and for patients with a variety of other solid epithelial cancers. Earlier detection and targeted therapy for hemangiosarcoma is already on the horizon. Treatments with antiangiogenesis agents including Thalidomide may provide some value in combating angiogenesis, although Thalidomide is costly and not readily available (Woods, Mathews, and Binnington 2004). There is interest in using histone deacetylase (HDAC) inhibitors such as: Vrinostat (suberoylanilide hydroxamic acid, SAHA) and valproic acid. SAHA was given orally with no adverse events by Leonard Cohen, MD, to his 8-year-old Rhodesian Ridgeback named Molly, who survived hemangiosarcoma for 3 years (Cohen et al. 2004). SAHA was unable to help one of my patients, a 12-year-old intact Siberian Husky named Tushka with hepatic and splenic hemangiosarcoma, survive past 4 months. Researchers at Colorado State University (CSU) evaluated the antiproliferative and chemosensitizing effects of valproic acid (Thamm et al. 2006).

Treatments that target marrow-derived host cells and signaling mechanisms for angiogenesis and micrometastasis may help hemangiosarcoma and other vascular tumor patients survive longer after surgery. Small molecule inhibitors such as Gleevec or multiple kinase inhibitors such as toceranib and masitinib may help increase survival times following surgery (London 2004).

A "liquid biopsy" screening test for circulating hemangioblasts will identify hemangiosarcoma dogs before they become clinical and collapse. This test becomes clinically valuable because Modiano and his research colleagues have developed a targeted treatment using e-BAT, a toxin that targets two receptors that will destroy the circulating hemangioblasts in dogs that test positive (Schappa et al. 2013).

Transitional Cell Carcinoma and Surgery

Transitional cell carcinoma (TCC) of the bladder mimics cystitis and urinary tract infection (UTI) syndrome. High risk breeds and dogs with hematuria will benefit with early diagnosis using the CADET[SM] BRAF Detection Screening Assay developed at Dr. Matthew Breen's laboratories at NCSU and Sentinel Biomedical. This molecular assay can identify bladder cancer cells with the mutated BRAF gene using a free catch urine sample and may detect TCC up to 4 months before it becomes clinical. TCC is generally seeded extensively in the mucosal lining of the bladder, causing hematuria and stranguria. Most TCCs are located in the trigone area and generally have been too advanced at the time of diagnosis to expect surgery to be helpful. In fact, surgery is often unhelpful unless the mass is focal and located near the apex of the bladder. Because surgery may actually seed malignant transitional cells along the incision site, the surgeon must take great care to make a new surgical glove change and to use new clean instruments to close the incision. Otherwise the patient is at risk for contamination of the incision site with TCC cells that will grow in and along the abdominal incision.

Tumors at the apex of the bladder may be successfully operable. Some may be benign polyps but most often the masses are TCC infiltrating extensively into the bladder wall. On ultrasound examination, a thickened appearance of the bladder wall adjacent to a primary mass indicates tumor infiltration, which hinders surgical success.

TCC patients that seem to be candidates for surgery would benefit from presurgical cystoscopy to verify the diagnosis and to determine whether the mass can be completely removed. Areas of neovascularization can be sampled to determine the extent of TCC infiltration. It is very difficult for attending surgeons to determine the true extent of the TCC infiltration at the time of exploratory cystotomy. Selected TCC patients with tumors confined to the apex of the bladder may benefit from surgery if the margins are free of TCC cells. Using technology that illuminates malignant tissue at surgery would be very helpful in bladder cancer surgery.

Cystoscopy to examine the bladder wall may be the most useful tool following ultrasound to actually determine whether surgery would be the right or the wrong approach. Procedures that remove the bladder and route the ureters into the distal colon have not yielded satisfactory clinical results. This procedure has failed to increase overall survival times due to metastatic disease.

Creating a stoma for urine to exit the bladder has been helpful in selected cases with outflow obstruction of the urethral lumen from trigonal and urethral TCC. The procedure for use of low-profile cystostomy tubes was described in four dogs and one cat. The patients were more comfortable and had more mobility with the low profile tubes (Stiffler et al. 2003). The pet owner evacuates urine on a regular basis. I believe that cystostomy is a viable palliative option to offer selected TCC patients because it provides relief and clearly solves a life-threatening dilemma. Ureteral and urethral stenting are sophisticated procedures, which are potentially life-extending options for TCC patients.

Prostate Cancer and Surgery

Prostate surgery has been considered unhelpful in dogs because the canine prostate gland is intimately involved with the prostatic urethra. Prostatectomy can benefit selected cases where neoplastic tissue is confined within the capsule and there is minimal to no urethral involvement. Imaging technology and exploratory surgery are both required to determine if the patient has an operable prostatic tumor. The surgeon must use caution to avoid complications and incontinence (Henderson 2004). Stereotactic radiosurgery (SRS), also known as CyberKnife Radio Surgery, may be very helpful in sparing local tissues.

Male cats have tiny prostate glands that rarely develop malignancy and are generally not operable. I have only cared for two cats with prostate cancer in 45 years of practicing oncology. For one 13-year-old DSH cat, Shakespeare Rapheal, a debulking surgery and an open cystostomy, that permitted the drainage of urine, was lifesaving. Chemotherapy with mitoxantrone and piroxicam cytoreduced a 3cm recurrence, allowing Shakespeare a 1-year survival. The second case was Boukie Cohen, a 16-year-old DSH with a heart murmur. Boukie developed urinary obstruction from a malignant prostate tumor. Urine outflow was reestablished with urinary catheter placement. Surgery was not attempted. Chemotherapy with mitoxantrone every 21 days and piroxicam 1mg daily reduced the prostatic mass and allowed normal urine outflow after 7 days. After 6 treatments, he was switched to carboplatin. Boukie developed splenomegaly, reactive lymphadenopathy, and extensive non-painful cutaneous metastases from his prostatic carcinoma during the last 6 months of his 1-year survival in Pawspice care.

Detailed descriptions for surgical oncology excisions of various tumor types and locations are described elsewhere in numerous texts. Please refer to Chapters 18, 19, and 20 by Dr. Kathleen Salisbury in W.B. Morrison's (2002) book *Cancer in Dogs and Cats: Medical and Surgical Management*, and to related texts for in-depth information.

Freddy's Case (Control Multifocal Mast Cell Tumors without Surgery)

Freddy, a 9-year-old M/N Golden Retriever–German Shepherd Dog mix, with a history of colitis and inflammatory bowel disease, suddenly developed multifocal skin tumors extending over his neck, shoulders, and back. His attending veterinarian removed most of the tumors. They ranged from 1 to 3cm in size. Histology diagnosed the tumors to be moderately to poorly differentiated, multifocal mast cell tumors (MCTs) with moderate to marked mitotic activity (high grade). The lateral and deep margins were complete but narrowly excised at less than 0.1cm, and therefore inadequate. The prognosis was fair to guarded. When Freddy came in for his first oncology consultation, he had sprouted 20 new tumors and some were growing in between the sutures. Multiple cutaneous MCTs in dogs are generally associated with a low rate of metastasis and a good prognosis with adequate excision (Mullins et al. 2006).

All of Freddy's tumors regressed rapidly following one treatment with 2mg/m^2 of vinblastine IV, oral prednisone at 40mg/m^2 PO daily for 7 days, tapering to every other day. He also received chlorambucil 6mg every other day PO. Freddy received weekly injections for 2 months, tapering to monthly maintenance. Freddy's caregivers elected to discontinue his maintenance protocol after he remained tumor free for 8 months. Freddy remained in complete remission for 1 year, at which time he developed inoperable intestinal carcinoma.

Sage's Case (Aggressive Surgery and RTx Curative for Five-Time Recurrent Hemangiopericytoma)

Sage, a 12-year-old M/N Whippet, had five surgeries on his left front leg for hemangiopericytoma. Sage's owner was determined to save the leg due to chronic arthritis. We approached this as a three-step multimodality procedure. Step 1 was to surgically remove the recurrent mass with a deep wide excision, followed by intraoperative radiation therapy. The wound was wrapped with a wet-to-dry bandage daily and left as an open wound to await the histology report. The biopsy reported clean but narrow margins. Step 2 followed a week later, when the wound was debrided and closed with an axial pattern flap graft. Step 3 was provided as follow-up external beam radiation therapy delivered in 10 fractions. Sage had no further recurrence over a 3-year follow-up period.

A Letter to Every Surgeon (Please Read Before Recommending Surgery)

I have often thought of writing the ideal letter to members of our profession who are planning to remove a potentially malignant tumor from a geriatric patient. I will take this opportunity to realize that wish. I hope that every surgeon will heed the advice in the following letter.

Dear Colleague,

This geriatric cancer patient would benefit if you were actually able to completely excise the mass with your first surgery. If your intention is not to provide definitive surgery (such as mandibulectomy for an oral melanoma or a wide and deep excisional biopsy for a mast cell tumor or vaccine-associated sarcoma), your client must be made aware of this.

Would this pet be better off if you perform an incisional biopsy of the primary mass and regional lymph nodes today as a diagnostic, grading, and staging procedure? If so, please do so at this time. Rather than upsetting the tissue planes infiltrated by the mass with an inadequate excisional procedure, please consult with an oncologist and refer the case to a board certified surgeon for definitive en block resection. This plan is more likely to provide the patient a greater tumor-free interval.

If you decide to proceed, then do so with wide and deep margins around the mass. If you consider the following oncologic procedures, your patients may survive longer and your success rate in curing certain cancers may soar.

Please perform an FNA cytology or impression smear of the mass, stain it with new methylene blue, and examine the cells. This takes 2 minutes of your time, but it is worth it because you will then know if you are dealing with a mast cell tumor or a sarcoma. Draw a line around the mass with ink and pre-place deep sutures to keep your margins intact during the excision. Remove the mass and a cuff of normal tissue on all planes around it without cutting into the mass itself. Mark the deep margin with India ink. For large masses, slice them at 1cm intervals for fixation and place each margin in a separate well-marked biopsy bottle.

Provide the pathologist with information about the mass and the surgical margins. Illustrate the location and size of the mass on a cartoon map for the pathologist and for the medical record and also write down the size of the deep and lateral margin excision around the tumor. Leave metal clips in place to show the complete extent of the borders of your excision in the event the pet is referred for radiation therapy. This information is vital because the entire surgical field is considered to be potentially seeded with cancer cells if the mass is incompletely resected. This information will also help to determine shrinkage. Margins around the excised tumor may have been 2cm on the gross cut, but they may be reported as a third to a half of the actual operative margin due to shrinkage in formalin.

A new gold standard for all veterinary surgeons might be to create, around a mass, surgical margins that are, at the very least, the same size as the tumor itself. This means a 2cm diameter tumor would have 2cm wide margins. If margins are questionable, and it is feasible to use open wound management, then do not perform wound closure/reconstruction until the pathology report is accessible. Once again, please be certain to clearly illustrate and document the extent of the operative margins in the medical chart as part of the surgery report. Send the pathologist a copy of the surgical report as well as a cartoon map indicating the location and size of the mass. Mark the tissue's cranial, caudal, dorsal, ventral, or deep margins with sutures or India ink to provide orientation and a marking code for the pathologist, especially with large tumors.

Please do not send your pathologist a large tissue section in a small bottle. Avoid placing samples that are over 1cm in thickness into small formalin containers. Please slice large tissue samples as if you were cutting a loaf of bread into 1cm slices. Use a larger bottle to send large tumor tissues to the lab in a 1:10 ratio of tissue to formalin.

If you prefer to use only the small formalin bottles provided from your diagnostic laboratory, then follow this margin evaluation method: cut a rim of tissue from the periphery of the mass and wind it flat on a gauze pad like an onion or cinnamon roll, starting with the cranial end on the inside of the roll. Place this rolled sample in formalin and send it to the pathologist along with samples of the mass.

Another technique to satisfy the curious oncologist is to cut new strips of tissue from the peripheral and deep margin of the tumor bed following excision of the mass. Be sure to mark the strips well with suture or India ink for orientation markers as well. These extra steps provide an excellent method for your pathologist to survey the cutaneous and deep margins. Then, when an oncologist or radiation therapist is asked to consult for follow-up therapy on the case, he or she will be able to review the pathology report and understand the patient's exact situation.

If you don't want to prepare samples in this way, most pathologists will accept larger samples. Keep the entire specimen refrigerated and properly packaged in a chilled container. Arrange for same-day transport and arrival of the sample at the laboratory. Be sure to mark the medial and anterior edges of the sample for orientation.

Lymph Node Cytology
For assessment of the local lymph nodes, perform FNA cytology on the draining lymph nodes before surgery. The FNA may be performed during surgery (intraoperative cytology) as well. If the lymph

node(s) cytology is positive, removal is indicated. If a lymph node is not enlarged and is FNA negative, then it is recommended to leave it in place. Please remove the local draining lymph node for staging of all oral and lip malignant melanoma cases. If you are performing a radical mastectomy, please locate and remove the inguinal and axillary nodes. Remove these nodes if you are removing the fifth or first mammary glands in a partial chain mastectomy for staging and prognostic purposes.

Exploratory Celiotomy
During exploratory laparotomy, please take samples of the liver and other involved organs and of enlarged lymph nodes during surgery. If the patient is a lymphoma suspect, consider examining or sending an impression smear for cytology for an immediate answer (intraoperative cytology). This may assist patient support while the confirmation from the biopsy specimen is pending.

As soon as the biopsy report comes in, especially if it is lymphoma, seek consultation from an advising veterinary oncologist to formulate a treatment plan. In some cases, especially with lymphoma, the patient will need immediate follow-up treatment to control and/or downstage the malignancy so that it will not skip to a higher stage. Make every attempt to prevent recurrence and deterioration of the patient during the postoperative recovery phase.

If a geriatric patient is sick from the effects of abdominal neoplasia, and if there is no access to ultrasound or if ultrasound is not affordable, the attending veterinarian is justified in making the recommendation for exploratory laparotomy. In cases like this, secure a written agreement with the family that allows euthanasia if the mass is considered inoperable. We do this in the geriatric patient's best interest to avoid struggling with recovery and to bypass the expected difficulties of recovery and poor quality of life for the geriatric oncology patient as the malignancy progresses.

Lola's Case (An Inoperable Abdominal Mass Was Tamed)

Lola, an 8-year-old F/S Bassett Hound, presented with weight loss, anorexia, and vomiting. On physical exam, a huge mesenteric mass was palpated. Radiographs showed no involvement with intestines and no other organomegaly. Initial FNAs were non-diagnostic on cytology slides. Exploratory laparotomy was recommended. The attending surgeon felt the mass was inoperable due to endangerment of the mesenteric vasculature feeding a large section of intestine. There was no obstruction. Samples were taken for histopathology. Lola's family did not want euthanasia at the time of the exploratory. Wound closure was routine and Lola recovered uneventfully except for vomiting, which was treated symptomatically. The biopsy report diagnosed lymphoma. Lola received combination chemotherapy and lived 4 wonderful years in complete remission. Three years into her remission, Lola was featured as a cancer survivor in a local magazine article.

Reconstructive Surgery

Wide surgical margins are necessary to excise the tentacles of neoplastic lesions (see Figure 5.7). Due to improved anesthesia techniques and perioperative pain control, geriatric dogs and cats are able to better survive prolonged surgical procedures. The reconstructive procedure necessary to cover large defects may be as challenging as the primary excision itself. Radical, aggressive excisional surgery that employs reconstruction techniques is the most effective procedure for cure of localized and slow-to-metastasize neoplasms. Tension-free wound closure using Z-plasty and staggered parallel incisions can be very helpful. Axial pattern flaps can be used to cover large areas left open by radical surgical excisions of large tumors. Full-thickness mesh grafts are excellent options to cover open wound beds located in difficult to close areas where the wound is uneven or requires movement (Tobias et al. 2004). The use of engineered tissue products such as extracellular matrix bioscafold technology may be very helpful to stimulate healing for wound closure at difficult sites (Norsworthy 2005). The most important consideration for tumor removal in the geriatric oncology patient is for the surgeon to do the first surgery correctly. This approach requires knowledge of the tumor type, its anatomical extent, and careful presurgical planning with reconstruction techniques for viable wound closure.

Summary: The Role of Surgery in Cancer Management

The Veterinary Society of Surgical Oncologists (www.vsso.org) held its first meeting to honor Dr. Steven Withrow's retirement from his long leadership career at the Animal Cancer Center at CSU. The 2012 book, *Veterinary Surgical Oncology*, provides comprehensive coverage of surgical treatments for cancer and is an invaluable decision-making tool and an essential reference. Well-planned surgical oncology with careful hemostasis and gentle tissue handling is life-saving for many geriatric cancer patients. Anesthesia recovery and healing may be prolonged in older animals due to paraneoplastic syndromes, reduced functional reserve, and comorbidities associated with aging and senescence. Surgical intervention leaves geriatric cancer patients more challenged with the issues of recovery and tissue healing. Excellent perioperative support and decision making regarding intraoperative and interventional procedures, adjuvant chemotherapy, or radiation therapy are imperative so that the geriatric cancer patient may have the best chance for a good quality of life. The attending doctor must provide the timeliest options for follow-up management of high grade neoplasia, especially high grade lymphoma. For more information read "Thinking Surgeon or Cutting Surgeon: To Be or Not to Be?" (Osborne 2001). Look for clinical trials that may benefit the patient at the AVMA Animal Health Studies Database at https://ebusiness.avma.org/aahsd/study_search.aspx/.

Chemotherapy in the Management of Geriatric Cancer

> Wisdom is a blend of many attributes in addition to knowledge. They include understanding, discernment, thinking ability, intelligence, experience, diligence, shrewdness and good judgment.

Dr. Carl A. Osborne, DVM, PhD, ACVIM

Chemotherapy is the use of agents with the intention to kill viable cancer cells to retain quality of life and increase survival. It is currently the standard treatment used for control of many types of cancers, especially those that constantly shed cells that contribute to the metastatic process. Aging is associated with the progressive decline of physiologic organ system reserves, total body water, circulating plasma proteins, and hemoglobin concentration. These factors affect the pharmacokinetics and pharmacodynamics of the various chemotherapy drugs used in older cancer patients. The attending doctor must be knowledgeable and flexible with the dosing and administration of chemotherapy drugs for all geriatric pets. The clinician must have a working diagnosis and staging information and be mindful of the variability and vulnerability of the individual geriatric dog or cat. An older animal's physiologic age, chronologic age, body condition, and overall performance and health status must be evaluated and stabilized to minimize drug toxicity.

Chemotherapy dose adjustments are recommended for older patients with concurrent renal disease, cardiac compromise, and/or severe hepatic insufficiency, since the liver is the main site of drug metabolism. Geriatric pets fare best with a strategy that is mindful of using drugs offering dose flexibility. If we spread the total dose of oral and IV chemotherapy over 4 to 8 days, we can maximize absorption and minimize toxicity for the geriatric patient (Cova and Balducci 2004).

Handling Chemotherapy Drugs Safely

In general, caution must be taken with staff and surroundings when chemotherapeutic agents are being used. Safety glasses, chemotherapy gloves, gowns, and masks must be worn by all personnel who handle the preparations or hold the patient for administration. Precautions to prevent aerosolizing chemotherapy drugs should be used. Place gauze at the neck of drug vials or use a special aspiration filter (PhaSeal™) when aspirating chemotherapy agents into syringes. Laminar flow hoods are required in pharmacies and clinics that dispense large volumes of chemotherapeutic agents (Takada 2003).

Special containers are needed for disposal of used drug vials, needles, and syringes. A chemotherapy spill kit should be readily available to the entire staff. The drug material safety data (MSD) sheets must be available to all staff. Occupational Safety and Health Administration (OSHA) regulations and recommendations must be carefully observed when using chemotherapeutic agents. (See instructions for handling chemotherapy drugs in the "Suggested Reading for Medical Oncology" section at the end of this chapter.)

Classification of Chemotherapy Drugs

Chemotherapy drugs are classified as alkylating agents, antimetabolites (analogs), antibiotics, anthracyclines, enzymes, hormones, plant alkaloids, taxanes, Platinol®-containing drugs, topoisomerase inhibitors, metalloproteinase inhibitors, telomerase inhibitors, protein kinase inhibitors, angiogenesis inhibitors, small molecules, and so forth. A growing number of drugs, such as NSAIDs, tamoxifen, metformin, and rapamycin, are often considered as chemoprevention drugs, and some for their antiangiogenic action, pathway signaling inhibition action, cytostatic activities, etc. These drugs may be used in combination with conventional and metronomic chemotherapy agents. A growing number of natural extracts, compounds, and supplements, considered as immunonutrition agents, have demonstrated the ability to enhance macrophage, natural killer cell, and cytokine activity, and they may also fall into the category of chemoprevention agents. A new class of drug therapy that may prevent hemangiosarcoma is being developed by Dr. Jaime Modiano, PhD and researchers at the University of Minnesota for treatment of dogs that have tested positive with early detection testing (Shine On Project) or have had surgery for hemangiosarcoma. The drug is a bispecific ligand-targeted bacterial toxin (BST, e-BAT) that eliminates circulating tumor initiating hemangioblasts. Enrollment for clinical trials on-site will be accessible via the AVMA Clinical Trials Database at: https://ebusiness.avma.org/aahsd/study/_search.aspx.

Terminology for Applied Chemotherapy

Clinicians should be familiar with the basic use and terminology for the various methods and routes in the application of chemotherapy.

The initial use of chemotherapy for responsive tumors such as lymphoma is called the *induction* phase. It generally requires more intense and more frequent dosing with the goal of achieving a complete remission (CR). The patient's response may be described as achieving CR, partial remission (PR), stable disease (SD), or progressive disease (PD). The next phase of chemotherapy is called the *consolidation* phase, which aims to destroy cancer cells that remain after induction.

Maintenance therapy is the use of pulsed doses or lower doses at less frequent intervals to sustain remission. When the patient relapses, the original induction protocol is given as *reinduction* chemotherapy. *Rescue* or *salvage* chemotherapy employs different drugs and/or protocols after frontline chemotherapy has failed the patient. The use of maintenance chemotherapy for lymphoma is controversial (Simon et al. 2005; Rosenthal 2001). Long term maintenance chemotherapy has always been my preference for lymphoma management as we are able to monitor patients more carefully.

Rescue therapy is the use of induction drug protocols or the use of other drugs to treat relapsed lymphoma patients. There are many rescue protocols to offer clients as options, but the first remission is considered the longest and second remission is expected to be half as long as the first remission, and so forth. Rabacfosadine (Tanovea™), a small molecule that inserts into tumor cell DNA, became widely available in 2017 as a 30 minute IV infusion every 21 days for dogs with resistant lymphoma. It may also be used as first-line therapy in lymphoma, multiple myeloma, and cutaneous lymphoma. Carers are cautioned to take extra care when handling and cleaning up after their dog for five days after treatment.

Each chemotherapy drug has a specific *nadir*, the period when the drug exerts its maximum myelosuppressive effect, which is manifested by low white blood cells, low platelets, or anemia. The nadir is the time when we expect leukopenia and it may span for several days. The nadir starts at a certain point such as 7 or 10–12 days following administration of a specific drug (Chun, Garrett, and MacEwen 2001; Morrison 2002). Some cancer patients may develop a prolonged thrombocytopenia from drugs such as lomustine, chlorambucil, or carboplatin. When a cancer patient develops pancytopenia, it is important to determine if the marrow hypoplasia is caused by the chemotherapy or a neoplastic or immune-mediated mechanism (Kearns and Ewing 2006).

Adverse events (AEs) are unfavorable and unintended side effects, problems, or reactions associated with treatment. A consensus document from the Veterinary Cooperative Oncology Group describing common terminology for AEs (VCOG-CTCAE) was reprinted in the December 2016 issue of *Veterinary and Comparative Oncology*. It employs a clinical grading scale of severity from 1 to 5. AEs are graded as mild (1), moderate (2), severe (3), life-threatening/disabling (4), or death related to AE (5), within various categories such as GI, blood/bone marrow, cardiac, renal/genitourinary, metabolic, and so forth (Vail et al. 2004, 2011).

Combination Chemotherapy in Geriatric Pets

It is well understood that combination chemotherapy is more effective in gaining remission and cure than treatment with a single-agent protocol. Most geriatric pets are able to tolerate combination chemotherapy if the oncologist is careful to adjust the dose to avoid toxicity and AEs. The selection and sequencing interval of drugs included in various combinatorial protocols are designed to accomplish three goals that are not possible with single-agent therapy: (1) To maximize cell kill without toxicity to the host; (2) to provide a broader range of coverage to heterogeneous, mutant/resistant cells; and (3) to prevent and slow the emergence of resistant clones. The dose–toxicity relationship and the nadir of each drug selected for a protocol should be known by the attending doctor who orders the administration of the drugs. Proper client education will help prepare caregivers to anticipate and offset adverse events using the items (thermometer, antinausea Rx, antidiarrhea Rx, and antibiotics) in their "Cancer Care Package". Geriatric patients generally benefit from combination chemotherapy. However, the protocols should be tailored to their specific body condition and functional reserves.

For Dogs

At best, chemotherapy has an 85–94% chance of creating remission in lymphoma and myeloma, and just over 50% efficacy in mast cell tumors. For most other tumor types, it yields only 20–33% response or is considered palliative. Despite treatment with combination chemotherapy, most high-grade malignancies such as hemangiosarcoma and osteosarcoma patients do not achieve long term survival. Hemangiosarcoma dogs develop early resistance and metastasis with median survival from 3 to 6 months (Sorenmo et al. 2000). This situation may change after the Shine On Project is complete.

Most dogs and cats handle chemotherapy very well. The veterinarian administering chemotherapy must be mindful of potential side effects and prepare pet owners to recognize them and treat them properly. Poodles, Scottish and other long hair Terriers, Maltese, and Shih Tzu breeds have a continuously growing (anagen phase) hair cycle and may develop alopecia (especially with the use of Adriamycin). The hair coat generally grows back 2 months after discontinuation of chemotherapy.

For Cats

At best, chemotherapy achieves remission in up to 87% of cats with lymphoma (Milner et al. 2005). Response can only be assessed during treatment. There is a need to identify indicators that will allow for prognostication for response before treatment (Limmer et al. 2016). Chemotherapy only provides 20–33% improvement in other types of cancer. In general, cats handle chemotherapy very well but they ***cannot*** tolerate cisplatin, 5-FU, or capecitabine (Xeloda®). Cats may have anorexia following chemotherapy but exhibit less nausea and vomiting than dogs, and they do not lose their fur. In shaved areas, the fur will grow back very slowly and may be a darker color. After 1 year of chemotherapy, cats have a velvety texture to their coat and their whiskers fall out. Whiskers will not grow back until chemotherapy is discontinued.

Neoadjuvant Chemotherapy

Neoadjuvant therapy is the use of chemotherapy at the earliest possible time in a treatment plan to cytoreduce a mass. It is most often used prior to surgery or perioperatively. In addition to cytoreduction, neoadjuvant therapy may reduce the metastatic potential of a tumor as it is manipulated during surgery. Neoadjuvant therapy given prior to surgery is difficult to justify in geriatric oncology. A major concern would be that the older patient might be overburdened with the stress of anesthesia, surgery, and immunosuppression from the drug, resulting in complications. It is very helpful and life-saving in high grade lymphoma following surgery if the patient has a good recovery.

Directed Chemotherapy

Special uses and delivery of chemotherapy are particularly appealing for geriatric patients. Directed chemotherapy, for example, is the delivery of drugs by one of the following methods: into the tumor (intralesional, intratumoral), into the tumor bed (intracavitary), intraperitoneal, intrathoracic, intrathecal, intraluminal, inhalational, organ-directed therapy such as liver-directed therapy, and so forth. Some chemotherapy drugs are encapsulated into STEALTH® liposomes such as Doxil®. It accumulates in tumor tissue and extravasates to deliver doxorubicin HCL into a leaky vascular tumor bed. Some liposomes will keep a drug active for a longer period of time. Liposome encapsulation may reduce the toxicity of some drugs.

Electrochemotherapy also known as electroporation, is a technology that uses specific electrical impulses to cause cancer cells to absorb circulating or intralesional bleomycin 1,000 times. It also causes cancer cells to absorb intralesional cisplatin 10 times. This chemoablative technology results in cell necrosis. See the section below written by Dr. Robson Pasquale of Brazil, which describes this technology in greater detail.

HylaPlat™ is cisplatin conjugated with hyaluronan, a polymer occurring naturally in the body, to create nanoparticles. When injected directly into tumors in dogs, many experienced tumor reduction or regression. HylaPlat spreads into the lymphatics and adheres to CD44 hyaluronan receptors on metastatic tumor cells that slowly take up the cisplatin. This conjugated nanotechnology can be used with docetaxol or doxorubricin (HylaDox™) to treat various tumor types while confining the chemotherapy drug to the tumor and lymphatics and avoiding adverse events (HylaPharm.com 2016).

Yittrium 90 (Y-90) is an affordable isotope that has been used by interventional oncologists for transarterial radioembolization and angiosomal (segmental) ablation for liver tumors in humans (Toskich 2016). Y-90 has been formulated into a microsphere solution that can be mixed with a polymer solution immediately prior to intralesional injection of accessible tumors. The patient's body temperature causes the polymer to transform to a gel that traps the Y-90 microspheres in place (IsoPetSolutions.com 2016).

A multimodality protocol may have patients receiving intracavitary chemotherapy and high fraction intraoperative radiation therapy before surgical closure. After a 10–14 day waiting period, the patient may receive follow-up external beam radiation therapy to the tumor field along with systemic chemotherapy, concurrently or in sequence. Some patients may receive intralesional chemotherapy prior to radiation therapy in a series of treatments to cytoreduce tumors, especially oral, head, and neck tumors. Dogs with carcinomatosis, sarcomatosis, or mesothelioma (with or without malignant effusion) that were given intraperitoneal or intrathoracic mitoxantrone and/or carboplatin survived 10 months longer than untreated cases (Charney et al. 2005).

Intralesional Chemotherapy

Many geriatric cancer patients will not be allowed to have general anesthesia for definitive surgery or receive systemic chemotherapy to control their tumors. However, their caregivers may be willing to try other convenient, less toxic options such as intralesional chemotherapy. We can use this technique to infiltrate surgical excision sites of incompletely resected masses. The most common tumors and tumor beds that we inject are mast cell tumors, hemangiopericytomas, fibrosarcomas, and squamous cell carcinoma (SCC).

Direct local delivery is accomplished with syringe injection to infiltrate chemotherapy along closely spaced gridlines to evenly infiltrate the mass and the area surrounding it. Jet guns, which use air pressure to drive the drug through the skin into the mass, are also feasible for intralesional delivery of chemotherapy at an estimated depth. Local hyperthermia may also be used to enhance the effect of intralesional or regional chemotherapy.

Chemotherapy agents are emulsified with various matrix vehicles to keep the drug in the tumor tissue. Matrix agents commonly used for intralesional injections of tumors include medical grade bovine collagen, sesame seed oil, safflower oil, and autologous serum. Intralesional chemotherapy is an excellent palliative option for geriatric cancer patients, although it yields variable results (Kitchell 1993; Theon 1990–1994; Weisse 2004; Goldstein 2004; Hahn 2005).

Carboplatin and 5-FU are the most common chemotherapy agents used for intralesional chemotherapy in our practice. In the past, we have used other agents such as BCG vaccine (for malignant melanoma), cisplatin, linoleic acid, inositol hexaphosphate (for fibrosarcomas), and, more recently, *Agaricus* extract (from *Agaricus blasei* mushroom) for hemangiopericytoma, various other sarcomas, melanoma, and mammary carcinoma, with some surprising successes.

Topical and Intralesional Immunotherapy

Intralesional delivery techniques may also be used to deliver agents that may help the immune system recognize and destroy tumor cells. For decades, the anticancer biologic response modifier, *Bacillus Calmette-Guerin* (BCG), was applied over scarified skin and directly on malignant melanomas in people, with some sporadic responses. BCG is currently used in people with early stage bladder cancer as a weekly infusion into the bladder for 6 weeks and then monthly for 6–12 months. My mentor, Dr. Gordon Theilen, conducted a clinical trial using BCG applied by scarification for canine lymphoma and osteosarcoma in the 1970s. Imiquimod, tacrolimus, and sirolimus (rapamycin) are topical ointments with immunomodulator effects. They can be used on superficial lesions of carcinoma in situ, squamous cell carcinoma, and basal cell carcinoma for their local antitumor effects. One clinical trial at Northwestern used imiquimod topically on accessible metastatic malignant melanomas twice daily followed by 6 joules of cold laser treatment (using a MicroLight 830 nm laser) applied every other week to enhance its antitumor effect. Preparations may be diluted and given intralesionally or topically.

Intralesional injections with agents that can stimulate a local response may be helpful. Immunocidin™ is a non-specific immunotherapy product with DNA from a non-pathogenic strain of a mycobacterium cell wall fraction. It has the potential to cause regression of mammary and squamous cell carcinomas and melanomas and it may be infused into the bladder of patients with transitional cell carcinoma (TCC) as BCG is used to treat human bladder cancer. Immunocidin induces a strong cell mediated response and may be given into tumors before surgical excision and/or after (www.immunocidin.com). Since the CADETSM® free catch urine test may identify patients with TCC up to 4 months before they show clinical signs, treatment with Immunocidin makes sense. It would be difficult for me to rationalize giving chemotherapy to these patients when there is not yet any tumor growth.

Merial has a recombinant canarypox virus that expresses feline interleukin 2 (ALVAC IL-2™). It is used as adjuvant immunotherapy when given SQ at postsurgical tumor sites. It was shown to significantly increase time to relapse in cats that had excision of feline injection site sarcoma (FISS) and treated with iridium-based brachytherapy. Intralesional gene therapy and cancer vaccines may also help tumors regress. Immunomodulation products administered via the intralesional approach may benefit geriatric cancer patients with other tumor types.

Lymphocyte T-cell Immunomodulator (LTCI®), also known as T-Cyte™ (tcyte.com), is a signaling protein for T-cells. It was first approved for use to help cats with FeLV and FIV by increasing CD-4 lymphocyte numbers and function and *IL-2* production and hematopoiesis. T-Cyte can also be injected into warts and cutaneous mycosis fungoides lesions, resulting in regression. Patients on

T-Cyte should not be given steroids or NSAIDs. In 2016, T-Cyte was approved for alleviation of osteoarthritis symptoms. Therefore, LTCI may provide a dual benefit for geriatric cancer patients with arthritis as it did for $13^1/_2$-year-old yellow Lab, Lotus Phan.

Lotus' Case (Combinatorial Therapy for STS and OA)

Lotus Phan had several multiple soft tissue sarcomas (STSs) that were not treated for over 2 years due to family reluctance to use chemotherapy and aggressive surgery. We offered a non-aggressive surgical plan for the large STS on her right foreleg. We gave intralesional T-Cyte before surgery with a plan to make IFx® vaccine from her excised tumor. We used T-Cyte given intralesionally in predebulking surgery. Our plan was to give it SQ postop while waiting for her IFx vaccine to arrive. The large STS on her right front leg was debulked along with her other STSs and all the tumor beds were treated with electroporation. The tumor tissue was sent for IFx vaccine production. Lotus was treated with T-Cyte SQ weekly along with cold laser therapy using the MicroLight 830 nm laser. Four weeks postop, she received 4 weekly doses of IFx vaccine and laser therapy to the electroporation wound sites to facilitate healing. Lotus became more active at each follow-up visit. At her 2 month recheck, for her 5th IFx vaccine, her carer reported that Lotus had more energy and wanted to take longer walks. Lotus Phan achieved a very successful result using combinatorial treatment, which had a dual effect: to help her immune system and to treat her arthritis. These options helped the carers treat their beloved Lotus without using conventional chemotherapy.

Further investigation using immunomodulators and immunotherapy is warranted, especially since the CancerMoonShot2020 is promoting immunotherapy. It is not unusual to find that some anticancer treatments also have other actions that will benefit geriatric patients, such is the case with the use of low dose rapamycin, a drug used to suppress the immune system to attenuate organ transplant rejection, which also has anticancer action via the mTOR pathways. Rapamycin is being evaluated in a large clinical trial through the Dog Aging Project (see more details below). We must be vigilant and aware that immunotoxicities may result from using any form of immunotherapy and/or immunomodulators. Adverse events may generate grade 1–5 severity and often need prompt attention.

Locoregional Tumor Treatments with Interventional Radiology

Interventional radiology (IR) is increasingly being used in veterinary medicine. Minimally invasive surgery with interventional techniques yields less morbidity and mortality and may treat tumors that are difficult to access. This holds promise for geriatric patients. Interventional oncology is called the fourth pillar of human oncology therapy because of the vast array of new options (Weisse 2014). Interventional oncologists collaborate with surgical oncologists, medical oncologists, and radiation oncologists playing a role that spans from neoadjuvant to definitive to palliative applications. Often these procedures can be performed safely with negligible morbidity (Toskich 2016).

This outpatient technology can be very beneficial for the geriatric cancer patient. IR uses 3-D imaging, fluoroscopy, or ultrasound to guide the delivery of antitumor agents into the vasculature of non-resectable and metastatic tumors. The agents are designed or compounded to cause tumor embolization (embolotherapy) and localized cell death. With this growing sub-specialty, geriatric cancer patients have another option for locoregional tumor cell kill at lower overall systemic doses. Ultrasound imaging is also used to provide direct visualization of inoperable nodules that can be treated with percutaneous injections with various agents. The agents used with IR are creative and include nanoparticles, ethanol, brachytherapy particles, magnetic particles, gene therapy, Y-90 based brachytherapy devices, and so forth (Weisse 2004; Goldstein 2004: www.IsoPetSolutions.com/ products/ 2016).

Chemotherapy with Rapamycin May Provide Antiaging Benefits

There is a lot of media interest in the dual role that rapamycin (sirolimus) may have in antiaging in addition to its anticancer action. Rapamycin was first isolated from *Streptomyces hygroscopicus* on Easter Island in the mid-1970s. It was initially characterized as an antifungal and antimicrobial agent but was found to have immunosuppressant and anticancer properties. The mechanistic target of rapamycin (mTOR) pathway acts as the nutrient sensor of the cell and integrates signals to regulate cell growth and metabolism. The dose and toxicity for long term use needs to be clarified. Oral administration may potentially benefit geriatric cancer patients with osteosarcoma, hemangiosarcoma, and malignant melanoma as cell lines of these malignancies express the mTOR pathway (Larson et al. 2016). Rapamycin at various doses inhibits mTOR, which blocks the pathways required for cell-cycle progression, proliferation, and angiogenesis. Its evaluation in clinical trials for its anticancer action in patients with these malignancies will be very interesting and potentially useful.

Given to dogs at low doses, rapamycin also has the potential ability to provide improvement in cardiac function and energy in older dogs and may extend life span (DogAgingProject.com). It is also immunosuppressive and has its toxicity profile; therefore more information is needed. I welcome this work if reliable repeatable clinical trials demonstrate evidence-based efficacy. Early media reports about "wonder drugs" and supplements on small numbers of cases have mislead millions. A large number of patients in well-designed clinical trials is needed to demonstrate reliable data. I have always been interested in extending the quality of life and longevity for my geriatric patients. It has always been distressing for us to lose our geriatric cancer patients to old age issues if we have cured or controlled their cancer. We should think of using rapamycin in terms of a dual role chemo drug that treats the cancer while delaying the onset of diseases of aging, such as dementia or heart disease, therefore giving our geriatric cancer patients more longevity with a better quality of life.

Protocols for Various Tumor Types

There are literally hundreds of chemotherapy protocols used in cancer management. Each university teaches its favored protocols to resident students, who then modify them according to their preferences and their geriatric patients' needs. Every oncologist has his or her own favorite protocols and drugs. Appendix 1 has protocols that are currently used at my clinics to treat specific tumors in our geriatric oncology patients. Use good clinical judgment to select a working protocol and modify it to accommodate the individual geriatric oncology patient's requirements.

The drugs most commonly used for common tumors are presented in chart form in Table 6.1. When providing chemotherapy, it is important for the practitioner to check up-to-date information regularly, to learn of innovative protocols that improve patient survival. Look at a wide range of protocols to see which one fits your geriatric patient's unique set of concurrent conditions and polypharmacy to avoid interactions and side effects. Research the methods that other oncologists use for the particular malignancy and the issues that your geriatric patient is dealing with.

Table 6.1. Common Chemotherapy Drugs and the Animal Cancers in Which They Are Useful or Potentially Useful

Drug Name	MCT	LSA	OSA	AC	MMel	SA	CNS	Miscellaneous Notes
Prednisone (hormone)	*	*	HO				*	Plasma cell, histiocytosis
COX-2 Inhibitors								Pain and palliation
Piroxicam, Meloxicam			*	*		*		TCC, SCC Anticancer effect
Deracoxib, Carprofen, etc.			*			*		Pain control Anticancer effect
Plant-Derived								Vinca alkaloids, taxanes
Vincristine (Oncovin®)	*	*				*		TVT
Vinblastine (Velban®)	*	*						Vasosclerotic
Vinoralbine								Lung metastases
Taxol				*		*		Acute GI toxicity
Alkylating Agents								
Lomustine, carmustine	*	*					*	T-cell LSA, histiocytosis, metronomic chemo
Cyclophosphamide (Cytoxan®)		*		*	*	*		Hemorrhagic cystitis
Ifosfamide		*		*	*	*		Cystitis Must use Mensa
Chlorambucil (Leukeran®)	*	*		*				M. Myeloma
Melphalan (Alkeran®)		*r		*				M. Myeloma
Dacarbazine (DTIC))		*r			*			4–5 days
Procarbazine		*r					*	Lung cancer
Mechlorethamine		*r						T-cell LSA
Temozolomide		*r			*		*	Used with Adria for *rLSA
Antitumor Antibiotics								
Doxorubicin (Adriamycin), Epirubicin, Anthracyclines, Doxil, daunorubicin		*	*	*		*		Cardiotoxic, vasosclerotic hypersensitivity reactions MTD causes 25% toxicity
Mitoxantrone		*r		*		*		RTx sensitizer, expensive!
Actinomycin-D		*r						Vasosclerotic
Bleomycin		*r		*e	*e	*e		SCC, used IV, IL with *e
Doxy/minocycline	*	*	*	*	*	*	*	Antiangiogenic
Antimetabolites		*						L-asparaginase for LSA
Cytosine Arabinoside		*					*	4 h drip or SQ over 2-4 days
Methotrexate		*					*	Folic acid *r
5-FU, Xeloda® (***never in cats***)				*				Abdominal carcinomas, SCC
Hydroxyurea								Polycythemia
Gemcitabine (Gemzar®)				*				Pancreatic AC
L-asparaginase (enzyme)		*						Potential allergic reactions
Tanovea® rabacfosadine		*, *r		+/−				Cutaneous LSA, MultipleM

(continued)

Table 6.1. *(Continued)*

Drug Name	MCT	LSA	OSA	AC	MMel	SA	CNS	Miscellaneous Notes
Heavy Metal Platinol								
Cisplatin (***never in cats***)			*	*e	*e	*e		Nephrotoxic given IV, IL *e *Never use in cats*
Carboplatin			*	*	*	*	*	Safe in cats
Antiangiogenesis Agents								
MMP inhibitors	*	*	*	*	*	*	*	Investigational
Thalidomide	*	+/−	*	*	*	*	*	Birth defects
Tamoxifen (Hormone)				*	*	*		MGAC
NSAIDs,			*	*	*	*		GI side effects
Avastin®, etc.				*		*		Monoclonal antibody
Targeted Therapy **Checkpoint Inhibitors** **(TBA)**								Adjunctive antisense therapy, novel drugs
Interferon		*		*	*	*	*	Retrovirus
Monoclonal antibodies		*						Target antigens on cancer cells: many actions
Gene therapy		*		*	*	*	*	Investigational, personalized
Tyrosine kinase inhibitors	*	*	*	*		*		Small molecules: toceranib, masitinib, flavopiridol *r
Gleevec®, SAHA, bispecific ligand targeted toxin BST						*		Hemangiosarcoma Other sarcomas TBA

*r Rescue drugs used in resistant lymphoma protocols.
*e Used in electroporation/electrochemotherapy.
* Drug commonly used.
+/− May or may not be used depending on the attending doctor.

Since it is impossible to present all of the protocols and clinical trials from the vast and vibrant field of veterinary oncology in these pages, please reference specialty textbooks, proceedings, journal articles, and online resources (www.veterinarycancersociety.org, https://ebusiness.avma.org/aahsd/ study/_search.aspx and www.Medscape.com), including membership resources through www. vetfolio.com and www.vetstream.com. Veterinary Information Network (VIN, www.vin.com) provides a free online information site for your clients, with helpful articles (www.veterinarypartner. com). A web site hosted by Drs. Anthony Moore and Angela Frimberger (www.oncologypartners. com) contains insightful and up-to-date information for clinicians. Oncura Partners offers DVM case management consultations for members (www.oncurapartners.com). Consultations for stereotactic radiosurgery (SRS) are accessible online (Petcureoncology.com). In addition, most major clinical laboratories provide consultations with staff oncologists at no charge for clinicians who use their services.

Table 6.2 is a list of protocols used at Ohio State University Veterinary Oncology Service when Guillermo Couto, DVM, ACVIM (hematology–oncology) was director. These protocols represent one of the most highly respected teaching hospitals that offer oncology services in the US. Chemotherapy protocols vary from one institution to the next and they are constantly changing. The protocol and drug doses that you select for your geriatric oncology patients should be verified as current through one of the given references and/or a consulting oncologist and adjusted to the patient's body condition.

Table 6.2.   Protocols Used at the Ohio State University Veterinary Oncology Service

I.   Lymphoma * **Monoclonal antibody immunotherapy may improve treatment outcomes.**

   A. Induction of remission
      1. COAP protocol
         Cyclophosphamide (Cytoxan®): 50mg/m² BSA, PO, every other day for 8 weeks in **dogs**;
            (200–300mg/m², PO, every 3 weeks in **cats**).
         Vincristine (Oncovin®): 0.5mg/m² BSA, IV, once a week, for 8 weeks.
         Cytosine arabinoside (Cytosar®): 100mg/m² BSA, IV, or SQ, divided BID, for 4 days.
         Prednisone: 40–50mg/m² BSA, PO, SID for a week; then 20–25mg/m² BSA, PO, every other
            day for 7 weeks.
         In cats, cytosine arabinoside is used for only 2 days, and the remaining 3 drugs
            (cyclophosphamide, vincristine, prednisone) for 6 weeks rather than 8 weeks.
      2. COP protocol
         Cyclophosphamide (Cytoxan®): 50mg/m² BSA, PO, every other day dogs; or 300mg/m² BSA,
            PO, every 3 weeks (dogs or cats)*.
         Vincristine (Oncovin®): 0.5mg/m² BSA, IV, once a week.
         Prednisone: 40–50mg/m² BSA, PO, SID for a week; then 20–25mg/m² BSA, PO, every
            other day.
         *The duration of chemotherapy using this protocol is variable.
      3. CLOP protocol
         As in COP, but with the addition of L-asparaginase (Elspar®), at a dose of 10,000–20,000IU/m²
            BSA, SQ, once every 4–6 weeks.
      4. CHOP protocol (21-day cycle)
         Cyclophosphamide (Cytoxan®): 200–300mg/m² BSA, IV, day 10.
         Doxorubicin (Adriamycin): 30mg/m² BSA, IV, day 1.
         Vincristine (Oncovin®): 0.75mg/m² BSA, IV, days 8, 15.
         Prednisone: 40–50mg/m² BSA, PO, SID days 1–7; then 20–25mg/m² BSA, PO, QOD,
            days 8–21.
         Sulfa-trimethoprim: 15mg/kg, PO, BID.
   B. Maintenance
      1. Chlorambucil (Leukeran®): 20mg/m² BSA, PO, every other week;
         Prednisone: 20–25mg/m² BSA, PO, every other day.
      2. LMP protocol
         Chlorambucil (Leukeran®) and prednisone as above, plus methotrexate 2.5–5mg/m² BSA, PO,
            twice or 3 times a week.
      3. LAP protocol
         Chlorambucil (Leukeran®): 20mg/m² BSA, PO, every other week.
         Prednisone: 20–25mg/m² BSA, PO, every other day.
         Cytosine arabinoside (Cytosar®): 200–400mg/m², SQ, every 2 weeks, alternating with
            Leukeran®.
      4. COP protocol used every other week for 6 cycles; then every third week for 6 cycles; and once
         a month thereafter.

(continued)

Table 6.2. (*Continued*)

I.   **Lymphoma** * **Monoclonal antibody immunotherapy may improve treatment outcomes.** (*continued*)

    C. "Rescue"
       DOGS
       *Rabacfosadine (Tanovea™), a novel acyclic nucleotide for IV injection by a 30-minute infusion in 5% dextrose, for injection at 1mg/kg, given every 21 days. Released in 2017.
       * Flavopiridol (cyclin-dependent kinase (CDK) inhibitor), a potential therapy (Ema et al. 2016)
       1. D-MAC protocol (repeat continuously for 10–16 weeks)
         Dexamethasone: 0.5mg/lb, PO or SQ on days 1 and 8.
         Actinomycin D (Cosmegen®): 0.75mg/m^2, IV push on day 1.
         Cytosine arabinoside (Cytosar®): 200–300mg/m^2, IV drip over 4 hours, on day 1.
         Melphalan (Alkeran®): 20mg/m^2, PO, on day 8 (AFTER 2–3 DOSES OF MELPHALAN, SUBSTITUTE IN LEUKERAN® AT THE SAME DOSE).
       2. ADIC protocol
         Doxorubicin (Adriamycin): 30mg/m^2 BSA IV, Q/3 weeks.
         Dacarbazine(DTIC-Dome®): 1,000mg/m^2 BSA, IV drip for 6–8 hours, once every 3 weeks.
       3. L-Asparaginase (Elspar®): 10,000–30,000IU/m^2 BSA, IM, Q/2 or 3 weeks.
       4. CHOP protocol if second relapse on COAP or if good response to Adriamycin was previously observed in the patient.
       CATS
       1. Cytosine arabinoside (Cytosar®): 100–200mg/m^2 BSA/day, IV drip for 6–24 hours.
         Mitoxantrone (Novantrone®): 4mg/m^2, IV drip, mixed in the bag with the Cytosar®.
         Dexamethasone: 0.5–1mg/lb, PO, once a week. Repeat every 3 weeks.

II.   **Acute lymphoid leukemia (ALL)**
    COAP, CLOP, or COP.

III. **Chronic lymphocytic leukemia (CLL)**
    1. Chlorambucil (Leukeran®): 20mg/m^2 BSA, PO, every other week (with or without prednisone 20mg/m^2 BSA, PO, every other day).
    2. Cyclophosphamide (Cytoxan®): 50mg/m^2 BSA, PO, 4 days a week.
    Prednisone 20mg/m^2 BSA, PO, every other day.

IV.   **Acute myelogenous leukemia (AML)**
    1. Cytosine arabinoside (Cytosar®): 100mg/m^2 BSA/day, IV drip or SQ (divided BID) for 4 days.
      6-Thioguanine (6-TG®) 40–50mg/m^2 BSA, PO, SID, or QOD.
    2. Cytosar® and 6-TG® plus Adriamycin (10mg/m^2 BSA, IV, on days 2 and 4 of the cycle).
    3. Cytosine arabinoside (Cytosar®): 100–200mg/m^2 BSA/day, IV drip for 1–2 days.
    Mitoxantrone (Novantrone®): 4mg/m^2, IV drip, mixed in the bag with the Cytosar®.
    Repeat every 3 weeks.

V.   **Chronic myelogenous leukemia (CML)**
    1. Hydroxurea (Hydrea®): 50mg/kg, PO, divided BID, daily or QOD until normal white blood count.

VI.   **Multiple myeloma**
    1. Melphalan (Alkeran®): 2mg/m^2 BSA, PO, SID × 1 week; then QOD.
    Prednisone: 40–50mg/m^2 BSA, PO, SID × 1 week; then 20mg/m^2 BSA, PO, QOD. Can also be used at 6–8mg/m^2, PO, for 5 days, repeating every 21 days.
    2. CHOP protocol.

(*continued*)

Table 6.2. *(Continued)*

VII. Mast cell tumors (systemic)

1. Prednisone: 40–50mg/m² BSA, PO, SID for a week; then 20–25mg/m² BSA, PO, QOD.
2. Prednisone: 40–50mg/m² BSA, PO, SID for a week; then 20–25mg/m² BSA, PO, QOD. Cimetidine (Tagamet®): 10mg/kg, PO, QID (optional).
3. Prednisone: 40–50mg/m² BSA, PO, SID for a week; then 20–25mg/m² BSA, PO, QOD. CCNU (lomustine): 60–100mg/m², PO, q/3–4 weeks
4. CVP protocol
   Vinblastine (Velban®): 2mg/m² BSA, IV, once a week.
   Cyclophosphamide (Cytoxan®): 50mg/m² BSA, PO, QOD or 4 days a week.
   Prednisone: 20–25mg/m² BSA, PO, QOD.
*5. Toceranib (Palladia™): 2.25–2.75mg/kg M-W-F. Dose escalated to 3.25mg/kg if well tolerated.
*6. Masitinib (Kinavet™, Masivet™): 12.5mg/kg BID.

VIII. Soft tissue sarcomas – Dog

1. ADIC protocol (for spindle cell sarcomas)
   Doxorubicin (Adriamycin): 30mg/m² BSA, IV, Q/3 weeks.
   DTIC-Dome® (Dacarbazine): 1,000mg/m² BSA, IV drip for 6–8 hours; repeat Q/3 weeks.
   Sulfa-trimethoprim: 15mg/kg, PO, BID.
2. VAC protocol (21-day cycle) (for other sarcomas)
   Vincristine (Oncovin®): 0.75mg/m² BSA, IV, days 8 and 15.
   Doxorubicin (Adriamycin): 30mg/m² BSA, IV, day 1.
   Cyclophosphamide (Cytoxan®): 200–300mg/m² BSA, PO, day 10.
   Sulfa-trimethoprim: 15mg/kg, PO, BID.

IX. Soft tissue sarcomas – Cat

1. Carboplatin (Paraplatin®): 200–280mg/m², IV, every 3–4 weeks.
2. AC protocol (21-day cycle)
   Doxorubicin (Adriamycin): 1mg/kg, IV, day 1.
   Cyclophosphamide (Cytoxan®): 100–150mg/m² BSA on days 10 and 11.
3. VAC protocol (28-day cycle)
   Vincristine (Oncovin®): 0.5–0.75mg/m² BSA, IV, days 8, 15, and 22.
   Doxorubicin (adriamycin): 1mg/kg, IV, day 1.
   Cyclophosphamide (Cytoxan®): 100–150mg/m² BSA on days 10 and 11.
4. MiC protocol (21-day cycle)
   Mitoxantrone (Novantrone®): 4–6mg/m², IV drip over 4 hours, on day 1.
   Cyclophosphamide (Cytoxan®): 200–300mg/m², PO, on day 10.
5. MiCO protocol (21-day cycle)
   Mitoxantrone (Novantrone®): 4–6mg/m², IV drip over 4 hours, on day 1.
   Cyclophosphamide (Cytoxan®): 200–300mg/m², PO, on day 10.
   Vincristine (Oncovin®): 0.5 to 0.6mg/m², IV, on days 8 and 15.

X. Osteosarcoma—Dog: amputation of affected limb

1. Cisplatin (Platinol®): Rarely used: 50–70mg/m² BSA, IV drip over 2 hours, q21d. Prior intensive diuresis is required. Not for geriatric dogs, nephrotoxic! Carboplatin is preferred.
2. Carboplatin (Paraplatin®): 300mg/m², IV, Q/3–4 weeks.
3. Doxorubicin (Adriamycin): 30mg/m², IV, every 2 weeks, for 6 doses.
*4. Bisphosphonates have been shown to reduce pain and decrease tumor invasion in bone.
*5. Consider using immunotherapy with osteosarcoma vaccine once efficacy is established.

(continued)

Table 6.2. *(Continued)*

XI. **Carcinomas – Dog**
  1. Carboplatin (Paraplatin®): 300mg/m^2, IV, Q/3–4 weeks.
  2. CMF protocol
     Fluorouracil (5-FU): 150mg/m^2 BSA, IV, once a week.
     Cyclophosphamide (Cytoxan®): 50mg/m^2 BSA, PO, 4 days a week or QOD.
     Methotrexate: 2.5mg/m^2 BSA, PO, 2 or 3 times a week.
  3. FAC protocol
     5-Fluorouracil (5-FU): 150mg/m^2 BSA, IV, days 8 and 15.
     Doxorubicin (Adriamycin): 30mg/m^2 BSA, IV, day 1.
     Cyclophosphamide (Cytoxan®): 200–300mg/m^2 BSA, PO, day 10.
     Sulfa-trimethoprim: 15mg/kg, PO, BID.
  4. Cisplatin (Platinol®): 60–70mg/m^2 BSA, IV drip, Q/3 weeks. Prior intensive diuresis is required.
  5. VAF protocol
     Vincristine (Oncovin®): 0.75mg/m^2 BSA, IV, days 8 and 15.
     Doxorubicin (Adriamycin): 30mg/m^2 BSA, IV, day 1.
     5-Fluorouracil (5-FU): 150mg/m^2 BSA, IV, days 1, 8, and 15.
  6. VAC protocol
  7. 5-Fluorouracil (5-FU): 150mg/m^2 BSA, IV, once a week.
     Cyclophosphamide (Cytoxan®): 50mg/m^2 BSA, PO, 4 days a week or QOD.
  *8. Toceranib and masitinib at recommended dosage may have efficacy.
  *9. Paccal-Vet® CA-1: 150mg/m^2 BSA, IV diluted over 15–30 min q21 days × 4.

XII. **Carcinomas—Cat**
  5-Fluorouracil is toxic for the cat, producing severe and often fatal CNS signs. Cisplatin is also extremely toxic, causing acute pulmonary toxicity in this species.
  1. Carboplatin (Paraplatin®) 200–240mg/m^2, IV, every 3–4 weeks.
  2. AC protocol (28-day cycle)
     Doxorubicin (Adriamycin): 1mg/kg, IV, day 1.
     Cyclophosphamide (Cytoxan®): 100–150mg/m^2 BSA on days 10 and 11.
  3. VAC protocol (28-day cycle)
     Vincristine (Oncovin®): 0.5–0.75mg/m^2 BSA, IV, days 8, 15, and 22.
     Doxorubicin (Adriamycin): 1mg/kg, IV, day 1.
     Cyclophosphamide (Cytoxan®): 100–150mg/m^2 BSA on days 10 and 11.
  4. Vincristine (Oncovin®): 0.5mg/m^2 BSA, IV, once a week.
     Cyclophosphamide (Cytoxan®): 50mg/m^2 BSA, PO, 4 days a week or QOD.
  5. MiC protocol (21-day cycle)
     Mitoxantrone (Novantrone®): 4–6mg/m^2, IV drip over 4 hours, on day 1.
     Cyclophosphamide (Cytoxan®): 200–300mg/m^2, PO, on day 10.
     *I prefer to give mitoxantrone diluted IV over 15 min and divide Cytoxan over 2–3 days.
  6. MiCO protocol (21-day cycle)
     Mitoxantrone (Novantrone®): 4–6mg/m^2, IV drip over 4 hours, on day 1.
     Cyclophosphamide (Cytoxan®): 200–300mg/m^2, PO, on day 10.
     Vincristine (Oncovin®): 0.5–0.6mg/m^2, IV, on days 8 and 15.
  *7. Tyrosine-kinase inhibitors (small molecules): toceranib (Palladia®): 2.5mg/kg PO, MWF.
     Masitinib (Kinavet®, Masivet®): 12.5mg/kg PO, BID or 50mg per cat BID.

*New drugs, agents, or immunotherapy added to be used as first-line therapy, rescue, or adjuvant (AV).

Precautions with Specific Chemotherapy Agents

You have the ultimate responsibility for your geriatric cancer patients. Conversions, calculations, and decimal placement for all dosages should be double-checked and confirmed prior to use, including chemotherapy drugs that are dispensed. Be sure to use an overweight patient's lean body mass for all calculations. Adjust all drug doses and selections for species-specific toxicity, obesity, chronic kidney disease, cardiac disease, liver disease, cancer cachexia, sarcopenia, leukopenia, thrombocytopenia, anemia, and other concurrent medical conditions and polypharmacy that may affect each particular geriatric patient. Use the dose escalation system for geriatric cancer patients, starting with the lowest dose first and then increasing the dose to the known maximally tolerated dose (MTD) if the patient shows no adverse side effects.

Always provide the Cancer Care Package for patients receiving IV chemotherapy to offset expected adverse events. Some oncologists always recommend antinausea Rx such as Cerneia or ondansetron for one week following the use of anthracyclines.

An example of using specific precautions applies to the use of ifosfamide (Ifex®) for treating sarcomas. It is an alkylating agent that shares similar pathways with Cytoxan to produce metabolites that release acrolein, which causes hemorrhagic cystitis. A 6-hour Mesna-diuresis protocol is required to prevent the adverse effects of acrolein-induced damage to uroepithelium and nephrotoxicosis. The MTD dose for dogs is $375mg/m^2$, whereas cats tolerated dose escalations to an MTD of $900mg/m^2$ in a phase I study (Rassnick et al. 2006a). Ifex is not considered nephrotoxic in dogs but caused acute renal failure in 7% (2/27) of cats in a phase II study (Rassnick et al. 2006b).

The following precautions have become incorporated into our protocols to avoid toxicity for geriatric and frail cancer patients:

Avoid Cytoxan-induced hemorrhagic cystitis. Advise clients to increase the pet's fluid intake when using Cytoxan. We give prednisone at $20mg/m^2$ on the days of oral Cytoxan and recommend feeding broth or soup. This strategy has reduced the incidence of Cytoxan-induced hemorrhagic cystitis in our practice to almost zero. We do not use Cytoxan IV. Our preference is to spread out the dose PO over 2 or 3 days with broth and prednisone on the same day to increase water intake to avoid toxicity.

Avoid Adriamycin toxicity and underdosing in large-breed dogs. Split the delivery of Adriamycin in large-breed dogs by giving $20mg/m^2$ and repeat in 4–8 days. This technique provides a higher overall total dose. It avoids using the MTD of $30mg/m^2$, which may cause adverse events yet is considered an underdose in large dogs.

Avoid lomustine nadir. Divide the MTD of 50–$90mg/m^2$ by three to four and give that dose over 4–8 days. Repeat every 21 days in dogs. We never give 10mg capsules of lomustine to cats. We divide that dose, give it over 4–5 days, and repeat every 30–42 days, depending on CBC results. We prefer metronomic lomustine.

Avoid toxicity in frail geriatric patients. Consider metronomic (low continuous daily dose) therapy. For example, instead of giving capecitabine (Xeloda®) in a pulse cycle PO twice a day for 10 days on and 10 days off for canine carcinoma cases, give it once a day or once every other day on a continuous basis at the metronomic dose of $250mg/m^2$ per day. Never use Xeloda or any 5-FU derivative in cats!

The Treatment Calendar

Carers are often emotionally overwhelmed by the news that their geriatric pet has cancer. They are additionally overwhelmed by the list of treatments, medications, tests, and supplements that will be used to help their pet survive. A treatment calendar helps the family to get organized at home. Having a daily treatment schedule that needs to be checked off every time medications and supplements are given helps the pet stay on schedule.

When we give clients their treatment calendar, we explain the entire chemotherapy protocol as well as supportive drugs and supplements. The calendar includes recheck dates and the type of blood test needed for monitoring. At recheck visits, our technicians check the calendar and draw the patient's blood accordingly. They run the tests while the caregiver is waiting for the exam.

The top line of the treatment calendar reads: *"Always bring this calendar and your Rx bottles with you on your next appointment"* (Figure 6.1). We read this top line to the caregivers and remind them to bring the chemotherapy chart and their medication bottles for each visit. This gives us the opportunity to see if the medications are being used.

Encourage clients to keep notes on the treatment calendar about how the pet seems to feel after each chemotherapy visit and any adverse events that occur. We carefully review this calendar with the client at every recheck.

This calendar is important as it quickly shows us what medications the patient has received and what drug is next. By taking the time to go over the previous month's chemotherapy calendar and outline the drugs for the new calendar, we can catch mistakes made by the pet owner and look for potential drug interactions.

Our nursing staff looks at the bottles and sometimes we count the tablets to see if they are being used properly. It is important to take these precautions, especially for senior citizen clients who may

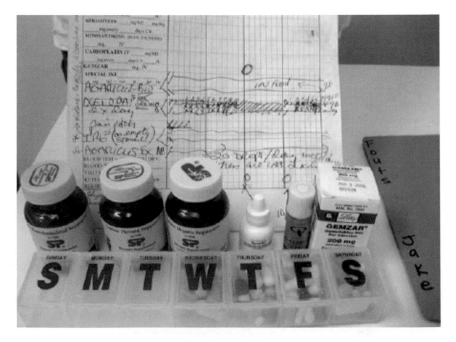

Figure 6.1.   The treatment calendar and Rx bottles are reviewed at each visit.

have some confusion. It is not unusual to discover something that needs to be adjusted. This inspection is a review for the client on the importance and purpose of the medications and to see if the pet is having any problems accepting them.

It is surprising how many people make mistakes. The May 2005 issue of *Veterinary Economics* focused on servicing a growing segment of senior clients. It quoted from the American Animal Hospital Association (AAHA) 2004 Pet Owner Survey that 7% of active clients are 65 or older and that this segment may increase to 35% by 2020. Some elderly people may have trouble understanding and remembering what they are told. Some forget instructions and get confused with the medications. Sometimes a mistake can be fatal, as in Pookie's case, which follows. Common sense is an ingredient that we are unable to add to our client's thinking. However, we must do the best we can to give clear and written instructions and then carefully check the use of potent chemotherapy drugs in order to prevent mistakes.

Pookie's Case (A Senseless Senior Moment Overdose)

Pookie, a 12-year-old F/S Scottish Terrier mix, belonged to a senior couple. She was referred for treatment of residual grade II–III mast cell cancer. The family elected to use oral alternate day prednisone and lomustine. Their instructions were to give one 10mg capsule of lomustine once a day for 2 consecutive days only. We dispensed two capsules per visit. They were instructed to repeat the cycle for lomustine every 21 days after recheck blood tests to monitor platelets and liver enzymes. They wanted to save money and learned that their daughter could get the lomustine at a friend's pharmacy. The directions and dose were clearly outlined in the chemotherapy treatment calendar and the clients had used lomustine properly according to instructions for over 2 months. We issued a written prescription for the lomustine to be used as directed on the chemotherapy treatment calendar.

Three weeks later, Pookie was presented in very poor condition for a recheck. The CBC revealed profound neutropenia and thrombocytopenia. These low values were totally unexpected. We reviewed the chemotherapy treatment calendar with the couple and found no errors. I asked the family to show me their Rx bottles and show me exactly what pills they were giving on a daily basis. We found that the new prescription of lomustine was being given improperly at the rate of one 10mg capsule once a day, every day! This represented a fatal overdose for poor Pookie.

We explained to the clients that Pookie needed to be hospitalized on an emergency basis and that she needed intense monitoring and nursing for over 6 weeks because lomustine has a prolonged effect. We offered options for treatment with Neupogen® and multiple transfusions to help restore red cells and white cells but we had no way to restore her platelet count. We explained that Pookie's platelets would most likely not regenerate following the magnitude of her lomustine toxicity. For these reasons, we knew that the damage to Pookie's bone marrow was most likely irreversible. She would probably die even with the best of supportive treatment even if the family could afford the expense.

Summary: Chemotherapy in the Management of Geriatric Cancer

Geriatric dogs and cats undergo a progressive decline in the functional reserve of their major organ systems. They may be less able to cope with chemotherapy following the stress of surgery and radiation in a multimodality protocol. The presence of comorbidities associated with aging necessitates modifications to the drug dosages and timing of standard chemotherapy protocols. Astute clinical and home monitoring of the geriatric patient is needed, as well as accessible, compassionate doctor–client communication.

Combination chemotherapy offers better efficacy for treating cancer; however, dose modification is important to minimize toxicity for geriatric patients. The attending doctor can research and offer other less toxic options, such as split dose chemotherapy (as I have described) at $20mg/m^2$ given one week apart when using Adriamycin, intralesional and regional chemotherapy delivery, or metronomic (low dose) continuous therapy, or pulse therapy. Successful pulse therapy was reported for 14 dogs with apocrine anal sac adenocarcinoma following surgery. They were given melphalan at $7mg/m^2$ orally over a 5-day period followed by 16 days off for life (Emms 2005).

In the coming years, cancer patients may have the option to routinely receive immunotherapy, small molecule therapy, and chemoprevention as part of a permanent maintenance program. This would add yet another maintenance modality of therapy, sequenced after the initial treatment.

Adverse Effects of Cancer Therapy in Geriatric Pets

We must never lose sight of the fact that there are some patients we cannot help; there are none we cannot harm.

Dr. Carl A. Osborne, DVM, PhD, ACVIM

The treatment of cancer in geriatric pets bears a risk-to-benefit ratio that includes the possibility of experiencing a wide range of adverse events (AEs) from the use of surgery, radiation, chemotherapy, and immunotherapy. The adverse effects from surgery and radiation therapy are discussed in previous sections of this chapter. The AEs encountered using immunotherapy will need to be addressed differently. The global immune-related adverse reactions may cause immunotoxicities ranging from relatively minor conditions, such as skin depigmentation, to severe toxicities against crucial organ systems, such as liver, bowel, and lung. This section focuses mainly on the various adverse events associated with chemotherapy and its multiple applications. The caregiver needs education regarding what and when to expect adverse events. A user-friendly list of AEs may be very helpful to educate caregivers (Table 6.3).

The Veterinary Cancer Society has a clinical trials arm known as the Veterinary Co-operative Oncology Group (VCOG). VCOG created a consensus document known as Common Terminology Criteria for Adverse Events (CTCAE), which parallels the National Cancer Institute (NCI) evaluation program, available at http://ctep.cancer.gov/. The VCOG-CTCAE tables are adapted for dogs and cats and are intended to standardize the reporting of adverse effects for clinical trials using the grade 1–5 system described in the "Chemotherapy in the Management of Geriatric Cancer" section of this chapter. Most oncologists use the 0–4 grading system for chemotherapy-related toxicities (Table 6.4).

Chemotherapy agents, along with the support drugs used in cancer management, are well known for causing physical side effects such as polydypsia, polyuria, nausea, vomiting, colitis, and diarrhea. More insidiously, chemotherapy may cause bone marrow suppression with severe leukopenia, which may result in life-threatening sepsis. Thrombocytopenia may be induced by chemotherapy drugs, especially the platinum-based drugs and lomustine. The long term use (>6 months) of metronomic chlorambucil may cause cumulative irreversible thrombocytopenia (de Lorimier 2014). Renal failure

Table 6.3. Chemotherapy Agent Clearance and Adverse Events

Generic Name	Brand Name®	Cleared Via	Clearance Time	Route of Therapy	Adverse Events
Actinomycin-D	Cosmegen	Urine, feces	7 days	IV	Vessels, marrow, GI
Doxorubicin	Adriamycin	Feces	7 days	IV infusion	Marrow, GI, heart, anaphylaxis, severe vesicant
Asparaginase	Elspar			IM or SQ	Allergy, marrow
Azathioprine	Imuran	Urine	8 hours	PO	Marrow, GI
Carmustine	BCNU	Urine	4 days	IV	Marrow, lungs, GI, nephrotoxic
Lomustine	CCNU	Degradation	1 day	PO, IV	GI, marrow, lungs, liver
Carboplatin	Paraplatin	Urine	1 day	IV infusion	Marrow, GI, allergy
Cisplatin	Platinol	Urine	1 day	IV, IV infusion	Nephrotoxic, GI, marrow, KILLS CATS
Capecitabine	Xeloda (oral prodrug of 5-FU below)	Urine	1 day	PO	Marrow, GI, CNS, KILLS CATS!
Fluorouracil	5-FU	Urine	1 day	IV, IL	Marrow, GI, CNS, KILLS CATS!
Chlorambucil	Leukeran	Urine	1 day	PO	Marrow, GI
Cyclophosphamide	Cytoxan	Urine	3 days	PO, IV	Marrow, nephrotoxic, GI
Cytosine arabinoside	Cytosar-U	Urine	1 day	IV, SQ	Marrow, GI
Etoposide/VP-16	VePesid	Urine	1 day	PO, IV	Marrow, GI
Gemcitabine	Gemzar	Urine	3–4 days	IV	Marrow, GI, flu syndrome
Ifosfamide	Ifex	Urine	7 days	IV infusion	Urotoxic without mesna, CNS, myelosuppression
Interferon, interleukin, etc.	(Many cytokines)	Urine	1 day	SQ, IV, IM, PO	Lethargy, fever prostration
Mechlorethamine	Mustargen	Urine	5 minutes	IV	Toxic contact, vesicant, amyloidosis
Melphalan	Alkeran	Urine	7 days	PO, IV	Marrow
Methotrexate	Trexsol	Urine	1 day	PO, IV	GI, marrow
Mitoxantrone	Novantrone	Urine, feces	7 days	Slow IV	GI, marrow
Paclitaxel	Taxol Paccal-Vet-CA1	Feces	5 days	IV	Marrow, GI, anaphylaxis
Prednisone		Urine	12 hours	PO	PUPD, weakness, panting, Cushings
Procarbazine	Matulane	Urine	1 day	PO	Marrow, GI, liver, CNS, drug interactions
Small molecules	Masivet Palladia, etc.	Variable	Variable	PO, IV, IL	Variable
Rabacfosadine	Tanovea	Urine, feces	5 days	IV	Marrow, GI, Skin
Vinblastine	Velban	Urine	3 days	IV	Vessels, marrow, GI, vesicant
Vincristine	Oncovin	Urine, feces	7 days	IV	Vessels, nerves, GI marrow, vesicant
Vinorelbine	Navelbine	Urine	5–8 days	Slow IV	Marrow, vesicant

Source: Reprinted with permission of Laurie Kaplan from the book *Help Your Dog Fight Cancer*, and adapted by Alice Villalobos DVM for the First Edition in 2008 and Second Edition in 2016 (JanGen Press, Briarcliff Manor, NY).

Table 6.4.   Toxic Effect and Grade for Chemotherapy-Related Toxicities, Adapted from the NCI Toxicity Table

Toxic Effect and Grade for Chemotherapy-Related Toxicities, Adapted from the NCI Toxicity Table						
Grades **Effects**	**0**	**1**	**2**	**3**	**4**	**5**
Neutropenia	None	1,500–2,500	1,000–1,500	500–1,000	< 500	Death
Diarrhea	None	Soft stools, response to diet change	< 2 days	2–5 days	> 5 days	Death
Vomiting	None	Nausea	Sporadic, self-limiting	< 2 days	> 5 days or requires hospitalization	Death
Anorexia	None	Inappetence	< 3 days	3–5 days	> 5 days	Death

Note: Grade 5 toxicity is listed as "Death" in all new references.

Source: Veterinary and Comparative Oncology, Vol. 2, No. 3, September 2004 with permission of Blackwell Publishing. Newly reprinted: *VCO,* Vol. 14, No. 4, December 2016: lists Grade 5 as Death.

is notorious with nephrotoxic cisplatin. This agent is not used intravenously in my clinics. It is only used in very small doses, as an intralesional injection prior to electroporation or electrochemotherapy. Cats are intolerant of certain chemotherapy drugs, specifically 5-FU and cisplatin. Cardiomyopathy is a well-known adverse effect in dogs receiving the maximum tolerated dose (MTD) of doxorubicin (Adriamycin), which is cardiotoxic. Familiarize yourself to know what drugs can injure which susceptible tissues, resulting in the specific adverse effect (Table 6.5).

Some multimodality treatment protocols call for the concurrent use of chemotherapy and immunotherapy during the radiation therapy cycle (Table 6.6). Multimodality treatment may increase tumor kill but also places the geriatric oncology patient at greater risk for adverse events (AEs) related to chemotherapy and radiation-related acute toxicity (Gustafson et al. 2004). In addition, the patient may experience AEs of allergic immunologic reactions related to immunotherapy ranging from mild to life-threatening. Radiation therapy predictably causes immediate and delayed effects with variable levels of toxicity. Acute effects from radiation therapy include erythema, pain, desquamation, mucositis, lethargy, and diarrhea (Table 6.7). Radiation toxicity is related to the dosimetry and fraction scheme. The reduced number of treatments in stereotactic radiation protocols will be a welcome change for geriatric cancer patients. When evaluating chemotherapy-related radiation toxicity, use the grade 0–4 Radiation Morbidity Scoring Schema (Table 6.8).

Some chemotherapy agents are synergistic or radiomimetic with radiation and may cause increased local tissue necrosis and discomfort. Radiation oncologists use this synergism to benefit the geriatric oncology patient. Mast cell tumors have the potential to release histamine during surgery or radiation therapy, causing localized inflammatory swelling and systemic effects. Preemptive treatment with Benadryl and famotidine reduces these adverse events. Clients must always be educated and informed about potential side effects so that they can be watchful and prepared.

Medications used for pain control, such as NSAIDs and narcotics, may cause GI ulceration, hemorrhage, constipation, and sedation. It is essential to teach carers how to take their pet's temperature and to monitor, recognize, and be prepared to deal with any type of adverse side effects as soon as possible. This is particularly important for carers of older, more fragile geriatric cancer patients. Human

Table 6.5. Common Adverse Effects from Various Chemotherapy and ImTx Agents

Name of Drug	Susceptible Tissue	Adverse Effects
Anthracyclines	Heart	Arrhythmias
Doxorubicin (Adriamycin®)	Bone marrow	Cardiomyopathy
Daunorubicin	Gut, kidneys (in cats)	Congestive heart failure, death
Doxil (liposome compound)	Perivascular tissues (Vasoclerotic)	emesis, colitis, azotemia (cats)
		Myelosuppression
Mitoxantrone (less cardiotoxic)	Skin-hand-foot, axilla, groin	Severe, deep, fungating necrosis if extravasated (read section)
Vincristine (Oncovin®)	Bone marrow	Mild bone marrow suppression
Vinblastine (Velban®)	Peripheral nerves	Mild tingling of nerves, ileus
Vinorelbine (Navelbine®)	Ulcers if extravasated	Vomiting, colitis, constipation
		Peripheral neuropathy
Cyclophosphamide (Cytoxan®)	Bladder mucosa	Low WBC, hematuria, chronic
Ifosfamide (Ifex®)	Bone marrow	hemorrhagic cystitis, sterility
	Gonads	Bladder cancer (late onset)
	Renotoxic (cats)	Mensa-diuretic protocol needed
Prednisone, prednisolone	Hunger/thirst center	Increased water intake and
Dexamethasone (all steroids)	Muscle	urination, restlessness
	Gut	Muscle wasting, bleeding ulcers,
	Skin and coat	obesity, thin skin
	Endocrine	Diabetes mellitus, hepatopathy
Chlorambucil (Leukeran®)	Bone marrow	Mild-moderate myelosuppression
Carboplatin (Paraplatin®)	Bone marrow, kidneys	Myelosuppression
Cisplatin (Platinol®) (I do not use this	Nephrotoxic w/o IV fluids	Acute kidney failure and death
drug IV only for electroporation)	Bone marrow	Myelosuppression, colitis, hearing
Must be given during intense diuresis	Gut, acoustic nerves	loss
(25ml/kg/hour)	(Lungs – KILLS CATS)	Cats: Pulmonary edema, death
Cytarabine (Cytosar®)	Bone marrow (if given IV)	Low WBC
Dacarbazine (DTIC-Dome®)	Gut, bone marrow	Low WBC, vomiting, seizures
Mitoxantrone (Novantrone®)	Bone marrow	Low WBC
Fluorouracil (5-FU, Xeloda®)	Gut, CNS (*Kills cats*)	Seizures, ataxia
Bleomycin	Lungs	Fibrosis, poor diffusion
Lomustine (CeeNu)	Bone marrow, liver, eyes	Low platelets/white cells
Methotrexate	Kidneys, liver	Vomiting
Mechlorethamine (Mustargen®)	GI tract, vasosclerotic	Vomiting, myelosuppression
Piroxicam/thalidomide NSAIDs	Gut, liver, kidneys, coagulation system	Bleeding ulcers, vomiting, anemia, coagulation problems
Melphalan (Alkeran®)	Bone marrow	Myelosuppression
Taxol®, Taxotere®, paclitaxel	GI tract	Myelosuppression, CNS, tingling
Paccal-Vet CA-1 (less toxic form)		Vomiting (FDA withdrew 2017)
Capecitabine (Gemzar®) is the IV form, Xeloda® is the oral form	GI tract, liver, bone marrow, hand and foot syndrome	Myelosuppression, vomiting, diarrhea at MTD; used mCTx
Imitinab (Gleevec®)	Liver	Bone marrow suppression, GI
Antiangiogenesis drugs	Gastrointestinal	Multiple pathways
Targeted therapy drugs	Specific proteins in cells	Multiple pathways
Gene therapy	Specific features in cells	Multiple pathways, Sense and antisense
Tyrosine kinase inhibitors	Bone marrow, GI, kidneys	Cytopenias, low serum protein
New drugs: to be announced (TBA)	Tanovea: marrow, skin, mild	Tanovea: pulmonary fibrosis
Tanovea® (rabacfosadine)	AEs self-limiting	reported in some cases, West Highland White Terriers
BST, bispecific targeted ligand toxin (e-BAT), www.Modianolab.com	Hemangiosarcoma early diagnosis, post Sx	BST toxicities unknown, TBA
Protocols: lymphoma-leukemias	Malignant blast cells	Tumor breakdown syndrome
Immunotherapy agents, cytokines, etc.	Multiple tumor types can	Allergic Immunologic Events:
See table: *VCO*, Vol. 14, No. 4, Dec.	have precision made	Anaphylaxis, Autoimmune Dz,
2016, p. 420. VCOG-CTCAE v1.1	targeted vaccines	Serum Sickness, Vasculitis

Table 6.6.   The Most Frequently Recommended Treatments for the Most Common Tumors

Type of Cancer	Type of Multimodality Treatment			
	Surgery	Chemotherapy	Radiation	Adjuvant Tx
Mast cell tumor	*	*	*	H-$_2$ blockers
Skin cancer, SCC	*/*EP	+/−	*	Cryotherapy
				Laser therapy
Lymphoma	−/+	*	+/−	Monoclonal antibody vaccines
Breast cancer	*	*	+/−	Vaccines
Anal, sweat AC	*/*EP	*	*	Check serum calcium
STS	*	*	*	IFx, gene therapy
FVAS	*	*	*	IFx, gene therapy
OSA	*	*	*Samarium	Limb sparing
Head/neck	*/*EP	*	*	Brachytherapy, HyalPlat™
Malignant melanoma	*/*EP	*	*	Oncept™, IFx, vaccines
Oral cancer	*/*EP	*	*	Brachytherapy
Nasal cancer		+/−	−/+	Post-RTx Sx for residual disease, Cryoablation
Brain tumor	+/−	*	*	Steroids
Endocrine tumor	*	*	+/−	Iodine 131
Abdominal tumor	*	*		Second look Sx
Bladder/prostate cancer	−/+	*	+/− SRS	Piroxicam
Hemangiosarcoma	*	*	−	Antiangiogenesis Tx, Ligand-targeted toxin
Liver cancer	+/−	*	Y-90	Percutaneous injection with Y-90 brachytherapy (IsoPet)
Intestinal AC	*	+/−	−	Downstage with chemo or radiation before surgery
Colorectal AC				
Pancreatic AC				
Primary lung cancer or metastatic disease	*	*	−/+	Vinorelbine, nebulized liposomes containing *IL-2*
Multiple tumor types	+/−	+/−	+/−	Precision immunotherapy

*EP, electroporation/electrochemotherapy: read the section on "Electrochemotherapy (ECT)/Electroporation (ET)" at the end of this chapter.

medical texts refer to the very old and frail as "the oldest of the old." I have referred to terminally ill patients as "TIPs."

Adverse Events Related to Chemotherapy

The drugs used in cancer management may cause polydypsia, polyuria, panting, nausea, vomiting, diarrhea, anorexia, bone marrow suppression, alopecia, acute renal failure (cisplatin, ifosfamide), cardiac arrhythmias, heart failure (Adriamycin), hepatopathy, pancreatitis, urticaria, rash, anaphylaxis, blindness, neuropathy, erythema multiforme, toxic epidermal necrolysis, and so forth. Patients treated for advanced stage lymphoma-leukemia may experience acute tumor lysis syndrome. The list of adverse effects related to chemotherapy is extensive and must include the possibility of unforeseen death. The December 2016 issue of *Veterinary and Comparative Oncology* reprinted the entire consensus document from the Veterinary Cooperative Oncology Group – *Common Terminology Criteria for Adverse Events* (VCOG-CTCAE) v1.1, published July 2011.

Table 6.7.   List of Typical Short and Long Term Adverse Events and Risks of External Beam Radiation Therapy (Teletherapy) Directed at Specific Locations of the Body

Radiation Therapy Field (Tumor Bed)	Short Term Side Effects	Long Term Effects and Late Onset Risks
Brain, cranium	Dermatitis, conjunctivitis mucositis, acute otitis	Cataracts, hearing loss, mental dullness, necrosis
Nasal passage	Mucositis, dermatitis	Dental problems, cataracts
Frontal sinus	Oral sensitivity	Skin necrosis over bone
Throat, oral cavity, mandible, maxilla	Mucositis, pain (most severe if pet has not had dental prophylaxis)	Hypothyroidism Dental problems, xerostomia Bone necrosis, sequestrum
Chest/thorax	Dermatitis, esophagitis	Fibrosis of lungs and heart
Skin	Dermatitis, hair loss	Hair loss, scar formation, thin skin, later malignancy
Mast cell cancer	Local desquamation	
Soft tissue sarcoma	Degranulation reaction dermatitis, self-injury	Scarring, permanent hair loss Need for skin graft
Legs/extremities, bone	Dermatitis, lameness Anemia, lymphocytopenia	Demineralization, necrosis, ligament failure, sequestrum
Abdomen and pelvic area	Colitis, indigestion	Liver, gut, kidney problems
Anus	Mucositis, colitis	Stricture, loss of function

The degree of neutropenia, diarrhea, vomiting, and anorexia induced by chemotherapy can be more objectively evaluated using the grade 0–4 scale adapted from the NCI chemotherapy-related toxicity table (Table 6.4).

A unique ulcerative plantar-palmar rash called hand–foot syndrome occurs with Doxil, a liposome encapsulated Adriamycin preparation, and with Xeloda®. The rash may also appear in the axilla and groin and cause self-mutilation. Using pyridoxine (vitamin B6) supplements helps to alleviate this rash as well as the rash associated with radiation sickness (Kisseberth and MacEwen 2001; Morrison 2002).

Iatrogenic Cushing's Disease and Polypharmacy

Long term use of steroids, as in some lymphoma and mast cell cancer protocols, may cause iatrogenic Cushing's disease. Dogs are more prone to this effect than are cats. The use of immunosuppressive drugs may injure the function of and reduce the number of white cells and occasionally platelets as well. Many geriatric cancer patients are on polypharmacy for pre-existing problems. If these patients develop leukopenia and/or thrombocytopenia from chemotherapy, they are more prone to infection and hemorrhage. The concept of supporting the immune system is popular with pet caregivers and they are very interested in using supplements that may offset immunosuppression (see the "Chemo-prevention and Immunonutrition for Cancer Patients" section of this chapter).

Bone Marrow Toxicity

Explain to pet owners that the bone marrow is made up of rapidly dividing cells, which are therefore highly susceptible to the effects of chemotherapy. For this reason, it is important to monitor the CBC and make decisions for dose adjustment before each chemotherapy treatment. Educate caregivers

Table 6.8. Radiation Toxicity

Tissue	Grade 0	Grade 1	Grade 2	Grade 3	Grade 4
Acute radiation morbidity scoring scheme (RTOG)					
Skin	No change over baseline	Follicular, faint or dull erythema, epilation, dry desquamation, decreased sweating	Tender or bright erythema, patchy moist desquamation, moderate edema	Confluent, moist desquamation other than skin fold, pitting edema	Ulceration, hemorrhage, or necrosis
Mucous membrane	No change over baseline	Injection may experience mild pain not requiring analgesic	Patchy mucositis, which may produce an inflammatory serosanguineous discharge, may experience moderate pain requiring analgesic	Confluent fibrinous mucositis, may include severe pain requiring narcotic	Ulceration, hemorrhage, or necrosis
Late radiation morbidity scoring scheme (EORTC/RTOG)					
Skin	No change over baseline change, some hair loss	Slight atrophy, pigmentation, total hair loss	Patchy atrophy, moderate teleangiectasis	Marked atrophy, gross teleangiectasis	Ulceration or necrosis

Source: Dobson, J., S. Cohen, and S. Gould. 2004. Treatment of canine mast cell tumors with prednisolone and radiotherapy. *Veterinary and Comparative Oncology* 2 (3):141. Blackwell Publishing Ltd.

Note: The Radiation Morbidity Scoring Schema may be found on the RTOC web site, http://www.rtog.org.

*EORTC = European Organization for Research and Treatment of Cancer; RTOG = Radiation Therapy Oncology Group.

about the function of the bone marrow as the manufacturing plant for white blood cells, platelets, and red blood cells.

It is natural for the bone marrow to experience some suppression with chemotherapy. The suppression can be more dramatic in geriatric patients due to fibrosis and reduced stem cell function. Since the red cell count is often on the low side of normal in elderly animals, we must make every attempt to avoid severe myelosuppression. See the table on "Blood/Bone Marrow Adverse Events" on p. 421 of *VCO*, Vol.14, No.4, December 2016.

Neutropenia

Neutropenia becomes the most common dose-limiting factor for most of the chemotherapy drugs used in animals. Instruct the client to expect that his or her pet's white cell count will be lowest during the drug's nadir, which generally occurs 7–10 days after administration. Teach the client to take the pet's temperature and to be alert for the signs of sepsis.

If the absolute neutrophil count drops below one thousand, the pet is at great risk for life-threatening sepsis, with signs including fever, anorexia, weakness, lethargy, general malaise, and collapse. Some dogs develop aspiration pneumonia from inhaling vomitus.

No matter how prepared we think clients are for a crisis, they still feel better if they have ready access to their oncologist for advice. They must be ready and able to admit their sick pet for urgent care at a local hospital or emergency clinic.

The treatment for sepsis is standard supportive care that includes IV fluids, broad-spectrum antibiotics, correction of electrolytes, Neupogen®, and granulocyte colony stimulating factor (G-CSF) at 5µg/kg SQ BID for the first day; if the WBC is below 1,500 then follow once daily for 2 more days. The effect from Neupogen® is dramatic and this may only be needed for 1–2 days. Because we have access only to human recombinant G-CSF, it is expected that animals will mount a cross-reactive antibody response. Therefore, we use it when necessary rather than prophylactically.

Thrombocytopenia

Thrombocytopenia most commonly occurs with the Platinol drugs and lomustine but may be induced by long term chlorambucil and any combination of chemotherapy drugs. The long term effect of lomustine and chlorambucil may cause a prolonged period before platelet rebound. Patients are usually asymptomatic until the platelet count falls below 20,000. It is generally safe to continue the protocol in the face of thrombocytopenia, as long as the platelet count does not drop below 60,000. Platelet growth factor products that will help dogs and cats may be soon be available.

Anemia

Some chemotherapy agents and protocols, especially when used for several weeks or more, may cause low-grade anemia. Chemotherapy may be responsible for a dip in the hematocrit as low as 20. It is important to establish anemia and other hematologic effects as having been caused either by the cancer or by the treatment (see the section "How Cancer Causes Anemia" in Chapter 3).

Regardless of the cause, anemia creates weakness, decreased appetite, tachycardia, bounding pulses, and tachypnea in the geriatric oncology patient. It must be addressed with proper precautions. Withdrawal of chemotherapy or increasing the interval between treatments will often correct chemotherapy-related anemia but in the geriatric oncology patient this may increase the risk for coming out of remission. Help your clients to understand that you are walking a tightrope to find the very elusive line between treatment toxicity and maintaining remission. These clients will deeply appreciate your expressed concern and your efforts. Red blood cell growth factors may be effective. However, the patient may mount an antibody response that will cancel efficacy.

Susceptible Tissues and Species Sensitivities

Organ toxicity is often related to a specific drug's characteristics and a specific pet's unique and unpredictable sensitivities. It is very important to know which drugs endanger which organs (Table 6.5). It is also important to know which drugs cannot be given to cats. For instance, cisplatin is nephrotoxic and should not be used in dogs with CRF and *NEVER* in cats. I would never use cisplatin in geriatric cancer patients because their aging kidneys have less functional reserve. The risk is just not worth it, in my book! I exclusively use carboplatin for geriatric animals, including cats that need a Platinol drug. Cats are unable to handle 5-FU in any form. It is also important to know that the therapeutic index and the maximum tolerated dose for a drug may be different between dogs versus cats. Cats may require lower doses of a drug than dogs. Expect to find further variability linked to the individual geriatric oncology patient's health and hydration status.

If a geriatric cancer patient has pre-existing heart disease, or is a breed that is prone to dilated cardiomyopathy, such as the Doberman Pinscher, or is a geriatric cat with renal disease, such as CRF or glomerulonephritis, then it is best not to use Adriamycin and other anthracyclines. I prefer to use mitoxantrone versus Adriamycin in Doberman Pinschers with lymphoma when needed in the CHOP protocols.

Cats and small dogs weighing less than 20 pounds should be dosed at 1mg/kg. The meter squared (m^2) body surface area (BSA) graph is not appropriate for small patients because they often experience unacceptable toxicity. Large dogs over 80 pounds may be underdosed using the BSA formula. I have found that splitting the dose for large dogs minimizes side effects without compromising efficacy. When we need to use Adriamycin for compromised or large canine geriatric patients, we divide it into two doses of $20mg/m^2$ each. We administer the first half, diluted in sterile saline to 1ml/pound, and administer it as a 15-minute IV bolus and then give the second half the following week. The patient endures a longer duration of effect with this split dose technique without the risk of the MTD.

Splitting Adriamycin has spared our large canine geriatric lymphoma patients from unwanted adverse events, while providing an overall higher therapeutic dose. We feel this method safely treats cardiomyopathy-prone breeds and geriatric cancer dogs with less risk for side effects, while remaining efficacious. Adriamycin-induced cardiomyopathy can occur at any dose but the risk is greater in dogs as they exceed a cumulative dose of $240mg/m^2$.

Cats are resistant to clinical cardiotoxic effects of Adriamycin, but they develop adverse histologic changes in the myocardium. Some cats experience elevation of their creatinine and BUN levels. All cats developed histologic evidence of renal disease following administration at $30mg/m^2$ to a total cumulative dose of $300mg/m^2$. Based on this information, the feline dose for Adriamycin has been reduced to 1mg/kg or $25mg/m^2$ (O'Keef et al. 1993). Adriamycin-induced cardiac and renal toxicity should be anticipated when treating cancer in geriatric cats with heart disease and/or pre-existing CRF.

Organs Sensitive to Chemotherapeutic Agents

Know your chemotherapy drugs backward and forward. Be familiar with how the drugs are metabolized and excreted by the body. Know which drugs cause fatal toxicity in cats versus dogs. Be aware that Collies, Shelties, Australian Shepherds, and Long-Haired Whippets are at risk for toxicity from Adriamycin, vinca alkaloids, taxanes, dactinomycin, and etoposide due to the prevalence of multidrug resistance (MDR1) gene mutation and poor P-glycoprotein production. Small molecules may affect serum albumin and cause cytopenia. The following list will get you up to speed on this important issue. Also, be sure to check these details with new drugs as they come on the market.

Bone marrow: Most chemotherapeutic drugs have the potential for myelosuppression.

GI tract: Most chemotherapeutic drugs at higher doses cause nausea, vomiting, and colitis. Steroids and NSAIDs cause ulceration, hemorrhage, and reduced gastric cytoprotection.

Heart: Adriamycin, daunorubricin, all anthracyclines (cumulative dose).

Lungs: Bleomycin may cause fibrosis. *Cisplatin KILLS CATS* by causing pulmonary edema/effusion. Tanovea® may cause serious and sometimes fatal respiratory complications, including pulmonary fibrosis in some cases. Do not use in West Highland White Terriers and use with caution in other terrier breeds.

Liver: NSAIDs, steroids, lomustine, miscellaneous other drugs.

Kidneys: Cisplatin nephrotoxicity – requires intense diuresis, *KILLS CATS*, Adriamycin (cats).

Bladder: Cyclophosphamide (Cytoxan) and ifosfamide cause sterile hemorrhagic cystitis.

CNS: Vinca alkaloid induced neuropathy, cisplatin-induced hearing loss, 5-FU may induce seizures in dogs and *KILLS CATS*.

Eyes: Cisplatin may cause blindness; one of my geriatric canine mast cell cancer patients developed blindness with lomustine (very rare).

Skin: Hypersensitivity (rash, angioedema, urticaria, facial edema): L-asparaginase, Adriamycin, paclitaxel, Paccal-Vet® CA-1, Tanovea®, immunotherapy agents. Palmar-plantar erythrodyesthesia syndrome (PPES) may appear in the axilla, groin, and footpads of dogs given Doxil and various other drugs. Using vitamin B6 at 50mg PO TID abates PPES. Immunotherapy may bring about skin rashes, flushing, flu-like syndrome, asthma like reactions and inflammation of organs: immunotoxicities.

Hair follicles: Delayed growth – most drugs, Adriamycin alopecia in Poodles, Old English Sheepdogs, and Terriers; cats develop a velvet-like coat after long term chemotherapy.

Whiskers: Fall out with no replacement due to long term chemotherapy in cats.

Herding Breeds, Collie breeds: Drugs that are actively transported by the p-glycoprotein pump induce toxicity due to a pharmacogenetic mutation of the MDR1 allele. Some Collies are adversely affected by Platinol-related drugs. Vincristine, Vinblastine, Doxorubicin (Adriamycin), and Paclitaxel (Paccal-Vet) are chemotherapy drugs that require dose reductions to avoid SEVERE toxicity. Loperamide (Imodium®) and butorphanol also need dose reductions for affected dogs. To identify homozygous dogs at greatest risk, send cheek swabs for a special PCR assay c/o Dr. Katrina Mealey at Washington State University Veterinary School (Vail 2006b). http://vcpl.vetmed.wsu.edu/http://vcpl.vetmed.wsu.edu/problem-drugs.

Cats: Some chemotherapeutics are fatal in cats. Do not use cisplatin in cats. Do not use 5-FU, capecitabine (Xeloda), or any other 5-FU derivatives by any route in cats.

Coaching Caregivers (Carers) to Deal with Adverse Events: Cancer Care Package

We coach carers to be on patrol for adverse events and side effects with a 25% expectation rate in healthy pets and 25–35% in geriatric pets. Instruct caregivers to use a strategic plan for detection and handling of the most common chemotherapy side effects: GI tract and bone marrow toxicity. Make sure that the family knows how to take their pet's temperature and that they understand the significance of fever. Make sure that they know when the drug will typically nadir. At the slightest sign of anorexia or lethargy, instruct carers to take their pet's temperature. If it is above 102.5 degrees, advise them to start oral antibiotics for a minimum of 5 days. If the pet is listless for 6–12 hours, advise the client to visit the doctor ASAP for a CBC and assessment for sepsis.

Medications used to control inflammation and pain may also produce adverse events. Steroids and all NSAIDs may cause vomiting, GI ulceration, and hemorrhage. I recommend oral famotidine (Pepcid®) on an empty stomach daily for geriatric cancer patients taking steroids and NSAIDs. This will reduce the potential for GI ulceration. Warn clients that narcotics, including all morphine-related pain control drugs, may cause sedation, disorientation, drooling, loss of appetite, and constipation.

Prepare a "Cancer Care Package" for your clients, containing specific medications to manage anticipated side effects. Each medication bottle should be clearly labeled with the name of the medication, dosage, and its purpose. This enables the owner to immediately begin treating the adverse problem and possibly offset a visit to the emergency room. Explain to carers that if the problem persists or worsens, the geriatric cancer patient should be seen by their local veterinarian for evaluation or taken to an emergency clinic.

Because we anticipate that the cancer patient may encounter some degree of nausea, vomiting, or diarrhea during treatment, we send two or three prescriptions home with the carers after the very first visit. For control of nausea and vomiting, we send home metoclopramide (Reglan®). Metoclopramide is effective to offset nausea and emesis for most cases and most clients are willing to learn to give subcutaneous injections of it to help their pet feel better around chemotherapy treatment time. Some dogs may not respond to or tolerate metoclopramide. We have found that antiemetic therapy is effective with oral maropitant (Cerenia™), ondansetron (Zofran®), dolansetron mesylate (Anzemet®), or granisetron HCL (Kytril®). These antiemetics are excellent for refractory vomiting and may also be used on a pre-emptive basis against nausea and vomiting. A good choice for treatment of diarrhea and colitis is sulfasalazine (Azulfidine®) or metronidazole (Flagyl®).

We also inform clients about the potential need for using oral famotidine (Pepcid®) or sucralfate (Carafate®) to help their pet avoid nausea and feel better during chemotherapy. If the pet experiences nausea and vomiting with metoclopramide tablets, we instruct the client to crush the pills and blend the powder with honey, then rub the compound on to the pet's lips. Clients can also crush tablets, mix the powder with butter, and then shape the compound into bullets. Instruct clients to put these "butter bullets" in the freezer until they are firm. Medicated butter bullets can be administered rectally as a suppository.

For colitis or diarrhea, we send home metronidazole or sulfasalazine. We also recommend using oral kaolin-pectin products to help control diarrhea. Stay away from the newer formulations of Kaopectate® because these products now contain bismuth subsalicylate, which is essentially an NSAID. Since many of our lymphoma and mast cell cancer patients are on steroids, we must avoid NSAIDs. We also recommend loperamide (Imodium®) and RxClay® to help control diarrhea when metronidazole or sulfasalazine are not helpful. Loperamide was shown to have anticancer effects on several cancer cell lines, so it may have a dual benefit effect. We use other products that contain intestinal protectants and probiotics such as: BioSponge®, NutriGest®, and FortiFlora® to support the gastrointestinal tract and reduce diarrhea. We also recommend Diggin-Your-Dog FirmUp®, an antioxidant-rich blend of pumpkin and apple fiber that may help reduce chronic diarrhea and dietary change issues.

Oncology clients must have access to their oncologist, attending doctor, or a good emergency clinic for after-hours advice. It is important that caregivers are properly educated to anticipate that an adverse event may escalate and if not treated properly, it may lead to death. If the client does not take proper action and is not controlling or reversing the problem, or if the pet fails to respond to treatment, they must see their referring veterinarian or take their pet to an emergency clinic for help. Educate your clients to evaluate their geriatric pet for dehydration, fever, and sepsis. Remember to send the client home with a thermometer and antibiotics as part of the cancer care package (CCP) to keep on reserve so they can treat mild fevers at home.

The carers of a geriatric pet on chemotherapy with serious adverse events should not wait 2–3 days before calling a veterinarian or going to an emergency clinic. When the pet is taken to the hospital, evaluation and treatment for leukopenia, sepsis, and GI disease is empirical. The attending doctor must use antibiotics aggressively to deal with sepsis. Filgrastin (Neupogen®) at 5 mcg/kg, given SQ BID on day one, then once daily for 3 more days, may be life saving for patients with severe leukopenia, where the WBC is below 1,000.

A Word of Caution About Vesicants

Some of the most important chemotherapy drugs routinely administered as intravenous injections are vesicants. This means that the drug may cause a variable degree of localized tissue injury if there is a perivascular leak. The problem is compounded if the extravasation goes undetected and untreated. The most notorious vesicants are drugs in the anthracycline family, of which Adriamycin is the most commonly used. In my opinion, there is no equal to the damage that even small amounts of this extremely potent vesicant can cause to a patient's limb.

Adriamycin and vincristine, the most commonly used vinca alkaloid in dogs and cats, rank as severe and moderate vesicants, respectively. Taxanes and Actinomycin D rank with the anthracyclines as severe vesicants. Vinblastine, vinorelbine, and mechlorethamine (Mustargen®) are moderate vesicants. Cisplatin, mitoxantrone, dacarbazine (DTIC), 5-fluorouracil, mithramycin, etoposide, streptozotocin, and Bleomycin are considered mild vesicants. They pale in their perivascular toxicity when compared to the irreversible indolent tissue damage inflicted by drugs in the potent vesicant group. Plastic surgeons are asked to repair the tissue damage that occurs from chemotherapy extravasation in human cancer patients.

Other anthracyclines, such as daunorubicin, epirubicin, and idarubicin, are potent vesicants (Doroshow 1996). Doxil (STEALTH liposome encapsulated doxorubicin hydrochloride) is an irritant. If Adriamycin is extravasated into perivascular tissue of your patient, the results may turn into one of your worst nightmares (Figure 6.2). In my opinion, there is no equal to the tissue necrosis that even small amounts of Adriamycin can cause to a limb. We always emphasize my favorite descriptive term, "vasosclerotic," on our chemotherapy work order forms to warn our technical staff that localized tissue injury will result if there is a spill.

Most perivascular leaks are noticed right away as a "bleb" or swelling immediately adjacent to the venipuncture site. Alternatively, the pet may experience overt immediate discomfort, crying out or struggling against the person restraining the animal for the injection. If a cancer patient fights restraint, recommend sedation for the safe administration of any caustic chemotherapy agent, especially Adriamycin. We insist on sedation to protect nervous and upset cancer patients from the nightmare of extravasation. I educate pet owners that "If we do not use sedation and your pet struggles, he may cause a mishap that could literally lead to the loss of his leg!" We rely on the attending staff to be vigilant in deciding which patients need sedation.

It is recommended not to use acepromazine and phenothiazines (or any drug that causes arrhythmias or vasodilation) as a sedation drug when using Adriamycin. We prefer to use the low dose

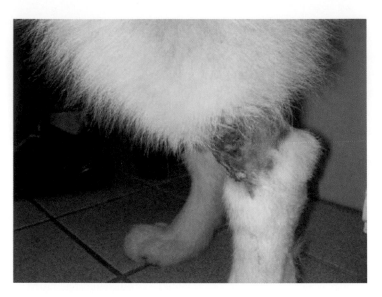

Figure 6.2.   Extravasated Adriamycin site at 10 days showing early tissue necrosis. This lesion worsened over several months, exposing muscle, tendons, and bone.

combination of Dexdomitor® and butorphanol IM with Antisedan® reversal for healthy cancer patients: www.dexdomitorcalculator.com. Some clinicians prefer Telazol® for immobilization of healthy fractious dogs. For patients with heart disease or advanced age, and for frail patients, we use a combination of fentanyl, a short-acting opioid, and midazolam, a short-acting benzodiazepine IV, or a combination of butorphanol and diazepam IM or IV. The preferred method for many clinicians is the use of sevoflurane inhalation anesthesia for masking or closed-chamber sedation/anesthesia, particularly for geriatric feline cancer patients. The objective is to make patients be still, for their own safety, during the administration of severe vasosclerotic chemotherapy drugs.

I came up with the theory that either the physical presence of the drug had to be altered or else we had to do much more to get the spilled drug out of the site. We rely on our nursing staff to point out loud and clear when even small, suspected extravasations occur.

The attending chemotherapy nurse and clinician must be on immediate alert. They must team up and act vigorously to literally remove every drop of the spilled drug from the perivascular site. Unfortunately, there is not much written on how to effectively do just that! Most textbooks say that whatever is done probably will not make a real difference anyway. So there was a sense of gloom and doom when vasosclerotics like Adriamycin were extravasated. That situation was unacceptable for me when looking at the risk–benefit ratio for my patients. It made me rethink the situation.

Occasionally, a spill may go undetected and untreated only to be noticed anywhere from 1 to 10 days after treatment. The caregiver calls the office with complaints that the pet has pain, is limping, has swelling or desquamation, or is licking the venipuncture site.

The extravasation site may not look threatening at first, even after the first 3–10 days or well into the second week. Vincristine sloughs are evident within the first 1–7 days. The damaged tissue forms necrotic crusts, causing the injured skin to stiffen like leather. The patient will lick the site and may exhibit pain by holding up the leg or limping. When the dead tissue sloughs off, it may leave a deeper ulcer, which eventually heals over a 6-week period.

Adriamycin sloughs may begin to show only after 7–10 days. The spill area appears inflamed for another 1–3 weeks. The lesion then slowly worsens as the weeks and months wear on. The ulceration and tissue necrosis from Adriamycin will gradually infiltrate and spread deeper and deeper, exposing muscle, tendons, and bone. The area of eschar (a slough produced by a thermal burn or corrosive agent or gangrene) enlarges and deepens, forming necrotic sequestration of tissue that may become infected and then this case turns into the worst nightmare that one can imagine.

Why the tissue damage spreads is poorly understood but be sure to understand that the eschar from an Adriamycin spill will continue to fungate for longer than 3–4 weeks (the time frame given in most textbooks). In actual fact, the effects of an Adriamycin extravasation will persist for months – more than 3 months, in my experience – and will involve an area much larger than that affected by the initial spill. Be sure to understand that tissue damage will continue to worsen over these months. The injured tissues will not heal or regenerate. There is tremendous and severe pain, swelling, and corruption of the tissues of the entire limb.

In most cases, amputation becomes the only option, due to the extensive and irreversible nature of the tissue necrosis. Do we continue the futile nursing care, despite the pain, because the pet's primary problem is cancer? There is no easy way out of this situation. Deciding whether or not to recommend amputation of a geriatric patient's leg when the patient may die from cancer in the near future is truly a nightmare. After your recommendation, the nightmare of making the decision is passed along to your client.

Inexperienced clinicians and nursing staff may not fully understand the consequences of an Adriamycin spill because it does not really look so bad at the beginning. It is easy to initially understate the ramifications to pet owners, especially when trying to comfort them. In my opinion, Adriamycin spills must be accurately and honestly described to clients from the start. The client must be carefully counseled and warned of the fact that the wound will most likely get worse with time despite the best bandage-changing and nursing care. To explain the gravity of the situation to a client, I say, "Unfortunately, we had an accident while administering chemotherapy today. Some of the drug leaked outside of the vein. This is called 'extravasation' or a 'spill,' and is, unfortunately, always a danger when using these drugs. Although this drug is very good at killing cancer cells, when it is in direct contact with tissue it behaves like an acid. The drug may continue to destroy tissue relentlessly, despite our best efforts to halt it. In the worst-case scenario, we may, regrettably, have to recommend amputation to stop the pain."

Please compassionately explain extravasation to clients who want to know why you insist on suggesting sedation for their uncooperative pets for each Adriamycin treatment.

Can We Prevent Extravasation?

Prevention of disaster is the very best control. First, set your staff up to prevent extravasation of any chemotherapy drug. The chemotherapy room should be quiet and free of distractions. The nurses should be focused and should not be given cross-orders or be pressured to hurry through the procedure. There must be a clean stick into the vein when placing the catheter. There must be constant visual and hands-on monitoring of the intravenous injection site to ensure that the needle is still in the vein during the entire administration of every drop of the drug.

Some oncologists propose the use of an indwelling catheter and dilution of the Adriamycin into a small bag of saline that is infused over a 30–45 minute period. This technique may yield the largest extravasations. Other oncologists prefer to run the Adriamycin IV through a well-placed indwelling catheter simultaneously with rapidly flowing saline over a period of 15–20 minutes. The oncologists and oncology nurses I have spoken to feel most comfortable with direct, close supervision of every drop of Adriamycin using very small gauge butterfly catheters (no larger than 23 gauge).

The total calculated dose of Adriamycin is diluted in a 12 cc syringe with sterile saline to 10ml for the average cat. We dilute the dose for dogs to approximately 1ml/lb with sterile saline or sterile water, for injection using a 35ml syringe for small dogs and a 60ml syringe for large dogs. The carefully placed butterfly catheter is flushed with saline. The Adriamycin solution is administered while frequently pulling the syringe back just enough to see blood in the hub of the syringe. This verifies that the catheter remains well positioned and not up against the wall of the vein. We administer Adriamycin to cats over a slow bolus over 5–7 minutes and to dogs at a slow, steady infusion rate over 15–20 minutes. In our experience, the intense, hands-on, direct visual supervision during the administration of diluted solutions of Adriamycin to well-behaved or sedated patients works best to avoid the nightmare of extravasation.

An excellent suggestion to prevent extravasation appeared in the "Tech Talk" section of the *Veterinary Cancer Society Newsletter* (Rose 2004). Rose recommends using a small gauge butterfly catheter with 12-inch tubing. She attaches a three-way stopcock to the catheter and places a 12ml Luer–Lock syringe with 0.9% saline solution at one port and the chemotherapeutic drug at the other port. Flushing before and after drug administration is easily performed without switching from one syringe to another. The chemotherapy nurse monitors flow by continuous aspiration of small amounts of blood to verify placement of the catheter in the vein during the entire administration of the drug (Figure 6.3).

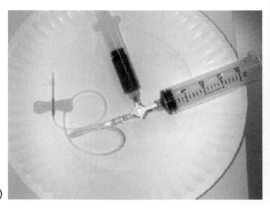

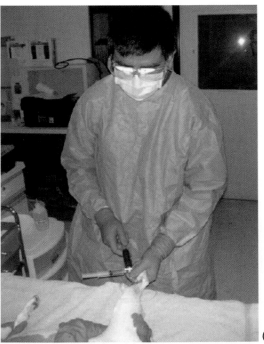

(A)   (B)

Figure 6.3.   A small gauge butterfly catheter with 12-inch tubing attached to a three-way stopcock (A). This setup can be used for convenient flushing with a 12ml Luer–Lock syringe filled with 0.9% saline solution. This technique facilitates flushing and delivery of chemotherapy without changing syringes (B).

Extravasation Site Treatment in the Literature

All references instruct the attending doctor to act immediately. They recommend not removing the catheter, but rather keeping it in place to cleanse it before withdrawing it. Use a syringe to remove as much drug as possible from the catheter, tubing, and tissue. Removal of 5–6ml of blood in a cat and 10ml in a dog should be adequate. Insert a 27-gauge needle into the spill bleb and aspirate as much of the drug as possible to minimize the amount of drug at the site. Some references then say to administer the "appropriate antidote" or flush saline through the catheter to dilute residual drug, then to use ice cold packs or cold compresses for Adriamycin, actinomycin-D, and mechlorethamine spills. The compresses are recommended for 6–10 hours.

All references agree that warm compresses should be placed on vinca alkaloid and etoposide spills for the first 3–4 hours. These procedures are recommended to minimize the vesicant's toxicity. The objective is to spread the vinca alkaloid with warm compresses to disperse the drug into the circulatory system. The opposite idea is to use cold compresses to localize Adriamycin spills to reduce its toxicity. Are you thoroughly confused yet by this? The most disheartening thing to read in the literature is that all experts agree that nothing, including the recommended "antidotes" in the following section, seems to work when dealing with anthracyclines extravasations! I could not accept this hopelessness and still get to sleep at night.

Recommended "Antidotes" for Extravasations

Most references suggest using a compound called DHM3 or the timely use of dexrazoxane (Zinecard®) injected directly into the tissue area of the spill within 3 hours of the accident. Some oncologists use IV Zinecard at 10 times the Adriamycin dose within 3 hours and at 24 and 48 hours after a spill (Vail 2006b). These measures are anecdotally reported to help offset the damage from anthracycline spills.

This may indeed help if the compounds are readily available and used in time. Unfortunately, some spills are not detected until the patient has begun to exhibit a slough lesion. The price of Zinecard is $250.00 and $350.00 for the 250mg and 500mg vial, respectively. Zinecard is used in humans to reduce the cardiotoxic effects of anthracycline drugs. Some references say that using 1ml of 1/6 molar isotonic sodium thiosulfate for each ml of extravasated cisplatin can inactivate it. This antidote is recommended only if a large amount of cisplatin is extravasated. Hyaluronidase at 150 units/ml is recommended at 1ml for every ml of extravasated vinca alkaloid or etoposide. This is purported to enhance absorption and disperse the extravasated drug. Topical dimethyl sulfoxide (DMSO) or infiltration of the area with 1mg/kg of hydrocortisone or using intralesional dexamethasone is considered controversial and most references say that using these anti-inflammatory agents is probably a waste of time. Since the consequences of extravasation add up to an iatrogenic event, I was still dissatisfied with this information.

Dr. Steven F. Swaim, Professor Emeritus at Auburn University, specializes in wound management. Dr. Swaim suggested to me that hydrophilic wound dressings be used over extravasation sites, because these dressings act to pull the body's homeostatic fluids up through the tissues to bathe the wound tissues from the inside out. This may help to reduce edema and bathe the wound with antibiotic-containing fluids if the patient is on systemic antibiotics. Theoretically, hydrophilic dressings should also help remove the caustic agent from the tissues and stimulate the healing process. Dr. Swaim prefers to use Carrington Carrasyn Hydrogel Wound Dressing®, a product containing acemannan (derived from aloe vera). It stimulates macrophages to produce cytokines and growth factors needed for indolent wounds. Using this product may have potential benefit, but there are no clinical studies to assess its value in managing extravasations.

Overall, in my practice there was a feeling of dread, helplessness, and hopelessness surrounding the situation of extravasation. We felt that if we were going to work every day with these drugs for our entire careers, we needed to do something more to challenge and offset this potentially devastating problem. I decided to treat Adriamycin spills as if they were very nasty poisonous snakebites.

An Aggressive Approach to Extravasation: "The Villalobos Modified Snakebite Slit Technique"

The literature makes only fleeting mention about flushing extravasation sites with saline and mentions caution for this procedure, as it may indeed spread the drug to a deeper or wider area. I was determined to find a better technique for flushing the drug OUT.

There is only one way for me to sleep without nightmares when dealing with Adriamycin extravasations. We treat every Adriamycin spill like the worst snakebite on earth and we treat it immediately. First of all, there is no blame or anxiety placed on the technician who observes and/or reports the spill. Rather than putting tension in the air, there should be only encouragement and gratitude for the informant. The attending doctor needs to know if there is even a suspicion of extravasation because the patient's well-being is clearly the first priority. Accidents happen and pride and feelings are hurt, but those issues need to be set aside to rescue the patient from the nightmare that extravasation can become.

After the initial aspiration from the catheter and the bleb are completed, we infiltrate saline into the site as described earlier. The team preps the leg for surgical incision and at this point I take charge.

Using the bevel of a sterile 18-gauge needle, I make at least 10–30 vertical, deep skin incisions (slits). The slits extend into the perivascular SQ tissues in a "lettuce bag" pattern as staggered parallel incisions. The slits should extend beyond the entire extravasation site and 360 degrees around the entire limb (Figure 6.4). We then run copious amounts of saline or isolyte solution through the entire site and around the limb with the philosophy of flush, flush, and flush and then flush some more.

We gently squeeze or "milk" the tissue bleb site during the entire time that we are flushing. I may poke the 18-gauge needle into deeper parts of the limb, into muscle and fat, to let solution infiltrate deeper and allow the vesicant drug to ooze out. Hopefully, every drop of the offending vesicant will percolate out through the skin slits in a diluted fashion. On one occasion, we were pleased to see the distinctive red color of Adriamycin as it exited the tissue. In a typical 60-pound dog, we may flush 1–2 liters through the extravasation site over a 30–45 minute period, depending on which drug was spilled.

I recommend using nothing short of this extreme measure to get every drop of vesicant drug out of the spill area, especially if the spill involves Adriamycin. We send the patient home with a light wrap and instructions for the family to apply cold compresses 20 minutes on, 20 off for the next 24 hours. The patient is rechecked weekly for 3 weeks to monitor for tissue damage, infection, and healing of the skin incisions.

As soon as we started using this technique at our clinics, we were able to completely avoid the nightmares that are so predictable with extravasations of any type, but especially with Adriamycin. We have shared this procedure with many colleagues (because it works), christening it the "Villalobos Modified Snakebite Slit Technique." I feel confident that you will find similar success when dealing with extravasations using this practical technique. It has the potential to minimize unnecessary suffering for the patient, the pet owner, and the practitioner.

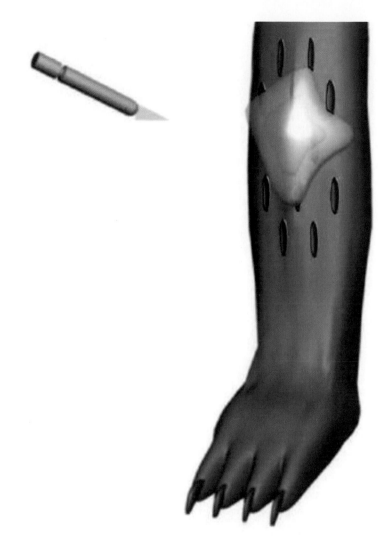

Figure 6.4.   Cartoon showing the "lettuce bag" or the staggered parallel incision pattern used over the extravasation site in the "Villalobos Modified Snakebite Slit Technique." Saline is run into the site and milked out through the incisions. This flushing process allows spilled Adriamycin and other spilled vasosclerotic drugs to exit the perivascular tissue. Figure contributed by David Perrot.

Judd's Case (Everybody Loses with Extravasations)

Judd Dow, a 13-year-old M/N Malamute, was receiving Adriamycin for anal sac adenocarcinoma with medial iliac and lumbar node metastases. Judd was a huge Malamute with pre-existing degenerative myelopathy and weakness in his hind limbs. Judd was doing well until a hind leg extravasation occurred. The spill involved the recurrent tarsal vein in Judd's hind limb. This spill was a nightmare case for the owner and for a young attending oncologist, who may never before have experienced the full extent of necrosis that a large Adriamycin spill can cause.

Judd's owner came to me for a second opinion. I did everything in my power to keep the client from targeting her anger at the well-meaning attending doctors and staff. I encouraged her to continue seeing her original oncologist and staff for wound care. I told her to retain confidence in the practice because they are dedicated, have a very good reputation, and are highly respected in the veterinary community. I mentioned that they might be gracious enough to absorb some of the expense for the long term wound care that Judd would most likely need.

As the ordeal of wound care wore on, the oncologist asked two board certified surgeons to look at the wound. They attempted to debride the necrotic tissue twice and helped set up the wound management program for daily bandage changes and inspections. At one time, Judd was hospitalized for 3 weeks on IV antibiotics and extra wound-care sessions to deal with sepsis. This effort dragged on over 3 months. Judd had the best wound-care management, but to no avail. The festering wound extended down through the muscle and to bone. The ligaments became detached after months of wound care, expense, and discomfort.

The surgical specialist ultimately recommended amputation rather than reconstruction. This was a great disappointment to the owner, after an earlier promise of reconstruction and after the extended and extensive hardship of treating the wound. Of course, chemotherapy was discontinued during the months of wound care and the cancer progressed.

Judd's carers could not fathom an amputation along with the degenerative myelopathy and the fact that Judd had progressive metastatic cancer in his abdomen from primary anal sac adenocarcinoma. The family regretfully elected euthanasia.

Later on, Judd's primary carer needed to vent. I became the listener that she needed. She told me that she was angry and inconsolable because Judd had been doing well in chemotherapy until the spill occurred. She felt that the attending doctor was not truthful with her about the situation from the start. I explained to her that the young doctor may have never seen an extravasation before and may have been unaware of the extent or of what was ahead, because not much detail has been written about it. Ultimately, all parties concerned suffered. She understandably wanted to pursue litigation despite my discouragement and despite the valiant efforts of the practice where the extravasation occurred.

With over 45 years of experience in oncology, I have seen just about everything there is to see. Extravasation is an accident. If it is not spotted at the time and not treated aggressively, it spells disappointment, disaster, and nightmare. There is no winner here. The attending doctors and staff need to offer a sincere apology for the accident and its repercussions and absorb the costs. Insurance companies have been teaching physicians to apologize to their patients and families for complications and for adverse events. Insurance companies found that patients appreciated their attending doctor's apology. If people felt their doctor was sincere and sorry for what happened, and expressed empathy and compassion, they were much less likely to pursue with malpractice litigation.

Extravasation Summary

Client communication and public relations (PR) is very touchy in this type of situation. The best you can do is to apologize and provide support and remain understanding of the caregivers' grief and resentment. Be sure to tell the family that you feel terrible about the situation and that it is one of the risks that the field of oncology endures. Tell them that it takes courage to use chemotherapy drugs to treat cancer in geriatric pets but that, like penicillin, it saves lives despite the risk of adverse events.

At each recheck, apologize and sympathize with the client's grief and dismay. Some clients will be able to resolve their anger and blame and others will not. It is important to remain in partnership with the client and commit to dealing with the immediate issues of pain control, extended care, or a decision to debride or amputate.

It is because of scenarios like Judd's that I am compelled to write so extensively about potent vesicants and extravasation. This is an extremely important issue and I hope that you will avoid extravasation in your practice. In the best interest of the patient, most oncologists recommend that general practices using Adriamycin should not allow technicians to perform the infusions. Chemotherapy nurses at specialty practices are highly trained and competent for this procedure, but the consequences of a spill are so dire that technicians in general practice should not be asked to take this responsibility. It may be best for the attending doctor to administer all chemotherapy drugs in the general practice setting. Again, chemotherapy should be done with no other activity going on in the area. Some doctors prefer to give all vesicant chemotherapy to cats while they are under Isoflurane or Sevoflurane sedation/anesthesia.

Treatment for Chemotherapy Toxicity

The treatment of toxicity and adverse events from chemotherapy is fundamentally a common-sense approach based on empirical medicine. When patients are given IV chemotherapy, we send home a "Cancer Care Package" (CCP) that contains a thermometer, antinausea, antidiarrheal, and antibiotic medications. Clients need to be educated to take action and use the medications in their CCP at the first sign of toxicity.

For mild gastrointestinal reactions, such as: inappetence, nausea, and vomiting, we routinely used metoclopramide (Reglan®) for many years and it is still effective. Reglan is a gastric prokinetic drug that also has central antiemetic effect. It is more effective in dogs than in cats. As first choice, we now routinely use more potent central acting antiemetics such as maropitant (Cerenia™) or ondansetron (Zofran®), which has become affordable. We also use oral dolansetron (Anzemet®) and granisetron (Kytril®). Chlorpromazine (Thorazine®) acts on the emetic center, chemoreceptor trigger zone, and on peripheral receptors at 0.1 to 0.25mg/lb IM or SQ SID–TID as needed. We use a compounding pharmacy for many of our patients or write a prescription and instruct clients to purchase the drugs at a pharmacy. This avoids having to keep so many drugs in stock at our clinics.

For dogs and cats with poor appetite, consider using capromorelin oral suspension (Entyce®) to stimulate the appetite. Capromorelin is a selective ghrelin receptor agonist that binds to receptors that stimulate appetite. Consider using oral mirtazapine (Remeron®) to restore appetite in dogs and cats. Mirtazapine has antidepressant, anxiolytic, and hyperphagic action. Use $\frac{1}{8}$–$\frac{1}{4}$ of a 15mg mirtazapine tablet every 72 hours for cats and $\frac{1}{8}$–1 tablet every 24 hours for dogs (Cahill 2006). See package inserts for empirical doses and precautions. Cyproheptadine is another option for appetite stimulation. It is an antihistamine with antiserotonin effects and may take 2–7 days to take effect and is effective in both dogs and cats.

To treat diarrhea and colitis, use sulfasalizine (Azulfidine®), sulfadimethoxine, metronidazole (Flagyl), and Tylosin®. We may instruct clients to use over-the-counter kaopectolin (Kaolin/Pectin®) at 1–2ml/kg orally 4–6 times daily as needed, and/or Immodium as needed. We also recommend FirmUp® for dogs, which is an antioxidant-rich blend of pumpkin and apple fiber that may help reduce chronic diarrhea and dietary change issues. Please note that Kaopectate® no longer contains kaolin and the US product contains aspirin, an NSAID.

If a geriatric oncology patient exhibits any adverse event over grade 2 (moderate) with GI signs accompanied by listlessness, then it is best for the patient to be examined by a veterinarian who may recommend outpatient supportive care or hospitalization until the patient is stabilized.

Hypersensitivity reactions such as rash, pruritis, urticaria, hives, and wheals may occur during or following chemotherapy administration or immunotherapy vaccines and preparations. Acute anaphylaxis or anaphylactoid reactions require immediate attention. Some patients may develop fever, difficulty breathing, and GI upset with the new precision medicine preparations. These adverse reactions respond quite well to diphenhydramine (Benadryl®) at 2–4mg/kg IM and dexamethasone at

0.5–1mg/kg IV.When pretreatment is recommended, we give our canine cancer patients IM Benadryl at 1mg per pound and both canine and feline patients with SQ or IM or IV dexamethasone at 4mg/m². IV pretreatment precedes IV drug administration while IM or SQ pretreatment is given 5–20 minutes prior to administration of all predictably allergenic drugs such as L-asparaginase and Adriamycin. Paccal Vet®-CA1 is paclitaxel injection for dogs. It is a taxane that has been developed for dogs to avoid severe toxicity. Do not use the human dose or formulations (Paxil® or DOCEtaxel) because it is toxic to dogs and requires an astute pretreatment protocol to minimize GI, CNS, cardiovascular, and anaphylactoid reactions. Prepare patients the night before with oral prednisone at 2 m/kg. Pretreat with Benadryl at 4mg/kg IM, cimetidine at 4mg/kg IV, and dexamethasone SP at 2mg/kg 30–60 minutes before using Paccal Vet®, which must be administered IV slowly over a 3-4-hour infusion. The US Food and Drug Administration withdrew the conditional approval for Paccal Vet-CA1 at the request of the drug's manufacturer in February 2017. Further studies regarding toxicity and efficacy will be conducted on a conditional use permit basis.

Sepsis and tumor breakdown syndrome are true oncologic emergencies. The treatment is empirical with IV fluid support, electrolyte balancing, antibiotics, symptomatic care for vomiting and diarrhea, and supportive care in the hospital. Anthracycline-related cardiomyopathy and heart failure is poorly responsive to therapy and has a poor prognosis. It is best to avoid cardiotoxicity by proper patient selection, slowing down the rate of infusion and splitting the dose as described above to avoid giving the MDT dose to dogs over 50–60 pounds. Use an EKG and monitor cardiac function with echocardiography before each administration of Adriamycin if using the MTD dose in large dogs. Be aware that cardiotoxicity develops more often in breeds predisposed to dilated cardiomyopathy and in patients that approach the cumulative toxicity dose, which ranges from 180mg/m² to 240mg/m². Consider using dexrazoxane (Zinecard) as a cardio protectant when Adriamycin is the best option or the only effective agent, or the pet relapses without it. Zinecard at a 10:1 dose ratio is given as a slow IV bolus starting 30 minutes prior to administration of Adriamycin (Vail 2006b).

Summary: Adverse Events of Cancer Therapy in Geriatric Pets

Adverse effects are an unintended but not unexpected sequelae in the management of geriatric cancer patients. Surgery, radiation, chemotherapy, and immunotherapy induce specific adverse events that can be graded from 0–5 according to severity, with grade 5 resulting in death of the patient. Carers need education and information sheets regarding what to expect and when to expect adverse events. The care and management of adverse effects should be prompt to spare the geriatric oncology patient further stress by use of the cancer care package, which contains medications to treat the adverse symptoms. Be sure to avoid extravasations by having a strict protocol for administration of vasosclerotics, especially when using Adriamycin in nervous or fractious patients. Empathize with caregivers and be sure to apologize whenever an adverse event or complication occurs.

The Role of Radiation Therapy in Cancer Management

Education is going from cocksure ignorance to thoughtful uncertainty.

Donald E. Thrall, DVM, PhD, DAVCR NC State University College of Veterinary Medicine

The specialty board of veterinary radiation oncology was established in 1994 and offers residency programs in radiation oncology (see Thrall 2004). Veterinary oncology became more sophisticated during the 1970s. Many veterinary radiologists and oncologists, myself included, incorporated RTx into their practices to palliate and control tumors with used equipment from the human side. Radiation therapy is involved in the management of 40–62% of all human cancers. Approximately 8,500 radiation therapy machines are in use for people worldwide with a disparity in low income countries. As of 2016, 190 countries have RTx and 40 countries have no facilities. There is a need for 7,000 more units in the world to treat human cancer patients, according to the Global Task Force on Cancer Care and Control (www.cancercontrol.info). A world standard of access would be 4–8 radiotherapy units per one million people. This may never be achieved for companion animals!

The Hi-Art® TomoTherapy unit, developed by researchers in Wisconsin, was considered to be the biggest innovation in RTx since the 1950s. Introducing image-guided radiation therapy (IGRT) it combined a linac and a CT scanner. The linac is mounted in a large doughnut (gander) and rotates around the patient in a helical fashion, while the CT scanner provides on-the-spot imaging. Its radiation beam is computerized to avoid healthy organs while striking the tumor from a variety of angles.Stereotactic radiation surgery (SRS) is also known as CyberKnife radiosurgery. Both names are misnomers because the applications are from an external source and are not actually surgery because there is no incision. SRS/CyberKnife uses a robotic arm to focus an intense dose fraction of radiation delivery precisely to the tumor over 1–5 treatments. SRS may be used to treat inoperable tumors and it spares at-risk geriatric oncology patients the stress of surgery. SRS bypasses the need for multiple daily or every other day anesthesia for low fractionated delivery of conventional radiation, which requires over 18–21 sessions.

These fusion units and newer and improved machines have $3.2 million price tags for installation at major hospitals with ongoing service contracts.

Veterinary specialty radiation oncology facilities in the United States and Europe installed previously owned and new linear accelerators (linacs) over the past several decades. As prices dropped, and if maintenance contracts were reasonably priced, veterinary cancer patients gained more access to linear accelerators and IGRT facilities. There are approximately 70 RTx facilities devoted to the treatment of companion animal tumors in the United States and Europe and we can expect more in the future, as graduates from the residency programs enter practice. PetCure™ offers a new concept in radiation oncology for animals. It combines on-site RTx facilities with remotely administered dosimetry, metrics, and treatment planning protocol. The PetCure™ Scientific Advisory Board consists of human and veterinary radiation oncologists, physicians, radiobiologists, and consultants (Mauldin 2016).

The average age of household dogs and cats in the United States has increased from 4 to 6 years old in 2006. The average life span of dogs is between 8 and 12 years. The aging of America's pets will produce a huge number of geriatric oncology patients. About 12 million dogs and cats will be diagnosed with cancer in the US per year according to the Morris Animal Foundation. If we go by an estimate that there are 65 million dogs in the US today, that half of them die of cancer, and that hemangiosarcoma composes 7% of cancers in dogs, we can estimate that this cancer will affect up to 2.5 million of the dogs currently owned in the country. The percentage rises when we focus on breeds with predilection such as German Shepherd Dogs and Golden Retrievers (Lamerato-Kozicki et al. 2005).

We estimated the number of feline injection site sarcomas (FISS) to be as many as 22,000 cats per year (Ford 2004). However, our profession was able to initiate preventative measures and reduced the occurrence of FISS. A rising percentage of pet caregivers will seek help from your clinic, asking for specialty care for their pets with cancer. Many of these cases will need RTx.

The lack of available facilities, risk to critical tissues, and the requirement for general anesthesia have always been limitations for electing RTx as an option. Cost and transportation logistics are additional factors for many pet owners. These reasons kept RTx in the background as a seldom-used modality in veterinary cancer medicine. Today, we use safer anesthetics or heavy sedation for geriatric cancer patients. The new generation of RTx machines is safer; linear accelerators cause less damage to tissues surrounding tumors than cobalt and orthovoltage machines and are ideal for use in small dogs and cats. IGRT and SRS will become more available at veterinary teaching facilities and at customized veterinary facilities in major cities. Palliative RTx protocols offer 3–4 fractions and stereotactic radiosurgery (SRS) can be completed in only 1–5 treatments.

New graduates are familiar with RTx because most contemporary veterinary schools have state-of-the-art equipment and offer radiation oncology services. New graduates are also familiar with the risk-to-benefit ratio of RTx for geriatric patients. In short, RTx, IGRT, and SRS are becoming a realistic and available option for pet owners who can access a facility and afford the cost.

When recommending RTx for a geriatric cancer patient, first investigate the type of RTx facilities that are available and, second, establish if the elderly pet is a good candidate for RTx. Do a thorough evaluation of the patient for tolerance to multiple anesthetic procedures and a thorough evaluation of the malignancy, to rule out metastatic disease prior to RTx. Many geriatric oncology patients will be eliminated as candidates for low fraction RTx due to compromised organ function. They may benefit with palliative radiation therapy using 3–4 fractions. If SRS is available, it would be the most advanced form of RTx for the patient. Chief concerns would be renal, hepatic, cardiac disease, and body condition. If the tumor is staged as localized, if it is not highly metastatic and is potentially responsive to radiation, then RTx is a good option for treatment.

At the initial stages of the workup, the attending doctor needs to decide about imaging with CT or MRI. Newer imaging machines are able to complete studies in under 7 minutes and provide three dimensional (3D) views. Some calm patients may only need mild sedation instead of anesthesia. The radiation oncologist may prefer CT for initial imaging because it is also used for computer-assisted treatment planning and thus accomplishes two steps. Initial imaging with MRI may provide valuable information but it may not integrate with CT-based dosimetry treatment planning. Requiring CT as a second step is unnecessarily costly for clients and creates more stress for older patients. Cancer patients receiving RTx for oral or nasal cancer must have complete dental cleaning and extraction of all loose teeth to completely eliminate plaque and clear up infection, which becomes a third step.

Uses of Radiation Therapy

RTx is used principally for local tumor control and palliation (treatment with non-curative intent). RTx is most successful when used in truly localized radiation-responsive neoplasia. RTx is most often used postoperatively to sterilize residual disease in surgical fields. It may be used preoperatively to shrink large tumors, making them more amenable to surgical excision or as a single modality to save structures in cases where the cancer is staged as local and believed to have low metastatic potential. RTx is used in combination with chemotherapy, hyperthermia, targeted therapy, immunotherapy, and so forth, to enhance local control. Because RTx is strictly a localized treatment, other modalities are needed to address the metastatic potential of the particular cancer being treated. Novel triple therapy is being used at UC Davis for RTx cases with metastatic disease, combining oral therapy to reduce T-regulatory cells and intratumor injections that enhance a local immune response against the tumor.

If your client is considering RTx as an option, an early referral for consultation will save steps. CT scans are programmed to interface with and reconstruct images for 3D computerized treatment planning in place of MRI. The closer the CT scan is to the time of treatment, the more accuracy there is because tumors change shape and size over time. This has been a major problem in human RTx. This is addressed with new combination units such as the Hi-Art TomoTherapy unit and the SRS PetCure™ equipment, which combines CT with radiation therapy.

Price is always a consideration. SRS will be 2–3 times more costly than conventional radiation therapy, which many clients cannot afford in the first place. It is important to know about another option if radiation therapy is impossible to finance. Electrochemotherapy (electroporation) is an excellent option in selected accessible tumors and most oral tumors. Read the section at the end of Chapter 6 for this practical and affordable technology as an option to offer clients who cannot afford RTx.

Radiation Therapy as a Curative Measure

To sterilize clean, narrow, or dirty margins in a sarcoma or carcinoma field as postsurgical follow-up.

As primary treatment for nasal tumors and facial squamous cell carcinoma (SCC).

As primary treatment for some brain tumors.

As local control of oral tumors (acanthomatous epulis, SCC, fibrosarcoma (FSA)).

As preoperative treatment of soft tissue sarcoma (STS) to decrease size and viability of the mass.

As intraoperative therapy (using a mega dose) to sterilize an open tumor bed (intracavitary) prior to skin closure.

As part of the induction protocol for anterior mediastinal lymphoma and as half-body RTx in some induction protocols for canine lymphoma.

As stereotactic radiosurgery (SRS) for tumors that were previously hard to access or considered untreatable due to location near a vital structure such as the spinal cord.

Radiation Therapy as a Palliative Measure

To reduce cancer pain and tumor growth with osteosarcoma.

To shrink bleeding facial and nasal SCC.

To shrink oral and pharyngeal masses (SCC, malignant melanoma, FSA, tonsillar SCC).

To treat inoperable brain tumors.

To shrink mediastinal masses and large lymph nodes in resistant lymphoma.

To reduce the size of large primary or metastatic lesions.

Very simply, radiation kills cells by crippling their ability to repopulate. The energy beam breaks chemical bonds in DNA directly by ionization or indirectly by ionizing cellular water (Figure 6.5). This results in the formation of charged free radicals and active oxygen species that transfer energy to and damage DNA. Tumor tissue is more sensitive to RTx than normal tissue but adjacent local tissue still suffers from the standby effect. Acute and late toxicity may develop.

The dose of radiation is measured in units of energy deposited per mass of tissue. The units were originally called rads and are now called the gray (Gy). One hundred rads = 1 Gy = 1 joule/kg. The

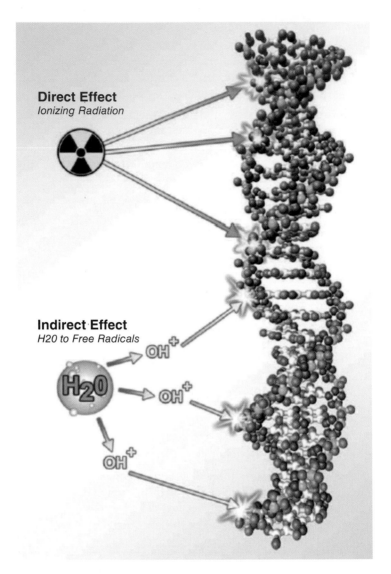

Figure 6.5.   The radiation energy beam breaks chemical bonds in DNA directly by ionization or indirectly by ionizing cellular water, which results in the formation of charged free radicals and active oxygen species that transfer energy to and damage DNA. Figure contributed by Andrew Hoffman.

dose–response curve for RTx has a sigmoidal shape with curves at the bottom and top like a stretched-out S-curve. The curve rises rapidly in a steep incline between the dose for tumor control and the dose for patient tissue toxicity (Figure 6.6). If treatment stops at a threshold dose of 40 Gy for a particular tumor and does not finish the total prescribed dose of 50 to 55 Gy, the probability of tumor control remains at the low end of the sigmoidal curve and minimal toxicity is expected. Conversely, if this patient receives more than 60 Gy, the side effects at the top end of the curve will be more likely to occur in the form of tissue morbidity.

RTx doses generally range from 30 to 60 Gy, delivered in 4–30 treatment fractions over a period of 3–6 weeks depending on the intent of treatment (palliative or curative). If SRS is available for the patient, the dose is generally delivered in 1–3 fractions over 1–3 days. Some tumors may require 5 fractions with SRS.

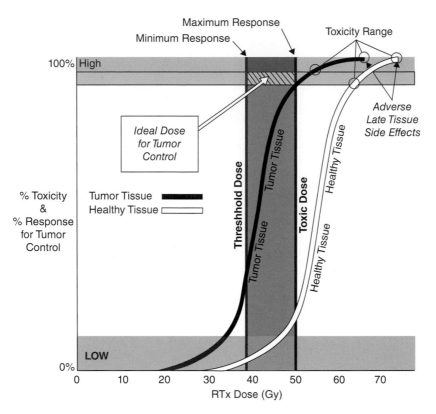

Figure 6.6. The dose–response curve for RTx has a sigmoidal shape with curves at the bottom and top like a stretched-out S-curve. The steep part of the curve rises rapidly between the dose for tumor control and the dose for patient tissue toxicity. Figure contributed by Andrew Hoffman.

The goal of the radiation therapist (radiation oncologist) is to deliver the safest dose over the least amount of time so that the patient has the highest antitumor benefit and the lowest risk of immediate and delayed radiation side effects. RTx is delivered via external beam (teletherapy) via implantation of radioactive beads inside and around the mass (brachytherapy) or via radiochemicals (radioisotopes) that localize in specific sites (such as iodine-131 in hyperthyroid cats or samarium-153 for osteosarcoma in dogs).Preparations of yittrium-90 are delivered by intralesional/intratumor injections into liver tumors in people with good results. Y-90 can be injected directly into accessible tumors on an outpatient basis in companion animals (IsoPetSolutions.com).

Adverse Events Related to Radiation Therapy

RTx is notorious for producing short term and long term side effects or adverse events (see Table 6.7). Most people know someone who has had radiation therapy. Clients often state their personal bias about RTx, based on their own experience with it through friends, family members, or self. Proper client education is the key to opening the door for the pet geriatric oncology patient to gain the benefits that RTx may offer.

Sensitivity of skin, mucous membranes of the oral cavity, eyelids, genitourinary, and the GI tract becomes the dose-limiting factor in external beam RTx. The hair coat in the RTx field generally falls out after 8–10 treatments. At this time, desquamation may appear and the area may remain alopecic

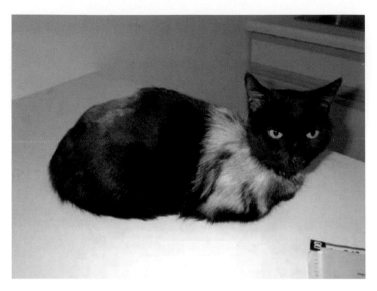

Figure 6.7. Notice the white patch over the radiation field in this patient, 3 years after treatment for FVAS. If higher doses of RTx are delivered to the skin, hair follicles may be completely damaged, causing desquamation and permanent alopecia. This cat was being treated for a new FVAS, which developed several months after a 3-year booster vaccination was administered in the left flank.

for 1 or 2 months, following healing of the skin surface. Fur growth may be prolonged if the patient is having concurrent chemotherapy and it may grow back in a different color than the pet's normal coat. New hair growth in Siamese cats is black but generally grows back as white or gray hair in most other cats (Figure 6.7). Higher doses of RTx to the skin may completely damage hair follicles and in this case the fur never grows back.

When one or both eyes are included in the RTx field, conjunctivitis, keratoconjunctivitis sicca (KCS), and cataract formation are commonly encountered. This occurs most often when treating nasal, retro-orbital, and brain tumors. Radiation toxicity can be more objectively graded by using a scoring system ranging from grade 0 to 4, according to the Radiation Morbidity Scoring Schema (see Table 6.8).

To review the Depth Acute and Late Radiation Morbidity Scoring Scheme, visit: www.acvr.org/sites/default/files/scoring_scheme.pdf.

Immediate or acute reactions occur in tissues that normally undergo mitosis, such as skin, gut, and bone marrow. Late reactions occur in tissues that have low regeneration rates, such as bone, nerves, brain, and the ocular lens. The skin undergoes desquamation both dry and moist and may exhibit pruritus, erythema, and a rash similar to a burn. Mucositis with odoriferous salivation and secondary anorexia and weight loss often develop in those patients being irradiated for oral and nasal tumors. The symptoms begin when the patient is three-quarters of the way to completion of the RTx schedule.

At this stage, if pet owners were not prepared for the expression of side effects in their pet, they may wish to terminate treatment. Proper education and supportive care for each of their concerns is essential.

Support from the referring veterinarian is very important to help pets and their families endure the difficult times that RTx may impose. If the client stops treatments early, the rate of tumor response drops dramatically. We counsel pet owners during their times of frustration, especially when the patient has lost weight and is dealing with the adverse effects of mucositis. Some geriatric patients, especially those with concurrent disease, need more supportive care than others during the course of therapy. They may need daily SQ fluids, hand feeding, or tube feeding. We remind the client of the steep shoulder on the radiation response curve. This encourages the family to allow their pet to finish the prescribed treatment dose.

Pneumonitis and pericarditis with effusion may develop following radiation to the lung field. This is especially worrisome when cats were treated with cobalt therapy units to control recurrence of FISS. Cats developed cardiac and respiratory problems 4–6 months following the completion of RTx and may have to face pericardiectomy with fibrotic lungs. Colitis, tenesmus, and bleeding may result if the colon and rectum are included in the treatment field. Fibrosis and loss of elasticity of the bladder are potential side effects of radiation to the sub-lumbar nodes. These side effects are inherent with the use of cobalt radiation therapy because the exit dose is the same as the entry dose. A bolus was used to offset this, but cats and small dogs were at risk for unwanted side effects from cobalt therapy units. Linear accelerators are able to mitigate the dose at a set depth. This is ideal for RTx treatment of mast cell tumors in dogs and injection site sarcomas in cats. Image-guided radiation therapy IGRT utilize a rotating gander that delivers the dose to the target tissue and reduces the dose to normal tissues.

Anemia and lymphocytopenia or general bone marrow suppression may occur when significant bone lies within the therapy field. Bones are subject to the delayed effect of necrotic sequestrum and this may occur years after treatment. Delayed effects such as xerostomia (no saliva) may appear after radiation therapy of the oral cavity. Adverse events from the treatment of brain tumors with RTx are rare in dogs and cats but may induce nausea, vomiting, pain, papilledema, and unresponsive neurologic problems related to late effect necrosis and myelomalacia of CNS tissue (nerve, spinal cord, brain).

Treatment of Radiation Adverse Events

Patience and good nursing care are required to treat radiation-induced adverse events or side effects. It is paramount to provide the best pain control possible for the patient. Without this, pet owners are likely to terminate treatment too early for their pet to receive any benefit. Counseling must be provided for frustrated pet owners, being sure to point out the steep shoulder on the dose–response curve. I tell pet owners that if they quit RTx before the protocol has been completed, they will have unwittingly put their pet through the first treatments for nothing.

The RTx site should be kept clean and treated with water-soluble aloe vera gel or the new topical preparations used for burn patients, which target the formation of oxidative free radicals in the cell's mitochondria, to prevent inflammation and cell death. Oral mucositis is best treated by frequent oral lavage with saline and green tea. The patient must be fed a bland, soft-food diet. If anorexia prevails, the placement of a feeding tube to keep up the caloric intake becomes essential, especially in geriatric cats. Water-soluble ophthalmic steroid preparations may help manage conjunctivitis, provided there is no corneal ulceration. Artificial tears are indicated for dry eye (KCS). For radiation-induced colitis, use bland diet and the recommended low residue diet; steroid enemas and stool softeners may also help. Steroids and antiemetics and steroid-containing otic solutions help to alleviate side effects from CNS radiation, but there is no effective treatment for late effects such as myelomalacia. Bone sequestra must be surgically removed.

Multimodality–Multidisciplinary–Combinatorial Therapy

Geriatric oncology patients may require more than one modality of therapy to gain survival advantage (see Table 6.6). The sequencing of surgery, radiation, chemotherapy, and immunotherapy treatments is critical. Proper spacing of the various therapeutic modalities to attack the cancer at the onset is preferable to treating a recurrence. The choices made early in the treatment plan generally impact the geriatric oncology patient's overall quality of life and survival time.

Cancer Drug Resistance and Genomics

In human medicine, only 25% of cancer patients respond to and benefit from the first drugs selected for their treatment. This results in treatment switching. New technology aims to help select effective drugs based on tumor genomics. Drug resistance is a major cause of relapse and death for human and animal cancer patients. In the US, it is estimated that 600,000 human cancer patients die annually due to drug resistance. Patients with lymphoma who were also on metformin were found to gain survival benefit from its action to inhibit the multi-drug-resistance (*MDR1*) gene. Tumor sequencing, followed by analysis of the genetic alterations and mutations, will generate reports that guide personalized treatment. A major effort to decode drug resistance pathways is underway with collaborative research, combining the machine-learning capabilities (artificial intelligence) of IMB Watson Health and the Broad Institute of MIT and Harvard. Researchers will generate tumor genome sequence data from responders and follow them over five years when their cancers become drug-resistant. New genome-editing methods that combine cognitive computing with genomic tumor sequencing will help to identify tumors' vulnerabilities and to predict sensitivity and resistance. This information will guide precision cancer treatment options customized for individual patients. Once the mechanisms of resistance are identified, targeted therapies may suspend or offset drug resistance and increase patient survival (http://www.healthcareitnews.com/news/ibm-watson-health-partners-mit-harvard-5-year-cancer-initiative).

Immunotherapy, Cancer Vaccines, and Gene Therapy

> Cancer is particularly difficult to treat because the body does not recognize the diseased cells as foreign and does not create a significant immune response against the cancerous cells.
>
> *Phillip Bergman, DVM, MS, PhD*

Immunotherapy in cancer medicine is the stimulation or arousal of the patient's own defense system to recognize antigens on cancer cell membranes and kill cancer cells. Immunotherapy can treat almost any type of cancer and is being touted as the 4th Pillar of cancer therapy, joining the "Three musketeers", surgery, chemotherapy, and radiation therapy.

The implementation of the CancerMoonShot2020 program is bringing together huge data sets for a worldwide oncology knowledge base. By employing artificial intelligence learning of tumor cell genomics, scientists will get reports that will generate tumor-specific molecular targets for precision or personalized medicine for an individual person or animal patient's cancer care. The Cancer MoonShot plans to lift regulatory restrictions to help scientists get their research from the bench to the trench by enrolling 20,000 patients, both human and animal, in clinical trials by 2020.

The immune system (antigen presenting cells, dendritic cells, macrophages, eosinophils, neutrophils, natural killer (NK) cells, T-cells (helper1,2, cytotoxic), B-cells, plasma cells, cytokines, etc.) responds to multiple stop and go switch signals and ligand pathways. T-regulatory cells negatively suppress the body's immunosurveillance against cancer and contribute to the milieu of cancer cell evade and escape mechanisms.

Immunotherapy requires the identification of tumor-specific antigen(s) that can become therapeutic targets. These targets may be antigens, growth factors or signaling proteins. The next step involves the cultivation, activation, and production of binding agents, or effector cells, to target the specific antigen(s). Another important component of immunotherapy is the reduction of endogenous and iatrogenic immune suppression using a new class of antibodies known as checkpoint inhibitors. There are multiple checkpoints for targeting. The most famous are antiprogramed death 1 (anti-PD-1) and anticytotoxic T-lymphocyte antigen 4 (ant-CTLA-4). An immune checkpoint blockade will be used in sequence and in combinatorial protocols that include antiangiogenesis agents, chemotherapy, and immunotherapy, to simultaneously attack cancer at various points. The immune system can be activated, unleashed, and trained to target cancer antigens with specificity, memory, and adaptability. Immunotherapy may become first-line therapy for some cancers or combined with standard therapy for the majority of cancers. Immunotherapy can generate flu-like adverse events (colitis, pneumonitis, endocrinopathies, etc.) that are generally treatable with steroids.

Active and passive immunotherapy play a role in cancer management. There are numerous products on the market that claim to support the immune system in a general fashion. Most of these active immunotherapy agents are classified as non-specific immunostimulants such as bacterial agents, cytokines, NSAIDs, glycoproteins, supplements, and so forth (see the "Chemoprevention and Immunonutrition for Cancer Patients" section of this chapter).

An example of an active specific immunotherapy agent would be a specific tumor cell vaccine or a vaccine made from the cancer patient's own tumor cells. Unfortunately, tumor cells contain many antigens that are shared with the host. Tumor cells and their selected antigenic fragments have been used as vaccines with some success in malignant melanoma and renal carcinoma cases in humans. This type of vaccine technology, or molecular adaptations of it, have translated to veterinary cancer medicine, particularly in the research and development of DNA tumor vaccines against malignant melanoma in dogs.

Researchers at the University of Wisconsin and the Animal Medical Center in collaboration with Sloan Kettering in New York City worked in this exciting area. From the AMC study, Merial brought Oncept™ to the veterinary market as an orthologous (different species) DNA vaccine against tyrosinase, an enzyme needed for melanin synthesis, which is overexpressed in malignant melanomas. It is most efficacious when the primary tumor has been adequately removed along with involved nodes, or removed before metastasis (www.petcancervaccine.com).

Researchers at Morphogenesis developed a technology that cultivates the patient's own cancer cells and inserts DNA that stimulates a dendritic cell response. IFx-VET® is their dendritic cell vaccine, which can be created from all tumor tissue types and given to the cancer patient as immunotherapy (www.veterinaryoncologyservices.com).

Vaccines for Cancer Therapy and Gene Therapy

Scientists have been able to create genetically altered tumor cells and effector cells that can be used to treat diseases including cancer. As gene mapping for humans and animals progresses, opportunities are emerging to harness gene therapy for veterinary cancer patients. Gene therapy, with its expanded applications, may become available to pets with cancer on a routine basis within a few years.

Initially, the concept of gene therapy was developed to replace or repair defective or mutated genes. Genes are the biologic units of heredity situated at specific locations on chromosomes. Genes are self-reproducing segments of DNA arranged in coils of nucleotide protein molecules sequenced in double helix protein chains. Genes dictate the vast structure and function of cells.

Over the past decade, the field of gene therapy has expanded to include many new applications. Today, gene therapy is used to program cells to become susceptible, to become more resistant, and to produce large quantities of specific cell proteins (cytokines such as Amgen's Epogen®). Gene therapy is used to change immune responses, alter cellular functions, seek and destroy tumor cells, and promote other factors that favor survival of the recipient (Helfand 2003).

Genes are transferred to cells with vectors. Virus vectors are used to carry genes into proliferating cells (transfection). They convert their own ribonucleic acid (RNA) into DNA by transcription and then the DNA integrates into the cellular genome for replication of the desired gene. Selected retroviruses are engineered to enter proliferating cells and deliver therapeutic genes. Genes may also be delivered by other vectors, such as liposomes, or by direct injection into tumors, sometimes with the use of a jet gun or via electroporation.

Without using the complex jargon and terminology of genetics, proteomics, and immunology, I will describe how gene therapy could be used for our patients to manipulate and alter populations of renegade cancer cells to behave as we want them to. Essentially, we want cancer cells to quit growing, quit invading, and quit metastasizing. Ultimately, we want cancer cells to commit suicide.

Gene therapy is the special technology that can alter molecular function and signaling at the cell surface and affect downstream pathways. It is hoped that this technology will prove useful in combating certain tumors. Large molecules on the surface of cells (macromolecules) will serve as antigenic targets. One such macromolecule is a sialomucin known as CD34, existing on the surface of bone marrow cells. CD34 is used as a marker in assisting the selection of enriched cells for bone marrow transplants. Antibodies produced against CD34 bind to the population of enriched cells and isolate them from cells collected for bone marrow transplants. These isolated, enriched bone marrow cells can be used as the recipients of retroviral vector genes via transduction or transfection. The altered CD43 cells are then transplanted into the patient for treatment of various cancers and certain genetic diseases.

Gene therapy may also be used to manipulate the immune system cells of veterinary cancer patients, which would be programmed to internally recognize specific proteins and attack them or bind to receptor sites that disable cancer cell proliferation. This would tip the immune balance back in favor of the patient's survival. Theoretically, molecular chemotherapy will allow us to "program" certain immune cells such as T-cells, B-cells, or natural killer (NK) cells to transform into stealth killer cells that will locate, recognize, attack, and kill the patient's cancer cells (Helfand 2003).

Suicide Genes

Another targeted gene therapy approach involves the delivery of suicide genes using multiple delivery routes including viruses, non-viral vectors, liposomes, nanoparticles, and stem cells. Cells are recoded so that they will be programmed to die (apoptosis). Normal cells undergo a certain number of divisions before they die. Each time a cell divides, it snips off a timer protein (telomere) from the end of the chromosome. Cancer cells develop their own immortal phenotype by increased expression of the enzyme telomerase. Telomerase reattaches telomeres back on to chromosomes. This type of aberrant repair liberates the cell from its natural time-clock, blocking senescence and death by apoptosis. Increased telomerase activity protects cancer cells from programmed cell death. One can view telomerase as a mechanism somewhat analogous to the regrowth of a lizard's tail.

Because humans and animals share genetically similar telomerase, this translational research will benefit our patients as well. Telomerase is a promising target for gene therapy. Suicide genes that inhibit telomerase could potentially cause all types of cancer cells to die. Gene therapy can also confer susceptibility upon cancer cells to attract the influx of the patient's own immune cells, resulting in widespread host destruction of primary and metastatic tumor cells.

One of the most well-known normal tumor suppressor genes is the *p53* gene, which plays an important role in the control of apoptosis. When *p53* is deactivated or rendered non-functional, cells become immortal and neoplasia occurs. Correction of *p53* deficits can be achieved by the transfection of functional *p53* genes into tumors, directing the tumor cells to undergo apoptosis. According to this concept, suicide genes are delivered via genetic molecular therapy.

Another gene therapy approach is to kill bystander cells via "molecular chemotherapy." Transfected cells are engineered to activate certain cytotoxic agents within tumor cells. Transfected cells are delivered into tumors and genetically produce signals for tumor cells to leak toxins around neighboring cells, resulting in cell death. This is called the "bystander effect." An example of the "bystander effect" is the engineered herpes simplex virus. It is used to transfect tumor cells and deliver genes that produce an enzyme that activates a prodrug into ganciclovir, which kills bystander cells.

Antiangiogenic Gene Therapy

Gene therapy may also target the ability of cancer cells to create new blood vessels (angiogenesis) from molecules in the extracellular matrix (ECM) or tumor microenvironment. Endostatin, a collagen XVIII fragment, is the representative for endogenous inhibitors of angiogenesis derived from ECM. The inhibition of angiogenesis (antiangiogenesis) is big business for pharmaceutical companies that are developing targeted drugs. One day we may be able to offer gene therapy capable of encoding antiangiogenic genes to inhibit microvessel formation or destroy hemangioblasts or cancer stem cells that will shrink and kill tumors. Not all malignancies are completely dependent on angiogenesis, but the majority will be affected by these agents.

Humans and canines share an interesting gene called Canstatin, located in a small segment of the *a2* gene chain that belongs to type IV collagen. It is ten times more potent than endostatin. Collagen appears to be similar across many species of animals, including man. Canstatin acts as an angiostasis agent because it inhibits the proliferation, migration, and microvessel tube formation of endothelial cells (cells that form the walls of blood vessels) and induces apoptosis of endothelial cells. Cloning the Canstatin gene yields a product called recombinant Canstatin, or rcCanstatin®. Delivering therapeutic amounts of rcCanstatin to cancer patients may be developed as another way to use genetically engineered products as part of overall gene therapy. Cloning and sequencing Canstatin and/or inducing its expression by using a vector that transfects carrier cells may prove useful in the development of new therapies against cancer.Endostatin has a checkered history in cancer therapy but it was recently found to be a signaling agent for stabilization of the function and plasticity of neural circuits.

Clinical Trials in Gene Therapy

There are currently over five hundred gene therapy protocols being evaluated in human clinical trials that have the potential to treat everything from Alzheimer's to Parkinson's to immune and genetic disorders and cancer. Some veterinary facilities are using gene therapy on a clinical trial basis. It is important to keep up-to-date on the subject, since your clients will certainly ask you about it. New names and terminology make up the complex world of gene therapy. Cell surface macromolecules and the milieu of proteins and molecules within cells create an intricate and vast "alphabet soup." Explain to clients that gene therapy uses engineered bacteria, viruses, or liposomes as Trojan horses. These agents can penetrate into the target cells while secretly carrying weapons in the form of therapeutic genes.

Progress is on the horizon, but not without many setbacks and problems along the way. Ongoing and future clinical trials will attempt to evaluate efficacy and toxicity, using controlled double blind studies. Will veterinarians soon be using gene therapy in everyday practice? The answer is a robust "yes"! One such vaccine uses allogeneic tumor cells such as antigenically distinct melanoma cells from other patients of the same species. The canine melanoma cells are transfected with DNA encoded to produce human GM-CSF (an immunostimulatory cytokine similar to Neupogen). This vaccine technology is being developed to fight canine malignant melanoma and is currently available from the research facilities at the University of Wisconsin (Kurzman et al. 2005; for information go to http://www.news.wisc.edu/12063.html or contact Kurzman at kurzman@svmvetmed.wisc.edu).

Oncept is an orthologous or xenogeneic (different species) DNA-based melanoma vaccine. It codes for human tyrosinase, which is a glycoprotein essential in melanin synthesis. When the DNA vaccine places human tyrosinase into a canine or mouse melanoma patient, it is incorporated into the tumor but it is recognized as foreign by the patient's immune system. The xenogeneic vaccine could break host tolerance against a self-tumor differentiation antigen. It may also induce antibody, T-cell, and antitumor responses. 245 dogs with confirmed malignant melanoma were treated with xenogeneic DNA vaccinations from April 2000 to February 2006 at the Animal Medical Center (AMC) in New York City. The vaccine was determined to be safe and potentially therapeutic for dogs that had local-regional control, including some dogs with advanced stage disease. This xenogeneic DNA-based vaccine gained USDA approval for immunotherapy against canine malignant melanoma (Bergman 2006). For information go to the Merial web page (www.petcancervaccine.com).

Another method of gene therapy under study involves intratumoral injections delivering super antigens and certain cytokine (cell proteins that act as intercellular mediators) genes. Antigenic tumors such as malignant melanoma may be responsive to this type of gene therapy. In addition, combinations of gene therapy, checkpoint inhibitors and immunotherapy agents such as interleukin-2 may be added to chemotherapy protocols in the future to increase efficacy against metastatic disease.

We can imagine that one day in the future preventative oncology may exist in the form of gene therapy. We may order a product to be delivered to our hospitals, nicely packaged as preventative vaccines, to spur the immune response against various tumor types for patients at risk for lymphoma, melanoma, hemangiosarcoma, mammary adenocarcinoma, osteosarcoma, and soft tissue sarcomas.

Some types of gene therapy will offer genetic immunopotentiation (immunogene therapy). This technology may restore tumor suppressor (*p53*) function to improve and revive the sagging immuno-surveillance system of aging geriatric patients. Imagine the benefits of its application as a prophylactic vaccine to protect our highest risk patients from developing neoplasia.

Despite its failures and related side effects, gene therapy has ignited tremendous hope as a potential treatment for many poorly responsive and chronic degenerative diseases in addition to cancer. Adverse events may include abnormal buildup of antibodies or antigens. During developmental stages, gene therapy may be found to have irreversible consequences. Immunotherapy may create chaos in the immune system or death. We may encounter patients that develop immunotoxicities or a Herxheimer-like reaction, which is the release of a cascade of pyrogenic cytokines that cause fever and collapse and which may be irreversible and fatal.

The Cancer MoonShot 2020 coalition wants to gather data on 20,000 cancer patients in clinical trials, including dogs and cats, treated with various forms of immunotherapy by 2020. This goal solidifies the One Medicine, One Health Model. Our geriatric cancer patients may benefit greatly from the collaborative information generated by the Cancer MoonShot 2020 alliance. We may be able to routinely use gene therapy for our geriatric cancer patients in the near future. Stay in touch with developments in gene therapy to see how it may impact our veterinary cancer patients. Some feel that this technology can be used to protect high-risk breeds. Preventative oncology may be the most promising research focus, because it will reduce the heartache and loss foisted on society by cancer's fatal agenda.

Monoclonal Antibodies

Another type of targeted therapy is immunotherapy, which employs reactive B-cells harvested from the spleens and lymph nodes of mice that have been injected with intact tumor cells or cell membranes. These stimulated B-cells are fused with an immortal cell line and cultivated as hybrid clones for their monoclonal antibody (MoAb) production. The antibody is given to the patient in the hope that lysis or phagocytosis or destruction of target cells will occur. The patient must have the proper antigen(s) present on his or her tumor cells for the MoAb to work. The technique is fraught with problems with host response against the MoAb or mouse antibodies, cross-reactivity, tumor size, and heterogeneity, which hamper success. The most famous MoAb used in human medicine is the recombinant anti-HER2 monoclonal antibody (trastuzumab), Herceptin®. Herceptin targets the oncogene Her-2-neu, which is overexpressed in some malignant breast cancers. If the patient is Her-2-neu positive, Herceptin is the mainstay for treatment (Love 2000). Her2 is overexpressed in canine bone and bladder cancer and in feline breast cancers. A clinical trial using adenovirus vaccine delivery and plasmid DNA delivery via electroporation under anesthesia may yield mature data in 2018–2019 (www.petcancerinformation.com).

Rituxan® is a genetically engineered MoAb that is directed against the CD20 antigen found on the surface of normal and malignant B lymphocytes. Rituxan is used in CD20 positive non-Hodgkins lymphoma patients and has been found to be helpful against other tumors as well. Infusion reactions and lymphopenia are common in human patients.

Veterinary MoAbs are on their way back into practice. Dr. Ann Jegulm pioneered the first commercially available MoAb for canine lymphoma. Clinical trials with canine MoAb 231 for lymphoma found that dogs had geographically variable results. New MoAb T-cell and B-cell canine lymphoma vaccines are being developed by several biotech companies. Despite multiple initial setbacks, MoAb vaccines are expected to eventually improve survival time for dogs with T- and B-cell lymphoma.

Checkpoint Inhibitors, Programed Cell Death Ligands, and Adverse Events

Programed Death Ligand 1 (PDL-1) is a gene that normally serves as an "off switch" that keeps T-cells from attacking normal cells. In cancer, PDL-1 is upregulated and plays a key role in protecting cancer cells so they can evade T-cell mediated immune surveillance and destruction. PDLs have been of great interest because their homeostatic inhibitory role for T-cells is upregulated in the tumor microenvironment, allowing cancer to grow under the radar of the immune system. Inhibitors of PD-L1 are being studied that will block signaling, which allows the immune system to do its job and recognize malignant cells and destroy them. These promising agents are classified as checkpoint inhibitors and will be major players in future cancer therapy. Most checkpoint inhibitors will be monoclonal antibodies that target PDL-1 on cancer cells.

Despite important clinical benefits, checkpoint inhibition is associated with a unique spectrum of side effects termed immune-related adverse events (irAEs). IrAEs include dermatologic, gastrointestinal, hepatic, endocrinopathies, and other less common inflammatory events. IrAEs are believed to arise from general immunologic enhancement. Temporary immunosuppression with corticosteroids, tumor necrosis factor-alpha antagonists, mycophenolate mofetil (a drug used to prevent organ rejection), or other agents can be an effective treatment in most cases.

With all new immuno-oncology breakthroughs, there are immunotoxicities and related adverse events and we are obliged to educate our clients about them. The toxicity profile of sequencing and combinations of immune checkpoint-blocking antibodies and targeted agents is just beginning to be understood. Results suggest that combinations involving targeted agents and ipilimumab (Yervoy®) may significantly increase toxicity in people treated for advanced melanoma. Clinical trials using combination therapy with agents like Yervoy that target and block the cytotoxic T-lymphocyte-associated antigen 4 (CTLA-4), another "off switch" downregulator of T-cell activation, have variable and mixed results, both with some very good responses and with some immuotoxic reactions due to irAEs. Clinical trials using autologous T-cells engineered with chimeric antigen receptor (CAR) T-cells as cancer therapy demonstrated clinical responses in both hematological malignancies and solid tumors. However, this sophisticated adoptive cellular therapy for cancer has generated some severe immunotoxicities (http://www.uptodate.com/contents/toxicities-associated-with-checkpoint-inhibitor-immunotherapy).

Summary: Immunotherapy, Cancer Vaccines, and Gene Therapy

MoAbs, cancer vaccines, targeted gene therapy, and suicide gene therapy have the potential to enhance tumor inhibition. Selective blockade of inhibitory molecules, PD-1 and PD-2, via immunotherapeutic antibodies is being investigated. There are currently over five hundred gene therapy protocols being evaluated in human clinical trials that have the potential to treat everything from Alzheimer's to Parkinson's to immune and genetic disorders and cancer. Various receptors on cells have been used as targets for immunotherapy and suicide gene therapy and more will be identified by researchers. Our geriatric cancer patients may benefit from gene therapy in combinatorial protocols. Stay in touch with developments in immunotherapy and gene therapy to see how vaccines and delivery systems may expand our options for the treatment of veterinary cancer patients. Be aware that cancer immunotherapy may cause immune-related adverse events.

There is the potential opportunity that gene therapy will be used in preventing cancer development in high-risk dog breeds. It would be ideal if a panel or cocktail of anticancer vaccines could protect our Boxers, Golden Retrievers, Bernese Mountain Dogs, and German Shepherd Dogs from their breed-specific predilection for cancer. Imagine having a vaccine for all large-breed dogs that would protect them from osteosarcoma. For an excellent review of antitumor immunity and checkpoint inhibitors, see the video slide show by Jeffrey S. Weber, MD, PhD: Cancer Revealed: How the Immune System Sees and Destroys Tumors, https://www.youtube.com/watch?v=3hlGq-3F1uQ.

Antiangiogenesis Therapy with Metronomic Chemotherapy

Metronomic chemotherapy (mCTx) is the use of small daily doses of standard chemotherapy that reduces angiogenesis, the formation of new microvasculature, which is needed for new tumor growth.

Most oncologist feel that mCTx is one of the most preferred approaches for managing cancer in geriatric patients, because it is safe and relatively free of adverse events (Mutseares 2014). We use cyclophosphamide at: $10–12.5 mg/m^2$ per day, chlorambucil at: $4–6–8 mg/m^2/day$, and lomustine at: $4 mg/m^2/day$ in dogs and $3 mg/m^2/day$ in cats for lymphoma, mast cell tumors, and miscellaneous other tumors. We use capecitabine at: $250 mg/m^2/day$ (DOGS ONLY), for carcinomas and adenocarcinomas.

Chemotherapy drugs used at mCTx low daily dose protocols in combinations with either steroids or NSAIDs and other agents that have anticancer action (such as metformin) are generally well tolerated in geriatric cancer patients. We also introduce therapy with small molecules, masitinib and toceranib, at their lower dose range for their antiangiogenic effects. If the patient is doing well, we may dose escalate the small molecule therapy on a monthly basis until we reach the recommended therapeutic dose. Geriatric cancer patients on metronomic chemotherapy need monitoring every 4–6 weeks.

Comet's case: (2 year+ survival with pulmonary adenocarcinoma)

Dan Mabbot and his fiancée, Allison Rome, presented their 10 years 8 months old, neutered, male Chihuahua mix, Comet, on February 3, 2015 with a history of a hacking cough and pulmonary effusion secondary to an $8 \times 4 cm^2$ mass filling the anterior left thorax that pushed his heart to the right. FNA diagnosed pulmonary carcinoma. Comet's prognosis was 3–8 months with surgery and chemotherapy. The family was on a budget and requested medical management. Masitinb, meloxicam, and metronomic lomustine were prescribed. Four months later, Comet developed more pulmonary effusion, a cough, and a heart murmur. He was treated symptomatically with enalapril and furosemide. Six months later, Comet helped Dan when he had a heart attack. One year later, Comet was best man at the Mabbot wedding. We switched Comet to toceranib on August 9, 2016 after losing access to masitinib. Comet welcomed the couple's newborn daughter, Briar, on August 30,16. Follow-up X-rays show no regression or growth of the mass. Comet celebrated his 2-year anniversary in Pawspice and remains alive at this writing with stable disease and a good quality of life.

More information is given in the last section of this chapter on Metronomic Chemotherapy in Dogs.

Chemoprevention and Immunonutrition for Cancer Patients

To cure sometimes, to relieve often, to comfort always – This is the first and great commandment.

Hippocrates

Chemoprevention is the concept of providing natural or synthetic compounds to reduce cancer risk in susceptible patients. Immunonutrition is the concept of providing nutrients that enhance the immune system. Both therapies affect the microenvironment of the cancer cell to discourage proliferation. Since cancer is a major cause of death in older pets, chemoprevention and immunonutrition are very appealing to pet carers. The mechanisms of action of these compounds vary and many are not fully understood. They may reverse malignancy or intervene and suppress the multistep process of carcinogenesis. Some agents block or suppress mutagenesis, promotion, proliferation, angiogenesis, invasiveness, recurrence, or metastases. Other agents intervene with genetic mechanisms such as initiation, progression, and proliferation. Some agents induce differentiation of premalignant cells to prevent them from progressing toward malignancy (Bergman 1999).

Hundreds of natural compounds have been formulated as supplements or nutraceuticals with claims of anticancer effects. Some compounds have been shown to play a role in the cell cycle to reduce the risk of cancer. I like to call these natural compounds "foodaceuticals" as well as nutraceuticals to emphasize to clients that they are generally non-toxic and are found in nature.

Research shows that natural and synthetic substances augment the immune system, inhibit cancer, and yield positive clinical results in rodents and humans. Chemoprevention and immunonutrition are standard therapy at my clinics. They are an important arsenal in the way I conduct all levels of care in the battle against cancer for my geriatric oncology patients. Enhancing a patient's normal diet and adding special supplements is a useful modality that supports and improves the overall health of the geriatric cancer patient. Clients have repeatedly remarked that their geriatric pet was feeling younger, looking better, and playing with toys again. We give credit for these pleasing reports to the supplements because experience tells us that chemotherapy does not provide this effect. Immunonutrition is very important in our oncology service. It plays a priority role in our palliative cancer medicine and Pawspice care programs.

Confusion and Controversy about Chemoprevention and Immunonutrition

Cancer chemoprevention is defined as the use of agents able to delay, reverse, or inhibit tumor progression, in order to decrease the risk of developing invasive or clinically significant disease (Ruggiero et al. 2012). Immunonutrition refers to the study of nutrients including macronutrients, vitamins, minerals and trace elements on inflammation, the actions of white blood cells, the formation of antibodies, and the resistance to disease. We should experience no surprise to find confusion and conflicting data in this field. Many diet-derived molecules and agents have multiple effects. Some agents have potentially negative effects. Some agents under large-scale studies were stopped due to adverse events. For example, beta carotene was stopped early for smokers in the CARET study. When given with retinol, the incidence of lung cancer increased. Merck's NSAID, rofecoxib (Vioxx®) released in 1999, was pulled off the market in 2004 after a study found that it increased the risk for heart attacks, when it was used as a chemopreventive in colon cancer patients. In 2011, Merck agreed to pay $950 million and pleaded guilty to a federal misdemeanor charge related to questionable marketing and sales tactics. It seems that marketing, sales, and profits drive many drug and supplement companies, rather than the medical justifications and quality of their products. Perhaps this text is not the forum for making this point, but many ethical issues are involved in the supplement and vitamin industry, including quality control. Up to 38% of vitamins and supplements are found not to contain what the labels claim. In the past, skeptics went so far as to say that nutritional supplements and megavitamin therapy for cancer was a profitable health-fraud industry (Curt 1990).

The World Health Organization and the United Nations held a Global Health Summit in 2011 in New York. The Summit identified sugar, salt, tobacco, and drugs (legal and illegal) as the four main causes of global death due to lifestyle choices for people under the age of 60. It therefore makes sense to instruct and advise clients to make good dietary and lifestyle choices for themselves and their pets. Avoiding obesity would be a top priority.

A paper presented at the 2004 Veterinary Cancer Society (VCS) meeting reported that dogs given NSAIDs were less likely to develop cancer and that the medication was well tolerated (Oberthaler et al. 2004). Hansen et al. (2004) reported on similar health benefits from a study of 575 dogs given NSAIDs in the 2004 American College of Veterinary Internal Medicine (ACVIM) Forum. This is no surprise, since oncologists have been using piroxicam for its anticancer effects since the mid-1990s (Knapp et al. 1994). Despite renal, hepatic, and GI toxicity, it seems that the downside of using COX-2 selective NSAIDs in our veterinary cancer patients may be minimal when compared to people.

Exercise has also been shown to have a positive effect in longevity against cancer. A study found that women breast cancer patients who walk 3–5 hours a week are more likely to survive twice as long as similarly staged women with breast cancer who do not exercise. The same is probably true for geriatric dogs. Lifetime caloric restriction was found to delay chronic disease, cancer, and death by nearly 2 years in dogs (Lawler et al. 2005). We can presume that if geriatric oncology patients are entertained, exercised, and kept lean, they will actually live longer.

The Dog Aging Project is conducting a large clinical trial to evaluate the safety and dose schedule using low dose rapamycin for its restorative, cardioprotective, neuroprotective, and prolongevity effects in addition to its anticancer effects on dogs as they age. There is tremendous interest in the advantages that metformin bestows its recipients in the reduction of cancer risk when being used for its antihyperglycemic action. The concept of chemoprevention will develop further when clinical trials provide evidence-based medicine to inform the profession regarding the proper use of agents such as rapamycin and metformin for prolongevity purposes.

Pets at Risk

We know that Boxers, Golden Retrievers, Bernese Mountain Dogs, Flat-Coated Retrievers, and intact female dogs are at greater risk for developing cancer than other dogs. The risk for developing breast tumors in intact female dogs rises to 60% as they become geriatric. Dogs with osteosarcoma and hemangiosarcoma and cats with breast cancer that have had their malignant tumors removed are at very high risk for recurrence and pulmonary metastases. Cats operated on for injection site sarcoma and pets with solar-induced skin cancer are at high risk for recurrence in the vicinity of their tumors due to "field cancerization."

Exposure to lawn chemicals (2,4-D) puts dogs at risk for lymphoma. Scottish Terriers exposed to lawns treated with both herbicides and pesticides are at seven times the risk for transitional cell carcinoma than unexposed dogs. Scotties are 20 times more susceptible to TCC than other dogs, according to a study by Dr. Lawrence Glickman et al. from Purdue (2004). Workers at Tufts found that cats exposed to cigarette smoke are at higher risk of lymphoma. Cats living with smokers or wearing flea collars have an increased risk for oral SCC.

Genetic mutations and environmental factors may cause damage, activation, and/or overexpression of certain mechanisms in the normal functions of repair genes, tumor suppressor genes, and suicide genes. Cancer is a multistep process involving initiation and promotion by these factors that tips the cascade of molecular and cell membrane signals and events that transition cells toward malignancy. A perplexing activation and proliferation of dendritic cells creates the confusing group of disorders classified as histiocytic diseases (Rassnick 2006). We know obesity, poor diet, and lack of exercise result in a shorter life span and increased risk of cancer in animals. It is well known that poor diet, obesity, and self-destructive lifestyle choices such as being sedentary, smoking cigarettes and drinking alcohol, and environmental exposure play a significant role in the incidence of cancer in humans.

Imagine the steps toward cancer as part of an intricate molecular choreography. Mutated DNA performs its immortal death dance. Renegade cells multiply and bypass surface signals for homeostasis and issue checkpoint signals to inhibit the immune system from recognition. Cancer cells expand exponentially, creating chaos as they expand, twirling into neighboring cells, dissolving barriers, and ultimately killing the host. In my opinion, immunonutrition and chemoprevention may rechoreograph the microenvironment and trip cancer at some of its intricate steps. Attention to diet, maintaining a lean body mass, and exercise along with the sensible use of immunonutrition and chemoprevention may add cancer-free years and longevity for our geriatric veterinary patients.

Highly metastatic cancers and most high-grade sarcomas prevail to kill their victims despite a timely and complete excision of the primary tumor. This aggressive biologic behavior results from the early dissemination of "scout" cells into the lymphatic and circulatory system before detection of the primary tumor. These abnormal aggressive scout cells acquire an immortal nature, evade, and survive the body's immunosurveillance. They disseminate and wait in various and widespread locations in the body until they are enabled to divide in continuous mitosis and develop into immortal new clones of cells that accumulate into metastatic tumors. The new metastatic clones are often more resistant to treatment than the primary tumor due to the hardiness of their progenitor scout cancer stem cells.

It would be ideal if there were a safe way to fortify high-risk breeds, exposed animals, and aging pets and postop cancer patients against the ravages of cancer's death dance. It seems obvious to me and to thousands of others in research and clinical medicine that people and animals can and do benefit from immunonutrition and/or chemoprevention and a diet that is low in sugar-producing carbohydrates. I started using anticancer supplements and nutritional changes for my cancer patients in earnest about 30 years ago. The difference in my patients' physical condition, quality of life, and survival times has been impressive.

The scientific community is taking a closer look at natural substances that modify the differentiation of cells and the extracellular microenvironment of cells. Other agents affect proliferation or mutation of cells as they transition from inflammation to premalignancy toward malignancy. The medical and scientific community has found it difficult to reach a consensus about nutraceuticals because the field and the claims are not regulated. Unfortunately, 38% of the compounds evaluated in the past for content in the marketplace were found to not be trustworthy. One study found very few probiotic compounds to be reliable. Since it has been difficult to trust the available products, the supplement and nutraceutical field suffers. Some companies have set up self-regulating quality control programs. It is our responsibility to source reliable and ethical products.

The National Cancer Institute has a Chemoprevention Branch that funds studies to look at the efficacy of chemopreventive agents in populations of susceptible and high-risk patients. The results of these long term studies are published. No doubt there will be controversy over the data. For instance: Should you stop antioxidants during chemotherapy and radiation therapy or not (Vajdovich et al. 2005)? Is it better to drink a glass of wine three to four times a week for its resveratrol or should you get it from eating peanuts and raspberries instead? What effect do Vioxx®, Celebrex®, piroxicam, and other COX-2 inhibitors have on angiogenesis and apoptosis? Can NSAIDs be used to cytoreduce or palliate mammary tumors (Dank 2006a)? Can NSAIDs be used as prevention to lower the incidence or recurrence of various types of cancer (Dank, Aung, and Yudelevitch 2005; Dank 2006b)?

It took 70 years for the scientific community to accept that vitamin C cured scurvy. It may take repetitious studies and more time before flavonoids, vitamin C, beta carotene, NSAIDs, selenium, vitamin A (retinoids), inositol hexaphosphate, mannose, fucose (do not confuse this with fructose!), beta glucans, fatty acids, antioxidants, and so forth are credited for their roles in the battle against cancer.

A study led by Dr. Mark Levine from National Institutes of Health was reported on Medscape. Dr. Levine found that IV vitamin C has anticancer effects and selectively kills several different types of cancer cells while leaving normal cells unscathed. The cytotoxic effects of vitamin C did not depend on metal chelators but required hydrogen peroxide formation. Studies in the 1970s that first suggested the anticancer action of vitamin C were not duplicated properly in subsequent studies. The original work used a combination of oral and IV vitamin C at high levels and the subsequent studies only used oral vitamin C, which did not achieve adequate plasma levels. A phase 1 trial to establish the safety of IV ascorbate in patients with advanced cancer was run by Dr. Levine. Be sure to check www.Medscape.com.

Colleagues and members of our scientific community may dismiss, become indifferent, or discredit data about the efficacy and use of nutraceuticals and supplements and diet as being important in the comprehensive management of cancer. The training that many of our current physicians received was devoid of education in nutrition. It is not part of what they know. They cannot believe or will not accept the available information. The scientific method is used to criticize and dismiss the Eastern concept that "food is medicine." Most articles about nutrition for cancer patients merely discuss maintaining weight and caloric intake to avoid cancer cachexia.

Many clinicians choose to uphold a double standard. They are against using supplements or immunonutrition, but they will accept the concept of chemoprevention. This same double standard is enacted every day in the field of oncology. This is because we, as healers, constantly use medications that we hope will win back a remission. Most of the second and third choice drugs that we use to treat resistant and metastatic cancer have little effect. However, we give these drugs with a "let's see if this helps" attitude that may put us on that slippery slope towards practicing futile medicine. We are trying to make our patients better. The same holds true for any type of palliative therapy. We want to alleviate symptoms. If a treatment seems to be helping we are justified in continuing it.

The late Leslie R. Bennett, MD, and his colleagues Amos Norman, PhD, a nutritionist, and Kai Iwamoto, a PhD student, inspired my epiphany regarding the impact that diet may have on cancer in 1989. Dr. Bennett was Head of Nuclear Medicine at the UCLA School of Medicine. He was one of my research colleagues during the decade when I was affiliated with the Animal Tumor Resource Facility, under the direction of Hal Snow, DVM. Dr. Bennett investigated the role of linoleic acid in protecting the small intestine in the mid-1950s. He wanted to revive and continue this early work with linoleic acid as his Professor Emeritus project. He asked me to help him investigate the role of linoleic acid and other fatty acids in tumor-bearing animals. We found some anticancer benefit in dogs with mycosis fungoides (Iwamoto et al. 1992) and brain tumors. Dr. Bennett found that cats needed Evening Primrose Oil because they could not convert linoleic to linolenic acid. Two dogs with mast cell tumors had adverse reactions with unintended histamine release, presumably due to degranulation syndrome.

Hundreds of distinguished researchers have published more than three hundred thousand articles and papers that have looked at the effect that antioxidants, fatty acids, glycoproteins, and hundreds of other natural compounds have on cancer. Journals such as *Nutrition and Cancer* and the *Journal of the American Nutraceutical Association* have presented evidence that shows that we can place our geriatric oncology patients on a better plane of health through immunonutrition and dietary adjustments.

Pet owners are constantly searching for the best supplements and diets for their pets, especially when cancer strikes. It is not unusual to see pets that are being given 10–50 different supplements by the time they come in for oncology consultations.

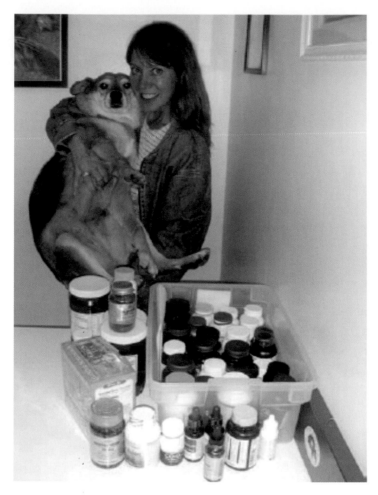

Figure 6.8. Mom Dog Artsis was given 51 supplements by her family following emergency surgery for hemoabdomen due to hepatic hemangiosarcoma. Six vials were in the box pictured in the lower right.

Mom Dog's Case (Help Clients Select Sensible Supplements)

Mom Dog Artsis, a 12-year-old F/S Shepherd Cross, was given a poor prognosis following splenectomy and liver lobectomy for hemorrhaging metastatic hemangiosarcoma lesions. Her family members, a nurse and neurologist, purchased a variety of supplements that added up to 51 items (Figure 6.8). The family did their research and felt compelled to try to beat the odds against Mom Dog's survival. She only survived a few weeks postop. I am sure that if Mom Dog's caregivers had known about suberoylanilide hydroxamic acid (SAHA), they would have searched for it as well. They would have used this histone deacetylase inhibitor based on Molly's case report in the December 2004 issue of *Veterinary and Comparative Oncology* by Leonard Cohen, MD (Cohen et al. 2004). SAHA failed to help one of my patients with hemangiosarcoma. A clinical trial is under way at the AMC to determine its efficacy.

Pet caregivers select available supplements based upon variable advice from the health food store-keepers, books, friends, the Internet, nutritional consultants, and animal communicators. It is time for contemporary veterinarians to look into the subject of immunonutrition and be able to recommend sensible supplements, which may benefit the geriatric cancer patient's health.

Immunonutrition Suggestions

There are hundreds of products and thousands of retail health food stores that market supplements. It is important to know and trust the quality of the product. We use the products mentioned in this section for our immunonutrition protocols because I know that the providers have proven in-house quality control. There are many other excellent providers that are not listed in this text. If you have confidence in the quality and consistency of their products, they can be used in your protocols.

Educate clients that it takes time for the supplements and nutraceuticals to show their beneficial effect and change the pet's physiology. Cancer patients on immunonutrition seem to handle chemotherapy treatments with fewer adverse events. We recommend continued use of the supplements long after the surgery, chemotherapy, or radiation therapy is completed, with the goal of supporting the immune system and chemoprevention to increase the time to recurrence of the patient's cancer.

Inositol hexaphosphate (IP-6), or phytic acid, is a glycoprotein derived from rice. It is also derived from soybeans, sesame seeds, beans, legumes, and cereals. IP-6 is a polysaccharide found in fiber that has potent antioxidant and anticarcinogenic action. It also enhances natural killer-cell activity and is beneficial for a wide range of metabolic conditions. For more information, visit www.phytopharmica.com and have your clients read the excellent book *IP-6: Nature's Revolutionary Cancer-Fighter* (Shamsuddin 1998).

Beta glucans are glycoproteins derived from medicinal mushrooms. Beta glucans stimulate macrophage activity to destroy viral, bacterial, and malignant cells. Beta glucans also increase the utilization of insulin. *Agaricus blasei* products are my preferred mushroom. Efficacy was validated in the research reported in *Medicinal Mushroom Review* by the UC Davis Department of Pharmacology. There are more than 50 medicinal mushrooms and they are used widely in Asia as a health supplement. Clients are often overwhelmed with the plethora of mushroom supplements available on the market, so I advise them to not overuse these products. Reliable scientific information on Agaricus Bio® is available at www.atlasworldusa.com.

Investigators at University of Penn believe that *Coriolis versicolor* mushroom increased the survival time of some dogs with hemangiosarcoma in a small study that was sponsored by the company. The study needs to be expanded to a larger clinical trial that includes at least 150–200 hemangiosarcoma dogs before conclusions can be made. However, there was a lot of press and product is being ordered to treat dogs. Every clinical study that I have conducted on hemangiosarcoma yielded 20% amazing long term survivors. However, the background long term survivors range from 10–15% for most follow-up studies, and 20% as stated during a talk at the World Veterinary Cancer Congress given by Dr. Cheryl London of OSU.

Advanced Protection Formula (APF) drops contain extracts from several types of Siberian ginseng. It is used mostly in equine performance as it enhances the body's ability to handle stress by increasing natural adaptogen activity during stress. Formulations of ginseng can be helpful for patients with cancer and related treatment. Cancer patients show increased energy and increased appetite and maintain higher white blood cell counts while on chemotherapy. APF drops may also help increase insulin utilization in diabetic patients and may be used to help stabilize hyperglycemic cats. This same effect may also be observed with *Agaricus blasei* products. Ginseng and Agaricus Bio should not be given to patients with insulinomas because this pancreatic islet cell neoplasia secretes excessive insulin, which lowers blood glucose. Enhancing insulin utilization in these patients would further lower blood glucose. For more information contact Dr. Mike Van Noy at www.auburnlabs.com.

The multitasking function of the liver is essential for metabolism and the detoxification of most chemotherapy drugs. It is one of the primary targets for metastatic disease and may give rise to primary neoplasms. Many geriatric cancer patients have acquired nodular hyperplasia, chronic fibrosis, cholestasis, fatty liver, and buildup of pigments in hepatocytes. The liver also undergoes SAMe deficiency and cellular damage with senescence. Evidence-based research has shown that SAMe is helpful in restoring hepatocellular function and membrane integrity. I recommend SAMe for its proven efficacy in restoring hepatic function and homeostasis. I also recommend milk thistle (silymarin) for its proven ability as a flavonoid to improve the solubility of bile and enhance the hepatic detoxification process. Milk thistle also prevents depletion of glutathione, raises glutathione levels by up to 35%, and protects the liver from damage. Used as a supplement for geriatric cancer patients receiving chemotherapy, milk thistle helps the liver process and to detoxify drugs. It is in several products designed for the liver such as Rx Vitamin's Hepato Support®, which contains a standardized extract of milk thistle along with a full complex of B vitamins and alpha lipoic acid to help promote normal liver function. The active bioflavonoid complex in milk thistle, silymarin, increases the uptake of hepatic glutathione and stimulates hepatocyte protein synthesis. The milk thistle used in these formulas has been standardized to contain 80% silymarin and 30% silybinin, the highest percentage available in any liver nutritional product. Rx Vitamins for Pets offers excellent high-quality supplements and support products formulated by Dr. Robert Silver. He asked me for suggestions in the formulation of OncoSupport® for cancer patients. It contains Hepato Support and NutriGest® with reliable probiotic agents and cell wall lysate of *Lactobacillus rhamnosus* and arabinogalactan. I suggested adding *Agaricus blasei* at 600mg per scoop. This formula reduces the number of supplements dispensed. For more information, visit www.rxvitamins.com/rxvitaminsforpet/.

My first-choice general supplement for geriatric cancer patients is Platinum Performance Plus® for dogs and PP Feline®, which contain over 40 nutrients and supplements that are chondroprotective for joint and ligament health. Some dogs may develop diarrhea due to the OM-3 fatty acids from flaxseed, so it should be introduced to the diet on a gradual basis over 2 weeks (www.platinumperformance.com). Standard Process, a well-known whole food supplement company, offers the veterinary market quality products such as Canine Musculoskeletal Support® and Canine Whole Body Support® and other products designed to provide nutritional support for various organs. For geriatric patients with anorexia, sarcopenia, or cancer cachexia and for patients receiving nutrition via feeding tubes, we also use L-glutamine powder and bovine colostrum powder (similar to whey protein or casein); seehttp://www.primaldose.com/.

The doses and special instructions that we use for most of the supplements discussed in this section are summarized for your convenience in Table 6.9.

Nutritional Support for Older Cancer Patients

It is important to assess the body condition (1–9 scale), the nutritional status (malnourished versus cachexia), and the appetite of the geriatric oncology patient, as discussed in previous chapters. For patients not requiring hospitalization and parenteral nutrition, educating the carers will help determine that cancer patient's intake and nutritional well-being. The composition of a diet, its nutrients, and the level of food intake can have a surprising impact in the body at the molecular and genetic level

Table 6.9.   Doses for Immunonutrition and Chemoprevention Protocol Used by the Author as Supplements for High-Risk Breeds, Senior, Geriatric, and Oncology Patients

Each geriatric cancer patient needs to be individualized. The one caution about nutraceuticals and holistic supplements is that many do not have specific doses. The maintenance dose is a reference but the providers may recommend more for pets with cancer. Below are the doses and recommendations for use that we have experienced as helpful for our geriatric cancer patients. Do not use escalated doses of a product or compound that you are not familiar with.

1.   Agaricus Bio® Capsules 600mg: one twice daily per 15–30 pounds.
       The capsule can be given directly by mouth or opened and placed in food or in gravy.
       For cats, we use the Agaricus SuperLiquid®, which is a liquid. Small dogs: 300mg capsule BID.
       For diabetic cats use Agaricus Eksimate. It is 300% more concentrated than the capsules.
       We start cats with 3–5 drops twice a day increasing to 10 drops twice a day for cats with severe
              advanced-stage cancer. There are 200 drops per vial. It can be used as a loading dose for dogs.
       The dose for advanced-stage cancer in dogs goes up to $1/_2$ vial per day for large dogs. Available
              from Atlas World USA. See https://www.mskcc.org/cancer-care/integrative-medicine/herbs/
              agaricus.
2.   IP-6: one capsule per 10–15 pounds per day (divided BID). It is best utilized on an empty stomach.
              Available from Integrative Therapeutics, Inc.
3.   Platinum Performance Plus® for Canines: gradually increase to 1 tbsp/30 pounds per day, divided.
       This compound is a great chondroprotective and general vitamin supplement for geriatric dogs.
       Mix in moist food such as yogurt, gravy, or canned food. Introduce to the diet over 2–3 weeks.
       Some dogs may develop loose stools and some will not accept it. Keep refrigerated.
       Platinum Performance Feline®: $1/_4$ teaspoon in canned or wet food per meal. Refrigerate.
4.   Advance Protection Formula (APF) drops: 3 drops per 10 pounds once per day in food. Contains
              Siberian ginseng. Available from Auburn Labs, http://www.auburnlabs.com.
5.   Onco Support: one scoop twice daily per 50 pounds. It also contains 600mg of Agaricus per scoop.
              Rx Vitamins for Pets sends a taste enhancer if the patient refuses it.
6.   Astragalus: enhances the action of some chemotherapy agents such as carboplatin, per the NCI.
7.   Musculoskeletal Support, Whole Body Support: helps combat weakness. Standard Process.
8.   CoQ10: acts as an antioxidant and specifically protects myocardium. We recommend using it to
              protect the heart from the cardiotoxic effects of Adriamycin.
9.   Fish oil is a source for OM-3 fatty acids. Use $1/_4$ of one teaspoon per 15 pounds per day if the
              patient can handle it without developing diarrhea. Use a high-quality product such as Ultra EFA®
              from Rx Vitamins for Pets. It is not needed for pets on Hill's n/d®.
10.   Vitality®: capsules contain a proprietary ratio of special extracts of panax ginseng, pomegranate,
              and *Cordyceps sinensis*. The formulation affects 92% of the 54 genes that regulate the numbers
              and function of mitochondria, most numerous in brain, cardiac, and skeletal tissue. It may help
              delay age-related changes in gene expression and biomarkers to increase endurance and
              cognitive ability. Pawspice.com/store.
11.   Astaxanthin: a carotenoid antioxidant, which may benefit dogs with OSA, at 2mg BID/large dog.

Instruct clients to introduce the supplements gradually over a period of 1–3 weeks to allow the patient to adjust to the supplements. Encourage clients to feed their geriatric pets high-quality food or homemade diets only. Try to get all cats off dry food completely as they often do better on canned food. If a dog is being fed Hill's n/d, we do not use Platinum Performance or fish oil. This combination often causes loose stools and/or diarrhea.

Note: Some clients are overwhelmed during the consultation that introduces both chemotherapy and supplements. It is best to introduce a few supplements at the first visit and add others at follow-up visits.

(nutrigenomics). Food nutrients influence genes to prevent or enhance certain diseases. An improper ratio of nutrients in pet food may adversely affect organs. For instance, taurine deficiency causes retinal detachment and cardiomyopathy in cats. Overfeeding shortens the life span of dogs and many other species. Some pet foods are formulated to offer clinical improvement in chronic conditions such as renal disease, diabetes, arthritis, and cognitive syndrome by altering the action of proteins and enzymes in the body that contribute to the degenerative condition.

Our profession has grown up with several dichotomies. For instance, we all know that the feline is an obligatory carnivore. However, our companion animal community has been trained to feed cats a high-carbohydrate diet and has become accustomed to fat cats and diabetes as part of the norm. According to feline specialist, Dr. Elizabeth Hodgkins, ACVIM, cats should not be fed dry food, because the short GI tract of the feline does not appreciate cellulose as a dietary ingredient. Cats need high protein, moderate fat, and low carbohydrate diets from birth to death. This would be their natural diet in the wild state. Obese cats tend to have more satiety and lose weight on a strictly canned food diet. Diabetic cats fed high protein diets may decrease or drop their need for insulin and become normalized. Some of my geriatric feline oncology patients, with concurrent diabetes, have normalized after they were taken off dry food, given a high protein canned food, and treated for their malignancies.

Can Diet Affect Geriatric Cancer Patients?

Clients frequently ask for recommendations about diet and nutrition. They search the Internet because they want to customize their pet's diet to fight cancer. They view nutrition as part of the therapy and ask questions about what to feed their pets. The Internet is replete with ideas and dietary suggestions to fight cancer and obesity. There will always be "food fads" and entrepreneurs and believers, who claim efficacy. The media often stirs up curiosity about various cancer diets and remedies as "miracles" and "breakthroughs" with hype, frenzy, and hoopla. It is best to check the validity of news articles that make sweeping claims for "cancer cures."Data reported in mice and cell lines only extrapolates to humans 10% of the time. Early findings reported by the media are not conclusive. It is important that veterinarians advise clients to seek balanced high quality diets for their geriatric cancer pets. It is always best to suggest a thorough look at the data and its source for its reliability, not the newspaper hype. Check these web sites: www.quackwatch.com, www.skeptic.com/naturalcancercures, and www.fda.gov/warning letters.

There is an ongoing revival of the 1931 Warburg theory that "cancer cells depend almost exclusively on glucose." Basically, Warburg (1931) felt that cancer cells could effectively be "starved" by using a high fat diet that would revert healthy cells to using ketones for aerobic energy metabolism, which cancer cells cannot utilize. This thinking evolved into the ketogenic diet and many of its permutations, including the Atkins diet.

The Paleolithic-type diets exclude grain. Then there is the alkaline diet and the macrobiotic diet. Other diets proposed by Drs. Gerson, Pritikin Ornish, Budwig, W.D. Kelly, Nicholas Gonzalez, and the Hoxsey herbal treatment, etc., have chimed in or flatly disagreed with the ketogenic diet theory. After ten years of trying, Atkins found that his diet did not help his cancer patients and he stopped accepting cancer patients for treatment. Most of the cancer diet data fails scientific scrutiny or is anecdotal, resulting in debate as to efficacy. However, the health benefits for people who improve their lifestyle choices, eat properly, maintain normal body weight, and exercise may obfuscate the data. Can we apply this to our companion animals?

"Caloric restriction" is an interesting and viable theory. A 14-year pivotal study in dogs clearly demonstrated that lifetime caloric restriction delayed cancer and osteoarthritis and extended life span by 2 years (Kealy et al. 2002). Metabonomics-based urine metabolite trajectories suggested that signals from gut microbiota may be involved in the longevity and health responses of caloric restricted dogs as per Dennis Lawler and colleagues (Lawler et al. 2008). Lifelong caloric restriction in dogs was found to delay immunosenescence (Greely et al. 2006). Caloric restriction lowers insulin and glucose levels, but it is not recommended for geriatric cancer patients who may often be or become easily malnourished. Carbohydrate restriction seems to mimic the metabolic state of caloric restriction. Ketogenic diets seem to mimic the condition of fasting. Metformin can be used to lower glucose.

Some pet owners are interested in trying to feed a ketogenic diet for their dogs with cancer. This is a high fat, moderate protein, very low carbohydrate diet that involves routine fasting. The goal is to achieve the Warburg theory to change the pet's physiology from burning carbohydrates and sugar to burning ketones, which are breakdown products from fat metabolism. This change is theoretically going to be hostile to cancer cells that utilize sugar and fermentation for energy. Since cancer cells do not use ketones from fat metabolism, the theory is that tumors present in the pet may be controlled and unable to metastasize. A ketogenic diet along with hyperbaric oxygen treatments was given to 50 dogs with various types and stages of cancer to see if it influenced progression. A summary of findings may be available at:www.ketopetsanctuary.com.

When Dr. Gregory Ogilvie, ACVIM, was at CSU, he employed the well-known and well-documented Warburg theory that cancer cells utilize sugars and carbohydrates more readily than fats, oils, and proteins. Dr. Ogilvie worked with Hill's Pet Nutrition, Inc., to formulate a diet with increased levels of fat, omega-3 fatty acids, protein, and arginine with reduced carbohydrates. The special diet was intended to "feed the patient and starve the cancer." Fifty lymphoma dogs were given the same chemotherapy protocol and divided into two groups. The group on the special diet had longer survival. The diet is available as Hill's Prescription Diet Canine n/d® (neoplasia diet), which contains 61.4% fat and 23.8% protein on a calorie weighted basis. Some oncologists recommend n/d for dogs with lymphoma and for dogs receiving radiation therapy. To avoid diarrhea, it is best to advise pet owners to gradually blend n/d into the patient's regular food until the majority of the intake becomes n/d. Seal remaining food in an airtight plastic bag to avoid oxidation. For more information visit www.hillspetnutrition.com.

Processed dry pet food has, by its very nature, lower protein and high processed carbohydrate content. I recommend a high-quality canned meaty food for cats and dogs with the addition of green vegetables. Lightly steam green vegetables with broth and place in a blender and store in a glass bowl to add to meals. Clients who want to try a ketogenic diet can prepare a homemade special diet that contains a 2:1 ratio of fats to protein and very low carbohydrate. The beneficial fats are from safflower oil, fish oils, butter, MCT oil, coconut oil, avocado oil, and flax seed oil. The protein should be fresh human grade meat and very low carbohydrates using only green vegetables such as asparagus, broccoli, brussels sprouts, kale, and string beans. The vegetables can be raw but chopped or diced finely or lightly steamed in beef or chicken broth and chopped in a food blender. Keep the steamed vegetable mixture in a glass container and add this to the food. Feed 15–30 calories per pound per day and monitor the blood glucose and ketone levels if possible at rechecks. For clients who are willing to prepare a homemade diet for their dog, I enthusiastically recommend the recipe in *Help Your Dog Fight Cancer: Empowerment for Dog Owners* by Laurie Kaplan and Alice Villalobos, which is now in its 3rd edition (2016). We keep office copies of this book for clients to explore. The book is available at www.helpyourdogfightcancer.com.

I generally avoid condoning homemade strict vegetarian and raw meat diets for my geriatric cancer patients due to the potential for nutritional imbalances, safe handling issues, and increased bacterial content. Bacterial contamination could be problematic for geriatric cancer patients struggling with cancer-induced and treatment-induced stress and immunosuppression. Some commercial vegetarian and raw diets are pre-sterilized and very carefully balanced and may meet the requirement for dogs and cats. The safest raw diets are prepared with USDA-inspected meat for human consumption, in high-quality kitchens, professionally sterilized, and immediately fresh frozen. If the packages are kept frozen properly and thawed just before feeding, the contamination issue should be less of a problem for cancer patients. Uneaten raw food should be discarded immediately. It is up to the doctor and the carers to verify that the chosen diet is nutritionally complete and tailored to the pet's level of activity, body condition score, and health status.

Summary: Chemoprevention and Immunonutrition for Cancer Patients

Chemoprevention, immunonutrition, and diet have become strong allies in the overall treatment of the geriatric oncology patient. During consultations, introduce the concept of chemoprevention, immunonutrition, and nutrition on general terms and then specifically for the geriatric oncology patient. Explain that dietary-derived phytochemicals and dietary supplements may influence the tumor microenvironment. It is no secret that Americans and their pets are suffering an epidemic of obesity and diabetes because of fast food, a high-carbohydrate diet, and minimal exercise. Feeding exclusively dry food on a free-choice basis to cats would be synonymous to giving them a total diet of "kitty fast food." Clients readily accept the theory of "starving the cancer cells and feeding the patient." This is an opportunity to improve the geriatric oncology patient's diet to a more calorie-dense, higher fat diet, moderate protein, very low carbohydrate diet, which may resemble a ketogenic diet. Some clients may choose Hill's n/d, a specially prepared diet, or a carefully made homemade diet. If the patient has a poor appetite or goes off food for 3 days, nutritional intervention and supportive care using appetite enhancers to maintain proper caloric intake is important. The quality of life for geriatric cancer patients diagnosed at early and at advanced stage cancer may benefit from thoughtful immunonutrition, chemoprevention, and dietary management.

Integrative and Alternative Medicine

Tis better to light one candle than curse the darkness.

Eleanor Roosevelt

When a geriatric cancer patient's family is told that there is nothing more that can be done, they often seek alternative, unconventional, and/or complementary medical therapies in the hope that the pet may benefit. It is admirable that so many of our highly bonded clients leave no stone unturned when it comes to caring for their older pets with cancer. We owe these questing clients courtesy and respect for their determination and efforts. We should discuss the considered options with a supportive, interested attitude and always offer end of life emotional support and guidance during their quest.

PP's Case (18-Year-Old Cat with Two Previous Brain Surgeries)

PP Roederick, an 18-year-old F/S Siamese cat, had two previous craniotomies for meningioma. PP developed recurrence of blindness, circling, anxiety, and weakness progressively over 2 months. The family declined further Sx and they did not want radiation therapy. PP was referred to us by chance. Her family was going to have her euthanized but their doctor was out of town. They went golfing and met a DVM colleague on the golf course who suggested a second opinion. That is how PP came to us. PP responded very well to our Pawspice care program using an integrative protocol for 6 months. Her medical management consisted of oral prednisone at 5mg BID, lomustine at 5mg on days 1 and 5 every 30–44 days depending on her CBC, oil of evening primrose capsules at 1–2 (538mg) BID (for linolenic acid), and Agaricus Extract Mate® (for beta glucans). We had conducted a clinical trial with medical colleagues at UCLA using linoleic acid in dogs. Dr. Leslie Bob Bennet, lead investigator, suggested using linolenic acid for cats because cats cannot convert linoleic to linolenic acid (Iwamoto et al. 1992). A survey of 356 human cancer patients who adopted complementary approaches for their treatment found them to be educated, intelligent, and unlikely to be persuaded that the therapy they employed is useless just because it has not been published in peer-reviewed journals (Cassileth et al. 1984). For a good source of reliable information, check https://www.cancerquest.org/patients/integrative-oncology.

Many practitioners do not agree with or know anything about the potentially adverse or beneficial effects of a particular complementary or alternative therapy or product chosen by clients to help their pet fight cancer (Lana 2006). We must avoid invalidating the client's search for non-conventional modalities to help a pet. The client may have invested great faith in a particular alternative therapy, and believing in a treatment is the preferred attitude for success. Crushing a person's hope is counterproductive and may turn them away from you. Therefore, it is best to incorporate the client's efforts into your treatment plan when possible and encourage the person to proceed with the benefit of your medical guidance.

Clients often tell me that they would do anything to save their pet. Many pet owners have embraced some aspect of holistic medicine for themselves or their pets. When the attending doctor makes jests, rolls back their eyes, dismisses, or disapproves of a client's choice to seek alternative therapy, the doctor alienates that client. If the pet shows a response to the dismissed therapy, the client is further alienated.

Cabo's Case: How and When Should One Stop Trying?

Cabo Greuel, a 12-year-old F/S Black Labrador Retriever, was diagnosed with end stage renal cell carcinoma (RCC) following signs of hematuria and "hobbling a bit." Elaine Greuel was determined to do everything possible for Cabo. Diagnostic imaging revealed that Cabo's left kidney was three times normal size and that she had five pulmonary metastases. Her BUN was 35 and her creatinine was 2.4. Cabo had a "great" response with deracoxib. Elaine searched the Internet, consulted with several oncologists, and brought in a stack of downloaded information. After our consultation, Elaine elected to enter Cabo into Pawspice with palliative chemotherapy. We used carboplatin, pain management, and our immunonutrition protocol including Onco Support and Renal Support® in an integrative approach.

Cabo experienced grade 3 adverse events from her first carboplatin treatment with lethargy, vomiting, and diarrhea, despite precautionary dose modification and using oral metoclopramide and sulfasalazine from her cancer care package. To avoid repeat toxicity, we opted to split her total dose over an 8-day period. Cabo's tumor growth stabilized with no progression for 3 months until the carboplatin failed to help. Her tumors enlarged as we tried other drugs to no avail. Elaine wanted to pursue further options despite my counsel to discontinue CTx and accept the sad fact that Cabo's days were numbered.

Elaine could not give up because Cabo remained in good spirits. I informed Elaine about small molecule research and that some agents had helped humans with RCC. Elaine wrote, "I tried to contact all of the pharmaceutical companies but no luck." She purchased three or four more alternative anticancer products during this time. She wrote, "Dr. Cheryl London called me back from Davis and felt very badly about Cabo, but said there is nothing out there and that she would take Cabo as one of her patients if there was. ... We decided to try the interferon therapy with Dr. Greg Ogilvie, being we didn't have too many options left so we wanted to give this a try. Cabo has been given five doses now and tolerates it very well with no side effects other than lethargy."

Elaine explained that she felt compelled to keep trying as long as Cabo was fighting the cancer. Her BUN was 39 and her creatinine was 2.9 when she was off piroxicam and on tramadol for the discomfort. She wrote, "At this point, there is not much to lose and maybe a little hope to gain, but we know that's slim."

Six days later, Elaine wrote, "Cabo was having trouble breathing all day yesterday and I noticed her gums were no longer pink and she was wobbly. As I was running her to Dr. Saunders, her primary veterinarian, she passed out in my arms. Dr. Saunders revived her. She fought like anything and even waited for Dave and Nikki to get home ... We even went back to bring Blaze to see her one last time and ... say goodbye ... I am so sad. Dave's heart is ripped out like mine ... We just wanted you to know how much we appreciate everything you have done for her and all your love and caring helped us tremendously. Please keep in touch with us."

When alternative therapies are used in combination with conventional therapies, they are considered to be complementary. If a treatment is used instead of or to replace conventional therapy, it is considered an alternative. Doctors that condone or use complementary therapies in concert with conventional treatment are involved with or practicing integrative therapy. The term "integrative oncology" describes an approach to treating cancer that combines standard Western treatments with other treatments or activities to further treat cancer, reduce side effects, and to improve patient wellbeing.

Accept Clients as Partners in Integrative Decision Making

The most important issue to clarify with your clients is that they should not forgo a known treatment for an unknown or, worse yet, an unsound therapy that lacks credibility (Miller 2005). Clients often feel that the alternative treatment is nurturing their pet. If that is the case, then blend this alternative into your protocol. A term commonly used to describe this fusion is "complementary and alternative medicine" (CAM). Complementary medicine refers to treatments or activities used in conjunction with standard Western treatments, while alternative medicine refers to treatments or activities that replace standard Western treatments. Go back to the old principle, "Do no harm." If the cancer patient is handling treatments with no innocuous or adverse side effects from a complementary medication, then the veterinarian should be willing to work with the regimen that the client has put together for their pet.

The most commonly used complementary therapies that have appealed to my clients to use for their pets include nutraceuticals, diet therapy, cannabinoids (CBD) from hemp (see "Cannabis Commentary" in Chapter 7), acupuncture, acupressure, massage therapy, chiropractic adjustment, herbal medicine, homeopathy (using very dilute solutions such as rescue remedy), energy field, and magnetic therapy. Metabolic therapy is based on the theory that cancer is caused by an accumulation of toxic substances in the body. Metabolic treatments include: megavitamin therapy, orthomolecular or high dose vitamin C therapy, enzyme therapy, cellular therapy, and detoxification therapy. There are many other types of alternative therapies, including immunoaugmentive therapy, oxygen, ozone, light, shock wave therapy, crystal, and aromatherapy. Most of these treatments are innocuous yet provide nurturing support. Some may be beneficial for some patients and some are probably ineffective.

The exception is with herbal medicine. Herbs have the potential to cause problems or create drug interactions, especially in geriatric patients on polypharmacy for concurrent conditions. The clinician must review herbal products to discover if there are any herb–drug interactions when given in combination with the patient's conventional medications.

Herb–Drug Interactions

Combining herbal products with conventional drugs and anticancer therapy may result in beneficial effects, no effect, or antagonistic interactions for the patient (Robinson 2006). There are two basic types of interactions between herbs and conventional drugs. A pharmacokinetic interaction affects the absorption, distribution, metabolism, or elimination of the herb(s) or drug(s), causing either an increase or a decrease in the amount of drug available to the patient. A pharmacodynamic interaction alters the way in which a drug or herb affects a tissue or organ system, causing either a synergistic or antagonistic herb–drug interaction (Carson 2002). Pharmacokinetic and pharmacodynamic herb–drug interactions may adversely affect the activity of antibiotics, cardiac glycosides, insulin, steroids, chemotherapy, and so forth, while exerting a protective and/or antioxidant effect for the liver, gut, kidney, heart, and immune system (Cassileth, Yeung, and Gubili 2010).

Antioxidants may be the most commonly used alternatives by owners of pets with cancer. Some oncologists prefer that herbs and antioxidants are not given to their cancer patients while they are receiving conventional chemotherapy and radiation therapy. The rationale for this precaution is based on the theory that part of the efficacy of the therapy is based on the generation of free radicals, especially true with Adriamycin. This recommendation is controversial and has been shown to be equivocal. My preference has always been to provide antioxidants to geriatric cancer patients so the patient receives their benefits during all types of conventional cancer treatments, including immunotherapy and gene therapy. For detailed information about the pros and cons regarding antioxidant therapy, please consult the suggested reading list for herb–drug interactions at the end of this chapter.

The introductory list of commonly used products and their potential drug interactions (Table 6.10) will acquaint you with how some commonly used herbs can interact, both positively and negatively, with some of the drugs that we employ in veterinary medicine (please note that the list is not complete). Clients will appreciate your acceptance of their contributions to their pet's care when you review the herbal products and supplements that they have chosen to give their pets. Keep in mind and inform clients that their aging pet may be more susceptible to herb–drug interactions due to decreased ability to absorb, metabolize, and excrete a polypharmacy of conventional drugs and herbal preparations.

For in-depth information, refer to *The Complete German Commission E. Monographs* and other suggested readings listed following the references at the end of this chapter. We as veterinary

Table 6.10. Drug–Herbal Interactions

Herb	May
Agaricus blazei	Counteract negative immunosuppression of steroids
	Increase insulin utilization, may lower glucose, and affect insulin dosage
Aloe vera	Increase potential toxicity with cardiac glycosides and antiarrhythmic agents
Astragalus	Impair immunosuppressive effects of cyclosporine, azathioprine, and methotrexate
	Increase immune stimulating effects of interleukin-2 and acyclovir
	Enhances the effect of carboplatin
Bromelain	Enhance some antibiotics
	Improve efficacy of some chemotherapeutic agents (vincristine and 5-fluorouracil)
Burdock	Necessitate adjustment of insulin dosage due to hypoglycemic effects
Cannabis (THC)	Unwanted psychotropic effects and toxicity, anorexia, listlessness: dose-dependent
Hemp (CBD)	Pain reduction, increased appetite, and well-being
Cayenne	Protect stomach from adverse effects of aspirin
	Enhance absorption of theophylline
Echinacea	Decrease effects of immunosuppressive drugs
	Enhance phagocytic immune function
Garlic	Behaves similarly to burdock with antiplatelet activity similar to ginkgo
Ginger	Help decrease nausea associated with chemotherapy
Ginkgo biloba	Increase antiplatelet effect of aspirin
Ginseng (APF®)	Regulate adaptogenic responses to stress, CTx, and RTx
	Potentiate corticosteroids
	Increase insulin utilization affecting insulin dosage
Goldenseal	Increase or decrease cardiac effect with cardiac glycosides
	Increase or decrease blood pressure effects of antihypertensive agents
Hawthorn	Behaves similarly to goldenseal for cardiac glycosides
Kava Kava	Potentiate substances acting on CNS
Licorice	Increase potassium loss with steroids and diuretics
	Increase sensitivity and potentiate toxicity with cardiac glycosides
	Reduce ulcer formation from aspirin
	Potentiate corticosteroids
MaHuang (ephedra)	Cause excessive nervous stimulation and weight loss with theophylline
	Cause dangerous hypertension with selegiline
	Increase clearance of dexamethasone
Marshmallow	Delay absorption of drugs taken simultaneously
Milk Thistle	Prevent liver damage
	Promote liver support with hepatoxic medications like acetaminophen and anticonvulsants
	Prevent nephrotoxicity from cisplatin
Nettles	Enhance anti-inflammatory effect of drugs
Rehmania	Antagonize suppressant effects of steroids
St. John's wort	Decrease digoxin, theophylline, and cyclosporine levels
Valerian	Potentiate effects of barbiturates
Not Herbs	
CoQ10 (Idebanone)	Protect heart from Adriamycin toxicity with antioxidant effect
IP-6	Regulate cell surface signaling to inhibit cancer, antioxidant activity

Source: Carson, K.M. 2002. *Veterinary Practice News* 16 (6):36, Amended by Villalobos in 2017 with permission.

practitioners need to educate ourselves on this subject and apply pressure to increase the number of useful scientific studies performed in the growing field of veterinary integrative medicine.

Summary: Integrative and Alternative Medicine

Advanced stage cancer and recurrence may preclude curative conventional therapy. Whether you agree or disagree about the efficacy of an alternative or complementary therapy, chosen by clients to help their pet fight cancer, we must respect their quest. We must avoid invalidating the clients' sincere efforts to help their geriatric cancer pet feel better. Believing in the alternative treatment is part of its prescription for success. It is not fair or courteous to crush a person's hope, but we must help clients realize what to expect from the patient's particular tumor type and stage of disease. Therefore, it is best to incorporate clients' efforts into your treatment plan when possible and encourage them to proceed with the benefit of your medical guidance.

When you integrate an alternative treatment into your conventional protocol, you turn it into a complementary therapy. Many of our deeply bonded clients would do anything to save their pet. If the pet shows a response to an alternative or complementary treatment, the client may feel less inclined to follow your advice in the future. Be sure to have a working knowledge of the basic alternative procedures and the products that are used in herbal medication and their potential adverse effects. In this way, you can integrate it as complementary care into your overall cancer treatment plan. You can oversee the patient's medical treatments to ensure that the patient avoids adverse herbal–drug interactions. Ultimately, the mutual goal of the veterinary–client relationship is to benefit the geriatric cancer patient's quality of life and support the emotional well-being of the carers.

Electrochemotherapy (ECT)/Electroporation (EP)

Robson Pasquale, DVM, and Marcelo Monte Mor Rangel, DVM

Electrochemotherapy (ECT), also known as electroporation (EP), is a form of local cancer therapy that is easier to apply than radiation therapy, but with much lower cost for the machine and facilities. Because of these characteristics, ECT/EP is another very viable weapon we can use against cancer. ECT/EP has emerged as one of the greatest options of therapy for localized cancer in some countries, such as Brazil, Slovenia, and Italy. It has a great potential to be used for battling cancer in companion animals throughout the world and in the US.

In the early 1980s, a researcher at the Institute Gustave Roussy in France, Luis Maria Mir, began to study a new technique to combat cancer. It would be later called electrochemotherapy (ECT) (Gehl 2003). Mir's first published papers regarding the principles of the technique date back to 1988 and the first publications of clinical studies date back to 1991 (Belehradek et al. 1991; Gehl 2003). After about two decades of research, in November of 2006, an exclusive edition devoted to the European Guidelines for ECT use in humans was published in the *European Journal of Cancer* (Mir et al. 2006). Since then, every year the technique has become more disseminated, predominantly in Europe and in human medicine.

ECT is now available in more than 140 European oncology centers, and in some countries, such as France, Denmark, Slovenia, and Ireland, among others, the government funds the treatment. A study evaluating the cost-effectiveness of ECT compared to the other forms of local therapy was performed and the results were favorable to ECT, encouraging its widespread use (Colombo et al. 2008). This applies very pertinently in veterinary medicine around the world. The country with the largest number of publications about ECT in veterinary medicine is Slovenia. Brazil, where more than 4,000 patients received ECT treatment before 2016, is the country with the largest number of patients treated.

Basic Principles

ECT associates two basic modalities: chemotherapy and electropermeabilization (also called electroporation (EP) (Mir and Orlowski 1999). In his research, Dr. Mir inferred that the increase in the reversible permeability of the cell membrane used for molecule insertion, such as DNA in gene transfection experiments, could also facilitate the entry of molecules into the cytoplasmic membrane, thus potentiating its action (Mir et al. 1991; Neumann et al. 1999; Miklavcic et al. 2000). ECT was tested for effectiveness *in vivo* with various anticancer drugs, including doxorubicin, cyclophosphamide, vincristine, vinblastine, carboplatin, 5-FU, paclitaxel, melphalan, mitomycin C, etoposide, gemcitabine, etc. The only agents that showed a good response were bleomycin and cisplatin. Using bleomycin in ECT, its absorption action is potentiated *in vitro* by up to 1,000 times. Using cisplatin, the absorption action is potentiated just a few dozen times (Miklavcic et al. 2014).

Mechanism of Action

The goal of the ECT technique is to facilitate the entry of the antineoplastic agent into cancer cells, thus increasing their potential action. The main mechanism of action of the technique is the chemotherapy itself. In the case of bleomycin, there are two mechanisms of death related with the drug, depending on the number of internalized molecules inside the cancer cells. When this number of molecules is smaller, it is observed as mitotic death. When the number of molecules is greater, a type of death is observed that is morphologically and biochemically similar to apoptosis, as in a pseudoapoptosis (Tounekti et al. 1993; Mir and Orlowski 1999). The mechanism of death related to cisplatin is apoptosis (Mir and Orlowski 1999; Rebersek et al. 2004).

Electrochemotherapy Technique

ECT/EP requires that the antineoplastic agent is present at the site to be treated when the electric field is applied (Gothelf et al. 2003). The drug is provided at the tumor tissue by the intravenous route or by intratumoral (intralesional) administration. Bleomycin is the only drug that demonstrated similar efficacy in clinical trials using either the intratumoral or the intravenous route. When ECT/EP is performed with cisplatin, only the intralesional route should be used.

In humans, the application of the electric field should be performed 7 minutes after intravenous administration of bleomycin, or immediately if the drug is administered intralesionally. When the intravenous technique is performed, it is recommended that the electric field be applied within 25 minutes after the 7-minute waiting time, so the total time after the administration of the drug and the ECT itself does not exceed 32 minutes. After this interval, sufficient drug concentration cannot be guaranteed for the technique to be effective (Gothelf et al. 2003; Campana et al. 2016). The application of the electric field must cover the entire area to be treated. Where there is no application of the electric field, there is no effective action (Mir et al. 1991).

It is very important to choose the optimal electrode type. Electrode configuration affects the electrical field distribution in the tissue. Two types of electrodes are used. Plate electrodes have parallel stainless steel plates. The inner distance between the electrodes depends on the size of the tumor and the capacity of the generator of electric pulses. The distance between the electrodes is usually 6–8mm. Needle electrodes can be arranged in rows (in a parallel array) or in hexagonal geometry. The hexagonal electrode has a central needle and 6 needles in a circular array. The pulses are applied between the electrodes in the circular array and between them and the central one. The pulses are applied in both directions between each pair of electrodes. In general, both types of electrodes, plate and needle, can be used for the treatment (Tozon et al. 2016).

Equipment, Devices, and Machines

The equipment available to perform ECT/EP was first developed as the Cliniporator™ from IGEA, a company associated with the University of Modena in Italy. This machine is currently used by the European medical community to treat cancer in human medicine (Mir et al. 2006).

A few machines have been developed exclusively for veterinary use. Two machines were developed by a French company, Leroy Biotech: ElectroVet S13™ and ElectroEZ Vet™;Vet Cancer of Brazil developed the VET CP 125™ electroporator, and BioPulse offers the OnkoDisruptor™ made in Italy: www.onkodisruptor.com. These devices are used exclusively in veterinary medicine and are in accordance with the criteria of the scientific literature to perform the technique with safety and efficacy.

There are still some electroporators that were developed for laboratory use that can produce the specific fields to perform ECT/EP, but they require the construction of special electrodes in order to be used in practice. The most widely used machine is the BTX ECM 830, produced by Harvard Apparatus.

Electrochemotherapy Protocol

The process requires heavy sedation or general anesthesia and is generally well tolerated. Many tumors can be treated in 1–3 treatment sessions. The most widely used protocol for ECT uses 800–1,300V/cm of electric field amplitude, 100µs of electrical pulse length, 8 pulses sequences, and frequencies ranging from 1 Hz to 5 kHz (according to the characteristics and limitations of each device) (Mir et al.1997; Heller 1995; Heller et al. 1996; Sersa et al. 1998; Lebar et al. 2002; Gothelf et al. 2003; Suzuki et al. 2015).

The drugs used in the ECT technique are bleomycin and cisplatin. Bleomycin is more enhanced by the technique and it is more widely used. It can be administered both intratumorally and intravenously. If used intravenously, the dose is $15,000IU/m^2$ or $15 U/m^2$. If used intralesionally, the dose is proportional to tumor volume, in accordance with Table 6.11.

Advantages

ECT is a very effective treatment for local tumors as well as for incompletely removed tumors. The technique is usually very well tolerated with generally no side effects observed, due to significant

Table 6.11.   Dose and Concentration of Bleomycin for Intratumoral Administration. Dose and Concentration of Cisplatin for Intratumoral Administration (Mir et al. 2006)

Tumor Volume ($V = ab\pi^2/6$)	$V < 0.5cm^3$	$0.5cm^3 < V < 1cm^3$	$V > 1cm^3$
Bleomycin dose concentration of 1,000IU/ml	1ml (1,000IU)/cm^3	0.5ml (500IU)/cm^3	0.25ml (250IU)/cm^3
Cisplatin dose concentration of 2mg/ml	1ml (2mg)/cm^3	0.5ml (1mg)/cm^3	0.25ml (0.5mg)/cm^3

reduction in chemotherapeutic doses. The targeted nature of the treatment, along with minimal damage caused to surrounding healthy tissue, makes ECT an exciting new weapon for clinicians to have in their armamentarium.

Larger tumors may require repeated treatments to obtain tumor control and a full remission. Despite the 4–6 week wound healing period post-ECT, which may concern some pet owners, there is generally minimal impact on the patient's quality of life.

ECT represents an alternative to surgical treatment for treating solid tumors. It is advantageous specifically in cases when owners do not consent to surgery. It is a great option for tumors are difficult to excise with adequate clean margins due to location, which is often the situation with oral and facial tumors.

ECT/EP Approach

The use of ECT in oncology should still be the subject of many additional scientific studies. However, its efficacy in association with traditional therapies has shown promising results. Among the most used combinations we can highlight monotherapy (ECT used as a sole therapy). In this approach, ECT is applied directly into the neoplasia without using other adjuvant therapies (Cemazar et al. 2008; Sersa et al. 2012; Campana et al. 2014; Spratt et al. 2014; Guida ct al. 2016; Montuori et al. 2016; Ribero et al. 2016; Tomassini et al. 2016; Zygogianni et al. 2016). When applied in this manner, there is a higher probability that more than one application will be needed, depending on the size of the neoplasia.

In smaller formations (e.g., Figure 6.9), the chances of local control in a single session are excellent, whereas in cases such as Figure 6.10 it was necessary to give 7 EP applications in order to get local control. The patient in Figure 6.10 survived 3.5 years without evidence of recurrence. In Figure 6.11 a patient with oral melanoma got only one ECT/EP treatment. The patient presented in complete remission with no evidence of gross disease 8 months later and died 20 months post-EP of unrelated causes.

Tita, a 7-year-old Boxer at 28kg, was diagnosed with MCT in the ear by cytopathological examination. The referring DVM suggested pinnectomy or electrochemotherapy as treatment options. The owner chose ECT because it was a more conservative treatment and because this allows the option of later amputating the ear, in case ECT fails. Only one ECT session was performed and complete remission was achieved. The patient was followed throughout his life, and died of other causes $2^1/_2$ years later.

ECT/EP can be used as a first step (neoadjuvant) treatment before surgical removal. In some cases, cytoreduction is necessary for the surgery to be technically feasible. EP can be used for this intent. It

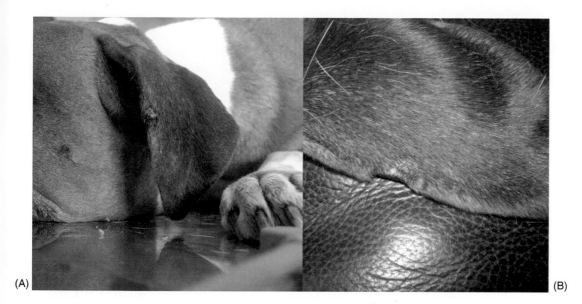

Figure 6.9.   Patient treated with ECT only, for MCT in the ear. (A) Before ECT–MCT with 0.8cm diameter; (B) 70 days after ECT, complete remission, and followed during 2 years, with no recurrence.

is very important to beware and consider in planning that the treated tumor tissue may respond to EP as an open wound undergoing necrosis.

ECT can be used as adjuvant surgery. In this approach, the technique is applied in the trans or in the postoperative period. With this approach, the main objective of the technique is to expand the surgical margins. This has been used in difficult cases when adequate surgical reconstruction is difficult or impossible, such as in regions such as the oral cavity, limbs, perianal region, head, and neck. The use of ECT can offer a more conservative surgery, and in some cases can avoid amputation

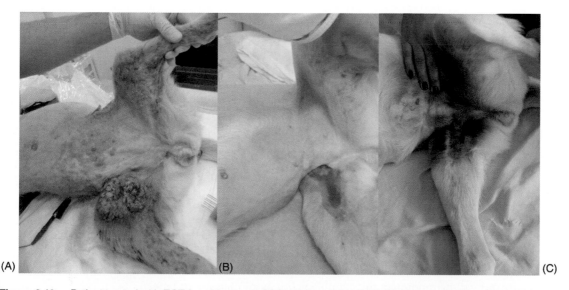

Figure 6.10.   Patient treated with ECT for widespread SCC. (A) Day of first ECT, (B) 25 days after her 7th session of ECT, with complete remission confirmed by biopsy, and (C) patient in complete remission 3 years after last ECT.

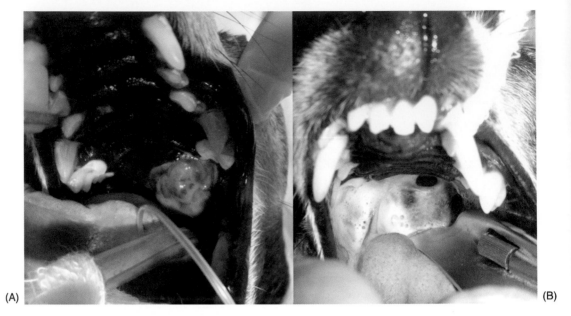

(A)   (B)

Figure 6.11.   Patient with diagnosis of soft palate melanoma treated with electrochemotherapy. A single session was sufficient for complete remission. (A) Immediately before ECT, 1.3cm oral melanoma on the soft palate region and (B) 28 days after with complete remission. An oronasal fistula developed, which was subsequently corrected with a surgical procedure. The patient died 20 months post-EP of other causes.

or more radical surgery. The combination may consequently yield better functional and cosmetic results than excisional surgery alone (Cemazar et al. 2008; Kodre et al. 2009; Muñoz Madero and Ortega Pérez 2011; Rangel Monte Mor et al. 2015; Lowe et al. 2016; Spugnini et al. 2016). Figure 6.12 shows a patient with a large tumor of approximately 17cm in the medial region of the elbow, with diagnosis of hemangiopericytoma. Marginal excision (conservative surgery) was performed, followed by ECT at the surgical bed. The ECT procedure effectively treated the margins that were compromised according to transoperative histological evaluation using the freezing technique. The patient was still alive 4 years after the procedure, without evidence of recurrence.

Indications

ECT can be performed on most neoplasms in geriatric dogs and cats. Unfortunately, there is a paucity of literature with prospective studies. There are few studies on the use of this technique for SCC, MCT, and others types of tumors in animals. In general, tumors need to be superficial. Debulked larger tumors allow access to the tumor bed so that ECT can be successful in controlling residual disease for wider margins.

The following are examples of tumor types that are amenable to ECT/EP:

- Fibrosarcoma in the mouth or eyelid
- Melanoma in the mouth, eyelid, or paw
- Squamous cell carcinoma in the mouth, eyelid, nasal planum, or paw
- Soft tissue sarcoma postdebulking surgery, when aggressive surgery would necessitate amputation

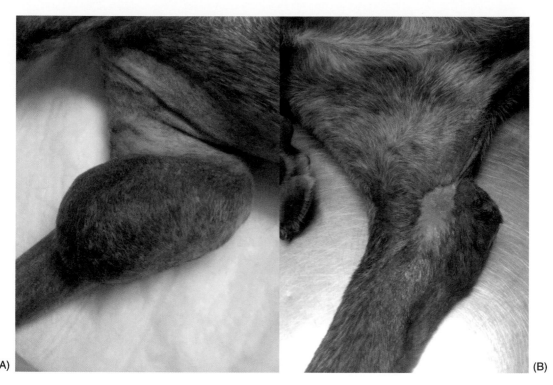

(A) (B)

Figure 6.12. Patient with STS with approximately 17cm in the medial region of the elbow. Conservative surgery was performed with transoperative ECT during the surgery. (A) STS in the medial region of the elbow. Patient was submitted to conservative surgery with transoperative ECT. (B) 70 days after the procedure, the patient had complete remission of the lesion. Four years and three months after the procedure, the patient was still alive with no evidence of local recurrence.

- Feline vaccine-associated fibrosarcoma after surgery
- Localized cutaneous lymphoma in dogs or cats
- Plasmacytic tumors of the footpad, lip, or skin
- Low to intermediate grade mast cell tumors on a distal limb, trunk, or face
- Perianal and rectal tumors
- Operation site margins when there is a significant risk of remaining tumor tissue
- Sarcoids and squamous cell carcinoma in horses
- Superficial tumor on exotics (small mammals, birds, and zoo animals)
- Some internal tumors such as tracheal and esophageal tumor (on a case by case and location basis) (Trip 2016)

Limitations

One important limitation of the ECT technique is when it is used in areas where it is difficult to introduce the electrodes, e.g., skull, abdominal and thoracic cavities, sinuses, ear canals, etc. In these situations, it is still feasible to apply the technique, but it is necessary to open a surgical access for the introduction of the electrodes. New electrodes and new approaches are being developed to overcome these limitations, e.g., intraluminal delivery by endoscopes, laparoscopic systems, or intravascular catheters (Kos et al. 2010; Lencioni et al. 2010; Miklavcic et al. 2010; Jahangeer et al. 2013; Mali et al. 2015; Miklavcic and Davalos 2015; Bianchi et al. 2016).

Metronomic Chemotherapy in Dogs

Hugo Gregório, DVM and Felisbina Queiroga, DVM

Key Points

- Metronomic chemotherapy (mCT) is a viable option for oncologic disease resistant to conventional therapeutic plans, especially in the advanced stage of disease.
- NSAIDs that inhibit COX-2 will interfere with carcinogenesis. Their analgesic properties improve the quality of life. NSAIDs can be used together with cytostatic drugs in metronomic chemotherapy protocols.
- Chlorambucil and cyclophosphamide are some of the most commonly used drugs used in metronomic protocols.

Introduction

Cancer has an elevated prevalence in older dogs, constituting the major cause of death in aged dogs.

Multimodal therapy, comprising surgery, chemotherapy, radiotherapy, and immunotherapy, has achieved control and even cure in some types of cancer. Priority is given to quality of life – not only the number of days survived.

Conventional Chemotherapy versus Metronomic Chemotherapy

Conventional chemotherapy protocols utilize the maximum tolerable dose (MTD) for the animal, with an interval or resting period between doses. This allows normal and healthy tissues to recover before repeating the treatment. Unfortunately, this resting period also allows disease progression, in which the tumor cells can recover and multiply.

This strategy of chemotherapy administration allows for a fixed percentage of dividing cancer cells to be killed at every administration and is most effective in patients that have a small tumor burden but a high percentage of tumor cells in active division. An example would be in the adjuvant setting when chemotherapy is given right after surgical tumor removal. This phenomenon also explains why conventional chemotherapy is usually not rewarding in the face of large tumor burdens and when tumors have a slow growth or grade.

In order to circumvent these pitfalls of classical chemotherapy protocols, a few strategies have been implemented. These include: using alternating different types of cytostatic drugs to minimize resistance; using PEGylated liposomal doxorubicin to minimize adverse events in non-target tissues; and maximizing the local effect of chemotherapy through local administration of chemotherapy agents such as Bleomycin for ameloblastoma, or carboplatin for pleural carcinomatosis, electrochemotherapy or electroporation, and chemotherapy under hyperthermia conditions. Despite these efforts, limited gains have been achieved in treatment response, and few therapeutic alternatives are available for patients with advanced macroscopic disease.

Metronomic Chemotherapy

Metronomic chemotherapy (mCT) uses a different approach from the MTD concept. Targeting the highly sensitive endothelial cells of new blood vessels formed by the tumor, smaller dosages of cytotoxic agents are administered daily instead of weekly or biweekly. This continuous low-dose treatment arrests angiogenesis, thus preventing new blood vessel formation and halting tumor progression. COX inhibitors are usually combined to potentiate cytostatic action, due to their proven antiangiogenic properties. With this approach, the relatively long resting periods of MTD chemotherapy are avoided. As endothelial cells are not true cancers cells, they are genetically stable and resistant to cytostatic drugs. This is not a recognized problem with some tumors that show response to lower-dose mCT treatment after failing to respond to the same agent in MTD schemes. Tumors eventually use escape pathways and angiogenesis ensues. Normal angiogenesis such as in healing and scar formation (cicatrization) is not affected.

Although angiogenesis inhibition is thought to be the main mechanism of action of mCT, other mechanisms are also implied that may contribute to the overall anticancer effect of mCT. Although dosages used are well below MTD dosages (10–20 times less), a direct cytotoxic effect is observed to some degree. Immune function may increase, as there may be a decreased number of T-regulatory lymphocytes in the tumor microenvironment.

Metronomic chemotherapy offers several advantages, including low toxicity, lower cost, and ease of administration.

Inflammation and Cancer

The close relationship between cancer and inflammation has been known for decades. Observational studies demonstrate that chronic inflammatory states can lead to cancer disease. This association was shown in feline injection site sarcoma (FISS) in cats and was suspected in orthopaedic implant associated osteosarcoma and in the progression of feline inflammatory bowel disease to gastrointestinal lymphoma.

In fact, PGE2, the main end product of COX-2 action, plays a major role in several carcinogenesis hallmarks such as proliferation, angiogenesis, invasion, metastasis, and apoptosis inhibition (Figure 6.13).

NSAIDs in Cancer Treatment

The first evidences of clinical applicability of NSAIDs in cancer treatment came from the human field. In the early 1980s, large cohort studies found that people who routinely took NSAIDs for a variety of conditions had a lower incidence of cancer and that patients with familial adenomatous polyposis showed regression of their intestinal lesions with Sulindac therapy, which supresses the COX-2 pathway.

In the veterinary field, early work from Debora Knapp in 1994 showed that piroxicam had an anticancer activity against transitional cell carcinoma (TCC) of the bladder in dogs, achieving two

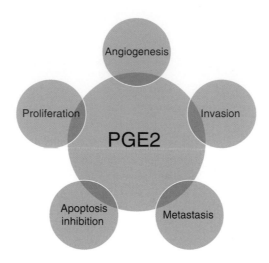

Figure 6.13.   Key steps of carcinogenesis.

complete remissions in 34 dogs treated with piroxicam alone. Since then, several other studies have documented clinical activity of NSAIDs against several oncologic diseases (Table 6.12).

Commonly Used Protocols

Due to its unspecific mechanism of action, mCT can potentially be used in treating several forms of cancer.

Currently, there are few studies showing evidence of clinical usefulness of metronomic protocols in dogs. One retrospective study demonstrated a prolonged disease-free interval in dogs with dirty margin sarcomas that were treated with cyclophosphamide and piroxicam, as compared to dogs treated with surgery alone (> 410 days versus 211 days). Another study found similar overall survival time in dogs with hemangiosarcoma treated with mCT after surgery, compared to an historic control group that was treated with surgery and conventional chemotherapy.

Interestingly, a recent study found a survival advantage in dogs with hemangiosarcoma treated with mCT after surgery and completion of a classical chemotherapy protocol. Chlorambucil was also found to be safe while providing clinical activity against TCC of the bladder and several other cancer forms (Table 6.13).

The alkylating agent cyclophosphamide (10–$15mg/m^2$/day) has been the most commonly used agent in early mCT studies. However, chlorambucil ($4mg/m^2$/day) has gained recognition because it offers a safer profile (absence of risk of developing hemorrhagic cystitis) and a larger clinical knowledge due to its use in chronic leukemia cases. It requires less drug compounding, commonly observed with cyclophosphamide. Lomustine ($2.84/m^2$/day) has also been evaluated. It has proven clinical activity against several tumors but has demonstrated higher toxicities.

Usually an NSAID is added at regular dosage. Piroxicam is still commonly used based on Knapp's early work in TCC. More recently specific COX-2 inhibitors such as deracoxib and firocoxib have also been evaluated due to their safer security profile.

Combining mCT with another antiangiogenic agent to prevent escape pathways is a logical approach. Combination with toceranib seems to be an option, but further studies are needed to evaluate its effectiveness and long-term safety.

Table 6.12. Clinical Studies on the Therapeutic Use of NSAIDs in Cancer in Dogs

Tumor Type	NSAID Used/Other Drugs	Comments	Reference
Transitional cell carcinoma	Piroxicam	$N = 34$; 2 CR; 4 PR; 18 SD; 10 PD	Knapp et al., 1994
Oral SCC	Piroxicam	$N = 17$; 1 CR; 2 PR; 5 SD; 9 PD	Schmidt et al., 2001
Oral SCC and oral melanoma	Piroxicam + Cisplatin	SCC	Boria et al., 2004
		$N = 9$ (2 CR; 3 PR; 3 SD; 1 PD)	
		OMM	
		$N = 11$ (2 CR; O PR; 1 SD; 8 PD)	
Nasal carcinoma	Piroxicam + alternating dosages of Carboplatin/Doxorubicine	$N = 8$; 4 CR; 2 PR; 2 PD	Langova et al., 2004
Transitional cell carcinoma	Piroxicam + Carboplatin	$N = 31$ (11 PR; 13 SD; 5 PD)	Boria et al., 2005
Transitional cell carcinoma	Deracoxib	$N = 26$ (0 CR; 4 PR; 17 SD; 3 PD; 2 N/A)	McMillan et al., 2011
Nasal carcinoma	Piroxicam + Carboplatin or Toceranib	$N = 3$; 2 CR; 1 PR	de Vos et al., 2012
Transitional cell Carcinoma	Firocoxib and/or Cisplatin	Firocoxib ($N = 15$)	Knapp et al., 2013
		0 CR; 3 PR; 5 SD; 4 PD; 3 N/A	
		Cisplatin ($N = 15$)	
		0 CR; 2 PR; 8 SD;4 PD; 1 N/A	
		Firocoxib+ Cisplatin ($N = 14$)	
		0 CR; 8 PR; 3 SD; 0 PD; 3 N/A	
Nasal carcinoma	Firocoxib + Radiotherapy	Firocoxib + Radiotherapy ($N = 12$)	Cancedda et al., 2015
		MST: 335 days	
		Radiotherapy ($N = 12$)	
		MST: 224 days	
		No statistical difference between treatments but quality of life improved in NSAID group ($p < 0.001$)	
Mammary carcinoma	Firocoxib or Mitoxantrone	$N = 28$	Arenas et al., 2016
		Mitoxantrone ($N = 8$)	
		MST: 18 ± 8.5 months	
		Firocoxib ($N = 7$)	
		MST: 19.4 ± 2.1 months	
		Control group ($N = 13$)	
		MST: 12.7 ± 1.7 months	
		MST of NSAID group statistically higher than control ($p = 0.048$)	

SCC, squamous cell carcinoma; OMM, oral malignant melanoma; SD, stable disease; PR, partial remission; CR, complete remission; N/A, information not available; MST, medium overall survival time.

Table 6.13. Review on Studies on Metronomic Chemotherapy in Dogs

Tumor Type	Protocol	Comments	Reference
Hemangiosarcoma	Cyclofosfamide + Piroxicam + Etoposide	N = 9 Comparable OS against doxorubicine: 178 d versus 133 d	Lana et al., 2007
Dirty margin sarcomas	Cyclophosfamide + Piroxicam	N = 85 Increased DFI in metronomic group versus surgery alone: 410 d versus 211 d	Elmslie et al., 2008
Various	Chlorambucil	N = 36 3 CR, 1 PR, 17 SD	Leach et al., 2012
Various	Lomustine	N = 64 4 PR, 19 SD	Tripp et al., 2011
Various	Cyclophosfamide + Celecoxib	N = 15 1 CR (oral melanoma), 5 SD	Marchetti et al., 2012
Transitional cell carcinoma	Chlorambucil	N = 31 1 PR, 20 SD	Schrempp et al., 2013
Various	Cyclophosphamide + Piroxicam +/− lansoprazol	N = 34 5 CR, 11 PR, 4 SD	Spugnini et al., 2014
Hemangiosarcoma	Cyclophosphamide	N = 208 Increased survival	Wendelburg et al., 2015
Hemangiosarcoma	Cyclophosphamide + NSAID +/− Thalidomide versus Doxorrubicine alone	N = 22 Increased survival on the mCT group	Finotello et al., 2017

One of the major difficulties in using mCT is finding biomarkers. Discovery of the biomarkers could help to evaluate treatment response, allow for dosage optimization, and facilitate the selection of optimum candidates for treatment.

Since angiogenesis inhibition is the major treatment goal of mCT, disease stabilization (rather than remission) is probably a more realistic treatment objective. This is difficult to establish without randomized clinical trials. Several biomarkers have been used, such as tumor microvessel density and circulating endothelial cells, to optimize treatment protocols and evaluate their efficacy.

Side effects

Low cytostatic dosages are used in mCT to offer protocols with a good safety profile. Even so, hemorrhagic cystitis is observed in about 10% of dogs treated with the higher metronomic dose range of cyclophosphamide. Renal failure and gastrointestinal toxicities remain a concern when NSAIDs are used, especially in older patients with comorbidities. Combination with other drugs such as tyrosine-kinase inhibitors appears to be an option, but special concerns regarding long term use and efficacy should be considered along with rigid monitoring and needs to be further investigated before being routinely used.

Clinical Case

This case concerned a male Bernese Mountain Dog (Bouvier Bernois), 8 years old with a subcutaneous hemangiosarcoma removed from the neck region: staging (abdominal ultrasound and thoracic X-rays) negative. The family declined adjuvant chemotherapy. Cutaneous and thoracic metastasis were detected on chest X-rays 6 months postsurgery. The dog was given oral mCT (firocoxib 5mg/kg/day + chlorambucil 4mg/m^2/day). The dog achieved a partial remission of both the cutaneous and the thoracic lesions lasting 5 months and with an overall survival of 19 months (see Figure 6.14).

During mCT, no relevant clinical or laboratorial adverse effects were noted. At 19 months after beginning treatment, the dog developed pulmonary metastasis with severe dyspnea and the family opted for euthanasia.

Conclusions

Metronomic chemotherapy protocols are attractive treatment options due to ease of use, low cost and safety profile. Early results show clinical efficacy against various types of cancers. These were mostly of advanced staging and heavily pretreated, making them less prone to respond to treatment. Several limitations exist regarding the use of mCT:

1. Difficulty calculating optimum dosages and evaluating their action.
2. Lack of high scientific evidence studies comparing its use with conventional therapies in tumors in early stage disease, limiting its application in such cases
3. Its use has been restricted to cases where alternative treatments are not available or have failed or where its higher safety profile proved to be advantageous for patients with comorbidities.

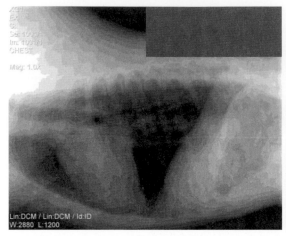

0 months after tumor removal

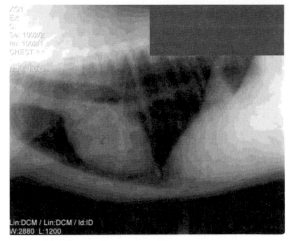

6 months after tumor removal
(before initiating metronomic chemotherapy)

10 months after tumor removal and 4 months after initiating
mCTremission after metronomic chemotherapy

Figure 6.14.   Various stages of the dog's treatment.

From the author's point of view, mCT will not substitute classic chemotherapy in the future. However, it will probably be used in combinatorial protocols. It may be used to control angiogenesis in the resting periods of MTD chemotherapy protocols. It may be used as a follow-up maintenance treatment after completion of classical chemotherapy protocols. It may be combined into cancer protocols via combination with specific molecular inhibitors and with immunotherapy. However, further studies are needed to ascertain its safety and efficacy.

References

Arenas, C., L. Peña, J.L. Granados-Soler, and M.D. Pérez-Alenza. 2016. Adjuvant therapy for highly malignant canine mammary tumours: Cox-2 inhibitor versus chemotherapy: a case-control prospective study. *Vet Rec* 179 (5):125.

AVMA News. 2005. Osborne honored for achievements in veterinary medical ethics. *JAVMA* 227 (5):685.

Belehradek, J., et al. 1991. Electrochemotherapy of spontaneous mammary tumours in mice. *European Journal of Cancer* 27 (1):73–76. ISSN 0959-8049. Online at: https://www.ncbi.nlm.nih.gov/pubmed/1707290.

Bergman, P.J. 1999. Differentiation and chemoprevention: Fact or fiction? *17th Annual ACVIM Forum Proceedings*, pp. 388–390.

Bergman, P.J. 2006. Immunotherapy options for canine malignant melanoma. *24th Annual ACVIM Forum Proceedings*.

Bianchi, G., et al. 2016. Electrochemotherapy in the treatment of bone metastases: A phase II trial. *World Journal of Surgery* July 2016. ISSN 1432-2323. Online at: https://www.ncbi.nlm.nih.gov/pubmed/27443372.

Boria, P.A., D.J. Murry, P.F. Bennett, et al. 2004. Evaluation of cisplatin combined with piroxicam for the treatment of oral malignant melanoma and oral squamous cell carcinoma in dogs. *JAVMA* 224 (3):388–394.

Boria, P.A., N.W. Glickman, B.R. Schmidt, et al. 2005. Carboplatin and piroxicam therapy in 31 dogs with transitional cell carcinoma of the urinary bladder. *Vet Comp Oncol* 3 (2):73–80.

Cahill, C. 2006. Mirtazapine as an antiemetic. Clinical Feature. *Veterinary Forum* 23 (2):34–37.

Campana, L.G., et al. 2014. Electrochemotherapy in non-melanoma head and neck cancers: a retrospective analysis of the treated cases. *British Journal of Oral Maxillofacial Surgury* 52 (10):957–964, December. ISSN 1532-1940. Online at: http://www.ncbi.nlm.nih.gov/pubmed/25183266.

Campana, L.G., et al. 2016. Electrochemotherapy: mechanism of action and clinical results in the locoregional treatment of patients with skin cancers and superficial metastases. *Recenti Prog Med* 107 (8), August:422–433. ISSN 2038-1840. Online at: https://www.ncbi.nlm.nih.gov/pubmed/27571558.

Cancedda, S., S. Sabattini, G. Bettini, et al. 2015. Combination of radiation therapy and firocoxib for the treatment of canine nasal carcinoma. *Vet Radiol Ultrasound*; 56 (3):335–343.

Carson, K.M. 2002. Drug-herbal interactions. *VPN* 14 (6):36.

Cassileth, B., E.J. Luck, D.S. Miller, et al. 1984. Psychosocial correlates of survival in advanced malignant disease. *New England Journal of Medicine* 312:1551–1555.

Cassileth, B.R., K.S. Yeung, and J. Gubili. 2010. *Herb–drug interactions in oncology*. Memorial Sloan-Kettering Cancer Center, Integrative Medicine Service. Peoples Medical Publishing House, CT, USA.

Cemazar, M., et al. 2008. Electrochemotherapy in veterinary oncology. *Journal of Veterinary Internal Medicine* 22 (4):826–831, July–August. ISSN 0891-6640. Online at: http://www.ncbi.nlm.nih.gov/pubmed/18537879.

Charney, S.C., P.J. Bergman, J.A. McKnight, J. Farrelly, C.A. Novosad, N.R. Leibman, and M.A. Camps-Palau. 2005. Evaluation of intracavitary mitoxantrone and carboplatin for treatment of carcinomatosis, sarcomatosis, and mesothelioma, with or without malignant effusions: A retrospective analysis of 12 cases (1997–2002). *Veterinary and Comparative Oncology* 3 (4):171–181.

Chun, R., L. Garrett, and E.G. MacEwen. 2001. "Cancer chemotherapy." In *Small animal clinical oncology*, 3rd edn, eds S.J. Withrow and E.G. MacEwen, pp. 92–118. Philadelphia, PA: Saunders.

Cohen, L.A., B. Powers, S. Amin, and D. Desai. 2004. Treatment of canine hemangiosarcoma with suberoylanilide hydroxamic acid, a histone deacetylase inhibitor. *Veterinary and Comparative Oncology* 2 (4):242–248.

Colombo, G.L., S.D., Matteo, and L.M. Mir. 2008. Cost-effectiveness analysis of electrochemotherapy with the Cliniporatortrade mark vs other methods for the control and treatment of cutaneous and subcutaneous tumors. *Therapy Clinical Risk Management* 4 (2):541–548, April. ISSN 1176-6336. Online at: http://www.ncbi.nlm.nih.gov/pubmed/18728828.

Cova, D., and L. Balducci. 2004. "Cancer chemotherapy in the older patient." In *Comprehensive geriatric oncology*, 2nd edn, eds L. Balducci, G.H. Lyman, W.B. Ershler, and M. Extermann, pp. 463–488. Oxon, UK: Taylor & Franks.

Curt, G.A. 1990. Unsound methods of cancer treatment. *Cancer Principles and Practice of Oncology, PPO Updates* 4 (12):1–10.

Dank, G. 2006a. The use of carprofen in canine mammary neoplasia: A prospective study. *24th ACVIM Forum Proceedings.*

Dank, G. 2006b. A critical overview of NSAID usage in veterinary oncology. *24th Annual ACVIM Forum Proceedings.*

Dank, G., A. Aung, and S. Yudelevitch. 2005. Preliminary results of the use of carprofen in canine mammary tumors. *15th ECVIM-CA Congress Abstracts*, p. 40, and *JVIM* 19 (6):941.

deLorimier, L.P. 2014. Thrombocytopenia associate with chronic administration of metronomic chlorambucil in dogs. *Proceedings of Veterinary Cancer Society Poster Presentations*, p. 114.

De Vos, J., S. Ramos Vega, E. Noorman, and P. De Vos 2012. Primary frontal sinus squamous cell carcinoma in three dogs treated with piroxicam combined with carboplatin or toceranib. *Vet Comp Onc* 10 (3):206–213.

Dobson, J., S. Cohen, and S. Gould. 2004. Treatment of canine mast cell tumors with prednisolone and radiotherapy. *Veterinary and Comparative Oncology* 2 (3):132–141.

Dobson, J., and D. Lascelles. 2003. *BSAVA manual of canine and feline oncology*, 2nd edn. Quedgeley, Gloucestershire, England: British Small Animal Veterinary Association.

Doroshow, J.H. 1996. "Anthracyclines and anthracenediones." In *Cancer chemotherapy and biotherapy*, eds B.A. Chabner and D.A. Longo, pp. 409–434. Philadelphia, PA: Lippincott-Raven Publishers.

Electrochemotherapy with cisplatin: potentiation of local cisplatin antitumour effectiveness by application of electric pulses in cancer patients. *European Journal of Cancer* 34 (8):1213–1218, July 1998. ISSN 0959-8049. Online at: http://www.ncbi.nlm.nih.gov/pubmed/9849482.

Electrochemotherapy: mechanism of action and clinical results in the locoregional treatment of patients with skin cancers and superficial metastases. *Recent Progress in Medicine* 107 8:422–433, August 2016. ISSN 2038-1840. Online at: https://www.ncbi.nlm.nih.gov/pubmed/27571558.

Elmslie, R.E., P. Glawe, and S.W. Dow. 2008. Metronomic therapy with cyclophosphamide and piroxicam effectively delays tumor recurrence in dogs with incompletely resected soft tissue sarcomas. *J Vet Intern Med* 22 (6): 1373–1379.

Emms, S. 2005. Anal sac tumors in dogs and their response to cytoreductive surgery and chemotherapy. *Australian Veterinary Journal* 83 (6):340–343.

Finotello, R., J. Henriques, S. Sabattini, et al. 2017. A retrospective analysis of chemotherapy switch suggests improved outcome in surgically removed, biologically aggressive canine haemangiosarcoma. *Vet Comp Oncol* 15 (2):493–503.

Gehl, J. 2003. Electroporation: theory and methods, perspectives for drug delivery, gene therapy and research. *Acta Physiology Scandinavia* 177 (4):437–447, April. ISSN 0001-6772. Online at: http://www.ncbi.nlm.nih.gov/pubmed/12648161.

Glickman, L.T., M. Raghavan, D.W. Knapp, M.H. Dawson, and P.L. Bonney. 2004. Herbicide exposure and the risk of transitional cell carcinoma of the urinary bladder in Scottish Terriers. *JAVMA* 224 (8):1290–1297.

Goldstein, R.E. 2004. Percutaneous ethanol injections (PEI) for the treatment of benign thyroid and parathyroid tumors. *AVMA Convention Notes.*

Gothelf, A., L. Mir, and J. Gehl. 2003. Electrochemotherapy: results of cancer treatment using enhanced delivery of bleomycin by electroporation. *Cancer Treatment Reviews* 29 (5) 371–387, October. ISSN 0305-7372. Online at: http://www.ncbi.nlm.nih.gov/entrez/query.fcgi?cmd=Retrieve&db=PubMed&dopt=Citation&list_uids=12972356.

Greeley, E.H., E. Spitznagel, D.F. Lawler, R.D. Kealy, and M. Segre. 2006. Modulation of canine immunosenescence by life-long caloric restriction. *Veterinary Immunology and Immunopathology* 111 (3–4):287–299 (http://dx.doi.org/10.1016/j.vetimm.2006.02.002).

Guida, M., et al. 2016. Local treatment with electrochemotherapy of superficial angiosarcomas: Efficacy and safety results from a multi-institutional retrospective study. *Journal of Surgical Oncology* May. ISSN 1096-9098. Online at: http://www.ncbi.nlm.nih.gov/pubmed/27156580.

Gustafson, N.R., S.E. Lana, M.N. Mayer, and S.M. LaRue. 2004. A preliminary assessment of whole-body radiotherapy interposed within a chemotherapy protocol for canine lymphoma. *Veterinary and Comparative Oncology* 2 (3):125–131.

Hahn, K.A. 2005. Consider intralesional chemo. *VPN*, June, pp. 20–21.

Hahn, K.A. 2006. CT can help avoid useless surgery. *VPN* 18 (4):20.

Hart, B.L., L.A. Hart, A.P. Thigpen, and N.H. Willits. 2014, Long-term health effects of neutering dogs: Comparison of Labrador Retrievers with Golden Retrievers. *PlosOne*.

Helfand, S.C. 2003. "Emerging approaches for cancer therapy." In *BSAVA manual of canine and feline oncology*, 2nd edn, eds J. Dobson and D. Lascelles, pp. 115–119. Quedgeley, Gloucestershire, England: British Small Animal Veterinary Association.

Heller, R. 1995. Treatment of cutaneous nodules using electrochemotherapy. *Journal of Fla Medical Association* 82 (2):147–150, February. ISSN 0015-4148. Online at: http://www.ncbi.nlm.nih.gov/entrez/query.fcgi?cmd=Retrieve&db=PubMed&dopt=Citation&list_uids=7535837.

Heller, R., et al. 1996. Phase I/II trial for the treatment of cutaneous and subcutaneous tumors using electrochemotherapy. *Cancer* 77 (5):964–971, March. ISSN 0008-543X. Online at: http://www.ncbi.nlm.nih.gov/entrez/query.fcgi?cmd=Retrieve&db=PubMed&dopt=Citation&list_uids=8608491.

Henderson, R.A. 2004. Prostatectomy: Is it time for a revisit? Personal Communication, *VCS NL* 28 (3).

Iwamoto, K.S., L.R. Bennett, A. Norman, A.E. Villalobos, and C.A. Hutson. 1992. Linoleate produces remission in canine mycosis fungoides. *Cancer Letters* 64:17–22.

Jahangeer, S., et al. 2013. Review of current thermal ablation treatment for lung cancer and the potential of electrochemotherapy as a means for treatment of lung tumours. *Cancer Treatment Reviews* 39 (8):862–871, December. ISSN 1532-1967. Online at: https://www.ncbi.nlm.nih.gov/pubmed/23601905.

Kaplan, R.N., and A.E. Villalobos (2016) *Help your dog fight cancer: Empowerment for dog owners*. Briarcliff, NY: JanGen Press.

Kaplan, R.N., R.D. Riba, S. Zacharoulis, et al. 2005. VEGFR1-positive haematopoietic bone marrow progenitors initiate the pre-metastatic niche. *Nature* 438:820–827.

Kealy, R.D., D.F. Lawler, J.M. Ballam, et al. 2002. Effects of diet restriction on the life span and age-related changes in dogs. *JAVMA* 220 (9):1315–1320.

Kearns, S.A., and P. Ewing. 2006. Causes of canine and feline pancytopenia. *Compendium* 28 (2):122–133.

Kisseberth, W.C., and E.G. MacEwen. 2001. "Complications of cancer and its treatment." In *Small animal clinical oncology*, 3rd edn, eds S.J. Withrow and E.G. MacEwen, pp. 198–219. Philadelphia, PA: Saunders.

Kitchell, B. 1993. Personal Communication regarding intralesional chemotherapy. VCS Annual Meeting.

Knapp, D.W., R.C. Richardson, T.C. Chan, et al. 1994. Piroxicam therapy in 34 dogs with transitional cell carcinoma of the urinary bladder. *JVIM* 8:723.

Knapp, D.W., R.C. Richardson, T.C. Chan, et al. 1994. Piroxicam therapy in 34 dogs with transitional cell carcinoma of the urinary bladder. *J Vet Intern Med* 8 (4):273–278.

Knapp, D.W., C.J. Henry, W.R. Widmer, et al. 2013. Randomized trial of cisplatin versus firocoxib versus cisplatin/firocoxib in dogs with transitional cell carcinoma of the urinary bladder. *J Vet Intern Med* 27 (1):126–133.

Kodre, V., et al. 2009. Electrochemotherapy compared to surgery for treatment of canine mast cell tumours. *In Vivo* 23 (1):55–62, January–February. ISSN 0258-851X. Online at: https://www.ncbi.nlm.nih.gov/pubmed/19368125.

Kos, B., et al. 2010. Robustness of treatment planning for electrochemotherapy of deep-seated tumors. *Journal of Membrane Biology* 236 (1):147–153, July. ISSN 1432-1424. Online at: http://www.ncbi.nlm.nih.gov/pubmed/20596859.

Kurzman, I.D., M.K. Huelsmeyer, D.H. Thamm, E.G. MacEwen, D.M. Vail, et al. 2005. Canine melanoma allogeneic tumor cell vaccine: Findings of the ongoing multicenter compassionate use study. *25th Annual Conference Proceedings of the Veterinary Cancer Society*, p. 80.

Lamerato-Kozicki, A.R., K. Helm, S.C. Helfand, and J.F. Modiano. 2005. Innovations in the diagnosis of canine hemangiosarcoma. *VCS NL* 29 (1):4–5.

Lana, S.E. 2006. Complementary and alternative therapies for cancer: Are they benign? *24th Annual ACVIM Forum Proceedings*.

Lana, S., L. U'ren, S. Plaza, et al. 2007. Continuous low-dose oral chemotherapy for adjuvant therapy of splenic hemangiosarcoma in dogs. *J Vet Intern Med* 21 (4):764–769.

Langova, V., A.J. Mutsaers, B, Phillips, and R. Straw 2004. Treatment of eight dogs with nasal tumours with alternating doses of doxorubicin and carboplatin in conjunction with oral piroxicam. *Aust Vet J.* 82 (11):676–680.

Larson, C.L., S.D. Allstadt, T.M. Fan, et al. 2016. Pharmacokinetics of orally administered low-dose rapamycin in healthy dogs *AJVR* 77 (1):January,65–71.

Lawler, D.F., R.H. Evans, B.T. Larson, E.L. Spitznagel, M.R. Ellersieck, and R.D. Kealy. 2005. Influence of lifetime food restriction on causes, time, and predictors of death in dogs. *JAVMA* 226:225–231.

Lawler, D.F., B.T. Larson, J.M. Ballam, and G.K. Smith. 2008. Diet restriction and ageing in the dog: major observations over two decades. *British Journal of Nutrition* 99 (4):793–805. doi: https://doi.org/10.1017/S0007114507871686.

Leach, T.N., M.O. Childress, S.N. Greene, et al. 2012. Prospective trial of metronomic chlorambucil chemotherapy in dogs with naturally occurring cancer. *Vet Comp Onc* 10(2):102–112.

Lebar, A.M., et al. 2002. Optimisation of pulse parameters *in vitro* for *in vivo* electrochemotherapy. *Anticancer Research* 22 (3):1731–1736, May–June. ISSN 0250-7005. Online at: http://www.ncbi.nlm.nih.gov/pubmed/12168862.

Lencioni, R., et al. 2010. Loco-regional interventional treatment of hepatocellular carcinoma: techniques, outcomes, and future prospects. *Transplant International* 23 (7):698–703, July. ISSN 1432-2277. Online at: http://www.ncbi.nlm.nih.gov/pubmed/20492618.

Limmer, S., N. Eberle, V. Nerschback, I. Nolte, and D. Betz. 2016. Treatment of feline lymphoma using a 12-week, maintenance-free combination chemotherapy protocol in 26 cats. *Veterinary and Comparative Oncology* 14 (S1)21–10. doi: 10.1111/vco.12082.

Liptak, J.M., W.S. Dernell, E. Monnet, et al. 2004. Massive hepatocellular carcinoma in dogs: 48 cases (1992–2002). *JAVMA* 225 (8).

London, C. 2004. Kinase inhibitors in cancer therapy. *Veterinary and Comparative Oncology* 2 (4):177–193.

Love, M.L. 2000. "Diagnosis and types of cancer." In *Dr. Susan Love's Breast Book*, pp. 324–335. New York: Perseus Publishing.

Lowe, R., et al. 2016. The treatment of canine mast cell tumours with electrochemotherapy with or without surgical excision. *Veterinary Composition of Oncology* March. ISSN 1476-5829. Online at: http://www.ncbi.nlm.nih.gov/pubmed/27001443.

Lowik, C. 2016. Helping surgeons visualize cancer, World Veterinary Cancer Congress, Brazil.

Mali, B., et al. 2015. Electrochemotherapy of colorectal liver metastases – an observational study of its effects on the electrocardiogram. *Biomedical Engineering Online* 14 (Suppl. 3):S5. ISSN 1475-925X. Online at: http://www.ncbi.nlm.nih.gov/pubmed/26356120.

Marchetti, V., M. Giorgi, A, Fioravanti, et al. 2012. First-line metronomic chemotherapy in a metastatic model of spontaneous canine tumours: a pilot study. *Invest New Drugs.* 30 (4):1725–1730.

Mauldin, N. 2016. Introduction to PetCure Oncology and Stereotactic Radiosurgery (SRS), Veterinary Cancer Society Breakfast Meeting.

Mayhew, P.D., R.W. Richardson, S.J. Mehler, D.E. Holt, and C.W. Weisse. 2006. Choledochal tube stenting for decompression of the extrahepatic portion of the biliary tract in dogs: 13 cases (2002–2005). *JAVMA* 228 (8):1209–1214.

McMillan, S.K., P. Boria, G.E. Moore, W.R. Widmer, P.L. Bonney, and D.W. Knapp. 2011. Antitumor effects of deracoxib treatment in 26 dogs with transitional cell carcinoma of the urinary bladder. *JAVMA* 239 (8):1084–1089.

Miklavcic, D., and R.V. Davalos. 2015. Electrochemotherapy (ECT) and irreversible electroporation (IRE)–advanced techniques for treating deep-seated tumors based on electroporation. *Biomedical Engineering Online* 14 (Suppl. 3):I1. ISSN 1475-925X. Online at: http://www.ncbi.nlm.nih.gov/pubmed/ 26355606.

Miklavcic, D., et al. 2000. A validated model of *in vivo* electric field distribution in tissues for electrochemotherapy and for DNA electrotransfer for gene therapy. *Biochim Biophys Acta* 1523 (1):73–83, September. ISSN 0006-3002. Online at: http://www.ncbi.nlm.nih.gov/pubmed/11099860.

Miklavcic, D., et al. 2010. Towards treatment planning and treatment of deep-seated solid tumors by electrochemotherapy. *Biomed Engng Online* 9:10. ISSN 1475-925X. Online at: http://www.ncbi. nlm.nih.gov/entrez/query.fcgi?cmd=Retrieve&db=PubMed&dopt=Citation&list_uids=20178589.

Miklavcic, D., et al. 2014. Electrochemotherapy: from the drawing board into medical practice. *Biomedical Engineering Online* 13 (1):29, March. ISSN 1475-925X. Online at: https://www.ncbi. nlm.nih.gov/pubmed/24621079.

Miller, R.M. 2005. Alternative therapies. In *The revolution in horsemanship and what it means to mankind*, pp. 304–311. Guilford, CT: Lyons Press.

Milner, R.J., J. Peyton, K. Cooke, L.E. Fox, A. Gallagher, P. Gordon, and J. Hester. 2005. Response rates and survival times for cats with lymphoma treated with the University of Wisconsin–Madison chemotherapy protocol: 38 cases (1996–2003). *JAVMA* 227 (7):1118–1121.

Mir, L.M., and S. Orlowski. 1999. Mechanisms of electrochemotherapy. *Advamces in Drug Delivery Reviews* 35 (1):107–118, January. ISSN 1872-8294. Online at: http://www.ncbi.nlm.nih.gov/ pubmed/10837692.

Mir, L.M., et al. 1991. Electrochemotherapy potentiation of antitumour effect of bleomycin by local electric pulses. *European Journal of Cancer* 27 (1):68–72. ISSN 0959-8049. Online at: https://www.ncbi. nlm.nih.gov/pubmed/1707289.

Mir, L.M., et al. 1997. First clinical trial of cat soft-tissue sarcomas treatment by electrochemotherapy. *British Journal of Cancer* 76 (12):1617–1622. ISSN 0007-0920. Online at: http://www.ncbi.nlm. nih.gov/pubmed/9413951.

Mir, L.M., et al. 2006. Standard operating procedures of the electrochemotherapy: Instructions for the use of bleomycin or cisplatin administered either systemically or locally and electric pulses delivered by the Cliniporator™ by means of invasive or non-invasive electrodes. *EJC Supplements* 4 (11):14–25. ISSN 1359-6349. Online at: http://dx.doi.org/10.1016/j.ejcsup.2006.08.003.

Modiano, J.F. 2016. Innovations in Cancer Treatment and Prevention, World Veterinary Cancer Congress, Foz do Iguassu, Brazil.

Montuori, M., et al. 2016. Electrochemotherapy for basocellular and squamocellular head and neck cancer: preliminary experience in day surgery unit. *G Italian Dermatology and Venereology* July. ISSN 1827-1820. Online at: https://www.ncbi.nlm.nih.gov/pubmed/27377142.

Morrison, W.B. 2002. Principles of treating chemotherapy complications. In *Cancer in dogs and cats: Medical and surgical management*, 2nd edn, pp. 365–374. Jackson, WY: Teton New Media.

Mullins, M.N., W.S. Dernell, S.J. Withrow, E.J. Erhart, D.H. Thamm, and S.E. Lana. 2006. Evaluation of prognostic factors associated with outcome in dogs with multiple cutaneous mast cell tumors treated with surgery with and without adjuvant treatment: 54 cases (1998–2004). *JAVMA* 228 (1): 91–95.

Munoz Madero, V., and G. Ortega Perez. 2011. Electrochemotherapy for treatment of skin and soft tissue tumours. Update and definition of its role in multimodal therapy. *Clinical Transl Oncology* 13 (1):18–24, January. ISSN 1699-3055. Online at: http://www.ncbi.nlm.nih.gov/pubmed/21239351.

Mutsaers, A.J. 2014. Metronomic chemotherapy: Theory and practice. State of the Art Presenter, *Proceedings Veterinary Cancer Society Annual Forum*, p. 56.

Neumann, E., S. Kakorin, and K. Toensing. 1999. Fundamentals of electroporative delivery of drugs and genes. *Bioelectrochemistry and Bioenergy* 48 (1):3–16, February. ISSN 0302-4598. Online at: http://www.ncbi.nlm.nih.gov/pubmed/10228565.

Norsworthy, G.D. 2005. Closure of difficult surgical defects using an extracellular matrix bioscafold. Veterinary Forum, July.

Oberthaler, K., F. Shofer, A. Bowden, K. Skorupski, and K. Sorenmo. 2004. Chemoprevention using NSAIDS in dogs: A preliminary epidemiological survey. *VCS 24th Annual Proceedings*, p. 23.

O'Keef, D.A., D.D. Sisson, H.B. Gelberg, and D.R. Krawic. 1993. Systemic toxicity associated with doxorubricin administration in cats. *JVIM* 7:309–317.

Osborne, C. 2001. Thinking surgeon or cutting surgeon: To be or not to be? *DVM Newsmagazine*, October.

Rangel Monte Mor, M., et al. 2015. 1st Vet Câncer. *Proceedings of II Brazilian Meeting on Veterinary Electrochemotherapy*, eds M. Rangel Monte Mor and D. Suzsuki Ota, p. 29, São Paulo, SP, Brazil,

Rassnick, K.M. 2006 Diagnosing and managing dogs with histiocytic diseases. *24th Annual ACVIM Proceedings*.

Rassnick, K.M., A.S. Moore, N.C. Northrup, O. Kristal, B.B. Beaulieu, L.D. Lewis, and R.L. Page. 2006a. Phase I trial and pharmacokinetic analysis of ifosfamide in cats with sarcomas. *AJVR* 67 (3):510–516.

Rassnick, K.M., C.O. Rodriguez, C. Khanna, M.P. Rosenberg, O. Kristal, K. Chaffin, and R.L. Page. 2006b. Results of a phase II clinical trial on the use of ifosfamide for treatment of cats with vaccine-associated sarcomas. *AJVR* 67 (3):517–523.

Rebersek, M., et al. 2004. Electrochemotherapy with cisplatin of cutaneous tumor lesions in breast cancer. *Anticancer Drugs* 15 (6):593–597, July. ISSN 0959-4973. Online at: http://www.ncbi.nlm.nih.gov/pubmed/15205602.

Ribero, S., et al. 2016. Metastatic sebaceous cell carcinoma, review of the literature and use of electrochemotherapy as possible new treatment modality. *Radiology and Oncology* 50 (3):308–312, September. ISSN 1318-2099. Online at: https://www.ncbi.nlm.nih.gov/pubmed/27679547.

Robinson, N.G. 2006. Watching out for interactions between complementary and alternative medical (CAM) and conventional cancer treatments. *VCS NL* 30 (1):7–14.

Rose, J. 2004. RVT. Tech Talk, *VCS News*, Spring.

Rosenthal, R.C. 2001. "Hemolymphatic disorders." In *Veterinary oncology secrets*, pp. 179–189. Philadelphia, PA: Hanley & Belfus.

Schappa, J.T., A.M. Frantz, B.H. Gorden, E.B. Dikerson, D.A. Vallera, and M.F. Modiano. 2013. Hemangiosarcoma and its cancer stem cell sub-population are effectively killed by a toxin targeted through epidermal growth factor and urokinase receptors. *International Journal of Cancer* October 15, 133 (8):1936–1944.

Schmidt, B.R., N.W. Glickman, D.B. Denicola, A.E. De Gortari, and D.W. Knapp. 2001. Evaluation of piroxicam for the treatment of oral squamous cell carcinoma in dogs. *JAVMA* 218 (11):1783–1786.

Schrempp, D.R., M.O. Childress, J.C. Stewart, et al. 2013. Metronomic administration of chlorambucil for treatment of dogs with urinary bladder transitional cell carcinoma. *JAVMA* 242 (11):1534–1538.

Sersa, G., et al. 2012. Electrochemotherapy of chest wall breast cancer recurrence. *Cancer Treatment Reviews* 38 (5):379–386, August. ISSN 1532-1967. Online at: https://www.ncbi.nlm.nih.gov/pubmed/21856080.

Shamsuddin, A.M. 1998. *IP-6: Nature's revolutionary cancer-fighter*. New York: Kensington Books.

Simon, D., N. Eberle, N. Abbrederis, J. Hirschberger, and I. Nolte. 2005. Malignant lymphoma in the dog: Results of treatment with a 12-week maintenance-free chemotherapy protocol. *15th ECVIM-CA Congress Abstracts*, p. 34, and *JVIM* 19 (6):939.

Sorenmo, K., L. Duda, L. Barber, et al. 2000. Canine hemangiosarcoma treated with standard chemotherapy and minocycline. *JVIM* 14:395–398.

Spratt, D.E., et al. 2014. Efficacy of skin-directed therapy for cutaneous metastases from advanced cancer: a meta-analysis. *Journal of Clinical Oncology* 32 (28):3144–3155, October. ISSN 1527-7755. Online at: http://www.ncbi.nlm.nih.gov/pubmed/25154827.

Spugnini, E.P., S. Buglioni, F. Carocci, et al. 2014. High dose lansoprazole combined with metronomic chemotherapy: a phase I/II study in companion animals with spontaneously occurring tumors. *J Transl Med* 21 (12):225.

Spungnini, E.P., et al. 2016. Electrochemotherapy as first line cancer treatment: experiences from veterinary medicine in developing novel protocols. *Current Cancer Drug Targets* 16 (1):43–52. ISSN 1873-5576. Online at: http://www.ncbi.nlm.nih.gov/pubmed/26712353.

Standard operating procedures of the electrochemotherapy: Instructions for the use of bleomycin or cisplatin administered either systemically or locally and electric pulses delivered by the Cliniporator™ by means of invasive or non-invasive electrodes. *EJC Supplements* 4 (11):14–25, October 17, 2016. ISSN 1359-6349. Online at: http://dx.doi.org/10.1016/j.ejcsup.2006.08.003.

Stiffler, K.S., M.A. McCrackin Stevenson, K.K. Cornell, L.E. Glerum, J.D. Smith, N.A. Miller, and C.A. Rawlings. 2003. Clinical use of low-profile cystostomy tubes in four dogs and a cat. *JAVMA* 223 (3):325–329.

Suzuki, D.O., et al. 2015. Numerical model of dog mast cell tumor treated by electrochemotherapy. *Artificial Organs* 39 (2):192–197, February. ISSN 1525-1594. Online at: https://www.ncbi.nlm.nih.gov/pubmed/25041415.

Takada, S. 2003. Principles of chemotherapy safety procedures. *Clinical Techniques in Small Animal Practice* 18 (2):73–74.

Thamm, D.H., L. Bisson, B. Rose, S. Dreitz, and L. Wittneberg. 2006. Histone deacetylase inhibition to enhance osteosarcoma chemosensitivity. Personal Communication, Symposium of Canine Osteosarcoma Syllabus, Veterinary Cancer Society, p. 28.

Theon, A. 1990–1994. Personal Communication, University of California visits, regarding intralesional therapy for nasal SCC in cats.

Thrall, D.E. 2004. An interview with Donald E. Thrall. *Veterinary Medicine*, August, pp. 636–638.

Tobias, K.M., S. Leonatti, A. Gibbs, and C. Bosworth. 2004. Symposium on skin reconstruction techniques. *Veterinary Medicine*, October, pp. 859–897.

Tomassini, G.M., et al. 2016. Electrochemotherapy with intravenous bleomycin for advanced non-melanoma skin cancers and for cutaneous and subcutaneous metastases from melanoma. *G Italian Dermatology and Venereology* 151 (5):499–506, October. ISSN 1827-1820. Online at: https://www.ncbi.nlm.nih.gov/pubmed/27595201.

Toskich, B. 2016. Angiosomal ablation of hepatic tumors with yttrium-90. Keynote Speaker, *Veterinary Cancer Society Proceedings*, October 20.

Tounekti, O., et al. 1993. Bleomycin, an apoptosis-mimetic drug that induces two types of cell death depending on the number of molecules internalized. *Cancer Research* 53 (22): 5462–5469, November. ISSN 0008-5472. Online at: https://www.ncbi.nlm.nih.gov/pubmed/7693342.

Towards treatment planning and treatment of deep-seated solid tumors by electrochemotherapy. *Biomedical Engineering Online* (9)10. ISSN 1475-925X. Online at: http://www.ncbi.nlm.nih.gov/entrez/query.fcgi?cmd=Retrieve&db=PubMed&dopt=Citation&list_uids=20178589.

Tozon, N., U. Lampreht Tratar, K. Znidar, G. Sersa, J. Teissie, and M. Cemazar. 2016. Procedures of the electrochemotherapy for treatment of tumor in dogs and cats. *Journal of Visual Experiments* (116), e54760. doi:10.3791/54760.

Tripp, C.D., J. Fidel, C.L. Anderson, et al. 2011. Tolerability of metronomic administration of lomustine in dogs with cancer. *J Vet Intern Med* 25 (2):278–284.

Trip, C. 2016. Electrochemotherapy in Private Practice – Scientific Session Comprehensive Review – ACVIM, June.

Vaden, S.L., J.F. Levine, G.E. Lees, R.P. Groman, G.F. Grauer, and S.D. Forrester. 2005. Renal biopsy: A retrospective study of methods and complications in 238 dogs and 65 cats. *JVIM* 19 (6):794–801.

Vail, D.M. 2006a. Molecular targets and osteosarcoma: The alphabet soup recipe. Symposium on Canine Osteosarcoma, *Veterinary Cancer Society Proceedings*, p. 55.

Vail, D.M. 2006b. New supportive therapies for cancer patients. *24th Annual ACVIM Forum Proceedings*.

Vail, D.M., et al. 2004. Consensus document: Veterinary Co-operative Oncology Group – Common terminology criteria for adverse events (VCOG-CTCAE) following chemotherapy or biological antineoplastic therapy in dogs and cats v. 1.0. *Veterinary and Comparative Oncology* 2 (4):194–213.

Vajdovich, P., P. Ribiczey, J. Jakus, et al. 2005. Changes of free radical and antioxidant parameters in blood of dogs with lymphoma during the course of treatment. *15th ECVIM-CA Congress Abstracts*, p. 35, and *JVIM* 19 (6):939–940.

Veterinary cooperative oncology group – common terminology criteria for adverse events (VCOG-CTCAE) following chemotherapy of biological antineoplastic therapy in dogs and cats v1.1, 2016 reprint from July 2011 publish date in *Veterinary and Comparative Oncology* 14 (4):December, 417–446.

Walter, C.U., B.J. Biller, S.E. Lana, A.M. Bachand, and S.W. Dow. 2006. Effects of chemotherapy on immune responses in dogs with cancer. *JVIM* 20 (2):342–347.

Weisse, C. 2014a. Interventional radiology: A trend in veterinary medicine. Clinicians Brief, October, pp. 61–66.

Weisse, C. 2004b. Regional tumor therapies: An approach to metastatic and nonresectable tumors. *AVMA Convention Notes.*

Wendelburg, K.M., L.L. Price, K.E. Burgess, J.A. Lyons, F.H. Lew, and J. Berg. 2015. Survival time of dogs with splenic hemangiosarcoma treated by splenectomy with or without adjuvant chemotherapy: 208 cases (2001–2012). *JAVMA* 247 (4):393–403.

Woods, J.P., K.A. Mathews, and A.B. Binnington. 2004. Thalidomide for the treatment of hemangiosarcoma in dogs. *Veterinary and Comparative Oncology* 2 (2):108–109.

Yang, T., J.B. Case, S. Boston, M.J. Dark, and B. Toskich. 2017. Microwave ablation for treatment of hepatic neoplasia in 5 dogs. *JAVMA* 250 (1):79–85.

Zygogianni, A., et al. 2016. Potential role of electrochemotherapy as anticancer treatment for cutaneous and subcutaneous lesions. *Asian Pacific Journal of Cancer Previews* 17 (8):3753–3757. ISSN 1513-7368. Online at: https://www.ncbi.nlm.nih.gov/pubmed/27644612.

Suggested Reading

Radiation Oncology

Gillette, T. 1987. "Principles of radiation therapy." In *Veterinary cancer medicine*, 2nd edn, eds G. Theilen and B. Madewell, pp. 137–143. Philadelphia, PA: Lea & Febiger.

LaRue, S.M., and T. Gillette. 2001. "Radiation therapy." In *Small animal clinical oncology*, 3rd edn, eds S.J. Withrow and E.G. MacEwen, pp. 119–137. Philadelphia, PA: Saunders.

McEntee, M. 2002. "Summary of results of cancer treatment with radiation therapy." In *Cancer in dogs and cats: Medical and surgical management*, 2nd edn, eds W.B. Morrison, pp. 389–424. Jackson, WY: Teton New Media.

McEntee, M. 2004. Radiation therapy. *AVMA 2004 Convention Notes.*

McNiel, E. 2003. "Radiation therapy." In *BSAVA manual of canine and feline oncology*, 2nd edn, eds J. Dobson and D. Lascelles, pp. 104–114. Quedgeley, Gloucestershire, England: British Small Animal Veterinary Association.

Meuten, D., and J. Moulton. 2002. "Radiation induced carcinogenesis." In *Tumors in domestic animals*, 4th edn, ed. D. Meuten, pp. 20–21. Ames, IA: Blackwell Publishing Professional.

Oglivie, G., and A. Moore. 1995. *Managing the veterinary cancer patient*, pp. 87–94. Trenton, NJ: Veterinary Learning Systems.

Oglivie, G., and A. Moore. 2001. "Radiation therapy-properties, uses, and patient management." In *Feline oncology*, pp. 77–81. Trenton, NJ: Veterinary Learning Systems.

Thrall, D.E. 2002. "Biologic principles of radiation therapy." In *Cancer in dogs and cats: Medical and surgical management*, 2nd edn, ed. W.B. Morrison, pp. 374–388. Jackson, WY: Teton New Media.

Withrow, S.J., D.M. Vail, and Page (eds). 2013. *Withrow and MacEwen's small animal clinical oncology*, 5th edn. Elsevier.
www.PetCureOncology.com.

Medical and Surgical Oncology

http://www.lib.ncsu.edu/vetmed/boards/ACVIM/oncology: 2017. Residency reading list.
Chabner, B.A., and D.L. Longo (eds. 2011). *Cancer chemotherapy and biotherapy: Principles and practice*, 5th edn. Philadelphia, PA: Lippincott Williams & Wilkins.
Dobson, J., and D. Lascelles. 2003. *BSAVA manual of canine and feline oncology*, 2nd edn. Gloucestershire, England: British Small Animal Veterinary Association.
Feldman, B.F. and C.A. Sink. 2006. *Practical transfusion medicine for the small animal practitioner*. Jackson, WY: Teton New Media.
Knapp, D.W. 2002. "Immunotherapy and biological response modifiers." In *Cancer in dogs and cats*, 2nd edn, ed. W.B. Morrison. Jackson, WY: Teton New Media.
Kudnig, S.T., and B. Seguin (eds). 2012. Veterinary Surgical Oncology, 604 pp. Wiley-Blackwell. ISBN 978-0-8138-0542-9.
Leibman, N. (guest ed.). 2003. Medical oncology. *Clinical Techniques in Small Animal Practice* 18 (2).
Meuten, D. 2002. *Tumors in domestic animals*, 4th edn. Ames, IA: Blackwell Publishing Professional.
Morrison, W.B. 2002. *Cancer in dogs and cats: Medical and surgical management*, 2nd edn. Jackson, WY: Teton New Media.
Ogilvie, G.K., and A.S. Moore. 1995. *Managing the veterinary cancer patient*. Trenton, NJ: Veterinary Learning Systems.
Ogilvie, G.K., and A.S. Moore. 2001. *Feline oncology*. Trenton, NJ: Veterinary Learning Systems.
Rosenthal, R. 2001. *Veterinary oncology secrets*. Philadelphia, PA: Hanley & Belfus.
Theilen, G., and B. Madewell. 1979. *Veterinary cancer medicine*. Philadelphia, PA: Lea & Febiger.
Theilen, G., and B. Madewell. 1987. *Veterinary cancer medicine*, 2nd edn. Philadelphia, PA: Lea & Febiger.
Withrow, S.J., and E.G. MacEwen. 2001. *Small animal clinical oncology*, 3rd edn. Philadelphia, PA: Saunders.
Withrow, S.J., and D.M. Vail. 2007. *Small animal clinical oncology*, 4th edn. Philadelphia, PA: Saunders.
Withrow, S.J., D.M. Vail, and Page (eds). 2013. *Withrow and MacEwen's small animal clinical oncology*, 5th edn. Elsevier. Elsevier

Herb–Drug Interactions

Blumenthal, M., W.R. Busse, A. Goldberg, J. Gruenwald, T. Hall, C.W. Riggins, and R.S. Rister (eds). 1998. *The complete German Commission E. monographs: Therapeutic guide to herbal medicines*, trans. S. Klein and R.S. Rister. Austin, TX: American Botanical Council; Boston: Integrative Medicine Communications.
Brinker, F.J. 1998. *Herb contraindications and drug interactions*. Sandy, OR: Eclectic Medical Publications.
Cassileth, B.R., K.S. Yeung, and J. Gubili. 2010. *Herb–drug interactions in oncology*, Memorial Sloan-Kettering Cancer Center, Integrative Medicine Service. Peoples Medical Publishing House, CT, USA.
http://homepage.eircom.net/~progers/herblink.htm. Dr. Phil Rogers' web site.
http://www.herbalgram.org/. American Botanical Council.
Lininger, Jr., D.C., and W. Schuyler (eds). 1999. *A–Z guide to drug–herb–vitamin interactions*. New York: Three Rivers Press.

McGuffin, J., C. Hobbs, R. Upton, et al. 1997. *American Herbal Products Association's botanical safety handbook*. Boca Raton, FL: CRC Press.

Medveckis, L.A. 2001. "A Discussion on Potential Drug–Herb Interactions." Herbal Crossroads, an information resource from Kan Herb Company, Scotts Valley, CA.

PDR for herbal medicines, 3rd ed. 2004. Montvale, NJ: Thomson PDR.

Wulff-Tilford, M.L., and G.L. Tilford. 2001. *Herbs for pets*. Irvine, CA: Bow-Tie Press.

Electrochemotherapy (ECT)/Electroporation (EP)

Tozon, N., U. Lampreht Tratar, K. Znidar, G. Sersa, J. Teissie, and M. Cemazar. 2016. Operating procedures of the electrochemotherapy for treatment of tumor in dogs and cats. *J Vis Exp* (116), e54760. doi: 10.3791/54760.

Metronomic Chemotherapy in Dogs

Burton, J.H., L. Mitchell, D.H. Thamm, S.W. Dow, and B.J. Biller 2011. Low-dose cyclophosphamide selectively decreases regulatory T cells and inhibits angiogenesis in dogs with soft tissue sarcoma. *J Vet Intern Med* 25 (4):920–926.

Carvalho, M.I., I. Pires, J. Prada, et al. 2016. High COX-2 expression is associated with increased angiogenesis, proliferation and tumoural inflammatory infiltrate in canine malignant mammary tumours: a multivariate survival study. *Vet Comp Oncol*. doi: 10.1111/vco.12206.

Colombo, C., D. Baratti, S. Kusamura, M. Deraco, and A. Gronchi 2015. The role of hyperthermic intraperitoneal chemotherapy (HIPEC) and isolated perfusion (ILP) interventions in sarcoma. *J Surg Oncol* 111 (5):570–579.

Emmenegger, U., S. Man, Y. Shaked, et al. 2004. A comparative analysis of low-dose metronomic cyclophosphamide reveals absent or low-grade toxicity on tissues highly sensitive to the toxic effects of maximum tolerated dose regimens. *Cancer Res* 64 (11): 3994–4000.

Gaspar, T.B., J. Henriques, L. Marconato, and F.L. Queiroga. 2017. The use of low-dose metronomic chemotherapy in dogs – insight into a modern cancer field. *Vet Comp Oncol*. doi: 10.1111/vco.12309.

Gregório, H., T.P. Raposo, F.L. Queiroga, J. Prada, and I. Pires. 2016. Investigating associations of cyclooxygenase-2 expression with angiogenesis, proliferation, macrophage and T-lymphocyte infiltration in canine melanocytic tumours. *Melanoma Res* 26 (4):338–347.

Harper, A. and L. Blackwood. 2017. Toxicity of metronomic cyclophosphamide chemotherapy in a UK population of cancer-bearing dogs: a retrospective study. *J Small Anim Pract* 58 (4):227–230.

Iliopoulou, M.A., B.E. Kitchell, and V. Yuzbasiyan-Gurkan. 2013. Development of a survey instrument to assess health-related quality of life in small animal cancer patients treated with chemotherapy. *J Am Vet Med Assoc* 242 (12):1679–1687.

Jergens, A.E. 2012. Feline idiopathic inflammatory bowel disease. *J Feline Med Surg* 14 (7):445–458.

Kelly, J.M., B.A. Belding, and A.K. Schaefer. 2010. Acanthomatous ameloblastoma in dogs treated with intralesional bleomycin. *Vet Comp Oncol* 8 (2):81–86.

Labayle, D., D. Fischer, P. Vielh, et al. 1991. Sulindac causes regression of rectal polyps in familial adenomatous polyposis. *Gastroenterology* 101 (3): 635–639.

London, C.A., H.L. Gardner, T. Mathie, et al. 2015. Impact of Toceranib/Piroxicam/Cyclophosphamide maintenance therapy on outcome of dogs with appendicular osteosarcoma following amputation and carboplatin chemotherapy: A multi-institutional study. *PLoS One* 10, e0124889.

Maiti, R. 2014. Metronomic chemotherapy. *J Pharmacol Pharmacother* 5(3):186–192.

Martano, M., E. Morello, and P. Buracco. 2011. Feline injection-site sarcoma: Past, present and future perspectives. *Vet J* 188 (2):136–141.

Mitchell, L., D.H. Thamm, and B.J. Biller. 2012. Clinical and immunomodulatory effects of toceranib combined with low-dose cyclophosphamide in dogs with cancer. *J Vet Intern Med* 26 (2):355–362.

Pasquier, E., M. Kavallaris, and N. Andre. 2010. Metronomic chemotherapy: New rationale for new directions. *Nat Rev Clin Oncol* 7 (8):455–465.

Queiroga, F.L., I. Pires, M. Parente, H. Gregório, and C.S. Lopes. 2011. COX-2 over-expression correlates with VEGF and tumour angiogenesis in canine mammary cancer. *Vet J* 189 (1):77–82.

Raposo, T.P., B.C.B. Beirão, L.Y. Pang, F.L. Queiroga, and D.J. Argyle. 2015. Inflammation and cancer: Till death tears them apart. *Vet J* 205 (2):161–174.

Shevchenko, I., S. Karakhanova, S. Soltek, et al. 2013. Low-dose gemcitabine depletes regulatory T cells and improves survival in the orthotopic Panc02 model of pancreatic cancer. *Int J Cancer* 133 (1):98–107.

Spugnini, E.P., Fais, S., Azzarito, T. and Baldi, A. 2017. Novel Instruments for the Implementation of Electrochemotherapy Protocols: From Bench Side to Veterinary Clinic. *J Cell Physiol.* 232 (3):490–495.

Stevenson, S. 1991. Fracture-associated sarcomas. *Vet Clin North Am Small Anim Pract* 21 (4):859–872.

Takkouche, B., C. Regueira-Mendez, and M. Etminan. 2008. Breast cancer and use of nonsteroidal anti-inflammatory drugs: A meta-analysis. *J Natl Cancer Inst* 100 (20):1439–1447.

Teske, E., G.R. Rutteman, J. Kirpenstein, and J. Hirschberger. 2011. A randomized controlled study into the efficacy and toxicity of pegylated liposome encapsulated doxorubicin as an adjuvant therapy in dogs with splenic haemangiosarcoma. *Vet Comp Oncol* 9 (4):283–289.

Wojciechowska, J.I., C.J. Hewson, H. Stryhn, N.C. Guy, G.J. Patronek, and V. Timmons. 2005. Development of a discriminative questionnaire to assess nonphysical aspects of quality of life of dogs. *Am J Vet Res* 66 (8):1453–1460.

Xu, X.L., F.J. Alexandro, J. Kruuv, and T.A. Waston. 1987. The biological foundation of the Gompertz model. *Int J Biomed Comput* 20 (1–2):35–39.

Zandvliet, M. and E. Teske. 2015. Mechanisms of drug resistance in veterinary oncology: A review with an emphasis on canine lymphoma. *Vet Sci* 2 (3):150–184.

Chapter 7
Pain Control for the Geriatric Cancer Patient

The question is not, "Can they Reason?" nor "Can they Talk?" The question is, "Can they Suffer?"

Jeremy Bentham

Your geriatric cancer patients experience pain on a regular basis. In the geriatric patient, cancer pain is often compounded on top of pre-existing concurrent chronic pain.

After completing a first generation oncology residency at UC Davis in 1972, in order to better help my own veterinary cancer patients, I visited human cancer patients and asked them to describe the sensations they were feeling. They discussed their pain and I then extrapolated this information to apply to my cancer patients. At that time, there was no information about cancer pain and pain management for pets. Ignorance about animal consciousness blocked intuitive realizations about the ability of animals to perceive and experience physical pain and emotional maltreatment (Dawkins 2005). Fears of creating addiction blanketed the professions against ministering to painful people and animals (Rollin 2005). Ideologically pure science did not accept that animals had consciousness and so it was acceptable to ignore a pet owner's plea to alleviate his or her pet's pain. Attending doctors simply passed over claims about pain with a counterclaim (Dawkins 2005).

That old thinking has changed radically. We now have the International Veterinary Academy for Pain Management (www.ivapm.org), which gives courses on pain management, publishes *Certified Veterinary Pain Practitioner* (CVPP), and uses the slogan, "Because their pain is our pain." IVAPM declares September as Veterinary Pain Awareness Month. Despite their efforts, there is still a paucity of papers about cancer pain in geriatric dogs and cats. Therefore, this chapter is written mostly from personal experience, paralleling the experience of esteemed colleagues and honoring the memory of thousands of my cancer patients.

It is up to you, the contemporary veterinarian and healer, to be attentive when clients feel or assume their geriatric companion animal is in pain. We cannot fully understand the dimensions of pain experienced by another person or being unless we have the misfortune of experiencing that same pain ourselves. Veterinarians need to trust and believe their clients' hunches about pain in their geriatric pets. Clients often sense their old pet's distress or notice behavior changes and need us to minister to the reality of the pain.

When a geriatric cancer patient does not display overtly painful behavior in the exam room, do not conclude that the pet is not in pain. Cancer pain may be more obvious in the home setting when the pet is quiet and not on guard. Cancer pain attacks people randomly and especially at night. Many pet caregivers experience their pet's whimpers and agitation from cancer pain during the night. A caregiver knows their pet intimately better than the veterinarian does and their observations should not be invalidated.

Canine and Feline Geriatric Oncology: Honoring the Human–Animal Bond, Second Edition. Alice Villalobos with Laurie Kaplan.
© 2018 John Wiley & Sons, Inc. Published 2018 by John Wiley & Sons, Inc.

The most painful cancers involve expanding lesions of the head and neck, bone, liver, GI, CNS, and urogenital tract. Invasive sarcomas, ulcerated skin tumors, inflammatory carcinoma, and any advanced stage visceral cancer, such as malignant histiocytosis, are also very painful (De Lorimier and Fan 2005). Anticipate, therefore, that almost all cancer patients have pain. Be proactive to alleviate it. Your job is not merely to treat the cancer but also to prevent pain, or treat the pain and restore quality of life to the patient.

Geriatric cancer patients often present in a double calamity with the unrelenting stress of pre-existing chronic pain overlaid by the onset of cancer pain. Age-related chronic pain causes stress and adversely affects the immune system, emotions, and overall health status of the patient.

Treating Pain Is Good Medicine

Inherent survival instincts dictate animal behavior to mask pain and keep moving with the pack. This survival instinct remains in domestic animals and is present even in our domesticated household pets. The stoic nature of animals persists well into their geriatric years. Dogs with chronic steady pain will still follow their family members from room to room. Dogs still want to go out for their walks and some will even run with their master or mistress despite chronic debilitating pain. They may be diagnosed with severe osteoarthritis or osteosarcoma or an abdominal mass within days of a sporting activity.

Geriatric dogs may simply slow down or not be able to go the normal walking distance, due to pain, without exhibiting overt signs of pain. Dogs and cats with primary or secondary orbital and brain tumors most likely experience moderate to severe headache pain but they cannot communicate this to us. It is often a shock for families to learn that their pet endured the pain and discomfort of bone cancer or a huge abdominal mass or a chest mass while keeping up nearly normal appearances.

Dogs, especially the working breeds, often have their carers completely fooled about their pain to the point where they may think that nothing is wrong. One minute we must trust the carer's intuition, believing that he or she knows more than we do about whether the pet has pain. Yet, we are faced with the reality that many times the carer is clueless about the pet's pain. This is not contradictory. It is simply that both situations are true. It may be due to breed and species variation, communication level, and intimacy of the bond shared between the pet (sending) and carer (receiving) pain signals.

I have consulted with some pet owners who sincerely felt that their osteosarcoma dog was not in pain despite the fact that their dog would not put weight on the cancerous leg. When we point out to them that not bearing weight on a leg is a screaming pain signal, they began to understand that they were not receiving the only communication that their pet could give them about bone cancer pain.

Most pet owners do not recognize the pain, discomfort, and disability of respiratory compromise. Many cats with anterior mediastinal lymphoma and dogs with pulmonary effusions must go into respiratory distress and crisis before their condition is realized. When I interviewed people with cancer, they listed respiratory distress at the top of their most stressful and painful experiences.

Geriatric dogs and cats are often presented with cancer pain, yet pain medication ranks low (if at all) on the attending doctor's priority list during the automatic workup for diagnosis. Develop a kneejerk response to provide pain relief medication from the very start for conditions that you can reasonably assume are painful. It is appropriate to give pain medication to a patient in pain even before subjecting the patient to the rigors of a workup. I call this attentive, responsive, caring palliative medicine.

Treating cancer pain is often the only option that we can offer for compromised geriatric patients, especially those with advanced stages of cancer. Do not miss the opportunity to treat pain. Clients have come to me for a second opinion after their veterinarian explicitly told them that their geriatric pet was in pain and should be euthanatized. In one case, in particular, this patient somehow left the doctor's office with absolutely no pain control medication. Pain was the prevailing diagnosis providing the rationale for the pet's euthanasia, and yet the doctor offered no options that would allay the pet's pain. The clients felt that their veterinarian had no concern or compassion for their pet and did not understand or respect the special relationship and the human–animal bond that they shared with their pet. This cry for help has spanned my entire career.

Drs. James Gaynor, Peter Hellyer, Robin Downing, and others helped to organize the International Veterinary Academy for Pain Management. They teach that pain management is good medicine (Hellyer and Gaynor 1998). When you recognize, acknowledge, and treat pain aggressively in your geriatric patients, you will create a higher quality of life for those patients and you will also create very grateful and loyal clients. Dr. Gaynor says, "Recognizing the close bond between pets and owners is crucial to understanding the importance of pain management. People suffer and become depressed when their pets suffer. Alleviating their pet's pain makes the owner feel better, too" (Gaynor 2004).

The veterinarian has two simple but obligatory tasks to perform regarding pain in a geriatric cancer patient: the first is to recognize pain and eliminate it, and the second is to anticipate when pain will occur and prevent it. Ask owners if they sense that their pet is in pain. Achieving proper pain control may initially require a combination of drugs. In the comprehensive treatment of geriatric cancer patients, the attending doctor addresses pain directly with a well-thought-out treatment plan that has been explained to the medical staff as well as the carers.

We can refer to well-thought-out management plans in specialized texts and articles for specific procedures and conditions (Tranquilli, Grimm, and Lamont 2004; Greene 2002). The World Health Organization Analgesia Ladder (Figure 7.1) serves as an excellent guide to assist decision making. A strategic plan against unnecessary pain in your clinic should include recognizing and treating acute pain, chronic pain, and cancer pain while treating induced iatrogenic pain related to surgery and procedures on a pre-emptive basis.

Pre-emptive pain control is the use of antipain drugs before a painful event, such as a biopsy or surgery or radiation therapy, with medications that allow the patient to avoid pain all together. If the patient is to receive chemotherapy, surgery, or radiation therapy, the attending doctor and team should work to control anticipated pain, fear, and emotional stress that results directly from the procedure or its side effects and related adverse events.

Topical anesthetics are used for all catheter placements. A "cancer care package," including: a thermometer, antiemetics, antibiotics, and diarrhea/colitis medications, should be provided for all chemotherapy cases. Some oncologists use antiemetics with chemotherapy drugs that are known to cause nausea. Always provide pre-emptive and postoperative pain control for surgery cases.

For the patient receiving radiation therapy, provide topical anesthetics and soothing creams. Instruct the client to apply the preparations on the radiation therapy field before the burn and desquamation lesion become visible. It is very important to provide pain control for the pruritus, pain, discomfort, stress, and anxiety caused by radiation therapy burns. I have consulted many clients who abandoned therapy for their pets due to inadequate pain control for chemotherapy reactions, extravasations, biopsy procedures, surgery, or radiation therapy. In short, if any one of these painful issues is not recognized and treated pre-emptively or directly after onset, the client may discontinue therapy in order to rescue the pet from suffering and, as a result, the patient's cancer may recur.

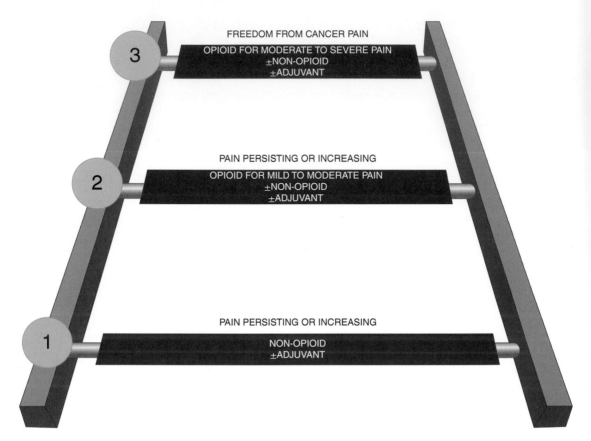

Figure 7.1.   World Health Organization Analgesia Ladder.

Pain Pathways

Be able to recognize all forms of pain and understand its mechanisms. This is important for the care and management of the geriatric oncology patient. The terms used to describe pain classify pain by its duration, intensity, and origin. Pain can be intermittent, chronic, or acute. It can be mild, moderate, or severe. It can originate from somatic, visceral, or nerve tissues and it can be generated from both central and peripheral sensitization. Because so many geriatric cancer patients have concurrent chronic pain from osteoarthritis and dental disease, they probably experience and endure all aspects of pain simultaneously while we are trying to guess about it. Feline pain is less recognized than canine pain due to the inherent silent and solitary nature of the feline personality.

The anatomic and physiologic functions that relay pain to the brain begin with a mechanical, thermal, or chemical stimulus. Tiny afferent nerve endings in the skin, muscles, joints, periosteum, viscera, and subcutaneous tissues transmit pain signals to myelinated A delta nerve fibers and unmyelinated C nerve fibers. These nerve fibers pass through the dorsal root ganglia and enter the dorsal horn of the spinal cord into the gray matter, where they synapse with second-order neurons and excitatory and inhibitory interneurons. The signal is transmitted to the brain along the spinothalamic tracts.

The tiny nerve endings that transmit and conduct pain are called "nociceptors." "Nociception" is the term used to describe how the body is alerted to and perceives pain. Myelinated A beta fibers transmit sensations such as touch, pressure, movement, vibration, and proprioception. In addition, a non-painful stimulus, such as touch, that is transmitted by the A beta fibers can become altered or sensitized in the dorsal horn neurons and thus be perceived by the patient as pain. This painful condition is called ***allodynia*** and it is very resistant to pain control medications. A dog may yelp and a cat may hiss in pain when touched or picked up. Other factors may influence pain perception, causing increased sensitivity to touch (hyperesthesia) or an exaggerated response (hyperalgesia) to a light pinch (Lascelles 2003).

Pain often has deeper roots in our senior and geriatric cancer patients because of the phenomenon of sensitization. This is the prolongation and exaggeration of pain. Sensitization occurs most often in untreated or undertreated painful patients. This hypersensitivity occurs peripherally along the spinal cord and centrally in the brain. Modulating cytokines such as the prostaglandins, histamine, serotonin, tumor necrosis factor (TNF), and bradykinin become unregulated as part of the inflammatory process and may contribute to the phenomenon of peripheral sensitization.

Spinal cord sensitization results when N-methyl-D-aspartate (NMDA) receptors on dorsal horn neurons are activated. NMDA receptors are located on the C fibers and, when stimulated, cause an additive spinal pain called "wind-up." Ketamine is an NMDA receptor antagonist which, when delivered as a constant rate infusion (CRI), has been proven to be effective in the prevention and correction of severe neuropathic pain and spinal cord wind-up. Sensitization also occurs in the brain by agents such as substance P and glutamate. Some dogs occasionally exhibit phantom pain after amputation of a leg. Because of these phenomena, the veterinarian must treat pain aggressively from the start with a combination of analgesics, tapering the dose later (De Lorimier and Fan 2005).

In a 1999 paper in *JAVMA*, Dr. Frank McMillan pointed out that opioid peptides activate receptors on lymphocytes and macrophages. Opioid receptors are also found in the GI tract, all through the body, and on certain cancer cells. The CNS has receptors for all sorts of immunopeptides and cytokines produced by lymphocytes and macrophages. This bidirectional communication between the immune system and the nervous system serves as a functional link among the body's cellular defense and repair mechanisms, endocrine glands, brain, behavior, mood, and emotions.

Cannabinoid receptors have been found on numerous tissues and on some cancer cells. This may explain the multiple responses to Cannabidiol (CBD) observed in cancer patients experiencing pain reduction, improved appetite, and ability to sleep. Clients come in with their own CBD products or they ask about it and expect a little knowledge and help from their veterinarian, regarding its use. Dr. Robert Silver of RxVitamins for Pets, has helped to formulate HempRx™, which contains a high percentage of CBD content (0.5mg/drop or 15mg/ml) with less than 0.3% THC. It is best to start with the low end of the dose range at 0.1mg/kg (1 drop/5kg) BID for 3 days. If no response, then escalate slowly to 2.5 drops/5kg and if no response, escalate slowly to 5 drops/kg to effect.

Pain causes anxiety, fear, and helplessness in animals. Stress and negative emotional states lower the body's immune resistance to cancer and enhances tumor cell growth and metastases. From the information available about pain, we can conclude that pain adversely affects the animal's quality of life, overall health, and survival. In short, pain is carcinogenic in our geriatric veterinary patients.

Cancer-Induced Pain

Cancer causes pain directly and indirectly, acutely, and chronically, in many ways and at any location in the body. Tumors cause pain directly as they expand due to pressure, tissue destruction, invasion of surrounding structures, and obstructing the normal flow of stool, urine, and bile. Cancer causes pain

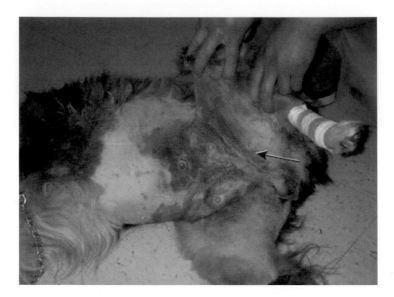

Figure 7.2.   Inflammatory adenocarcinoma.

indirectly via inducing stress and inflammation (Figure 7.2). This type of pain is most dramatic with inflammatory mammary adenocarcinoma (Figure 7.2) and mast cell tumors (Figure 7.3). Paraneoplastic syndromes cause pain indirectly by manifesting abnormal signs unrelated to the primary tumor, as with hypertrophic osteopathy, hypercalcemia, and peripheral neuropathies. Secondary metastatic nodules and lytic lesions may cause pain by invasion of bone, brain, lung, viscera, serosal capsules, digits, orbits, and so forth.

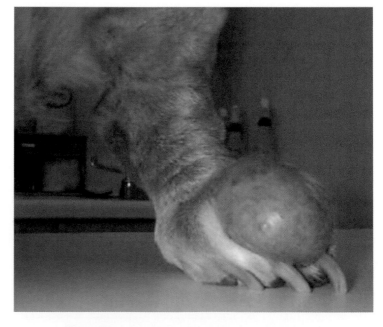

Figure 7.3.   Interdigital degranulating mast cell tumor.

Bone Pain

Bone tumors create primary and secondary lytic and proliferative lesions that can be very painful. Osteosarcoma (OSA) generally creates solitary lytic and blastic lesions that erode, expand, and stretch the periosteum of the appendicular skeleton. Lesions appear in the ribs, skull, and axial skeleton less commonly. OSA patients most likely experience chronic throbbing bone pain with episodes of acute aching that worsens on weight bearing and movement. Animals exhibit their appendicular bone pain by limping. However, because the forbearance of dogs is to remain cheerful, eat, and wag their tails despite pain, many pet owners do not understand the magnitude of their dog's malignant bone pain. Some stoic dogs are diagnosed with OSA only after a pathologic fracture. Malignant melanoma and squamous cell carcinoma that arises from the digits causes erosion of the digits and mimics painful osteomyelitis. Animal suffering has been and is still being underestimated because animals do not communicate their pain in the way that humans would expect them to.

Multiple myeloma causes multifocal painful, lytic lesions in the spine and long bones. Lesions may also cause painful compression of the spinal cord, resulting in paresis or paralysis. Synovial cell carcinoma and other tumors that involve joints cause pain by stretching the joint capsule, invasion of bone, disrupting ligaments and adjacent structures. Carcinomas and sarcomas that metastasize to bone, as a secondary target, cause pain most commonly in the lumbar spine, long bones, and digits. Intravenous bisphosphonates may help alleviate lytic malignant bone pain and inhibit osteoclast activity in geriatric dogs and cats with OSA (De Lorimier and Fan 2005).

Head and Neck Pain

Cancer mimics oral osteomyelitis when malignant melanoma and squamous cell carcinoma (SCC) efface the bone of the dental arcades. Oral cancer causes severe mandibular/maxillary pain as the tumor expands and as teeth become loosened (Figure 7.4). The patient may have halitosis, salivation, and dysphagia. The condition may go unnoticed or be tolerated by the family during the early stages. Fleshy oral tumors are often traumatized by teeth and infected with gingivitis organisms as they enlarge (Figure 7.4b). Feline lingual SCC causes difficulty eating and pain associated with hunger.

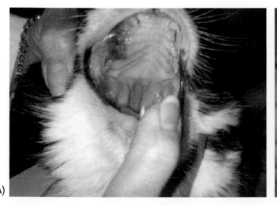 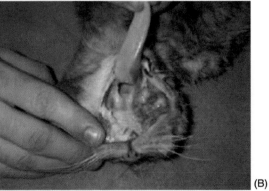

(A) (B)

Figure 7.4. Fleshy oral tumors are often traumatized by teeth and infected with gingivitis organisms as they enlarge. The lesion originally looks like infected teeth. It forms an ulcer in the location where teeth were extracted previously (A). Then over 60–90 days, it may develop into an invasive mass involving the maxilla and nasal cavity, such as the fleshy lesion shown here (B).

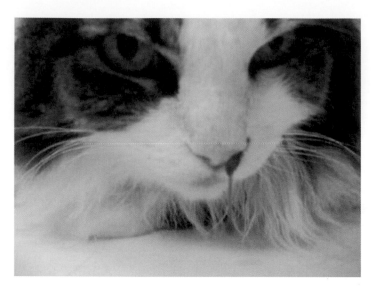

Figure 7.5. Fifi Vines, a 12-year-old, 20-pound cat, had nasal respiratory adenocarcinoma. Infected nasal tumors cause discomfort due to nasal discharge and obstructive stridor and pain due to turbinate destruction and facial deformity. Fifi responded well to IV carboplatin and supplements for one year.

Nasal passage tumors cause discomfort due to nasal discharge, infection and obstructive stridor (Figure 7.5). They cause pain due to turbinate and sinus destruction and facial deformity (Figure 7.6). Neoplastic tissue from primary nasal cancer may invade the cribriform plate of the ethmoid bone and invade the orbit and brain. This may cause exophthalmia, retrobulbar swelling, pain upon opening the mouth, localized meningitis and severe headaches, CNS signs, and seizures. Chondroma Rhodens originating at the ramus of the mandible, orbital tumors, middle ear tumors, and oral tumors that involve the temporomandibular joint may cause pain when opening the mouth (Figure 7.7). Tonsillar SCC, pharyngeal, laryngeal, and thyroid tumors cause respiratory discomfort and pain as they expand, causing esophageal and airway obstruction.

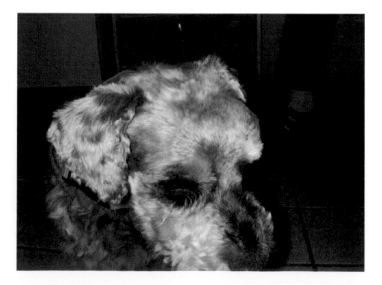

Figure 7.6. Frontal sinus tumors cause pain due to accumulation of mucus, bone destruction, and sinus headache.

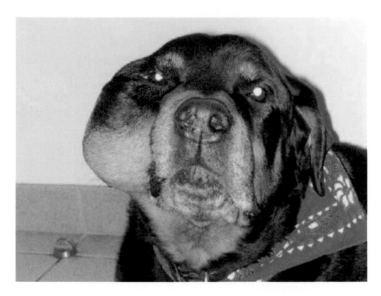

Figure 7.7.   Cabo Palmer, an 8-year-old Rottweiler with osteosarcoma, had pain when opening his mouth.

Abdominal Pain

Abdominal malignancies cause visceral pain directly due to tissue destruction, invasion, expansion of organ capsules, and distention of the peritoneum. Cancer causes abdominal pain indirectly by obstructing flow or pushing other organs aside, causing pain and discomfort.

Carcinomatosis is the condition of multiple metastases of a carcinoma or sarcoma throughout the entire abdominal or pleural cavity. Carcinomatosis lesions in the abdomen injure the serosal lining, causing abdominal effusions (ascites) and distension. These patients are in discomfort and have moderate to severe visceral pain (Figure 7.8).

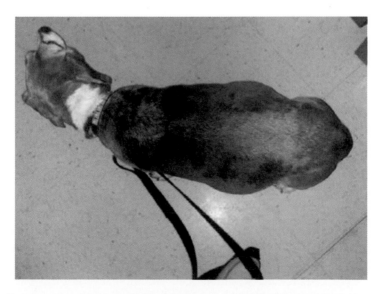

Figure 7.8.   Mitzie Karsch, a 13-year-old, spayed female Beagle, exhibiting abdominal distension and discomfort due to ascites caused by recurrent end stage hepatocellular carcinoma.

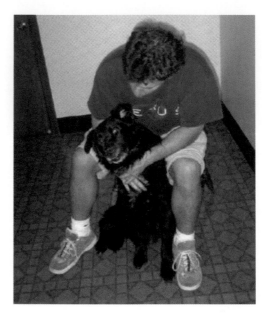

Figure 7.9. Bear Clinton, a 12-year-old Labrador Retriever, exhibiting head tilt and facial paralysis due to choroid plexus carcinoma of the brain stem. Bear responded to steroids, linoleic acid from safflower oil (3mg/kg PO given 3 consecutive days/week), and a supportive Pawspice care program with Roger for 1 year.

Abdominal neoplasia may invade and obstruct organs, vasculature, and lumens such as the intestines, the bile duct, ureters, or urethra. Abdominal cancer pain results from disrupted digestion, elimination, and urine outflow. The patient experiences visceral discomfort, nausea, vomiting, constipation or diarrhea, cramping, ataxia, and lethargy and may cry or grunt when lifted, when lying down, or when palpated. All of these visceral feelings need to be considered painful despite the stoic appearance of the geriatric pet.

CNS, Spinal Cord, and Nerve Pain

We need to presume that most of our brain tumor patients have headache pain prior to and in addition to exhibiting neurologic signs, behavior changes, ataxia, and seizures (Figure 7.9). We as caregivers can only guess at the magnitude of our patient's headache pain. Nerve sheath, spinal cord, and brachial plexus tumors are often very painful due to their tissue of origin causing neurogenic and neuropathic pain. Any tumor that compresses the spinal cord, such as multiple myeloma, lymphoma, and malignant melanoma, may induce severe agonizing pain.

Inflammation and Pain

Cancer pain is aggravated by inflammation and/or infection at the tumor site. Old animals often have chronic inflammation with dental disease and arthritis so their pain is compounded. We see this compounding effect commonly in oral, nasal, ear, canal, nail bed tumors, prostate carcinoma, transitional cell carcinoma, and most dramatically in inflammatory mammary adenocarcinoma (Figure 7.2). Malignant pain from inflammation and pruritus arises with ulcerated dermal tumors, especially degranulated mast cell tumors, squamous cell carcinomas, transmissible venereal tumors, inflammatory carcinomas, sweat gland and apocrine gland carcinomas, cutaneous hemangiosarcomas, epitheliotrophic lymphomas, cutaneous histiocytosis, and some soft tissue sarcomas.

Nervousness Plus Anxiety Equals Emotional Pain: Go Fear Free!

Many geriatric cancer patients exhibit nervousness and anxiety, which may be more pronounced at night due to their cancer. Some dogs and cats are very anxious during the car ride to each visit. Some cats are miserable during the entire visit and may defecate or vomit in their containers. These events are called situational stress and the patients' behaviors are indicators of emotional pain and should not be ignored. A pet's anxious behavior may lead clients to stop visiting your hospital for treatments. We need to be proactive to reduce this emotional pain.

The Fear Free Initiative was developed by Dr. Marty Becker to address this common problem. He encourages veterinarians and staff members to honor the emotional well-being of their patients. Through the Fear Free Certification program, hospitals can now become certified as Fear Free after being educated about how to prevent and reduce fear with positive behavioral coaxing techniques, pheromones, and medications as needed (http://www.fearfreepets.com/).

I suggest prescription relaxing medications be given to relax these nervous and upset patients so they can better cope with visits to the hospital. The client can administer the medication at home, an hour before the hospital visit. Oral medications including diphenhydramine (Benadryl®), butorphanol, diazepam, and/or Zilkene™ (a relaxing protein from milk) are effective. Cats respond very well and are relaxed with 100mg of gabapentin given one hour prior to visits. The owner can also give their pet formulations such as Rx Nutricalm™ and Rescue Remedy® to see if they help calm the pet. For patients that fight against being given oral medications, we suggest a transdermal gel preparation or an injectable relaxing agent instead. For willing clients, we provide instructions on how to give pills and injections until they are comfortable with the procedure that works best for their pet.

The client and pet may become demoralized if they have to constantly struggle with oral chemotherapy medications. Hard-to-medicate patients and fractious cats, or any cat with an oral tumor, feel less stressed and experience less pain when they are given injectable medications at home (antibiotics, steroids, analgesics, etc.).

We send injections home in prepared syringes at the proper dose for the client to administer as needed. Each syringe is capped and gets a fresh needle just before administration to avoid blockage. When a nervous pet must be hospitalized or have a procedure, we comfort the owner with the assurance that we will use an injection to relax the pet. On occasion, we may give diazepam and/or butorphanol IV to gain an immediate effect. We may give a follow-up dose in SQ fluids to extend the relaxation effect over a long car ride home.

My last choice for fractious or aggressive geriatric pets is acepromazine. Phenothiazine drugs are alpha-1 antagonists. They block vasoconstriction, cause vasodilation of arterioles, and lower blood pressure. They are not safe to use for aggressive or fractious patients or for patients receiving Adriamycin. However, since acepromazine has a prolonged tranquilizing effect, it may be the best choice for stressed, hypertensive, nervous patients that need to stay in the hospital all day. We occasionally dispense it, when necessary, for tranquilization as long as it is safe for that particular patient.

Short-Acting Immobilization for Chemotherapy

Our oncology staff strives to relax or immobilize nervous or rebellious cancer patients during the administration of all vasosclerotic chemotherapy agents. This allows us to avoid the issues of the patient struggling, the use of restraints, and the dangers of extravasations. When we administer Adriamycin chemotherapy, there are no exceptions to this rule. For healthy cancer patients under 8 years of age, we coadminister low dose dexmedetomidine hydrochloride (Dexdomitor®) or butorphanol IM or IV for relaxation. This combination is smooth, safe, and easily reversed with antipamezole (Antisedan®).

Occasionally, a patient has dysphoria (restlessness or malaise) or residual sedation effects following sedation. We suspect the dysphoria is due to butorphanol, so it is not used for these patients in subsequent visits.

For geriatric patients, and for any patient with suspected cardiac or renal problems, avoid the alpha-2 agonists dexmedetomidine (Dexdomitor®) and xylazine, because they cause reduced cardiac output by as much as 30–40%. This may adversely affect renal perfusion in geriatric patients with concurrent heart disease and/or chronic kidney disease (CKD) that cannot compensate for decreased cardiac output.

Some clinicians prefer sedation of geriatric patients with an opioid such as fentanyl at 20 to 40µg/kg IV, IM, or SQ with a short-acting benzodiazepine, such as midazolam at 0.05mg/kg or 0.1mg/lb IV, IM, or SQ for relaxation and analgesia. The effect of fentanyl is gone in 30–45 minutes. Atropine might still be used with this combination as a premedication to prevent bradycardia.

Fractious cats and aggressive miniature toy breed dogs need to be handled very gently. Take every precaution to avoid putting geriatric oncology patients into a state of catecholamine overload. If the IV, SQ, or IM route of sedation is too stressful for them, we gently place the patient into an inhalation chamber for induction with isoflurane or sevoflurane, and then transfer the patient to the procedure table and place a butterfly catheter while keeping the patient under light anesthesia with a face mask (Jaffe et al. 2003).

If the patient requires a procedure or prolonged chemotherapy infusion lasting over 10–15 minutes, or if administering a highly vasosclerotic drug, consider intubation. If the procedure takes only a short time, a mask and pulse oximeter monitoring are standard procedure. Patients return to full consciousness quickly and safely. Return nervous cats to their carrying cases as they start to awaken so that they feel secure. We have seen very positive results and benefits after administering SQ fluids and vitamins as supportive care for geriatric cancer patients during procedures that require sedation, anesthesia, and/or chemotherapy.

Confronting the Brutality of Pain

The veterinary profession has a huge historical deficit for not confronting pain in animals. Our lack of intuitive knowledge about recognizing and treating pain was brutal and almost unforgivable until our awakening and the inception of the organization called The International Veterinary Academy for Pain Management, www.ivapm.org.

Our profession is made up of clinicians who never intended to be brutal. However, most veterinarians who graduated more than 15–20 years ago confess ignorance of the reality and the amount of pain that their patients have experienced under their unknowing care.

It is hard to imagine that there was no formal training to recognize pain, evaluate its severity, and control it immediately or pre-emptively in veterinary schools previous to 2000–2005. Even today, during consultations, many oncology clients feel that their pet's cancer pain was passed over by their attending doctor. Unfortunately, in many instances, cancer pain is still not properly addressed by clinicians. We must admit to a profession-wide historical and ongoing failure in this area. The universities now actively educate students about the prevention and treatment of pain in all species and ages of veterinary patients.

Contemporary veterinarians must understand the science of pain and make every effort to recognize and confront pain in their geriatric patients. Patients recovering from surgery, minor procedures, and radiation therapy do experience pain. Chronic diseases in geriatric pets, such as arthritis, discospondylitis, and dental disease do cause pain.

We must anticipate cancer pain that attacks our geriatric oncology patients quietly, right under our noses. We must set up protocols to recognize and offset pain as a hospital service policy, especially cancer pain and postoperative pain.

Pain Scales and Scoring Charts

Various pain scales are proposed to measure factors such as heart rate, vocalization, restlessness, cramping, crying, hunching, thrashing, and agitation. Temperature, heart rate, respiratory rate, and pupil size are not reliable signs for assessing cancer pain or perioperative pain (Lascelles 2003). We are clearly at a disadvantage in recognizing the pain of oncology patients recovering from surgery.

Introduce your nursing staff to one of the proposed pain scales. Post a pain scale that they can use as a guide for on-the-spot decision making and to alert the doctor in charge for instructions to administer additional pain medication for the patient as needed. Studies have shown that no pain scale is reliable to assess pain accurately because the assessments are subjective. Proper assessment of pain requires focus, intuition, common sense, and interaction with the patient.

The pain scoring chart used at Colorado State University has a 0–24 point span (Table 7.1). Patients that rate over 14 points are considered painful enough to qualify for medication. When there is doubt, patients should always be given the benefit of pain medication. The patient's response to the analgesics can be used as a tool to evaluate the presence or absence of pain. Pre-emptive pain medication should always be given if you expect that a procedure or condition should be causing pain.

Agonist Opioids

The most effective agonist opioids work by blocking the conduction of pain signals. Opioids attach to mu receptors located in the superficial dorsal horn of the spinal tract. Two other types of opioid receptors, delta, and kappa, play a lesser role in pain management. Receptors are also found in the spinal cord, brain, and joints. Morphine is a pure mu receptor agonist. Opioids such as morphine, oxymorphone, hydromorphone, fentanyl, buprenorphine (a partial agonist), butorphanol and nalbuphine (agonist-antagonists), and tramadol (an opioid-like drug) are commonly used to alleviate cancer pain for veterinary patients.

Adverse events and side effects encountered are constipation, sedation, dysphoria, and respiratory depression. Opioid effects are difficult to monitor, especially in postoperative patients.

Opioids lower the heart rate for a longer period of time than their analgesic effect. After the opioid is no longer controlling pain, the heart rate may continue to be low. Therefore, a low heart rate should not be interpreted as a sign that the medication is still active. Instruct your staff to monitor the respiration rate rather than heart rate for patients on opioids to determine if the patient is experiencing pain.

Morphine

Morphine syrup at 0.5mg/kg every 4–6 hours PO may help relieve pain for dogs and cats. Codeine can be used at 0.5–2mg/kg. It can be prepared as a 5mg/ml transdermal lecithin gel or cream. Cats may benefit with 0.1ml of the gel rubbed in the pinna every 6–12 hours as needed.

Table 7.1.   Pain Scoring System at Colorado State University

Observation	Score	Criteria
Comfort	0	Patient asleep or calm
	1	Awake, interested in surroundings
	2	Mild agitation, or depressed and uninterested in surroundings
	3	Moderate agitation, restless and uncomfortable
	4	Extremely agitated, thrashing
Movement	0	Normal amount of movement
	1	Frequent position changes or reluctant to move
	2	Thrashing
Appearance	0	Normal
	1	Mild changes (eyelids partially closed, ears flattened or carried abnormally)
	2	Moderate changes (eyes sunken or glazed, unthrifty appearance)
	3	Severe changes (eyes pale, enlarged pupils, "grimacing" or other abnormal facial expressions, guarding, hunched-up position, legs in abnormal position, grunting before expiration, grinding of teeth)
Behavior (unprovoked)	0	Normal
	1	Minor changes
	2	Moderately abnormal: less mobile and less alert than normal, unaware of surroundings, very restless
	3	Markedly abnormal: very restless, vocalization, self-mutilation, grunting, facing back of cage
Interactive	0	Normal
Behaviors	1	Pulls away when surgical site touched, looking at wound, mobile
	2	Vocalizing when wound is touched, somewhat restless, or reluctant to move but will if coaxed
	3	Violent reactions to stimuli, vocalizes without touching the wound, snapping, growling, or hissing when approached; extremely restless or will not move when coaxed
Vocalization	0	Quiet
	1	Crying, responds to calm voice and stroking
	2	Intermittent crying or whimpering, no response to calm voice and stroking
	3	Continuous noise that is unusual for the animal
Heart Rate	0	0%–15% above preop/normal value
	1	16%–29% above preop/normal value
	2	30%–45% above preop/normal value
	3	>45% above preop/normal value
Respiratory Rate	1	16%–29% above preop/normal value
	2	30%–45% above preop/normal value
	3	>45% above preop/normal value

Source: www.colostate.edu/depts/lar/Pain_Assesment.doc.

Fentanyl: Injectable and Transdermal Preparations

Fentanyl is a mu opiate agonist that is 80–100 times more potent than morphine. It is a Class II opiate analgesic. The injectable form is short-acting. It is used for perioperative pain and for reducing inhalational anesthetic requirements. It may be used as a constant rate infusion (CRI) in critically painful patients. Cats have fewer adverse effects with fentanyl than with hydromorphone or morphine.

The transdermal fentanyl pain patch (Duragesic®) is an excellent choice for control of severe pain from surgical procedures and for severe cancer pain in end of life geriatric dogs and cats. Limb amputation, mandibulectomy, thoracotomy, celiotomy, and nosectomy cause great pain and discomfort in cats and dogs. The initial patch should be placed prior to surgery and, for most intense surgical oncology procedures, we recommend the placement of a follow-up fentanyl patch (or exposing the other half of the membrane of a 25µg/hour patch for cats) about 72 hours following the placement of the initial patch.

Fentanyl patches become effective 6–12 hours after application and may last up to 5 days in cats. Use a dose rate of 1–2µg per pound/hour, or 2–5µg/kg per hour, for dogs and cats. For cats under 7 pounds and small dogs, expose half of the membrane of a 25µg/h patch for the first 3 days and then expose the other half of the membrane for the second 3 days. Tramadol can be used while waiting for the pain patch to take effect. Tramadol may also be used at night for cancer patients that exhibit pain despite wearing a pain patch.

Instruct clients to leave the pain patch on until the first recheck or suture removal and then remove the patch painlessly and dispose of it properly. Early removal of the patch may pull skin and hurt, causing localized ulcers at the site. The potential adverse events associated with fentanyl patches are due to its opioid effects causing extreme sedation, bradycardia, nausea, ileus, or respiratory depression. Careful observation for levels of sedation, heart rate, respiratory rate, and nausea is essential to detect overdose. These signs are more likely to appear in smaller geriatric patients. The patch should be removed immediately if these adverse events are detected. Naloxone can be used to reverse the opioid effects while retaining the analgesic effect. Duragesic patches are not recommended if children or other pets are in the household in the event that they pull off the patch. Pain patches should not be allowed contact heating pads as it speeds up release of the fentanyl and can cause adverse events and possibly death.

Recuvyra® is a transdermal fentanyl solution, which is FDA approved for transdermal application in an inpatient setting for dogs only. It has high potential for human abuse and therefore the Risk Minimization Action Plan must be followed, along with the client reading the information sheet and signing the consent form. After application to the skin, it dries rapidly within 2–5 minutes and sequesters in the stratum corneum from where it is slowly absorbed into the systemic circulation over 4–7 days. The application site should not be touched by family members, especially children, for at least 3 days. Adverse events may be reversed with naloxone, naltrexone, trazadone, buprenorphine, or butorphanol. Adverse events should be reported to Elanco Animal Health at 1-888-545-5973 and to the FDA-CVM by phone at 1-888-FDA-VETS.

Oxymorphone or Hydromorphone

Oxymorphone or hydromorphone injections are helpful at 0.05–0.2mg/kg to control moderate to severe pain, but the effect only lasts for 2–4 hours. Buprenorphine is helpful in that it can be given at 0.02mg/kg sublingual every 6 hours for cats. Dogs can be given codeine at 1–2mg/kg PO every 8–24 hours for mild to moderate pain. Codeine has a shorter duration in cats.

Butorphanol

Butorphanol (Torbugesic®) is a synthetic agonist-antagonist opioid, which has antitussive and analgesic effects. It helps to settle patients down but does not alleviate moderate to severe pain. When given IV, its effect lasts only about 15–30 minutes in dogs and 15 minutes to 6 hours in cats. It may be adequate following minor procedures and superficial surgery but is unreliable when used in this manner. Butorphanol is a great antitussive but definitely not an adequate analgesic at low doses. It is inadequate and too short acting for moderate or severe pain relief, even when given at frequent and higher doses. Its sedation effect outlasts an analgesic effect by 2–4 hours. Therefore, many patients are suffering while still sedated. The patient may vocalize, but all too often the pain is not recognized or acknowledged due to the sedative effect. All too often, vocalizing, painful patients are chalked off as screamers because of dysphoria or an adverse excitement effect from butorphanol.

We no longer use or trust butorphanol as a primary analgesic. In the past, we relied on it for its antiemetic and sedation properties for dogs receiving cisplatin IV, but we no longer use cisplatin IV. We previously dispensed it to reduce stress in nervous patients or carsickness, utilizing its antiemetic and sedative effects. However, we use maropitant or ondansetron for carsickness. Butorphanol can be used in dogs at 0.5–2.0mg/kg every 8 hours and in cats at 0.2–1.0mg/kg every 6 hours.

Butorphanol can be very helpful to relax cancer patients at night for its sedation and antitussive effects. It can be helpful in combination with other more effective analgesics to relax painful or restless geriatric cancer patients experiencing discomfort associated with metastatic pulmonary disease. Butorphanol helps to diminish cancer-induced coughing and stridor as well as some forms of chemotherapy-induced nausea and vomiting. Zyprexa™ is now my first choice to palliate end of life patients who are suffering from primary or metastatic pulmonary cancer. It relieves stress and discomfort and stimulates the appetite and well-being. It is considered a higher bar of palliative treatment for human cancer patients. Read more on Zyprexa below.

Butorphanol should not be used in combination with a fentanyl pain patch because it is a mu receptor antagonist and reduces its effect. In injectable form, it can be used as a constant rate infusion during anesthesia and recovery for surgery patients where respiratory depression is a concern. It works synergistically with local analgesics and NSAIDs.

Dexdomitor™

In our practice, we routinely use butorphanol in combination with Dexdomitor™ as an IV combination for minor procedures in healthy patients using the package insert dose schedule. This combination is our chemical restraint of choice for healthy fractious patients needing chemotherapy. Patients are reversed with Antisedan™ and able to leave the office within minutes with minimal residual sedation effects. It is not recommended for use in geriatric oncology patients with cardiac, liver, kidney or respiratory disease, shock, and other debilitating conditions. Its action is similar to medetomidine, another alpha-2 agonist, which causes reduced cardiac output and potential perfusion problems for older dehydrated patients and for those with renal or cardiac disease.

Tramadol

Tramadol (Ultram®) is a mu receptor opiate-like agonist that also inhibits serotonin and norepinephrine uptake. It is an effective central acting opioid that can be used in dogs and cats as an analgesic and antitussive. It works quickly within 15–20 minutes and has a peak effect at 2–3 hours, which limits its efficacy for prolonged pain alleviation. It has a wide dose range for efficacy. If the initial dose is not effective, it is worth a try to double and triple the baseline dose of 1–4mg/kg BID or TID or QID administration. Even at 3mg/kg, oral tramadol was unable to help a geriatric Golden Retriever under my care who was suffering with anxiety from a skull tumor that applied pressure on the meninges and the brain.

There is a trend to move away from using tramadol in pain management protocols for severe pain due to its short duration of analgesia. Some pain management experts are using trazodone (see more information below) with tramadol and some recommend eliminating tramadol entirely.

Tramadol should not be used in epileptics or in patients that develop cancer-related seizures. It is available in 50mg scored tablets. It has a very bitter taste, which must be camouflaged for acceptance, especially with cats. Within the dose range, a 10-pound cat would need from one-eighth up to one-third of a 50mg tablet. Tramadol can be formulated by a compounding pharmacy as a 5mg/ml liquid to hide its bitter taste for use in small, frail geriatric cats. It might also be prepared as a transdermal gel but information is lacking in the effectiveness of this route.

Buprenorphine

Buprenorphine is 30 times as potent as morphine. It is a partial mu opiate agonist injectable. It may be given as a buccal transmucosal analgesic and IV, IM, or SQ to dogs at 5–20µg/kg and at 5–10µg/kg to cats every 6–8 hours. It seems to be more effective in cats than other opioids for analgesia when placed on the oral mucosa (Smith 2005). The oral route of buprenorphine is well absorbed and makes a good choice for home administration by carers. Simbadol® is buprenorphine labeled for postoperative pain in cats and FDA approved at 0.24mg/kg SQ. It should be given one hour before surgery and can be repeated daily for up to 3 days.

Ketamine

In addition to its use as an anesthetic agent, Ketamine is a critical medication used in pain management in animals. The mechanism of action of Ketamine (NMDA receptor antagonism) delivered as a constant rate infusion has been proven to be effective in the prevention and correction of severe neuropathic pain and spinal cord wind-up.

Trazodone

Trazodone is an antidepressant that potentiates serotonin. It is available in 50 and 100mg tablets. Dogs can be given 1.7–3.5mg/kg BID with tramadol or 7–10mg/kg BID or TID without tramadol. Adverse events include behavior changes, increased appetite, or anorexia and lethargy. It is best to start at 50% of the low end of the dose range for 3 days and dose-escalate to help the pet adjust to the medication. It can also be given at night to help reduce anxiety, restlessness, and breakthrough pain. It is not used in cats.

NSAIDs for Cancer Pain

There is good reason to use NSAIDs to alleviate cancer pain because of their added anticancer and chemoprevention advantage against many carcinomas, osteosarcoma, and melanoma (Boria et al. 2005). However, we must exercise thoughtful caution using NSAIDs in geriatric cancer patients, especially in the face of polypharmacy. Dogs metabolize NSAIDs readily, while cats metabolize them more slowly. This produces variable toxicity issues for cats. Many geriatric dogs presenting for cancer treatment have a history of long-term NSAID use for chronic osteoarthritis pain. There is no doubt that dogs with arthritis enjoy a better quality of life on NSAIDs.

While the more selective cyclooxygenase enzyme (COX-2) inhibitors such as meloxicam, firocoxib, deracoxib, carprofen, ketoprofen, and etodolac may be less toxic than aspirin, they are similar in their analgesic effects and they all have some COX-1 inhibitory effects. Therefore, any NSAID can cause GI and renal problems and more so in older, more frail geriatric cancer patients.

NSAIDs are contraindicated in patients with congestive heart failure due to their antidiuretic effects. NSAIDs are contraindicated in frail patients with poor hydration status and pets with impaired renal function. NSAIDs are more likely to induce GI, renal toxicity, hepatotoxicity, and drug interactions in compromised geriatric cancer patients.

The newer NSAIDs show less inhibition of COX-1 (the essential or constitutive prostaglandins needed for GI mucosal integrity) but they are *not* more protective of renal function. The kidneys uniquely express both COX-1 and COX-2 constitutively and can be injured by any type of NSAID. If the source of the patient's cancer pain is induced by inflammatory prostaglandins, then selective COX-2 NSAIDs are the best choice because they strike at the inflammatory mediators. If the cancer patient has visceral cancer pain from organomegaly, an opioid is a better choice to alleviate this type of pain. Inherently nephrotoxic NSAIDs are contraindicated for geriatric oncology patients with cancer-related blood dyscrasias, clotting abnormalities, von Willebrand's disease, poor perfusion, and concurrent steroid therapy.

Acetaminophen (Tylenol®) provides analgesia at 10–15mg/kg every 8 hours for 5 days and then 10mg/kg every 12 hours as needed for long-term therapy (for dogs only, *NEVER* cats). It is fatally toxic in cats at small doses, causing methemoglobinemia. COX-3 enzyme has been identified and found to be a site of action for acetaminophen (Lascelles 2003). Researchers may find that this COX-3 site plays a role in pain pathways or may play a role in explaining the feline's unique toxic reaction to this particular NSAID. Tylenol can be used alone or in combination with codeine. It has no renal toxicity and it is easy on the GI tract and may be a good choice for canine geriatric cancer patients. Some use it in combination with other COX-2 inhibitors but caution is advised.

Baby aspirin or buffered aspirin at 10mg/kg twice daily for dogs and at 48–72 hour intervals for cats is a helpful recommendation for cost-conscious clients. It is important to strongly recommend GI protectants for geriatric oncology patients receiving aspirin and other first generation non-selective NSAIDs to minimize the effect of gastric ulceration. I routinely recommend GI protectants such as famotidine (Pepcid®) for patients on chemotherapy, especially if they are also on any type of NSAID or steroid.

Onsior® (robenacoxib) is a safe NSAID approved for dogs and cats. It is packaged for cats as a 6mg tablet in a blister package containing 3 yeast-flavored tablets. There will always be new NSAID products released on the market. It is our responsibility to know about what is available.

Meloxicam

Meloxicam is a COX-2 preferential anti-inflammatory analgesic that alleviates pain very effectively in cats and dogs. For cats, the dose is variable depending on the experience of the attending clinicians. Cats can be given meloxicam daily for a short period of time not to exceed 4 days postop at 0.1mg/kg of lean body weight every 2–3 days. For chronic cancer pain in cats, it must be given only two to three times per week if using this higher dose.

Meloxiam oral suspension at 0.5mg/ml provides 0.02mg per drop. This preparation may be given to cats at one drop per 4 pounds per day for chronic cancer pain. Some clinicians use meloxicam liquid postoperatively for 2 weeks, on a tapering oral dose, to control pain in cats. They start with 0.2mg/kg on day 1, then split it to 0.1mg/kg for the following 4 days, then split again to 0.05mg/kg for 10 days. The dose can be split again down to 0.025mg/kg or one drop/4 lb of the 0.5mg/ml preparation, as described above as a daily maintenance dose for chronic pain if needed.

Meloxicam is a new generation NSAID that is FDA approved for a one-time injection for pain control in cats. It is ideal in the postoperative setting and as a supplement for the fentanyl pain patch.

Be sure to inform cat owners that only certain NSAIDs can be tolerated by cats and that each preparation must be used with specific instructions for proper dose and frequency. You must take every opportunity to inform and caution all cat owners never to use Tylenol® (acetaminophen) due to fatal methemoglobinemia. Cats do not have the hepatic glucuronidation enzyme systems to metabolize acetaminophen in a timely fashion. Some NSAIDs, such as baby aspirin, piroxicam, carprofen, meloxicam, and firocoxib, have been safely used in cats when spaced at alternate-day intervals or given at lower doses. This usage is off-label in the US.

Piroxicam

Piroxicam (Feldene®) is the first choice of many oncologists for the control of general cancer pain when renal function is normal. This non-selective COX inhibitor serves a dual role as a pain control drug that has anticancer effects. According to previous studies, piroxicam was an effective single agent in transitional cell carcinoma (Knapp et al. 1994). In combination protocols for bladder cancer, piroxicam helped remission rates increase from 20% to 70% when used with cisplatin and from 10% to 40% in combination with carboplatin (Boria et al. 2005). However, toxicity was objectionable and the authors do not recommend this protocol for therapy.

Piroxicam has also been helpful against osteosarcoma, squamous cell carcinoma, and some sarcomas. Thalidomide, the notorious NSAID that caused birth defects in humans, has antineoplastic properties but is costly and not widely available.

NSAIDs and Other Drugs used in Chemoprevention

The role that NSAIDs play against cancer is not completely understood. Inhibition of COX-2 seems to be the foremost anticancer mechanism attributed to NSAIDs. COX-2 is overexpressed in tissues exposed to carcinogens such as cigarette smoke and certain chemicals. NSAIDs may also play a role in antiangiogenesis.

The role that NSAIDs play in reducing COX-2 expression in tumors may justify their use as adjunct therapeutic and chemoprevention agents in the battle against cancer. The manufacturers of NSAIDs are very interested in establishing a database to define the actual benefits of using NSAIDs as chemoprevention agents and as therapeutic agents for the treatment of cancer. The Vioxx® fiasco and related lawsuits was a setback and discouraged further large-scale studies using NSAIDs in the chemoprevention arena.

Veterinarians must stay abreast of new data to stay up-to-date about NSAIDs and other non-anticancer drugs and supplements that can be used as chemoprevention for cancer management. The Dog Aging Project is studying rapamycin (which also has anticancer action) for its ability to delay age-related disease. Metformin, an antidiabetes drug, is another drug that will be interesting to follow for its chemoprevention action. Dual-purpose medications such as NSAIDs for their antipain and anticancer action are prioritized for their benefits in my practice for treatment of geriatric cancer patients.

Bisphosphonates for Bone Pain and Osteoclast Inhibition

Intravenous bisphosphonates (pamidronate, zolendronic acid, Aredia®, and Zometa®) inhibit osteo-clastic activity and reduce bone resorption and turnover. Injectable bisphosphonates are considered more potent than oral Fosamax®. Pamidronate at 1.4mg/kg IV may alleviate lytic bone pain in geriatric dogs and cats when administered IV on a monthly basis or as needed (De Lorimier and Fan 2005; Fan et al. 2007). It can be administered on the same day as chemotherapy. Clients should be instructed to be on high alert for the first signs of nausea or vomiting, and to use pre-emptive antiemetics. Check the Internet for current information about dosage and price if you plan to use bisphosphonates. These products are costly. Oral use has not been fully investigated but esophagitis and gastritis may present serious consequences. In selected cases, and only with highly compliant carers who agree to follow oral administration with a large liquid chaser, I have on occasion prescribed Fosamax® or the longer-acting risedronate at empirical doses. This choice is to help save clients' money and time. If the carer gives the water chaser and elevates the pet's front end so that the pills will pass down the esophagus and into the stomach, then their pet can have access to the potential benefits that these oral bisphosphonates provide in controlling cancer pain, refractory hypercalcemia, and bone protection.

Contraindications for NSAIDs with Concurrent Conditions

If you use NSAIDs in geriatric cancer patients with concurrent conditions, you may put them at risk for adverse events. NSAIDs are contraindicated with conditions such as chronic kidney disease (CKD), dehydration, hypotension, liver disease, GI ulceration, inflammatory bowel disease (IBD), coagulopathy, non-compressible bleeding (hemangiosarcoma), asthma, pulmonary disease, and shock. NSAIDs should not be used as preoperative analgesics; however, they can be safely used postoperatively. NSAIDs are contraindicated with other drugs such as steroids, diuretics for congestive heart failure (CHF), ace-inhibitors, and cyclosporine. There may be more drugs to add to this list after this writing, so be sure to check.

Using NSAIDs during surgery is dangerous for geriatric cancer patients due to adverse effects with renal compromise, CKD, congestive heart failure (CHF), hypovolemia, hypotension, and coagulation problems. Opioids are the best choice for geriatric cancer patients undergoing surgery. Opioids are more versatile, more effective against severe pain, and safer than NSAIDs.

GI Protectants

Famotidine, cimetidine, sucralfate, Prilosec, sucralfate, and other GI protectants are very helpful to minimize the side effects of gastrointestinal ulceration associated with the use of NSAIDs, especially for aspirin and piroxicam. The pain relief of all NSAIDs parallels the baseline relief provided by aspirin. We all have clients who feel that one product works miracles over another. Therefore, it is reasonable to recommend another NSAID to see if the patient has a better response.

Steroids

Never let a patient die or suffer without the silver bullet. Over the years, I have found steroids to be a great friend to end of life and geriatric cancer patients. Prednisone or dexamethasone alleviates mild to moderate inflammatory pain and can abate severe neuropathic pain. Injectable steroids can help alleviate swelling and inflammation for cats with oral neoplasia and also serve as appetite stimulators. Cancer patients with dysorexia due to oral, esophageal, or visceral neoplasia must experience severe hunger pangs and pain. It is our duty to do all that we can to compassionately alleviate the pain and discomfort of chronic anorexia in our cancer patients.

Oral, intravenous, and intratumoral (intralesional) injections of steroids for residual and inoperable mast cell tumors have been helpful to reduce pain, inflammation, and cytoreduction. Steroids have played an important role in the medical management of pain for most of my brain tumor patients.

Steroid hormones such as megestrol acetate (Depo-Provera®) and Nandrolone® injections may stimulate the appetite and create a sense of well-being. Some use the anabolic steroid Winstrol-V® for this purpose; however, in my experience, it does not increase appetite. I generally use megestrol acetate to increase appetite and to reverse catabolism. When combined with Zyprexa™, megestrol acetate may help increase the quality of life for many failing, anorectic geriatric cancer patients, especially those with respiratory disease. Entyce™ may be a great alternative instead of using steroids for appetite stimulation.

Bear's Case (Steroids Can Help Brain Tumor Patients)

Roger Clinton brought Bear, his 12-year-old male Labrador-Retriever mix, for a head tilt, circling to the left and ataxia with left-sided facial paralysis. An MRI identified a large, inoperable choroid plexus tumor. It was not amenable to radiation therapy or chemotherapy. Bear was given a very poor prognosis by our radiologist, who felt that euthanasia would be appropriate at any time. Roger was devastated and he entered Bear into our end of life Pawspice brain tumor program. Bear received palliative medical management with an initial injection of 8mg of dexamethasone IV followed by oral prednisone at $30mg/m^2$ and oral lomustine at $80mg/m^2$ in divided doses over 4 days q 21 days, and linoleic acid at 3mg/kg PO on 3 consecutive days each week. To our amazement, Roger returned with a normal-acting dog on the next recheck. Bear responded to injections of dexamethasone on an as-needed basis. Injections varied from once a month for the first 6–8 months and increased in frequency to weekly as we achieved Bear's 1-year anniversary with brain cancer (see Figure 7.9). I helped Roger and his son say farewell to Bear with the gift of euthanasia shortly after his one year anniversary.

Psychoactive Pharmaceuticals in Multimodal Therapy for Quality of Life

It often takes more than one class of pain medication to control cancer pain. Never hesitate to enlist adjunctive help, including acupuncture, to fully control your geriatric cancer patient's pain. When adequate analgesia is not given at the start of a painful event, the omission of control may allow the pain to progress and become chronic pain. Since animals are stoic about their initial pain, we can presume that a great deal of chronic pain in geriatric cancer patients goes untreated.

Using amitriptyline other tricyclic antidepressants to control pain is supported by a large body of literature. Using gabapentin (or other anticonvulsants), bisphosphonates, and/or amantadine (or other NMDA receptor antagonists) may further enhance your efforts to alleviate cancer pain. Pain has the physiological effect of creating intense anxiety and stress. Using benzodiazepine anxiolytics and selective serotonin reuptake inhibitors (SSRIs) can be very helpful to ease the tension for overtly anxious patients. Caution should be taken to not use SSRIs in patients on monoamine oxidase inhibitors such as L-deprenyl (selegiline, Anipryl™) for canine cognitive syndrome.

Zyprexa™ (olanzapine) is a second generation antipsychotic used for schizophrenia and bipolar disease in humans and causes weight gain. It is a dopamine antagonist and is classified as a thienobenzodiazepine. Studies found that olanzapine helps reduce the anxiety and discomfort that so commonly afflict end of life cancer patients, especially for those with the symptom burden of lung cancer, respiratory disease, metastases, and pulmonary effusion. It also increases the appetite. Its action antagonizes dopamine, which may explain these benefits. The dose is empirical for dogs. I use $^{1}/_{2}$ of a 5mg tablet BID for a 60–80 pound dog. Zyprexa combined with ondansetron can prevent chemotherapy-related immediate and delayed vomiting. It is also helpful in the treatment of cancer-related anorexia when combined with megestrol acetate (Gupta and Pal 2016). Since I have introduced Zyprexa™ to help my end of life geriatric cancer patients in distress, they have been able to recover a better quality of life. Some physicians feel that using olanzapine has set a new standard of care for human palliative medicine and hospice care.

Bentley's Case (Olanzapine and Megestrol Acetate Improved QoL)

Michelle Yabko, was concerned about Bentley, her 12-year-old neutered male Golden Retriever, who was being treated for multiple myeloma successfully for almost 2 years, using oral melphalan, prednisone, and supplements. Bentley developed pneumonia with subsequent chronic bronchitis and a cough that reduced his exercise tolerance and ability to sleep comfortably at night. Bentley's constant panting and coughing were ruining his quality of life. A combination of oral olanzapine 2.5mg BID and megestrol acetate weekly injections for 3 consecutive weeks improved Bentley's quality of life dramatically and gave him a new lease on life.

Integrate Complementary and Alternative Therapy

Complementary and alternative medicine (CAM) is popular with pet owners. Using acupuncture to alleviate pain can be very rewarding. Acupuncture and complementary medicine may alleviate pain, tension, and create a sense of well-being that offsets the negative aspects associated with uncontrolled pain. Acupuncture sessions can also be very nurturing for the cancer patient and may comfort and empower the carers as well.

Other modalities of alternative medicine and supportive care, such as chiropractic, cold packs, hot packs, electrical stimulation, low-level laser therapy (Shearer 2004), massage therapy, prolotherapy, and magnetic therapy, may complement pain control efforts and further alleviate cancer pain (Robinson 2005). If and when clients seek complementary and alternative care to alleviate their pet's pain, encourage them to give it a try. Anecdotally, the geriatric oncology patient may benefit and that is what matters most.

Fear Free Patient Visits

In 2011, the Bayer Veterinary Healthcare Usage Study found that 38% of dog owners and 58% of cat owners say their beloved pets hate going to the vet and 26% of dog owners and 38% of cat owners said that just thinking about going to the vet was stressful for them! It is ethical and reasonable to categorize fear and stress as anxiety and therefore as emotional pain. I am a member of the Fear Free Advisory Board that was founded by Dr. Marty Becker to solve this destructive fear problem that is pervasive in our profession. The Fear Free slogan is "Take the pet out of petrified."

Fear Free behaviorists advise that we consult with clients and plan ahead to see their pets when they are hungry and ready for a treat. They suggest giving pets a calming diet or "chill pill." For example, a client can be instructed to give a 100mg gabapentin capsule to relax their fearful or aggressive cat. Instruct clients to acclimate their pets to enjoy the car ride and to enjoy being in new generation carriers. At your clinic, consider playing comforting music. Synthetic pheromones can be released from electronic dispensers in exam rooms, treatment rooms, and on smocks and scrubs. Recommend the use of compression garments on the pets during their visit. Dr. Becker says, "We need both bookends in veterinary medicine – competent medical care and compassionate emotional care, not either or."

At our practice, we use Fear Free tactics and we have witnessed a relaxation response in many anxious patients and equally anxious clients who were simultaneously given the solution called Rescue Remedy®. We now routinely use RxNutricalm™ to relax our geriatric cancer patients and properly address their emotional pain.

Multimodality Pain Management

The combination of NSAIDs and opioids is very helpful for controlling moderate to severe pain. The fentanyl pain patch combines well with NSAIDs such as piroxicam or meloxicam for a postoperative nosectomy in a cat. Deracoxib or carprofen may be prescribed for a dog following amputation to supplement a fentanyl pain patch. The pain patch also combines well with gabapentin, oxymorphone and hydromorphone.

Naloxone reverses the pain patch's negative opioid side effects, such as respiratory depression, bradycardia, dysphoria, noise sensitivity, hypothermia, vomiting, and diarrhea. The analgesic effect of the pain patch remains intact while the opioid reaction is reversed.

Various NSAIDs complement the fentanyl patch and are routinely given to older dogs for severe postoperative pain and for chronic cancer pain control. Tramadol may also be coadministered with NSAIDs for improved control of cancer pain. The fentanyl pain patch or oral tramadol can be combined with steroids to achieve excellent pain control for moderate to severe pain in both cats and dogs. Amitriptyline or clomipramine may be helpful in reducing anxiety, stress, and pain when used in combination with NSAIDs, opioids, or steroids. Tricyclic antidepressants would be a good option for a patient like Bear Clinton, the dog just discussed. Bear was treated successfully for one year with steroids, lomustine, and linoleic acid for a large choroid plexus tumor. The steroids alleviated Bear's circling, head tilt, and facial paralysis. Using Zyprexa™ in combination with megestrol acetate may alleviate the symptom burden of patients with respiratory disease and lung cancer. When combined with ondansetron, Zyprexa™ may also reduce chemotherapy-related vomiting.

Cats and NSAIDs

Over 90% of cats over 12 years of age have some level of osteoarthritis and their pain is not being addressed. Meloxicam is one of the few approved NSAIDs for cats, although carprofen, ketoprofen, and aspirin are commonly used. Meloxicam is ideal in combination with the fentanyl patch to alleviate chronic oral cancer pain for cats. It is approved for one-time injection in cats. Administer meloxicam as the patient is recovering from anesthesia as a supplement to a freshly placed pain patch. It provides immediate pain relief for cancer patients undergoing painful surgical procedures such as mandibulectomy or thoracotomy. The effects of a meloxicam injection wear off over 24 hours while the fentanyl patch takes effect. This combination provides even, sustained pain control for feline patients that have normal hydration and renal function. Precautions should be taken as with all NSAIDs.

Meloxicam liquid can be used postoperatively for 2 weeks to control pain in cats on a tapering oral dose, starting with 0.2mg/kg on day 1. Half of this dose (0.1mg/kg) is given on each of the following 4 days and then it is halved again to 0.05mg/kg for 10 days. For further use, the dose is halved again to 0.025mg/kg once daily. Meloxicam oral suspension at 0.5mg/ml (0.02mg per drop) may be used long term at one drop per 4 pounds per day in cats.

The long term use of NSAIDs in cats has been studied for hazards and drug interactions. Experience using piroxicam and meloxicam for feline oral SCC cases has given myself and many oncologists confidence. The extra-label and judicious usage of NSAIDs can benefit the quality of life and the survival of geriatric feline oncology patients if the patient's hydration and renal function are maintained within normal limits.

Pre-emptive Analgesia for Surgery and Painful Procedures

Anticipate that any surgical procedure, including any type of biopsy, will create pain for the patient. Pre-emptive analgesia is an antinociceptive treatment that prevents establishment of altered processing of afferent input, which amplifies postoperative pain. If the cancer patient presents in pain, take measures to provide pain medication immediately. Alertness and attention to every level of pain is always greatly appreciated by the pet's family. Provide pain medication as a presedation treatment prior to placement of indwelling catheters and before beginning preparation for diagnostic and surgical procedures as described earlier.

The alpha-2 agonists, Dexdomitor™ and medetomidine (Domitor®), can be given IM to provide mild relaxation and sedation during the preparation process for healthy patients. Pretreatment or mixing it with atropine helps prevent bradycardia and emesis but it does not increase cardiac output, which is the reason to avoid using atropine in geriatric patients. Medetomidine has an opioid-sparing effect.

All alpha-2 agonists, especially xylazine, cause emesis in cats and bradycardia and hypertension in both dogs and cats and are contraindicated for geriatric patients with myocardial, liver, or renal disease. We prefer to mix the low dose of Dexdomitor™ with butorphanol (DB) as a combination for IV administration in healthy geriatric patients for its immediate sedation, analgesia, and immobilization effect. This combination is excellent for minor procedures in healthy geriatric cancer patients such as Tru-cut, punch and bone marrow biopsy, or wound debridement and cryotherapy. We use high dose DB if more analgesia is needed. It is best to avoid alpha-2 agonists for older geriatric patients and for any age patient with renal or cardiac problems. Read the updated information on these drugs in *Plumb's Veterinary Drug Handbook*, 8th edition, 2015.

My favorite systemic preemptive pain control for surgical oncology procedures in geriatric patients is the Duragesic™ fentanyl pain patch. It releases fentanyl from a transdermal membrane into the circulatory system over a 3-day period in dogs and a 3–5 day period in cats. It is safe and effective for moderate to severe levels of pain. The big problem with pain patches is the variation of time to effect from animal to animal and dog versus cat. It may take up to 24 hours for the full analgesic effect in some dogs, whereas 70% of cats experience the full effect within 6–8 hours.

We do not want 30% of our surgery patients to suffer perioperatively because their blood levels of analgesic are too low. That is why, when possible, we place the pain patch the night before surgery for dogs and the morning of the surgery for cats. Because of the variable delay in onset of analgesia, it is important to administer fentanyl by SQ injection at 20–40µg/kg hourly before and after surgery, until the fentanyl pain patch has reached its full effect.

Midazolam at 0.1mg/lb SQ, IM, or IV causes muscle relaxation and prolongs the relaxation effect of fentanyl injection. Benzodiazepine tranquilizers are the best choice to coadminister with fentanyl and other opioids, to relax geriatric or debilitated patients. This combination is safe for presedation and preanesthetic protocols in critical patients. Avoid using acepromazine in geriatric oncology patients.

The best choice for induction and anesthesia of geriatric cancer patients at this writing would be IV propofol, intubation, and sevoflurane or isoflurane inhalant anesthesia. The induction, anesthesia, postoperative pain control, and aftercare protocols for emergency, routine, and aggressive surgical oncology procedures described in Chapters 18 through 20 of W.B. Morrison's book *Cancer in Cats and Dogs* are excellent references (2002).

An injectable NSAID such as meloxicam or carprofen helps alleviate pain in the immediate postoperative period. A continuous rate infusion of microdose ketamine, which is an antagonist for NMDA receptors, can be very helpful during surgery and in the immediate postoperative period to complement the fentanyl patch as well as other opioids.

A contemporary multimodality approach for pre-emptive pain management has always been direly needed for aggressive surgical oncology procedures. Now we can successfully perform amputation, mandibulectomy, maxillectomy, thoracotomy, and so forth without hurting our patients. There is no longer any excuse for hurting our patients with definitive surgery that many tumors require for curative intent or palliation.

Remington's Case (Palliative Amputation for Pain Control)

Matthew Magsadia brought Remington, his 9-year-old intact male Bull Mastiff, for consultation. Remington has a history of lameness and arthritis of his right front shoulder that was being treated for 3 months by a holistic veterinarian. The lameness worsened and his shoulder started to swell rapidly. X-rays were diagnostic for osteosarcoma. Matt was very concerned about Remington's unrelenting pain, the enormous mass, and the late diagnosis when we discussed his options: palliative care or amputation followed by palliative care.

We prescribed multimodality pain management. One week later, the mass was larger and Remington was in agonizing pain as he tried to move. Matt elected amputation as the best option to provide immediate pain relief for his beloved dog. Despite clear chest X-rays, we could only offer 2–3 months survival time as a postop prognosis due to the late diagnosis, the enormity of the mass, and without conventional carboplatin chemotherapy. Presurgical imaging and postop carboplatin was not in the family budget.

Remington's amputation was very challenging. The cancer involved his brachial plexus and caused severe bleeding, which was fortunately controlled. His recovery was uneventful. We gave fentanyl injections every 2 hours postop. He went home that night after MicroLight 830 nm laser therapy along the incision and a 100mcg fentanyl patch, which was placed 8 hours previously. Matt was instructed to give high dose gabapentin every 4–6 hours as needed to keep Remington totally relaxed. He was instructed to also give amantadine and meloxicam (Mobic™) daily.

At our one week postop recheck Remington was a new dog in great spirits with his painful limb gone. I encouraged Matt to allow us to prescribe metronomic lomustine based upon data that it might help delay metastases and prolong survival time. To our surprise and delight, Remington's follow-up chest X-rays were clear at his 4 month "met" check and at his 6 month met check and he remained active for 9 months postamputation. Matt called me at 6:45 this Monday morning, January13, 2017, as I write, to tell me that Remington developed a mass on his abdomen and had difficulty standing over the weekend. I asked if Remington had difficulty breathing and the answer was, "Yes." We both knew it was time to let him go. Matt was thankful for the extra time that we gained for Remington despite the enormous odds against him.

Using Local Analgesics

We use topical lidocaine gel, refrigerant anesthetic spray, or local infusions of lidocaine directly on areas that we intend for venipuncture and for painful procedures. We use topical lidocaine gel at IV and FNA sites. We administer injectable lidocaine at biopsy sites and around superficial cutaneous tumors in addition to lidocaine gel before applying cryotherapy. The typical cryotherapy patient may be a white cat with facial SCC. Two percent lidocaine at 3–5mg/kg must be used with caution in cats due to its narrow margin of safety. It is safest to draw up the total dose ahead of time for small patients and dilute it if a larger volume is needed for infiltration of the surgical site. We perform cryotherapy most often in Whippets, Italian Greyhounds, and Pit Bull breeds with solar-induced superficial cutaneous hemangiosarcomas and SCC. Occasionally, we treat small superficial mast cell tumors with cryotherapy. Dogs with cutaneous solar-induced SCC and hemangiosarcoma have field cancerization, which means that they return periodically with new lesions needing cryotherapy.

We administer IV or IM sedation to relax most of our cryotherapy patients in addition to using topical and local anesthesia. Geriatric cancer patients need special attention paid to assuage their pain and anxiety, especially for repetitious procedures that have caused them pain in the past. We must anticipate their emotional state and pain levels and treat them resourcefully before they become agitated or fearful.

Epidurals and Local Pain Control

Local, regional, and epidural anesthesia can offset suffering from severely painful procedures that create tissue damage. This technique is underutilized in our profession. Researchers at Johns Hopkins found that opioid receptors are upregulated in inflamed tissues. Receptors will respond for up to 48 hours if the tissue is given intraoperative morphine at low doses. Butorphanol acts synergistically with local anesthetics. Use a nerve block with bupivacaine at 1.5–2mg/kg 10–15 minutes prior to digit and limb amputations. Epidural blocks, local nerve blocks, and regional blocks eliminate pain. Bupivacaine, or any other long-acting local anesthetic, infused along nerves and on to surgically traumatized tissue, blocks postsurgical suffering for 6–8 hours.

Perioperative Pain Control

From the time of hospitalization for surgery to the time of discharge, we owe the geriatric oncology patient as much comfort and protection from pain and emotional distress as possible. Aside from the humane benefits of perioperative analgesia, geriatric oncology patients undergoing surgical procedures have reduced requirements for anesthesia, smoother recovery, and shorter hospitalization periods as a plus. Improved anesthetics are safer than ever for geriatric patients and very helpful *but* their downside is a rapid return to awareness and perception of pain (McMillan 2005). Inhalation anesthetics that are eliminated rapidly leave the patient conscious and starkly devoid of analgesia. The patient recovers consciousness, is alert within moments, and is fully able to feel pain resulting from the surgical procedure. Therefore, pain control is needed during recovery and throughout the first night postop, on a set schedule. We must anticipate that all surgical patients will feel pain upon regaining consciousness. If a pain patch is placed just before the surgical procedure and has not yet reached a therapeutic blood level, it is important to provide preoperative and postoperative pain relief with the use of fentanyl or morphine or oxymorphone injections.

The goal is to make sure that the recovering patient is sleeping comfortably and is pain-free until the pain patch is fully effective. The attending doctor should leave written instructions to the nursing staff and prepare them to administer effective pain control medication on a set schedule or by constant-rate infusion. The goal is to allow the patient to sleep comfortably for 12–24 hours after intense surgical oncology procedures such as mastectomy, liver or lung lobectomy, splenectomy, large sarcoma excision, amputation, thoracotomy, rib resection, mandibulectomy, maxillectomy, enucleation, nosectomy, rhinotomy, and so forth.

Good postop pain control is essential. Monitor your geriatric cancer patients overnight with observant and caring nurses trained to assess pain. Train your staff to use the CSU pain chart as a standard reference (see Table 7.1). Train your nursing staff to look for increased panting and heart rate, crying, and restlessness in dogs. Cats exhibit pain with behaviors such as crouching, hiding, hunching, aggression, and holding the head in a down position. Since opioids slow the heart rate, this is not a valid parameter for patients on opioids. A veterinary staff properly trained to look for perioperative pain is invaluable to the clinician toward ensuring that no patient suffers needlessly.

Constant monitoring of the patient is the key to successful postoperative pain management. When the local infusion of bupivacaine wears off, the patient may suffer great pain. The nursing staff should be told when to expect the bupivacaine to wear off and should be on the alert to determine exactly when the patient needs additional pain control.

Discharge all postop cancer patients with some form of oral pain control medication. Carers expect to exit the hospital with the acknowledgement that their pet's procedure was painful and that you have the pain covered. Pain relief medications should be dispensed to them so that they can sustain analgesia at home at least for the following several days. I recommend sending a second pain relief drug as a backup for the carer to use in the event of breakthrough pain. This will limit patient suffering and client anxiety as well as phone calls of concern in the late hours of the night.

It is very important to provide enduring postoperative pain control medications effective enough to truly relieve pain and suffering for an appropriate period of time. All too often, clients have told me that they stayed up all night with a painful pet. Omitting control of some types of pain is inexcusable, such as a pet that is whimpering or crying after an amputation. Do not fail to provide your surgical oncology patients multimodality pain control to avoid the following scenario.

Sam's Case (Don't Fail to Provide Enough Analgesia)

Sam, a M/N 11-year-old Labrador Retriever, developed a large hemangiosarcoma originating in his left quadriceps muscle. His family reported that Sam cried and whimpered for hours after being sent home 1 day following his hind leg amputation. His surgeon was unavailable at night, so they took Sam to an emergency room at 2:00 a.m. for a pain injection. Sam got only 1–2 hours of relief from that injection and started crying again at 4:00 a.m. The clients were frustrated with the attending surgeon and the emergency room doctor because they did not provide more potent and longer-acting pain management. Somehow the amount of pain control dispensed did not acknowledge or address the severity of Sam's pain.

Compounding Pharmacies

Compounding pharmacies prepare palatable formulations that are easy and safe for carers to use at home. Pain control medications are formulated so that a measurable aliquot can be identified and given, especially for small dogs and cats. When engaging a compounding pharmacist, state clearly the desired dose and frequency of medication that the patient is to receive. For instance, the piroxicam dose for both dogs and cats is 0.3mg/kg. We use a 10mg capsule every 24 hours for a 60-pound dog and 1mg every 48 hours for a cat. To order compounded piroxicam for a cat, I specify: "Piroxicam, 1mg PO every 48 hours." This dose would be one-tenth of a 10mg capsule or tablet. Because cats generally do not mind the taste, liquid meloxicam packaged with a clearly marked dosing syringe is a very convenient NSAID for pet owners to use. Meloxicam oral suspension at 0.5mg/ml (0.02mg per drop) may be used long term at one drop per 4 pounds per day in cats.

Pain Control for Pawspice Care

Terminal geriatric cancer patients often live stoically with moderate to severe pain, even with hypertrophic osteopathy from pulmonary tumors. We counsel and encourage pet carers to enter our palliative end of life hospice care program, or "Pawspice." The Pawspice program places pain control as a top priority. We generally offer the pet owner the option of placing a fentanyl pain patch every 3 days. We shave both back legs of the patient and demonstrate the proper application and wrapping of the pain patches. The pet carers are asked to return their pet's used fentanyl patches at recheck for proper disposal. For cats and small dogs weighing less than 20 pounds, we instruct the carer to uncover half of the patch to provide adequate pain control for 72 hours and then to uncover the other half, which should provide analgesia for an additional 72 hours.

Nalbuphine

The generic form of nalbuphine is a convenient and inexpensive home care injectable pain medication. For many years, we used injectable nalbuphine SQ for cancer patients that fight oral medications, are intolerant of pain patches, or have resistant pain. It is a great option for dealing with resistant pain and/or for pet owners on a budget. Nalbuphine is a narcotic agonist-antagonist that provides pain relief for moderate to severe pain and calms the patient without a heavy sedative effect. Be sure to specify that you want the generic injectable nalbuphine when you order it to save money. Patients experiencing pain generally require subcutaneous nalbuphine injections every 6–8 hours.

Nalbuphine is a good choice for cats with oral tumor pain, especially lingual squamous cell carcinoma. The dose ranges from 0.2 to 0.5mg/kg given SQ as needed two or three times daily for dogs and 0.1–0.3mg/kg three to four times daily for cats. Nalbuphine may be sent home for SQ use without the typical narcotics precautions. Nalbuphine has fewer sedation effects than other similar analgesic compounds.

Alaska's Case (Nalbuphine Helped Us Say Goodbye)

I used nalbuphine occasionally to help Alaska, my own beloved $12\frac{1}{2}$-year-old Great Pyrenees, with arthritis and her 18-month end of life decline with degenerative myelopathy. Nalbuphine helped Alaska to sleep comfortably, yet she was able to get up and move to another resting spot when she wanted to.

When I knew that Alaska was nearing the end of her journey with us, it was very important to me that her final moments were free of pain or anxiety. I gave Alaska a 10-times dose of nalbuphine IM. She became very relaxed yet could still lift her head and look at us. She remained aware of our love and attention. The nalbuphine made Alaska's final moments painless and peaceful and allowed me to insert a butterfly catheter easily to prepare for our final farewell.

Adverse Drug Reactions and Interactions in Pain Control

The cadre of drugs used for pain control will continue to grow and become an everyday routine consideration for geriatric oncology patients. It is essential for the contemporary clinician to be familiar with polypharmacy and the potential for adverse reactions related to multimodal analgesics and adjunctive drugs used for comfort care in the geriatric oncology patient. We must distinguish the adverse effects of analgesics or their drug interactions with chemotherapy drugs from symptoms of progressive disease. Another problem with pain control drugs is that most strong analgesics also have sleep-inducing effects with uneven durations of activity. A geriatric oncology patient may be under sedation while being left without adequate analgesia.

Opioid Adverse Events

All opioids have the potential to cause constipation, ileus, urinary retention, and sedation. These physiologic effects may be more pronounced with polypharmacy. When giving a tranquilizer to a geriatric cancer patient on opioids, the initial dose should be reduced by 30–50% to avoid sedation. All opioids have a sparing effect for induction and anesthetic agents and caution is required to use these drugs to effect when coadministered with premed opioids. Atropine was routinely used in sedation and anesthetic protocols to prevent bradycardia. It also reduces GI motility and can act synergistically with opioids to induce ileus. Due to these adverse events, atropine is used much less frequently in contemporary practices.

Several of my geriatric oncology patients have exhibited adverse signs of opioid excess with fentanyl pain patches at the recommended dose. Do not use the full 25 micrograms of fentanyl/hour pain patch for old cats less than 10–15 pounds because it is an excessive dose. We expose one-half of the pain patch for all older patients under 12–15 pounds. The remaining half is exposed after 72 hours. Several of my older cancer patients also experienced bradycardia and dysphoria with fentanyl pain patches. We instruct clients to remove the patch if the patient exhibits adverse side effects. It may take up to 24 hours for the fentanyl level to drop and the patient to normalize.

Carmen's Case (Fentanyl Patches May Cause Adverse Events)

Carmen Ashlock, a 37-pound 11-year-old Springer Spaniel, needed pain control for hypertrophic pulmonary osteopathy (HO). One of her legs was very swollen and painful due to concurrent infection. HO was due to a large pulmonary metastasis from her 5-year battle with mammary adenocarcinoma (Figure 7.10). Carmen initially responded very well to pain alleviation, but on day 2 she became anorectic, then started whimpering the next morning. An emergency clinic diagnosed her with life-threatening ileus and urinary retention. These adverse events started 50–60 hours after placement of a 50mcg/hour fentanyl pain patch in a very sick geriatric oncology patient.

Steroids Plus NSAIDs Equals Trouble

Take every precaution to avoid adverse events that are notorious with the simultaneous use of steroids with NSAIDS. This combination invites severe, hemorrhagic GI ulceration and potential perforation. Although it would be ideal to be able to use both steroids and NSAIDs for pets with brain tumors, we must not use these two drugs simultaneously. On rare occasions, I may use this combination as a one-time-only initial dose along with injectable and oral famotidine and then discontinue the NSAID.

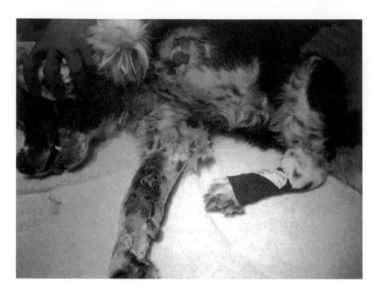

Figure 7.10.   Hypertrophic osteopathy due to pulmonary metastasis from a 5-year battle with mammary adenocarcinoma. Carmen Ashlock, an 11-year-old Springer Spaniel, needed pain control for her condition, which was complicated with concurrent infection of the left foreleg. There is a fentanyl patch on her left hind leg, which caused adverse events 50–60 hours after application.

The advantage of using steroids to reduce brain tumor swelling is clinically more valuable to the patient than the NSAID effects. Steroids may also relieve pain, create a sense of well-being, and increase appetite for cancer patients. For these reasons, I prefer to use steroids rather than NSAIDs for brain tumor patients. Mannitol, an osmotic diuretic, may be the best choice to reduce brain swelling in some brain tumor patients.

Adverse events such as: PUPD, restlessness, panting, weight gain, hepatopathy, and arousal caused by steroids may preclude their use in some geriatric oncology patients. NSAIDs inhibit platelet function and gastric acid inhibition, which erodes the prostaglandin-driven protective mucous layer of the stomach. This leads to GI ulceration and hemorrhage, which is poorly tolerated by most geriatric oncology patients with chronic anemia. NSAIDs may also interact with the clearance of chemotherapy drugs, especially hepatotoxic or nephrotoxic drugs such as cisplatin. For unresponsive pain, add gabapentin at 10mg/kg every 8 hours and tramadol at 4–10mg/kg every 6–8 hours. Trazodone can be given at 1.7–3.5mg/kg BID with tramadol or given at 7–10mg/kg BID or TID without tramadol.

Gabapentin and the "GAT" Protocol

Gabapentin (Neurontin®) is an anticonvulsant that alleviates chronic neuropathic pain in combination with NSAIDs or steroids at 10mg/kg every 6–12 hours. It may also relieve chronic headache and sinus pain. Evaluation of this effect would need to be a subjective observation made by the pet's carers. The dose may be increased to effect. It may be best to start gabapentin at night to observe if the pet will be drowsy. The dose can be lowered to avoid drowsiness during the day and increased at bed time to help the pet sleep better since cancer pain is worse at night. We use gabapentin routinely in the "GAT" protocol, which is Gabapentin, Amantadine, and Tramadol or Trazodone along with an NSAID. This multimodality approach provides effective management of cancer pain in the majority of our geriatric cancer patients. Cats respond well to Gabapentin and they may be given a 100mg capsule safely for pain control and for Fear Free hospital visits.

Summary

Pain management was not taught in veterinary schools until the 1990s, following the passing of the 1985 Federal Animal Welfare Law. This law recognized pain and distress in laboratory animals (Rollin 2005). Dr. Charles Short and Dr. Alan Van Posnak edited *Animal Pain*, one of the first veterinary books to influence how we address animal suffering (1992). Today, the International Veterinary Association of Pain Management offers education and a certification program (www.ivapm.org). The American Animal Hospital Association in conjunction with the American Association of Feline Practitioners issued the 2015 AAHA/AAFP Pain Management Guidelines for Dogs and Cats. The World Small Animal Veterinary Association's Global Pain Council issued the WSAVA Global Guidelines for Recognition, Assessment and Treatment of Pain in 2014.

The ravages of cancer pain destroy the geriatric cancer patient's immediate quality of life. If cancer pain is not properly addressed, the human–animal bond that holds our profession together will literally suffer a dead end. Pain has the power to short-circuit the human–animal bond because our historical answer to an animal in pain has been euthanasia. If the painful cancer patient is prematurely extinguished without the benefit of pain control, we have not served our patient's or our client's best interest.

Contemporary pain management in geriatric cancer patients enables cancer patients and their distraught families to regain quality of life and to have peace of mind at a very difficult time, which is end of life. Veterinarians and staff now have the tools to recognize and understand the complexity of chronic pain syndromes and their relation to cancer pain in geriatric patients. We can understand the biology of pain, and more specifically understand the mechanisms of cancer pain, and use the current pharmacology and complementary techniques such as acupuncture that are available to alleviate it. We can adopt management plans for specific procedures and conditions using the WHO pain management ladder (Figure 7.1) or we can turn the WHO ladder upside down and treat unbearable pain very aggressively from the start.

We have the obligation to create a more comfortable quality of life for our geriatric cancer patients while they live with cancer at the end of life. When cancer pain is unresponsive to our best contemporary efforts, then we can justifiably help our geriatric patients with more intense pain relief during a hospice vigil. We can help our end of life painful patients to find peace by way of providing final relief with the gift of euthanasia. If our clients feel satisfied with the quality of life that their companion animal experienced through our pain management program during their battle against cancer, then our job is well done.

Cannabis Commentary

Since approximately one in three of our new clients will answer "Yes" when I ask if they have given their geriatric cancer dog any cannabis products, it is important for veterinarians to know about its use, potential benefits, and misuse. "Cannabis" refers to plants of the genus *Cannabis* including products used for therapeutic applications. Preparations can be inhaled, or taken orally, sublingually, or topically. Hemp and marijuana originate from the *Cannabis sativa* L. plant. The plants contain dozens of cannabinoids, which act on the body's cannabinoid receptors that are found in many tissues in mammals, known as the endocannabinoid system. There are two basic subtypes of cannabinoid receptors (CB1 and CB2) in mammalian tissues. Agonists and antagonists selective for these receptors have been identified. Hemp has been used for its fiber and medicinal effects for centuries worldwide. Over

750 phytoconstituents have been identified in cannabis such as: terpenes, cannabinoids, flavonoids, non-cannabinoid phenols, nitrogenous compounds, and common plant compounds. Cannabis has a variable legal landscape.

Hemp yields cannabidiol (CBD), the most commonly used cannabinoid in pets. CBC offers benefits without causing the psychoactive effects. Marijuana refers to delta-9 tetrahydrocannabinol (THC), which is hallucinogenic and generally undesirable for pets. Both are extracted from various plant strains or manufactured synthetically. Many hemp strains have been cultivated to yield high levels of CBD and low levels of THC <0.3%. The main differences between hemp and marijuana are the ratio of THC to CBD. Hemp contains high levels of CBD and less than 0.3% of hallucinogenic THC. Dogs are very sensitive, especially to the effects of THC. Dogs develop toxicity signs of excessive panting, distress, and, in severe cases, static ataxia, after ingesting an overdose of THC in brownies and snacks. Marijuana is classified as a Schedule I drug and is illegal for veterinarians to prescribe. The FDA excludes CBD as a dietary supplement. The FDA sent warning letters to many companies about claims on websites and marketing materials that their hemp products could address problems as dietary supplements for pets. Analysis of many of the products by the FDA also found many hemp products to be fraudulent (www.fda.gov/WarningLetters).

Various cannabinoids have been used in human patients to reduce vomiting and nausea during the administration of chemotherapy, to improve appetite for HIV/AIDS patients, to treat chronic pain and inflammation, muscle spasms, and seizure control. It has been used to control cancer pain and to increase the appetite and weight gain and to improve well-being in cancer patients. The NCI has reported some anticancer and antiangiogenesis action in mice and in cancer cell lines, with conflicting data at times. There are no published clinical trials in people or pets to substantiate anticancer effectiveness, only anecdotal observations (https://www.cancer.gov/about-cancer/treatment/cam/hp/cannabis-pdq#section/_7).

There is public interest in using cannabis for pets. An anonymous online survey of 632 pet owners who purchased hemp products for their pets documented that most people found the CBD hemp products for their pets online, or a friend suggested it to them. They use it most often for pet dogs to treat arthritis pain, seizures, anxiety, and behavior problems (Kogan, Hellyer, and Robinson 2016). Other uses were to stimulate the appetite.

Restrictions on cannabis research for veterinary patients leaves us with very little research available to provide guidance about the use and dose of CBD for companion animals. We hear the trial and error anecdotal reports from clients and the online marketing from companies that claim to have the answer.

More states are legalizing medical cannabis for people and many states have made recreational cannabis legal as well. The market for legal cannabis is one of the fastest-growing industries in the United States. The Internet is vigorously marketing to pet owners, selling mostly low potency cannabis products extracted from hemp for its CBD activity, despite lack of testing for quality and contents. Marketing claims say that hemp products will help pets with arthritis, pain, poor appetite, cancer, and end of life situations, although there are no published clinical trials. With public interest being so high, there is no doubt that well-controlled clinical trials will be forthcoming. Dr. Narda Robinson of CSU is interested in conducting prospective double blind clinical trials to create evidence-based substantive data.

Connecticut Hospice is the first hospice to study end of life human patients taking cannabis capsules TID PO, evaluating whether it improves palliative care and symptom control. The goal of this study is to ease pain and enhance quality of life for patients at end of life, while reducing the costs of care. This is a federally approved medical marijuana study on 66 human patients for 6 months to see if it is an alternative to opioids. Data from this study may determine if medical cannabis is an option to curb the prescription opioid epidemic.

Robert J. Silver, DVM, MS, of RxVitamins for Pets, authored the book, *Medical Marijuana and Your Pet* (2015). He helped to formulate HempRx™, a liquid extract of organically grown hemp, for use in dogs and cats, that contains 15mg of phytocannabinoids per ml (0.5mg per drop), 375mg per 25ml bottle. HempRx has a high percentage of CBD and very low THC (less than 0.3%). Dr. Silver recommends that HempRx drops should be started at the low end of the dose and slowly increased when giving it to dogs because they are sensitive to its adverse effects. Start at the low dose of 0.05mg–0.1mg/kg (1 drop/5kg) BID for a few days. If there are no adverse events, and no beneficial effects, increase the dose gradually to 0.25mg/kg (2.5 drops/5kg). If no response or adverse events, it is safe to increase the dose gradually to as high as 5 drops/5kg for some pets. The dose in cats is not well established but it is best to start at the low dose range (one drop SID or BID per cat). I have used the HempRx formulation in my practice along with a group of ten oncologists organized by Dr. Silver to see if collectively we could evaluate responses. On questioning our clients, we found that HempRx had variable success in palliating our geriatric cancer patients. Occasionally, some dogs had adverse events and it was discontinued. When a beneficial effect was observed, the clients were pleased. The most beneficial effects were appetite increase and pain reduction.

Dr. Robin Downing, Past President of the International Veterinary Association for Pain Management, feels that it is unfair to use cannabis that contains THC in pet animals because they may react with fear, panic, and disorientation from the psychotropic cannabinoid receptor activity in the brain.

Overall, it is important for veterinarians to be aware of their state law regarding cannabis. It is best to address client concerns and to guide proper choices in their quest to provide the best of care for their geriatric dogs and cats. Knowing about cannabis and offering cautious guidance is better than taking a back seat. Dr. Silver says, "Certainly prescribing or dispensing cannabis that contains >0.3 percent THC is clearly illegal. The illegal status of hemp extracts is very vague. Ultimately, though, it is each veterinarian's responsibility to make the right decision for themselves regarding the use of this controversial plant."

References

Boria, P.A., N.W. Glickman, B.R. Schmidt, et al. 2005. Carboplatin and piroxicam therapy in 31 dogs with transitional cell carcinoma of the urinary bladder. *Veterinary and Comparative Oncology* 3 (2): 73–80.

Dawkins, M.S. 2005. "The science of suffering." In *Mental health and well-being in animals*, ed. F.D. McMillan, pp. 47–55. Ames, IA: Blackwell Publishing Professional.

De Lorimier, L.P., and T.M. Fan. 2005. Understanding and recognizing cancer pain in dogs and cats. *Veterinary Medicine*, May, pp. 352–377.

Gaynor, J.S., as quoted by J. McElhenny. 2004. Taking away the pain: A century of change. *Veterinary Medicine*, Special Supplement, January.

Fan, T.M., L.P. de Lorimier, K. O'Dell-Anderson, H.I. Lacoste, and S.C. Charney. 2007. Single-agent Pamidronate for palliative therapy of canine appendicular osteosarcoma bone pain. *Journal of Veterinary Internal Medicine* 21:431–439.

Greene, S. 2002. *Veterinary anesthesia and pain management secrets*. Philadelphia, PA: Hanley & Belfus.

Gupta, V., and S. Pal. 2016. Olanzapine eases treatment-related vomiting, nausea, disease-driven anorexia and lung cancer symptoms. ASCO Reading Room in collaboration with MedPage Today. September 16, 2016.

Hellyer, P.W., and J.S. Gaynor. 1998. Acute postsurgical pain in dogs and cats. *Compendium* 20 (2):140–153.

Jaffe, S.B., et al. 2003. Pain management in companion animals: A roundtable on butorphanol tartrate. A Supplement to *Veterinary Forum* 20 (5A):1–16.

Kogan, L.R., P.W. Hellyer, and N.G. Robinson. 2016. Consumer's perceptions of hemp products for animals. *Journal of the American Holistic Veterinary Medical Association* 42:40–48.

Knapp, D.W., R.C. Richardson, T.C. Chan, et al. 1994. Piroxicam therapy in 34 dogs with transitional cell carcinoma of the urinary bladder. *JVIM* 8:723.

Lascelles, B.D.X. 2003. "Relief of chronic cancer pain." In *BSAVA Manual of Canine and Feline Oncology*, 2nd edn, eds J. Dobson and D. Lascelles, pp. 137–151. Quedgeley, Gloucestershire, England: British Small Animal Veterinary Association.

McMillan, F.D. 1999. Influence of mental states on somatic health in animals. *JAVMA* 214 (8):121–125.

McMillan, F.D. 2005. "Emotional maltreatment in animals." In *Mental health and well-being in animals*, ed. F.D. McMillan, pp. 167–179. Ames, IA: Blackwell Publishing Professional.

Morrison, W.B. 2002. *Cancer in Dogs and Cats: Medical and Surgical Management*, 2nd edn. Jackson, WY: Teton New Media.

Robinson, N. 2005. Complementary medicine: Prolotherapy for pain entering mainstream. *Veterinary Practice News*, June, p. 19.

Rollin, B.E. 2005. "On understanding animal mentation." In *Mental health and well-being in animals*, ed. F.D. McMillan, pp. 3–14. Ames, IA: Blackwell Publishing Professional.

Shearer, T.S. 2004. *High-tech pain management for pets: Low-level laser therapy user's manual for veterinarians*. Columbus, OH: Ohio Distinctive Publishing.

Short, C., and A. Van Poznak. 1992. *Animal pain*. Philadelphia: Saunder.

Silver, R.J. 2015. *Medical marijuana and your pet: The definitive guide*. Lulu Publishing Services.

Smith, L.J. 2005. Practical analgesia in cats. *Veterinary Medicine*, August, pp. 602–609.

Tranquilli, W.J., K.A. Grimm, and L.A. Lamont. 2004. *Pain management for the small animal practitioner*, 2nd edn. Jackson, WY: Teton New Media.

www.colostate.edu/depts/lar/Pain_Assessment.doc.

Suggested Reading

AAHA/AAFP. 2015. *Pain management guidelines for dogs and cats*.

Cambridge, A.J., K.M. Tobias, R.C. Newberry, and D.K. Sarkar. 2000. Subjective and objective measurements of postoperative pain in cats. *JAVMA* 217 (5):685–690.

Conzemius, M.G., C.M. Hill, J.L. Sammarco, and S.Z. Perkowski. Correlation between subjective and objective measures used to determine severity of postoperative pain in dogs. *JAVMA* 210 (11):1619–1622.

Franks, J.N., H.W. Boothe, L. Taylor, S. Geller, G.L. Carroll, V. Cracas, and D.M. Boothe. 2000. Evaluation of transdermal fentanyl patches for analgesia in cats undergoing onchectomy. *JAVMA* 217 (7):1013–1020.

Gaynor, J.S. and WW Muir III. 2014. *Handbook of veterinary pain management*, 3rd edn, 627 pp. Elsevier.

Grimm, J., K. Grimm, S. Kneller, W. Tranquilli, S. Crochik, M. Bischoff, and J. Podolski. 2004. The effect of a combination of medetomidine-butorphanol and medetomidine, butorphanol, atropine on glomerular filtration rate in dogs. *Veterinary Radiology and Ultrasound* 42 (5):458–462.

Lemke, K.A. 2004. Perioperative use of selective alpha-2 agonists and antagonists in small animals. *Canadian Vet J* 45 (6):475–480.

Muir, W.W., J.L. Ford, G.E. Karpa, E.E. Harrison, and J.E. Gadawski. 1999. Effects of intramuscular administration of low doses of medetomidine and medetomidine-butorphanol in middle-aged and old dogs. *JAVMA* 215 (8):1116–1120.

Ogilvie, G.K., et al. 2001. *Proceedings, Golden State Veterinary Conference*, May.

Villalobos, A.E. 2000. Conceptualized end of life care: Pawspice program for terminal pets. *AVMA 2000 Convention Notes*, July, pp. 322–327.

Villalobos, A.E. 2001. Comprehensive pain management vital to oncology patients. *VPN* 13 (7).
WSAVA. 2014. *Global guidelines for recognition, assessment and treatment of pain.*

Cannabis Resources

Boothe, D.M. 2014. The high points of medical marijuana. *Proceedings of the Atlantic Coast Veterinary Conference.*
Cannabinoids in biology and medicine, Part 1, 2011. Themed Issue, *British Journal of Pharmacology* (http://dx.doi.org/10.1111/bph.2011.163.issue-7).
Guindon, J., and A.G. Hohmann. 2011. The endocannabinoid system and cancer: therapeutic implication. *British Journal of Pharmacology* 163:1447–1463.

Chapter 8
Decision Making with Advanced and Recurrent Cancer in the Geriatric Patient

No one should have to choose (in the either/or model of medical care) between fighting their cancer or receiving palliative or hospice care – care that offers comfort through prevention and relief of physical, psychological, social and spiritual distress. Patients nearing the end of life can, and should, receive both at once (in the new simultaneous care model).

Fred Meyers, MD, School of Medicine, University of California, Davis, California

Epidemiologic trends in our society show that both human and pet populations are aging. This means that veterinarians will encounter more cancer in older pets than ever before and they will be caring for them. Therefore, decision making for recurrence and relapse in geriatric oncology patients will become a more common clinical problem. Unfortunately, there is a paucity of literature, training, and experience to assist practitioners in the decision-making process for intervention against advanced and recurrent cancer for geriatric oncology patients. There is very little guidance in how to approach clients with palliative cancer medicine using the Pawspice concept that transitions to hospice when the geriatric cancer patient declines toward death. Pawspice works with geriatric patients that are diagnosed with advanced cancer. Pawspice embraces palliative cancer medicine, which is kinder and gentler to slow down the cancer and help pets live longer with quality of life. Hospice focuses on intense comfort care when a patient is in the final decline towards death.

Attitudes about aging pets are also changing. Carers are proud of their older pets and they want them to live as long as possible. People need and seek more services for their geriatric pets as they undergo normative aging. Aging is associated with reduced immune competence, thymic involution, T-cell deficiency, accumulated exposure to carcinogens, inflammation, and genetic damage (decreased DNA repair, defects in tumor suppressor genes, reduced numbers, and function of mitochondria, etc.), which are major factors increasing susceptibility to infection and cancer in the elderly (Kennedy 2004).

The contemporary pet owner is willing to deal with the pet's age-related medical conditions, such as arthritis, dental disease, renal disease, heart failure, endocrine disorders, neurologic problems, and so forth. These coexisting problems turn into threatening comorbidities when the geriatric patient is burdened with neoplasia. These comorbidities may worsen and become a more ominous hobble when dealing with advanced stage cancer, recurrence, or relapse in geriatric oncology patients. The geriatric oncology patient's coexisting problems are competing for treatment. The attending doctor must balance the patient's multiple pathologies against the risk–benefit ratio of the pending treatment

---

Canine and Feline Geriatric Oncology: Honoring the Human–Animal Bond, Second Edition. Alice Villalobos with Laurie Kaplan.
© 2018 John Wiley & Sons, Inc. Published 2018 by John Wiley & Sons, Inc.

and related adverse events (Iliopoulou, Kitchell, and Yuzbasiyan-Gurkan, 2013). Certain breeds are more sensitive to chemotherapy, such as Cocker Spaniels, West Highland White Terriers, Collies, and Old English Sheepdogs and their cross-breeds (Couto and Moreno 2013).

If the expected outcome is roughly comparable between two types of treatment, clinical judgment would elect the least stressful treatment for the geriatric oncology patient. There are no controlled clinical trials addressing advanced stage or recurrent cancer in geriatric pets. Therefore, the attending clinician must glean applicable information from available relevant data, blend this with common-sense and patient-specific, client-oriented decision making.

Linking Gene Expression to Decision Making for Personalized Cancer Care

There is a new option for submitting tissues that offers more detailed diagnostic and treatment information. Instead of sending samples for immunohistochemistry or flow cytometry or PCR to differentiate a particular tumor or to identify the phenotype of a canine lymphoma, we can order the Enlight Assay from Innogenics™. It differentiates B-cell, T-cell, or T-cell enhanced B-cell lymphoma using genomic markers. In addition, a personalized report informs the clinician about the genomic markers associated with a good or poor response to standard chemotherapy agents. This science links gene expression to our patient's molecular profile and guides the attending doctor(s) to select effective therapies. This technology helps the family and the clinician become partners in the decision-making process that will be most beneficial for the patient (www.innogenics.org).

If we can improve the outcomes and/or quality of life for older cancer patients challenged with advanced stage cancer or recurrence, we may satisfy our client's wishes for honoring their human–animal bond and gain a richly rewarding experience. Emotional issues surface when a geriatric cancer patient develops advanced stage cancer, recurrence, or relapse. The dread of recurrence beats upon the emotional heartstrings of the geriatric cancer patient's family. Issues with frustration, attachment, anticipatory grief, guilt, depression, and resignation as well as hope and determination strum upon the core fibers of the pet owner's character. These concerns and the decision-making process are very difficult to deal with. There is no perfect choice. This chapter offers guidance in helping you and your clients with the decision-making process and weighing probabilities when the odds are contradictory (Clary 2016a, 2016b; Villalobos 2016a, 2016b, 2016c).

During consultations, as the attending doctor, you must admit and remove your own personal preconceptions and biases regarding age and cancer treatment. Many pet owners have told me that they felt that their doctor was insensitive to their hope and grief or was fatalistic, impatient, or rushed. Sometimes there is too much control followed by too few options offered for management of advanced stage cancer or recurrence for the geriatric oncology patient. The client feels let down. He or she feels that the doctor gave up on their old pet just when the pet needed help the most.

The Need for Family Practice Skills

People of all personality types and means bring their personal pets to veterinarians for help. Pet owners openly define their pets, to themselves and others, as members of their family. The pet as part of the family has evolved into a social consensus ethic (Rollin 2005).

Most veterinary students in the United States are currently taught to parallel the pediatrician's model for small animal practice, whereby the pet is considered a member of the family. Graduates leave the university with excellent textbook and disciplinary knowledge. However, there is a big gap

Table 8.1. Veterinary Family Practice Skills and Knowledge

Animal abuse	Life span approach to health care systems
Animal welfare	Maintaining a culture of self-renewal (knowledge and skills)
Behavior	Managing referrals
Clinical genetics	Media interactions
Communication	Mentoring
Community issues	Nutrition
Community outreach	Pain management
Complementary medicine	Physical therapy
Conflict management	Preventative medicine
Disaster medicine	Principles of education
End of life issues	Risk assessment for companion animals
Financial issues	Service and performance animals, special needs
Information management	Shelter medicine
Jurisprudence	Understanding attachment
Leadership and teamwork skills	Zoonoses

The Program for Veterinary Family Practice recognizes that the relationship between companion animals and humans has evolved dramatically. Pets are likely to be treated like a member of the human family, and that family is demanding more sophisticated medical and surgical care for the pet. The Program for Veterinary Family Practice is a resource for teaching veterinary students, veterinary practitioners, and veterinary staff the knowledge and skills necessary to nurture the bond between pet and owner and to enhance the well-being of both.

between knowing how to act and what to do in situations of complexity and high client need and actually doing it.

People bring their four-legged family members to veterinarians, counting on their professionalism. Because people entrust us with their companion animals, veterinarians have the increased obligation to understand attachment and acquire good communication skills. Contemporary practitioners must keep apace and assume a multidimensional role as family practice veterinarians (Timmons 2005). Use as a checklist the proficiency skills proposed for the formation of the Society for Family Practice Veterinarians (Table 8.1).

Many graduates leave veterinary school with few acquired skills in communication and practical wisdom. If only we could strip down the communication barriers between veterinarians and pet owners. Often, clients experience profound insensitivity on the telephone or at the front desk, when speaking to hospital personnel. A busy hospital receptionist may place a client phone call on terminal hold. Staff workers often fumble with medical record keeping, bungle record transfers, or overbook appointments. The brisk attitude of a receptionist or an officious office manager can extinguish a client's loyalty to his or her veterinarian's animal hospital. Rushed 10-minute office visits limit oral narratives and leave carers deprived of valuable practical wisdom and advice that they so desperately need. Much remains unsaid. Oftentimes, the client feels abandoned with no positive support to deal with their geriatric pet's advanced stage cancer or recurrence problem.

Ethics, Economics, and Empathy Issues

Bernard E. Rollin, PhD, is a University Distinguished Professor and Professor Emeritus of Philosophy and Bioethics at Colorado State University. He is a well-known animal bioethics speaker who has addressed many basic ethics issues. In his papers "Oncology and Ethics" (2003, Blackwell Verlag, Berlin) and "Euthanasia and Quality of Life" (2006), *Journal of the American Veterinary Medical*

Association, Rollin exposes and ponders the following insightful questions: "What are the animals' best interests? Given the nature of animal consciousness and mentation limits, it is above all else not suffering, we need to realistically assess what the animal is experiencing and not prolong life at all costs. The oncologist must be careful not to put the client's interest in prolonging life above terminating the animal's suffering. In addition, currently trendy talk in veterinary circles may seduce the veterinarian away from that ideal; to wit, the claim that veterinarians serve the human–animal bond. This, in my view, is wrong and dangerous, for it treats an abstraction as a reified (enforced) entity. Veterinarians serve the animal and must work through the client. They do not serve, in the end, *the bond*."

Rollin asks every veterinarian to decide his or her answer to what he calls the "Fundamental Question of Veterinary Ethics": "To whom does the veterinarian owe primary allegiance; owner or animal?" (2004c). We can layer more issues from the rapidly growing field of geriatric oncology into Rollin's basic ethical questions about practice, such as: Has the demand for geriatric companion animal care been raised higher than seasoned practitioners are prepared or willing to offer? Can we properly educate caregivers to make informed decisions for treating recurrent cancer in their geriatric pets? Can we trust caregivers to know or want what is best for their aging pet? Should the veterinarian bear the burden of animal advocate? Should the veterinarian become the shoulder and the counselor for distraught pet caregivers who would do anything to save their aging pet from cancer? What can we do for pet owners who are caught in "analysis paralysis" or religious or cultural factors and cannot make a decision? What do we do about deeply bonded clients who want to continue treatment despite the veterinarian's recommendation to stop?

In 2003, I had the pleasure of presenting case reports in lectures titled "Ethics, Empathy, and Economics" alongside Dr. Rollin at Midwest and AVMA conferences. He believes that veterinarians owe primary allegiance to the animal. We bantered back and forth in our presentations. In contrast to his statements, I expressed my beliefs that veterinarians who are in private companion animal practices all around the world do, in fact, serve the human–animal bond, that veterinarians owe their primary allegiance to the human–animal bond ("The Bond" is often the real reason we entered our profession to begin with), and that The Bond is what confers a tremendous societal and personal value on a particular pet patient.

The Bond does not diminish with a pet's age or medical history. On the contrary, clients have told me that The Bond with their pet grew stronger as they nurtured the aging pet during an illness and especially during treatment for cancer. Honoring the human–animal bond inherently includes reverence and respect for quality of life as a personal ethic and as an appreciated and highly valued social aesthetic.

It is exactly that unique entity (the human–animal bond) and the fear of losing The Bond that motivates people to seek care for their pets. The Bond drives pet carers into our hospitals. The Bond is the force that created the demand that elevated our medicine to today's high-tech level. Our personal and professional ethics should always serve the patient's needs while honoring the human–animal bond of the unique family attached to that animal. We must balance these needs when dealing with recurrence, relapse, or metastasis in our geriatric oncology patients.

An Inherent Conflict of Interest

Rollin and various esteemed colleagues asked haunting questions in a series of lively panel discussions at major professional meetings across the nation. Rollin insists that we ask ourselves these revealing questions about conflict of interest (Rollin 2004a).

Has the high-tech megapractice ascended into a new realm of economics and ethics? Do doctors in superpractices that have the megafacilities and rotating schedules make decisions that favor the pet or the pet owner? Or do they make decisions that favor their practice's financial interests and their own personal percentage of gross income as per payroll arrangements? Are we redrawing the line of pet advocacy in the emergency room? When do veterinarians need to exert their professional authority and become the advocate for their patients to avoid unnecessary suffering, prolongation of life, and expense?

Veterinarians must constantly juggle ethical, economic, and empathy issues in daily practice. Conflict of interest is inherent in running a business and practicing medicine. This conflict of interest is unavoidable in the decision-making process for geriatric oncology patients needing treatment or Pawspice care.

All veterinarians in private practice have an inherent conflict of interest. We are caught up in the financial web of a "pay for services rendered" profession. Every hospital displays a sign saying "Payments are due when services are rendered." Essentially, we tell our clients "Pay as you go."

Veterinarians are often saddled with large student loans and living expenses. They are also carrying their own personal or normative ethics, evidence-based medicine, scientific references, and the limitations of an in-house pharmacy. These factors can all influence decision making. In practice, associates are often asked to "hurry up" in exam rooms and accept a double-booking appointment schedule. The associate's performance and average client transaction (ACT) is tracked on the practice computer for percentage income and contract negotiations. These factors easily create a conflict of interest that affects patient care.

Conflict of interest emerges between you as the healer and you as the wage earner, entrepreneur, and/or researcher. If you are running late or feel fatigued, these issues drift in and out of focus. These deep personal conflicts of interest and biases exist and they must, consciously or subconsciously, heckle every practitioner at one time or another. Your biases, personal baggage, and pressures impact every decision you make and have the potential of steering your decision-making process on to the wrong course.

As the attending doctor, you will have to wade through these issues concerning personal ethics, practice philosophy, multilevel economics, and empathy. If the atmosphere in your clinic is rushed, the result will be a lot of dissatisfaction on both sides of the exam table.

Yet another conflict of interest issue that places a layer of professional disconnect between associates and their clients is that some associates feel resentment against their private or corporate employers who care only about "the bottom line." Many associates have trouble integrating their ideal personal ethics into the established practice philosophy. Practice owners and associates, feeling overbooked and overworked, often reprioritize their time in ways that diminish client relations and patient care.

How do these conflicts of interest affect patient care when associates and seasoned veterinarians encounter an emotionally and ethically charged consultation? It takes time to help relieve client confusion and emotions in the area of decision making. "In the 1980s, Dr. Marvin Samuelson showed that ethics decision making occupies the single largest portion of a practitioner's time, yet education in ethics is scarce in veterinary schools" (Rollin 2004b). The American College of Veterinary Surgeons considered medicoethical decision making as a keynote topic for their 2016 annual Surgical Summit. The main questions they wanted me to address were, When is it too much surgery? What to do when the "chance to cut or treat" and the "chance to care" diverge? How do we identify and implement the pivot from curative intervention to comfort care? What was originally going to be a one hour keynote evolved into a full day surgical ethics track (Clary 2016a, 2016b; Villalobos 2016a, 2016b, 2016c).

Schedule enough time to carefully discuss all of the available options. For patients with recurrence, give your original level of care and concern. For patients with advanced-stage or an aggressive cancer, offer a wide range of options and referral for consultation with the appropriate specialists. Consider the needs, the physiologic condition, and the personality of the pet along with the wishes and financial ability of the owner. If you fail to consider all of these issues, you diminish the special doctor–client relationship that has the potential to work wonders.

How Far Is Too Far?

Many generalists, including veterinarians from other countries and specialists from other fields, feel that American veterinary oncologists in particular may go too far in the management of cancer (Rollin 2005). This would hold true in cases of recurrent cancer in geriatric pets. They may have entrenched feelings that it is wrong or inappropriate to treat cancer in animals, particularly if the animal is geriatric or if the cancer is advanced or disseminated. Others feel that older pets are too fragile or do not have the life expectancy to justify cancer treatment as worthwhile. These doctors may also eschew radical surgical oncology procedures such as amputation, nosectomy, or mandibulectomy for healthy cancer patients. They may feel that these procedures are disfiguring or unfair to the pet, especially if the cancer patient is older.

Nosey's Case (Old Pets Are Treasured as the Road Gets Bumpy)

Nosey Summers, a $13^1/_2$-year-old English Cocker Spaniel, was referred for consultation for management of chondrosarcoma, which caused a large painful swelling of her right distal radius. Her comorbidities were chronic bilateral purulent otitis, chronic ocular discharge, cardiomegaly with bradycardia (HR 60 bpm), and hepatomegaly with mild elevations of liver enzymes and mild anemia with 1+ spherocytosis. Chest radiographs were negative for metastatic disease. Despite the guarded prognosis, the family elected disarticulation and no follow-up chemotherapy. Supportive therapy was provided pre- and perioperatively and Nosey recovered uneventfully. Later that year, Nosey was attacked by a coyote and rushed to an emergency clinic, which saved her life. Nosey lived happily until age $15^1/_2$ when she reportedly had a "stroke," which left her back legs paralyzed; however, it might have been due to unverified recurrence.

Some veterinarians openly express negativity about recommending chemotherapy and/or radiation therapy for their cancer patients. They may not know about technology such as SRS or electroporation that may help reduce tumors that are difficult to resect. A high percentage of these same doctors are also less likely to promote home care support or the end of life hospice philosophy. They might not offer SQ fluids, feeding tubes, immunonutrition, mobility carts, or Pawspice care, which embraces palliative cancer care, for geriatric cancer patients and their families who want to support their beloved pets and improve quality of life despite the cancer.

Patriarchal Practitioners

It is crucial that practitioners refrain from insisting, pushing, converting, or controlling their clients with only two choices, either aggressive care or euthanasia. This patriarchal approach is dictatorial and sends the message, "I am practicing 'My way or the highway' medicine." It is not surprising that pet owners flee from this style of practice.

Patriarchal veterinarians unwittingly impose their biases on their clientele, claiming that their approach to medicine is down to earth and practical. They tell the pet owner what to think and what to do rather than helping clients make their own decisions. They often use expressions such as, "You should let nature take its course" or "You need to put him out of his misery."

More progressive doctors have termed this approach as "minimalist medicine." A minimalist doctor may be surprised when a client goes to the Internet or to some other animal hospital for a second opinion, palliative care, or Pawspice care services. Increasingly, pet owners want to keep their terminal pets comfortable at home. They want sophisticated supportive care until their pet passes away naturally or via at-home euthanasia.

It is understandable but not excusable that doctors may have difficulty scheduling enough time to weigh the issues and discuss all the options with their clients. A very narrow scope of options is provided for treatment of advanced stage cancer or recurrence in the geriatric pet when the doctor is indifferent, overwhelmed, rushed, patriarchal, or has a negative personal bias against treating cancer. People are aware that they must be their pet's advocates. It is no wonder that many pet owners seek second and third opinions and consult the Internet and the alternative medicine field for a more inclusive and supportive set of options.

Framework for Decision Making

For a helpful framework for ethical decision making, refer to the modified steps outlined in Table 8.2. Use these considerations as a guide to help associates and clients make decisions. Always ensure that all parties, including you as the attending doctor, the hospital staff, and the family, must have consensus and comfort with the final decision. If there is disagreement, work to provide the family with more options, such as palliation or Pawspice care. There is no perfect choice, but the course taken should feel reasonably acceptable by those involved under the circumstances (McDonald 2003).

Recurrence Bodes an Upset Lifestyle

Caregivers want to protect and defend their pets in the battle against cancer and its related health issues. They want their veterinary care team to go on the offensive and help them declare war against the advanced cancer or go into round 2 against a relapse or recurrence.

If the pet is a service animal for a blind, disabled, or wheelchair-dependent person or epileptic, the caretaker's quality of life is threatened. Apart from the emotional loss that many people with service dogs suffer, loss of the dog equals a loss of the person's independence, freedom, and security. It often takes months to years for a disabled person to receive and establish a working relationship with a new service dog.

Pets that participate in showing or agility or are involved in community service activities, such as Pet Partners or other animal-assisted therapy, share intense social connections with their caretakers. Many of these companion animals have a large fan club of school children and nursing home and hospital patients and their staff. Naturally, no deeply bonded family wants to see their geriatric pet die from cancer.

When recurrence appears, caregivers conjure up great fear that they will lose their special treasured relationship and their connection to the shared activities that represent and encompass their bond. These same feelings occurred with the initial diagnosis and treatment but they recur with tremendous disappointment due to the more ominous threat of recurrence or relapse.

Table 8.2.   A Framework for Ethical Decision Making

1.1	Be alert and sensitive to emotionally charged situations.
1.2	Identify what you know and don't know.
1.3	Summarize and discuss the decisions that need to be made.
1.4	Consider the context and clinical issues of the case.
1.5	Consider the patient's medical history/diagnosis/prognosis.
1.6	Consider if the problem is acute, chronic, critical, reversible.
1.7	Consider the goals of treatment and probabilities of success.
1.8	Consider the patient's quality of life with or without treatment.
1.9	Consider the merit for comfort and palliative care.
2.1	Consider the religious and cultural beliefs of the pet owner.
2.2	Consider the owner's financial situation.
2.3	Consider consequences of various decisions as they affect the pet.
3.1	Use the basic principles of ethics to guide decision making.
3.2	Ask if you are being loyal to a business concern or clinical study.
3.3	Ask if you are respecting the patient and family's wishes.
3.4	Ask if you are treating the client paternalistically or otherwise.
3.5	Ask co-workers and colleagues for their opinion and advice.
3.6	Always respect client confidentiality.
4.1	Propose and test possible resolutions.
4.2	Find the best alternative for the patient, all things considered.
4.3	Consider the impact on others involved in the case.
4.4	Maintain trust with the client.
4.5	Determine if you and others are comfortable with the choice.
5.1	Make your choice and accept responsibility for it.
5.2	Learn from the process knowing there is no perfect choice.

Source: From an article by Michael McDonald adapted for the *Society of Veterinary Medical Ethics* (SVME) *Newsletter*, September 2003. For this text, Villalobos modified the table to make it more relevant for geriatric oncology patient decision making, with permission from McDonald (www.ethics.ubc.ca/upload/a framework for ethical decision-making-pdf/).

Deeply bonded caregivers often lapse into anticipatory grief. This intense type of grief is the fear of loss. Often the caregiver feels unsettled but does not realize why. Some clients hide their grief or feel disenfranchised because their friends do not understand the importance of the bond they share with their geriatric pet (Meyers 2000; Corbin 2004).

Elements of anticipatory grief underlie the commitment and are the driving force that creates the demand for and recent proliferation of high-tech veterinary facilities. Commitment is the motivating reason that the pet-owning community has created an increasing demand for more specialized and sophisticated medical and supportive services for their pets. This increasing demand includes improved primary cancer care and earlier diagnosis of cancer and its recurrence. It certainly includes thinking that veterinarians would have an open mind to treating advanced stage cancer and recurrent cancer in geriatric patients.

Anticipatory grief also drives an increasing demand on attending doctors for improved monitoring for treated geriatric cancer patients so that adverse events or relapse or recurrence may be detected at its earliest stage. It drives the growing interest in metronomic chemotherapy, chemoprevention and immunonutrition for at-risk patients. This segment (fear of separation) of the human–animal bond drives the senior and geriatric health care and wellness programs that are becoming so well promoted in contemporary practices. It also drives the demand for improved effectiveness in palliative care. This includes the Pawspice concept of providing combinatorial palliative cancer medicine with prioritization on quality of life and transitions to hospice services when the pet declines towards death. Very simply, people do not want their geriatric pets to die sooner than need be. It is up to the veterinarian to identify which of their clients want nothing less than state-of-the-art services for their geriatric pet in the face of advanced stage cancer or recurrence. It is equally incumbent upon clients to make the attending doctor aware of the intensity and depth of their bond and their commitment to monitor for and treat advanced cancer in their geriatric cancer pet.

A short life expectancy is not a good reason for the clinician to turn the carer away and evaporate ongoing veterinary services. The attending veterinarian assessed the client's level of interest in sophisticated services when the geriatric oncology patient was first diagnosed. Upon recurrence, we must reassess the client's level of intent for further cancer therapy, which would include palliative cancer medicine. We need to find out if they want to discontinue cancer treatment and pursue palliative care and hospice for their pet. This information must be discovered dispassionately, in a non-judgmental fashion, with no attempt to impose the attending veterinarian's preferences on the client.

When treating geriatric oncology patients of deeply bonded families, the attending clinician must determine the level of service that will satisfy the owner yet still provide comfort and alleviation of cancer pain for the pet. These ethical issues have to be handled very delicately.

Veterinarians encounter dramatic highs and lows of human emotions on a daily basis. The doctor who jumps in and out of exam rooms like a rabbit is not dealing with his or her client's emotions. Most veterinarians practicing today received no training in this area in veterinary school, and so they avoid or deflect clients' emotions.

Many graduates and specialists are highly focused on the disease and its statistics and forget to notice, acknowledge, or serve the patient–client entity. They may be super technicians but lack interactive skills in communication, collaboration, interrelationships, and the needs of society. They may lack the perspective to learn about and understand the whole patient's attaché of family and environmental issues. Good communication skills are needed for these intimate consultations.

The aging pet population parallels the aging of the human baby boomer population. People expect their pets to have a longer and healthier life. The public is asking for our help and expertise and they are willing to pay for it even when cancer recurs.

Cricket's Case (Agility Dog Ages with Good Coat and Heart Despite Recurrences)

Shirley Russell wanted a second opinion on a guarded prognosis. She presented Cricket, her 5.5-year old Hungarian Pumi agility star, who was diagnosed with metastatic apocrine carcinoma of unknown origin effacing her right inguinal lymph node. Shirley was advised to allow Adriamycin IV therapy for Cricket but she was very concerned about alopecia and cardiotoxicity, since Cricket was an athlete and loved to compete. Shirley did not want Cricket to be disadvantaged in her agility competition or lose her quality of life. The Pumi is very similar to the Poodle with a continuously growing hair coat and was expected to develop alopecia from Adriamycin. I comforted Shirley and offered to treat Cricket with mitoxantrone IV injections × 6 q 21 days. We would also put Cricket on metronomic Cytoxan and capecitabine (Xeloda^{TM}) for maintenance chemotherapy along with immunonutrition. Shirley was pleased to have another option.

Cricket developed recurrence twice. The first was 8 months out and the second was a year after that. Both tumors were removed and each yielded guarded prognosis. We followed each recurrence with mitoxantrone IV × 6. One year later, Cricket started slowing down due to metastasis to her sub lumbar nodes, which responded to another round of mitoxantrone and rehab therapy. Cricket never missed a show! It has been over 4 years as I proof in August 2017, and 9.5-year-old Cricket enjoys her senior agility competitions despite recurrences.

Aesculapian Authority

As a profession, we must be wary of unscrupulous veterinarians. Our crooks are few and far between, but every profession has a sociopath here and there. They prey on the human–animal bond at the expense of the pet's quality of life and the pet carer's pocket book.

We must always remain true to the Veterinarian's Oath and remain ethical when helping the geriatric oncology patient's family make decisions. Personal ethics tell us not to lie, not to steal, not to take advantage of people, to be charitable, and to "do the right thing" for aging pets and their people.

Society has conferred trust upon veterinarians and other professionals, including priests and psychiatrists, via the Aesculapian authority. Aesculapius was the god of healing in Roman mythology. Aesculapius's staff, with its entwining snake, is the caduceus used as a symbol for the healing arts. The Aesculapian (Asclepiad) authority allows doctors to examine and make decisions for their patients. Society views violations of the Aesculapian authority as a heinous and serious crime of betrayal (Rollin 2000).

Since veterinarians are only human, a personal bias may show up in the way one steers a consultation (Yeates, Main 2010). When advising a client, always ask yourself, "Might another clinician advise differently?" and "Would a second opinion disagree with the approach that I recommended?" If so, how? And why? And might they be right?

Perhaps we neglect to provide a referral for a second opinion out of fear that a referral would enter our client and their geriatric oncology pet into the mindless machinery of high-tech medicine, causing them to spend more money than we think they can afford. However, the family veterinarian should not feel obligated to be an advocate of the client's pocket book. Are we being the pet's advocates or are we just trying to keep the client's business at our own hospital? Ask yourself these questions. Always examine and evaluate the methods you use. Look at the real reasons why you persuade clients to make decisions for or against caring for an aging pet's malignancies.

Rethinking Advanced Stage Cancer, Recurrence, and Age

I am in awe of the human–animal bond that ties a family to this particular dog or that special cat. This awe drives my philosophy in caring for geriatric cancer patients and dealing compassionately when they are challenged with advanced stage cancer or recurrence. As pets get older, *the bond* grows stronger. Pet lovers have a sincere longing to preserve their pet's life even in the face of recurrence, if the patient's quality of life can be maintained.

Geriatric patients are often denied conventional cancer care because of their perceived age rather than their physiologic age. This happens in human medicine as well. Geriatric patients are underrepresented in clinical trials. They are routinely excluded from studies due to comorbidities and short life expectancy. There is no doubt that our profession has discriminated against aging pets and withheld cancer care simply because they are old.

Treating geriatric oncology patients for a primary cancer is complex and more challenging than in non-geriatric patients because of the common coexistence of other chronic conditions. At recurrence, each concurrent problem needs to be reevaluated and compared to the patient's previous history. Any significant change deserves the full attention of the attending doctor. Testing for symmetrical dimethyl-larginine (SMDA) reveals chronic kidney disease (CKD) earlier than creatinine in thin hyperthyroid cats and older dogs (Relford 2016). Abdominal CT performed in older dogs with cancer reveals a prevalence rate of 15.9% for incidental adrenal gland masses (Baum, Boston, and Case (2016). Early and incidental comorbidities may or may not affect decision making.

There may be residual consequences from the previous cancer treatment. A reasonable treatment goal would be to provide at least a 50% alleviation of each unmanaged concurrent problem if definitive therapy is elected. Pay attention to all the conditions acquired over the lifetime of the geriatric patient with recurrent cancer to help that patient maintain a good quality of life.

We expect that recurrence, metastasis, concurrent disease, and/or organ failure will be progressive. Nevertheless, it is time to rethink how veterinarians can step up and partner with their deeply bonded clients to help them face these gripping issues and make their own choices. Are we going to help geriatric pets fight against advanced stage and recurrent cancer or will we abdicate without offering supportive care?

Many clients simply want support, basic advice, and training in end of life nursing and hospice care. Some of my clients have expressed that when they chose not to take the "high road" course of action recommended, their doctor became frustrated with them and lost interest in their pet. Many carers are told that conventional medicine cannot help their pet's situation but they are not offered Pawspice or hospice services. When told that nothing can be done, carers often leave the clinic and seek out other nurturing options such as palliation or complementary and alternative care.

Dilemmas During Decision Making

The acute hemoabdomen dog or the old cat with an abdominal mass presents a decision-making dilemma for all involved on both sides of the exam table. Veterinarians see animals of various species, breeds, and ages that may be diagnosed at advanced stages of disease and with diseases that have fatal agendas. The veterinary client embraces various personality types, nationalities, and religions, spanning every age group from children to millennials to baby boomers. Our clients' willingness and/or ability to pay for veterinary services will range from minimal to infinite. With all these factors weighing in, there is little wonder that decision making can take a great deal of time. Since more companion animals are aging, their attending veterinarians will encounter more geriatric disease, comorbidities, and cancer. The challenge of dealing with these comorbidities and the impact of cancer treatment will thrust veterinarians into the eye of an emotional whirlwind full of hasty deliberations and decision making.

General practitioners and specialists are increasingly interacting and collaborating with other specialists in the decision-making process for patients in their practice. What can generalists do to partner with their recession-battered clients and the "can do" specialists in a decision-making process that may involve end of life care? What can veterinarians do to make the right decision for each individual patient at the end of their life and ultimately prevent the frustration of under treatment or the regret of over treatment?

Because America is a youth-oriented culture, doctors are reluctant to talk about death and dying with their human patients. Most people suffering from terminal disease prefer to keep their hopes up and continue challenging their disease and their cancer as warriors, without ever giving up. Often the life of a terminally ill person ends with a horrible quality of life, and more pain and suffering than if they had entered palliative hospice care at the time of diagnosis. Studies show that advanced lung cancer patients receiving palliative care lived 3 months longer than those who chose standard care at the end of life (Temel 2010).

The Veterinarian's Role in Decision Making

Take the time to properly research and think about a geriatric oncology case and all of the unique features that may positively or negatively influence the patient's survival. Take the time to educate the client about the issues and the options in early, middle, and late stage recurrent cancer. Sadly, veterinary students are ill prepared to face these consultations and ethical issues when confronted by them in practice. Training is seldom provided and, when provided, it is often by unqualified personnel and delivered on the fly as an afterthought, in hallways or between exam room visits.

The issues of ethics, grief, and attachment education are generally not given formal curriculum time in veterinary colleges. Drills designed to teach students how to assist clients in decision making would prepare students to address clients properly, look them in the eye, answer their questions thoughtfully, communicate clearly, and get their point across in layman's language (Milani 2001).

Some pet owners have confided that they felt completely misunderstood by their attending veterinarian or specialist. They felt their doctors had an indifferent, "take it or leave it" attitude. One couple reported that their veterinarian proposed a difficult radiation therapy protocol for their dog and then rattled off statistics and percentages, but never listened to them or answered their questions and concerns about their aging pet's colitis and nervous personality.

Tiara's Case (Treat Clients as Decision-Making Partners)

Tiara, an 8-year-old, 100 pound, F/S German Shepherd Dog, had bilateral tonsillar squamous cell carcinoma and early degenerative myelopathy. The family knew the prognosis was poor from a previous oncology consultation. Tiara was very aggressive in the exam room, lunging and barking at us.

After our consultation, the client thanked me for discussing ways to deal with Tiara's obstreperous personality and for offering potential treatment options. She also thanked me for treating her as an intelligent person capable of making her own decision. Then she told me that she had battled breast cancer and that she was insulted when her own Los Angeles-based oncologist "talked over" her. After an evaluation, he spoke directly to her husband about her options without addressing her! She immediately changed oncologists and flew up to Stanford every 3 weeks for her treatments.

Because we showed no fear or dislike of Tiara for her aggressiveness, the family wanted us to treat her despite the poor prognosis. She was more than happy to sign an informed consent statement. Her signature verified the family's full awareness of the poor prognosis for Tiara, and their desire to provide treatment regardless.

Tiara received radiation therapy to both tonsils with concurrent mitoxantrone chemotherapy. This combination has a synergistic effect with radiation therapy against squamous cell carcinoma (SCC). We won excellent local control for more than 8 months. The SCC recurred in Tiara's trachea as a 2.5cm mass located 7cm caudal to her larynx. We suspected a poorly defined retropharyngeal mass as well. The family deliberated and decided that they felt very satisfied with the extra high-quality time that they had already gained. During her remission, Tiara's concurrent degenerative myelopathy became a mobility and incontinence problem. The family elected to provide Pawspice and hospice care for Tiara until her time came.

Veterinarians are expected to maintain the geriatric oncology patient's well-being, especially in the face of advanced stage cancer or recurrence. We are obligated to guard against unrecognized and unnecessary suffering in all of our cancer patients. We also have a social responsibility to ease the emotional pain of the pet's family members.

Clients are very needy during these difficult days of decision making. At the same time, they still have to go to work, perform their family obligations, and care for their ailing geriatric companion animal. We must ensure that the geriatric oncology patient's needs are met. Pain control and comfort must be the client's primary focus. To determine a pet's quality of life, carers may find it helpful to use the HHHHHMM Quality of Life Scale. The acronym stands for no Hurt, no Hunger, no Hydration problems, good Hygiene and Happiness, Mobility, and More good days than bad days (see Table 10.1).

The companion animal community needs its veterinarians to be aware of and deal effectively with the internal torment of decision making. Pet owners may experience a heart-wrenching ordeal and go into grief right in the doctor's office. They feel an acute emotional wound when they get the bad news that their geriatric oncology pet has "mets" (metastases) in the chest. The client projects the ravages of cancer as a threat to their pet and to their special human–animal bond. They are projecting nothing but heartbreak ahead.

The veterinarian needs to be aware that the client may not be rational during the appointment. The client may disconnect from reality and be in a daze. This complicates the tasks of educating the client and assisting with decision making. It stresses the relationship between the veterinarian and client.

Stress and confusion between veterinarian and client have a negative effect on the geriatric patient. The cancer progresses and the pet's health may decline during the time required for the client to seek other opinions. The best decision is to help the pet owner enter their pet into some level of defined care. That care may be to repeat another cycle of chemotherapy or another surgery or palliative radiation therapy, or to enter an end of life Pawspice care program. Pawspice embraces kinder, gentler palliative cancer medicine such as metronomic chemotherapy, immunonutrition, and chemoprevention. Pawspice simultaneously offers palliative medicine and transitions to hospice (comfort care) when the pet declines toward death.

Expect Recurrence and Look for It

A good strategy for dealing with recurrence is to have an active surveillance program for all cancer patients at risk. Upon achieving remission, I tell clients that we want to do everything we can to offset recurrence. We also tell them approximately when the literature warns to expect recurrence or metastatic disease. For example, when a cat or dog with hemangiosarcoma or osteosarcoma survives 4 months without signs of recurrence, we congratulate the client and celebrate the winning of extra quality time for their pet in the battle against cancer. At every recheck that yields clean radiographs and ultrasounds, I remind the clients that they have scored another run in the ninth inning and we are going into overtime. We congratulate the family for their success and celebrate the value and meaning of each "clean met check" (no metastasis). These are the joyful moments in oncology.

Ideally, when dealing with recurrence or relapse in a geriatric cancer patient, we would employ the basic principles of diagnosis and staging as outlined in Chapter 5. It is imperative to assess the patient's previous and recently acquired concurrent conditions. Define how these conditions will influence the patient's tolerance to rescue or salvage therapy. Take a fresh look at the geriatric oncology patient's current laboratory work, radiographs, and stage of disease and compare these data to the previous database.

Advanced stage cancer or recurrence may acutely impact the geriatric pet's function and create an emergency situation. The pet is often rushed to an emergency facility for stabilization and workup.

Many geriatric oncology patients are euthanized in emergency rooms due to acute manifestations of advanced stage cancer or recurrent cancer. Others are stabilized overnight so that the family can consult the pet's primary care veterinarian or oncologist about further evaluation and decision making. All of this causes the carers great distress and panic. They will look to you for help and wisdom in the decision-making process.

Make a complete set of radiographs to look for metastases in three views of the chest and two views of the abdomen. Evaluate organ function tests and urine analysis. Assess the patient's body condition (Figure 8.1). Document the geriatric cancer patient's basic performance level assessment. Further imaging with abdominal and/or thoracic ultrasound may be helpful to detect metastases. FNA cytology or Tru-cut tissue samples may confirm the diagnosis without more invasive techniques. Attempt to restage the geriatric oncology patient using the TNM scale discussed in Chapter 5 (Table 5.2).

Many geriatric patients with advanced or recurrent disease require further imaging under anesthesia for complete evaluation and staging. Before recommending any diagnostic test, determine the risk-to-benefit ratio of the test. How useful will the results be? How well do you expect the geriatric patient to tolerate the sedation or anesthesia required for additional diagnostic tests, such as CT, MRI, interventional radiography, or direct visualization with fiber optic scopes? If the test results will be useful for decision making, then the risk of general anesthesia for diagnostic procedures may be justified.

Physical Performance Assessment

Most veterinarians do not use scales such as the Karnofsky Performance Scale to evaluate their geriatric patients. It is time consuming, requires special equipment, and would have to be repeated periodically to gain value as a clinical tool for monitoring treatment success. The Modified Karnofsky Performance Scale measures patient activity from 0–4. In this scale, 0 is normal activity; 1 is acceptable function; 2 is compromised but able to eat, sleep, and eliminate properly (Activities of Daily Living (ADL)); 3 is disabled, anorectic, incontinent, or unable to get up to eliminate in acceptable areas; and 4 is moribund or deceased (Morrison 2002a).

We seldom conduct formal performance tests on geriatric cancer patients. However, we should discuss the patient's physical ability with the family and use their comments to document a basic performance assessment. Using terms such as slightly, moderately, or severely compromised with low, medium, or good levels of performance are adequate for performance assessments. We can also use a 0–10 scale for mobility assessment using the HHHHHMM Quality of Life Scale (see Table 10.1).

In human medicine, there is a simple test called "Get up and go" that is used to assess performance. If a person needs to use the arms of a chair to get up, and if he or she has dyspnea or trouble walking across a room, that individual is considered to be at a low performance level and this is associated with a poor prognosis (Balducci and Beghe 2004). This simple determination test applies to veterinary geriatric oncology patients as well. If a pet struggles to stand from a laying position and if the pet has dyspnea or trouble walking to designated areas for elimination, we can consider that pet to be at a low performance level.

Frailty, Sarcopenia, Aging, and Cachexia

The attending doctor should also determine if the recurrent geriatric cancer patient is frail or cachectic. Frailty is more often a chronic condition and related to sarcopenia, whereas cachexia is cancer related

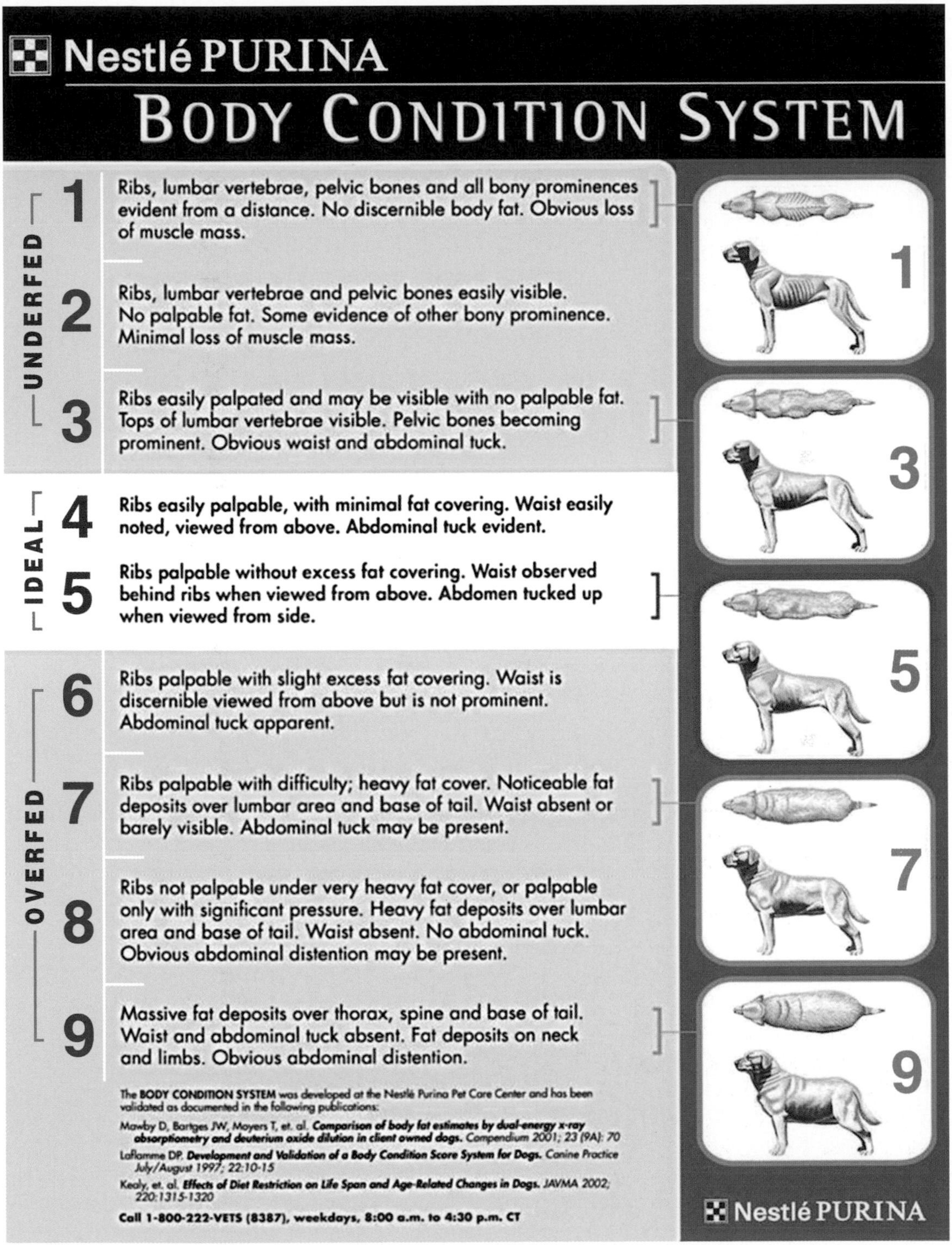

◫ Nestlé PURINA
BODY CONDITION SYSTEM

UNDERFED

1 Ribs, lumbar vertebrae, pelvic bones and all bony prominences evident from a distance. No discernible body fat. Obvious loss of muscle mass.

2 Ribs, lumbar vertebrae and pelvic bones easily visible. No palpable fat. Some evidence of other bony prominence. Minimal loss of muscle mass.

3 Ribs easily palpated and may be visible with no palpable fat. Tops of lumbar vertebrae visible. Pelvic bones becoming prominent. Obvious waist and abdominal tuck.

IDEAL

4 Ribs easily palpable, with minimal fat covering. Waist easily noted, viewed from above. Abdominal tuck evident.

5 Ribs palpable without excess fat covering. Waist observed behind ribs when viewed from above. Abdomen tucked up when viewed from side.

OVERFED

6 Ribs palpable with slight excess fat covering. Waist is discernible viewed from above but is not prominent. Abdominal tuck apparent.

7 Ribs palpable with difficulty; heavy fat cover. Noticeable fat deposits over lumbar area and base of tail. Waist absent or barely visible. Abdominal tuck may be present.

8 Ribs not palpable under very heavy fat cover, or palpable only with significant pressure. Heavy fat deposits over lumbar area and base of tail. Waist absent. No abdominal tuck. Obvious abdominal distention may be present.

9 Massive fat deposits over thorax, spine and base of tail. Waist and abdominal tuck absent. Fat deposits on neck and limbs. Obvious abdominal distention.

The BODY CONDITION SYSTEM was developed at the Nestlé Purina Pet Care Center and has been validated as documented in the following publications:

Mawby D, Bartges JW, Moyers T, et. al. *Comparison of body fat estimates by dual-energy x-ray absorptiometry and deuterium oxide dilution in client owned dogs.* Compendium 2001; 23 (9A): 70

Laflamme DP. *Development and Validation of a Body Condition Score System for Dogs.* Canine Practice July/August 1997; 22:10-15

Kealy, et. al. *Effects of Diet Restriction on Life Span and Age-Related Changes in Dogs.* JAVMA 2002; 220:1315-1320

Call 1-800-222-VETS (8387), weekdays, 8:00 a.m. to 4:30 p.m. CT

◫ Nestlé PURINA

Figure 8.1. Body Condition System chart for dogs. Reprinted courtesy of Nestle Purina PetCare. See www.purina.com/cats/health/BodyCondition.aspx for the chart for cats.

(Repetto, Venturino, and Gianni 2004). Frail and cachectic patients have little functional reserve and are not able to endure additional stress of surgery or chemotherapy without supportive care to counterbalance their condition.

We can assess biological aging by assessing the concept of frailty in our geriatric patients. Frailty is a biological syndrome demonstrating decreased reserves, an increase in vulnerability to stress, and the dysregulation of multiple physiologic systems. Frail dogs and cats are generally thin with sarcopenia, weak, prone to falling, and require careful attention. Large frail dogs often need burdensome care. The frailer a geriatric patient is found to be at the time of diagnosis of cancer, the less likely that patient will have a long term survival.

A very interesting article in *AJVR* titled "Assessment of frailty in aged dogs" described five core components of frailty: (1) sarcopenia, (2) exhaustion or exercise intolerance, (3) low activity, (4) poor mobility or gait, and (5) weakness. The study followed 116 aged guide dogs in France until death. If a geriatric dog had two or more core signs of frailty, they were at greater risk for death. The concept of evaluating frailty may help in decision making because if a dog has two or more core signs for frailty, it may indicate a worse prognosis (Hua et al. 2016).

There is tremendous interest in treatments that can safely delay the signs of aging. The Dog Aging Project is conducting a long term, large-scale study on rapamycin intervention in aging dogs to evaluate potential benefits. This study is intended to last 3–5 years and will monitor cognitive function, cardiac function, immunity, and cancer incidence. It would be ideal if this study could establish a matching cohort of dogs like the 116 French guide dogs and compare the data. It would be impressive if the study generated reliable prolongevity data about rapamycin intervention in aged dogs like the French guide dog group (mostly 9-year-old Labs and Golden Retrievers). It would be very interesting to see data using metformin together with rapamycin.

The first FDA approved drug to stimulate appetite in dogs is capromorelin (Entyce™) oral solution. It mimics the hunger-signaling hormone ghrelin and it binds to receptors that affect appetite signaling in the hypothalamus (Zollers et al. 2016). Ghrelin also affects the release of growth hormone and may help in weight gain.

Be sure to document the geriatric patient's physical appearance, body score, mentation, and physical performance in the medical record. These observations have a bearing on treatment selection and outcome. Immunonutrition, rehabilitation techniques, and age delay intervention therapies may help in decision making, treatment, care, and maintenance of frail geriatric cancer patients.

Dealing with Anemia and Chronic DIC

The presence of anemia is a major factor affecting the overall prognosis of geriatric oncology cases in human and veterinary medicine. Aging patients have reduced hematopoietic capabilities that are further stressed by the progression of cancer. Surgery, radiation, chemotherapy-associated anemia, and reduced helper T-cells (CD4 cells) aggravate an aging hematopoietic deficiency (Morrison 2002b). Anemia serves as a marker for recurrence in hemangiosarcoma patients. Disseminated intravascular coagulation (DIC), or consumptive coagulopathy, is associated with a number of diseases and cancer. DIC (particularly the acute form) is more common in dogs than in cats. Excessive activation of the coagulation cascade causes thromboses, ischemia, fibrinolysis, and paradoxical bleeding. If it is diagnosed and treated properly, up to 30–50% of patients may survive DIC (Couto and Moreno 2013).

Transfusions and/or hematopoietic growth factor therapy may be helpful to maintain the geriatric cancer patient's hematocrit at a level between 24% and 30%. Erythropoietin and its long acting analog, darbepoetin alfa, acts on late stage red blood cell precursors. As the precursor population is exhausted or the patient produces antibodies against it, the stimulatory effect of the growth factors runs out. Darbopoetin is worth using because it may increase the quality of life, especially for patients with anemia from chronic kidney disease or chemotherapy-associated anemia (Rowe and Avivi 2004). Clinicians may utilize new therapeutic developments in this field such as species specific erythropoietin or T-Cyte®, a thymic protein for SQ injection, which restores helper T-cells that may secondarily have hematinic effects in cats (Beardsley 2005).

Recurrent or highly metastatic tumors such as hemangiosarcoma are often diagnosed at advanced stages. Patients generally have anemia, thrombocytopenia, thrombosis, and coagulopathy. They may have sub-clinical peracute, acute, or chronic DIC. The prognosis for recovery with treatment is grim (Thomason, Calvert, and Green 2005). An early detection test for hemangiosarcoma was described at the 1016 World Veterinary Cancer Congress, which will detect circulating cancer stem cells (hemangioblasts). A novel toxin-based therapy (e-BAT), which selectively kills hemangioblasts, should soon be available for therapy and prevention of hemangiosarcoma in dogs (Modiano 2016).

Other Geriatric Syndromes

The attending doctor needs to probe the patient and ask questions to determine if the geriatric oncology patient has age-related syndromes such as: osteoarthritis, organ disease, cognitive disorders, mentation disorders, degenerative neuropathies, incontinence, hearing loss, visual deficits, depression, anxiety, and so forth. The family's ability to manage and/or tolerate pre-existing geriatric syndromes in their aging pet may create decision-making issues regarding treatment for advanced stage or recurrent cancer.

Diagnosing Recurrent Cancer

When dealing with the local recurrence of solid tumors or relapsing lymphoma, we first want to confirm the diagnosis with FNA cytology, incisional punch biopsy, or Tru-cut biopsy. For lymphoma, insert a 22-gauge needle into at least two lymph nodes using the standard non-aspiration technique. FNA is an excellent and reliable diagnostic tool if the primary mass is an exfoliative type of tumor such as mast cell tumor or lymphoma.

Routine FNA techniques will not confirm the diagnosis of recurrent sarcomas. To overcome this problem, we use a modified, more aggressive version of FNA. Insert an 18-gauge needle and angle it to chop off a core of tissue, then aspirate. Expel the tissue sample on to a slide and make smears for microscopic examination. This technique is described in detail in Chapter 5.

It is likely that thousands of primary and recurrent local sarcomas go undiagnosed because the attending doctor accepts a negative FNA report from a non-exfoliative tumor.

If only every graduate could have "situated knowledge" from the start. Situated knowledge is subjective knowledge drawn from practical experience of dealing with clients and patients. This knowledge is the missing piece or the gap in knowledge acquired in the classroom. It exists as practical wisdom, intuition, or good clinical judgment. The clinician must have it in order to do a good job, but there is no way to study it.

The attending doctor needs to approach each and every case using practical wisdom and commonsense. Practical wisdom and good clinical judgment are virtues that have much to do with on-the-spot decision making and can be studied and learned only by reviewing cases (Floersch 2002).

The attending doctor needs to distinguish each case using practical wisdom or "situated knowledge." If we suspect recurrence of a sarcoma, textbook knowledge tells us that they are non-exfoliative, but situated knowledge (from experience) tells us not to rely on simple FNA for diagnosis. Situated knowledge tells us to use the angle and chop FNA or a Tru-Cut.

This same situation occurs with vascular tumors such as hemangiopericytoma or hemangiosarcoma when the clinician attempts simple FNA and aspirates only blood. Practical knowledge tells us to look at the sample before sending it to the lab. The fact that only blood was aspirated from the mass indicates that you are dealing with a vascular tumor. Instead of wasting the client's time and money with a useless FNA, suggest the next diagnostic step. Confidently inform the client that you have a high index of suspicion that this particular mass may be a vascular tumor and that it needs tissue for biopsy and laboratory confirmation. The client will authorize the biopsy if a definitive diagnosis is needed for decision making.

Doobie's Case (Listen to Intuitive Carers)

I accepted an out-of-state phone consultation regarding an $11\frac{1}{2}$-year-old F/S Golden Retriever diagnosed with chondrosarcoma (CSA) on the skull. The owner discovered the primary mass. An initial FNA was negative for cancer cells. Doobie's owner intuitively insisted upon surgical removal. The mass was 3–4 mm in size and, according to the histopathology report, was completely removed. The family drove 5 hours to a university for consultation about treatment options. Three options were given: (1) tumor bed excision for wider, deeper margins, (2) radiation therapy, or (3) follow-up with monthly chest X-rays and abdominal ultrasound. The family selected option 3 and took Doobie dutifully for tests every month for the following 6 months.

At 3 months, the owner felt a thickening near the primary site. An attending clinician suggested FNA. Once again, the cytology report was negative with no significant cells. Doobie was given a clean bill of health at her 6-month recheck. The client asked about the swelling, which seemed to her to be larger. The oncologist looked at the record, cited the negative results of the previous FNA, and said that the results were not significant.

One week later, Doobie had a seizure. A neurologist ordered an MRI. The study identified a brain tumor and a large nasal tumor. The attending clinicians pondered whether Doobie's tumors were new or related to the original CSA. They all agreed that it would have been reasonable to follow up Doobie's case with CT or MRI of the skull at one of the monthly rechecks. The primary mass was located on her head and the intuitive owner had pointed out a new mass effect in the area of the primary tumor. The clinicians agreed that relying on FNA for diagnosis of non-exfoliating sarcomas such as chondrosarcoma could fail to rule out the presence or absence of malignant cells. Everyone on this case learned and gained experience and they all gained much more respect for the carer's intuition.

Using Technology for Monitoring Recurrent Cancer

The best way to deal with recurrence is to always be looking for it. Routine physical examinations, blood work, and imaging of the geriatric oncology patient all become an essential part of the treatment and follow-up protocol. Teach the client how to palpate all of the pet's lymph nodes and carefully examine the primary tumor site. This type of hands-on monitoring for recurrence can be called "tumor watch."

We can recruit clients to partner with us, so they will remind us to perform the specific exam that their pet needs at each recheck. Ask the clients to remind you to perform rectal exams on a monthly basis for their dog with excised anal sac tumors, for example. Ask the family whose pet has an abdominal mass to remind you about the follow-up radiographs or ultrasound for "met (metastasis) checks." Ask them to measure the pet's girth once a week at home, to monitor for abdominal distension. When the clients are in partnership with the tumor-watch monitoring program, they benefit emotionally as participants rather than remote spectators in the effort to save their pet. Enlist them to prompt you to stick to the recheck schedule and do your detective work.

Ultrasound is very useful for monitoring for recurrence of abdominal tumors, for monitoring bladder tumors, and to guide FNA or Tru-cut biopsy needles into organs and accessible masses. It is also helpful to monitor recurrent pleural effusions and to guide small gauge FNA needles into peripherally located thoracic cavity masses. FNA or Tru-cut samples may fall short of confirming the diagnosis, especially in the liver, due to lack of stroma, tumor heterogeneity, necrosis, and inflammation. It is good practice to look at the FNA cells immediately. If the sample does not contain representative cells, repeat the FNA procedure until you get a worthy sample (see Chapter 5).

There is a tendency toward overreliance on negative cytology reports. Consider FNA as a screening tool and depend on histopathology for the definitive diagnosis. When monitoring for recurrence, however, FNA results may fit the case history, yielding round cells or spindle cells that resemble the primary tumor.

There is good rationale to perform a second-look laparotomy (SLL) and surgical biopsy to accurately and definitively diagnose residual or recurrent tumor(s). Exploratory celiotomy is often the only sure way to definitively diagnose some cases of hepatic neoplasia and low-volume infiltrative GI lymphomas in cats. Mortality rates range from 17% to 27% and complication rates run from 16% to 30% for cancer patients surviving a first-time exploratory (Tobias 2005). However, these mortality statistics would be expected to be much greater when dealing with recurrence in geriatric oncology patients. It is reasonable to consider SLL as part of the monitoring program to evaluate the progress of treated primary or metastatic abdominal tumors, especially when secondary cytoreduction may be helpful (Stanclift and Gilson 2004).

The same residual disease monitoring consideration can be applied for patients with nasal passage cancer. MRI is used at routine checkpoints to locate residual or recurrent disease following radiation therapy (Henderson 2005).

A second-look endoscopy can be very helpful for viewing and sampling treated GI tract, respiratory tract, and bladder tumors. Laparoscopy and thoracoscopy can be used to visualize and diagnose metastatic and recurrent cancer. Follow-up imaging with ultrasound, CT, MRI, and PET is important. The newer imaging machines are faster, requiring only mild restraint or light sedation for compliant patients. Radiopharmaceuticals may be used to detect for occult cancer and recurrent tumors at early stages.

Routine ultrasound screening of the spleen every 6 months is reasonable for older dog breeds predisposed to hemangiosarcoma until "liquid biopsy" screening tests become available. This might detect tumors before rupture. Frequent tumor watch rechecks looking for expected metastatic or recurrent lesions may benefit cancer patients. It is hoped that earlier intervention could increase survival time.

It would be ideal to have a non-invasive, simple, inexpensive, and accurate test to detect early recurrent cancer in veterinary patients. The "Liquid Biopsy" via serology may reliably detect biological tumor markers. New tests will be proposed where a proteomic analysis can be completed with a 3–7 day turnaround. New screening tests such as one that detects circulating endothelial precursor cells (EPCs) may identify dogs at risk for hemangiosarcoma at sub-clinical stages (Modiano and Helfand 2005; Modiano 2016). Ask your laboratory's oncologist about these tests. Ask your consulting clinical oncologist. While one may be selling the test, the other may be trying to interpret the results and validate its clinical usefulness. Go online with Veterinary Information Network (VIN) chatrooms to learn if new serology tests are reliable and available to detect lymphoma, hemangiosarcoma, sarcoma, and carcinoma in dogs and cats. False positives are problematic and can cause a lot of distress and overscreening, overdiagnosis, and overtreatment, which are very common in the human medical field (Gawande 2014).

If the cancer patient's original tumor was associated with paraneoplastic hypercalcemia, a rise in the serum calcium level may serve as an inexpensive marker. This would apply most often for T-cell lymphoma, anal sac adenocarcinoma, and some miscellaneous tumors. Elevations in serum alkaline phosphatase levels may indicate metastatic lesions involving the liver and bone. This is associated with a poor prognosis in dogs with primary or metastatic osteosarcoma. Anemia and cancer cachexia-related weight loss would also indicate recurrence.

Advanced Stage and Relapsing Lymphoma

The most common recurrent cancer in our practice is relapsing lymphoma. Our typical relapsing lymphoma patients are older dogs that were in remission for over 1 year and dogs that come out of remission shortly after their induction. Decision making might be automatic to repeat the induction protocol again or the decision may be very difficult for the family due to financial constraints. This requires adjustment of the protocol to fit the family's budget and resourceful planning to achieve and maintain another remission.

The most common advanced stage cancer patients in our practice are dogs that present with advanced multicentric highgrade lymphoma. The clinician can request immunophenotyping of the patient's lymphoma for prognosis using special stains, flow cytometry, and PCR cloning. T-cell lymphomas are more resistant than B-cell lymphomas. One study found T-cell lymphomas to be more prevalent in Boxers (82%), followed by Rottweilers (68%) and Golden Retrievers (50%) (Lurie et al. 2004). The *Journal of Veterinary and Comparative Oncology*, Vol. 14, Supplement 1, is a special issue devoted to lymphoma in dogs and cats. This issue focused on characterization, understanding molecular events, and therapeutic strategies, such as the use of species-specific monoclonal antibodies and precision medicine to improve treatment outcomes in lymphoma.

Oncology clients need to know when to expect a relapse. We teach our lymphoma clients to check all of the patient's lymph nodes at least twice a week. We teach our feline lymphoma clients to be alert for warning signs of recurrence and to palpate the abdomen of their cats for recurrence. We want our clients to be alert and to detect relapse early on, before the tumor volume increases to an advanced stage.

Consultation for a relapsed lymphoma could go like this: "Bella's first remission has ended. It does not mean that she will die right now or very soon. We do know that the duration of the second remission is generally half of the first remission and the third remission is half of the second. Therefore, we will probably gain 6 months in this second remission since her first remission lasted 1 year. Bella has a good chance of achieving a second remission and she should feel well during her second remission. We must warn you that Bella could experience side effects to the reinduction protocol. Remember, we cautioned you about this possibility during her first induction protocol. Our plan is to start week 1 all over again and go from there for 6 weeks as before. Please look at your old treatment calendars to refresh your memory. How do you feel about starting week 1 over again? Can you bring Bella back for a CBC and chemotherapy in 2 weeks? Will you be able to afford this round of treatment?"

Generally, the family wants to try for another remission and consents to start the reinduction proto-col. In most cases, the second phase protocol duplicates the original protocol. The reinduction protocol should be modified if the geriatric patient had an adverse reaction to Adriamycin or vincristine dur-ing the previous induction. If Adriamycin was used as a single agent, the patient may be approaching the total cumulative dose range for Adriamycin ($280mg/m^2$). The patient may have developed heart disease, renal disease, or some other concurrent illness over the past year, which would increase the risk for side effects.

Rabacfosadine (Tanovea™) is a new double prodrug of the acyclic nucleotide phosphonate PMEG. It preferentially targets lymphoma cells with reduced systemic toxicity. It can be given IV over a 30-minute infusion at 1.0mg/kg for recurrent or resistant lymphoma or it can be used as a first-line chemotherapy agent (Vickery et al. 2016).

We routinely use metformin to reduce resistance to chemotherapy with its action to suppress mul-tidrug resistance genes. Most of the time, we settle for using other types of chemotherapy drugs for rescue or as palliative options. Patients may achieve a stable, partial, or complete remission that may last another 2–6 months. The most important goal is to maintain quality of life, avoid toxicity, and comfort the family during this round of chemotherapy.

When decision making for advanced stage first-time lymphoma cases, caregivers need consultation about the increased risk of tumor lysis syndrome, infections, and morbidity. Use the standard induc-tion protocols but administer the drugs over a 3–4-day period along with IV fluids, antibiotics, intense monitoring, nutritional support, and so forth, as described in the "Chemotherapy in the Management of Geriatric Cancer" section of Chapter 6.

Resistant Lymphoma

Decision making for geriatric patients with resistant lymphoma can be very challenging. The pri-mary treatment goals are to avoid adverse events, while trying for another remission, a stabilized partial remission, slow down progression of disease, and maintain quality of life. Multidrug resis-tance (MDR) is our biggest drawback. Metformin may be introduced early in the protocol to offset MDR activity but it is not known if it will help longevity if it is started after the patient develops resistant lymphoma. Diffusion gradients for drugs are variable in the interstitial matrix and extracel-lular microenvironment of lymphoma tissue. Drug concentration may be minimal in hypoxic under-perfused areas of the tumor. There are many valid reasons to abandon or alter standard reinduction protocols. The weary pet owner may not have the determination or the financial means to support another rescue protocol.

There are several useful single rescue drugs such as L-asparaginase given every 2–3 weeks, Adri-amycin rescue every 2–3 weeks (if appropriate), metronomic lomustine at $4mg/m^2$ daily, or lomustine at $40mg/m^2$ given on days 1 and 5 every 21 days. Metronomic chlorambucil at $4–8mg/m^2/day$ may also help. Rescue combinations D-MAC, ADIC, CHOP (Couto 2005), and MOPP (Vail, MacEwen, and Young 2001) are worth trying. (See the lymphoma rescue protocols used at the Ohio State Vet-erinary School for dogs and cats in section 1-C in Table 6.2.)

Rabacfosadine, administered IV every 3 weeks, demonstrated substantial response rates in a study of 50 first-time relapsed B-cell lymphoma dogs. The study dogs achieved 75% overall response rate with 45% complete remission. The median response duration was 172 days overall and 215 days for dogs that achieved complete remission (Vickery et al. 2016). Although this study was on first-time relapsed patients, Tanovea™ is expected to yield good results in dogs with resistant B-cell lymphoma because of its novel mode of action. Clinical trials using Tanovea for resistant lymphoma are needed.

It remains to be determined if novel treatments for resistant lymphoma will help dogs with B-cell and T-cell lymphoma pass the current plateau of survival. There is hope that one of the new canine monoclonal lymphoma vaccines will be efficacious; however, patients need to be in remission when the vaccines are administered. When cats develop resistance to chemotherapy, their prognosis worsens. Lymphoma generally responds well to radiation therapy but in a multicentric disease, radiation therapy is very difficult to deliver.

A Few Words on MOPP Rescue

The MOPP rescue protocol took a costly turn when procarbazine injectable became prohibitively expensive; however, the tablets are used with good efficacy. Resistant lymphoma patients may achieve remissions using Mustargen® IV at 3mg/kg and vincristine at 0.7mg/kg IV and oral prednisone and oral procarbazine tablets at 50mg/m² daily for 14 days. It may be used every other day if carers have financial constraints.

LoLuC-P: A Low-Cost Protocol for Lymphoma Maintenance

In relapse situations or where there are financial constraints, I try to provide one rescue dose of Adriamycin or, at the very least, vincristine at 0.7mg/m². Dexamethasone at 0.5–1mg/kg may also be very helpful for reinduction. If the client can afford L-asparaginase, we prefer to give it as well. For patients that are frail, sick, or have a high tumor burden, we recommend a reduced or a split dose schedule over 24–48 hours. We may give the vincristine on day 1 and L-asparaginase on day 2. We often split Adriamycin and give it at 20mg/m² IV two weeks in a row to gain remission.

For low-cost maintenance, a rotation of oral chemotherapy medications can be used in sequence. We have been successful in maintaining remissions for a number of relapsed lymphoma patients by rotation of oral lomustine followed by chlorambucil (Leukeran®) and then cyclophosphamide (Cytoxan®): We call this combination LoLuC-P protocol.

For dogs, the maximum tolerated dose (MTD) lomustine dose is 60–80mg/m² and for cats, it is 50–60mg/m²; however, I *always* divide the dose into 25% fractions and give it over 4–7 days to reduce nadir associated leukopenia and adverse events. The Leukeran dose is 1.4mg/kg divided a.m. and p.m. on day 21 or divided over two days. Cytoxan at 100mg/m² is given with a large amount of broth, 15–20 minutes before morning urination, on day 28 and 29. The increased intake of liquids with oral Cytoxan is essential to avoid hemorrhagic cystitis. I always describe the Cytoxan days as "Big Broth" days with a morning walk! This rotation cycle is repeated on day 35 after a CBC finds the WBC to be above 4,000 with neutrophils above 2,000.

If the client allows induction with vincristine and L-asparaginase, give the first divided dose of lomustine 4–5 days later. If only L-asparaginase was used, administer the dexamethasone IV or IM along with Benadryl; start giving the divided dose of lomustine on day 1. Divide the MTD dose into two to four (four doses are preferable, using 10mg capsules or a compounded capsule) equal amounts with instructions to administer 25% of the dose every 48 hours until finished.

Patients on lomustine need close monitoring for platelet counts and leukopenia and chemotherapy-induced anemia before each additional treatment. Liver function should also be checked periodically for lomustine hepatotoxicity. This protocol increases the interval between lomustine doses and, in my experience, seems to spare platelets when used long term. Cats often need intervals up to 6 weeks apart between doses of lomustine to avoid myelosuppression.

If prednisone has some efficacy for the resistant lymphoma patient, it is given concurrently on a tapered schedule as in the original induction protocol. It is given at 5mg twice daily long term for cats. Dogs are maintained on prednisone at 0.5–1mg/kg every other day, depending on the patient.

To ensure increased water intake with Cytoxan, we instruct clients to give prednisone on the days of Cytoxan along with a large offering of broth or chicken soup slurry. Since using this strategy for oral Cytoxan in the late 1970s, we have eliminated Cytoxan-induced hemorrhagic cystitis in our practice. I prefer *not* to use Cytoxan IV to avoid toxicity for geriatric cancer patients.

The LoLuC-P oral combination chemotherapy protocol has been helpful for achieving stable disease for many of our relapsed lymphoma dogs and cats. It has also been helpful as a low cost oral maintenance protocol for lymphoma dogs. Following an initial IV injection, lymphoma dogs may achieve and stay in remission or in stable partial remissions for variable periods with LoLuC-P. We may add subcutaneous cytosine arabinoside (Cytosar U®) injections at 250–300mg/m^2 on days 1 and 3 of each week (total 500–600mg/m^2) into this protocol for patients with CNS involvement or renal involvement, or to help sustain partial remissions in more resistant lymphomas.

Slim's Case (Life Was Good in Stable Partial Remission)

Slim Pancratz, a M/N Whippet, was diagnosed with multicentric lymphoma at 10 years of age. He received the modified Wisconsin protocol. Slim came out of remission at 10 months and received reinduction chemotherapy. He achieved only a partial remission. The Pancratz's needed to conserve funds and requested fewer visits and a less costly maintenance protocol. We placed Slim on a 10-day interval rotation schedule using oral lomustine, Leukeran, Cytoxan, and alternate-day prednisone. The Pancratz's brought Slim in every 2–3 months for a CBC recheck and IV vincristine. Slim gained weight and became lethargic. He was diagnosed with hypothyroidism and responded well to thyroid supplementation; he went back to his normal weight and vigor. Slim survived a total of 42 months with his lymphoma in a prolonged, stable, partial remission.

Options Beyond Chemotherapy for Cancer Recurrence

It was previously believed that the innate immune system ignored neoplastic cells because they are "homegrown" in the body. Molecular biology and proteomics has found that cancer cells have molecular signaling that inhibits or checks T-cells from recognizing and destroying cancer cells. Researchers have identified a gene that plays a key role in protecting cancer cells from T-cell mediated destruction. This gene is called programed death ligand 1 (PD-L1) and it has become a target for therapy. Some advanced cancers have been able to respond to this type of targeted therapy.

The mechanical and molecular signals for angiogenesis are unfolding and the trigger for lymphangiogenesis seems to be associated with inflammation. Lymphatic vessels are conduits for cells and they play a role in metastasis and organ rejection. Researchers in the field of proteomics (analysis of proteins and effector molecules) have identified tumor-specific signaling pathways. New drugs are being developed to target specific proteins that regulate immune checkpoint activity such as PD-L1, angiogenesis, and lymphangiogenesis pathways.

Targeted therapy may seek out and destroy cancer cells by finding a protein trigger, receptor, or a genetic switch to exploit. Inhibition of tyrosine kinase signaling, blocking growth receptors, and inhibition of angiogenesis hold promise as useful targeted therapies. New drugs may provide amazing results for relapsing and resistant geriatric lymphoma patients in the future. You may check new drugs and new protocols on the Internet at www.uptodate.com (Jain 2004).

Adverse reactions and high cost may restrict the use of targeted therapy drugs for use in our geriatric dog and cat patients. Gleevec® provided miraculous results for people with resistant CML. Gleevec may have some efficacy in hemangiosarcoma but it causes moderate grade 3 to severe grade 4 vomiting in dogs. It may be better tolerated physiologically by cats. It would cost $1,200.00 a month to maintain a 70-pound dog on Gleevec. It is recommended for daily use for CML in human patients until resistance develops.

When dealing with resistant lymphoma, the family may continue to ask if there is anything else to do. In situations like these, we educate the family about other potentially aggressive salvage therapies. Options to pursue would be to try half-body radiation therapy or bone marrow transplant (Tremayne and Sullivan 2005). At times, we recommend metronomic (low dose) therapy that involves using low doses of Cytoxan, Leukeran, and lomustine concurrently. Deeply bonded clients may readily accept these options. At this point, if the cancer is progressive, most Pawspice clients have begun to accept that their geriatric oncology pet has received a noble effort by all concerned and that they must accept the final part of their pet's end of life journey.

Metronomic Chemotherapy

Metronomic chemotherapy (mCTx) is the use of anticancer drugs at a lower dose and a higher frequency. Due to its low toxicity, there is no break period. Metronomic protocols are aimed at inhibiting the antiangiogenic mechanisms and immune modulation to boost antitumor immunity by changing the tumor microenvironment (Mutsaers 2014). It is a viable palliative option for geriatric cancer patients with resistant, inoperable, advanced, and recurrent cancer. Often, the geriatric oncology patient's family declines standard recommendations for salvage surgery, rescue chemotherapy, or radiation therapy. They fear that their aging pet cannot tolerate further definitive or aggressive treatment. Metronomic therapy may use any combination of NSAIDs along with chlorambucil, cyclophosphamide, lomustine, capecitabine, etoposide, tamoxifen, and doxycycline for their reported antitumor effects.

Metronomic therapy incorporates an evidence-based and scientific method of therapy, although the exact mechanisms of action are not fully understood. It is very well tolerated (Liptak et al. 2004; Mutsaers et al. 2001). Metronomic cyclophosphamide reduces the number and function of circulating regulatory T-cells and improved antitumor immunity (Oleinika 2013). It may enhance protective antitumor responses when used in triple therapy combinations with debulking radiotherapy along with immunotherapy in patients with metastatic melanoma or sarcoma (Monjazeb and Kent 2013).

I have frequently used low dose, increased frequency therapy as a kinder, gentler way to approach recurrence in my geriatric cancer patients. It is also helpful for frail geriatric oncology patients with concurrent illness or malnourishment and in patients with reduced renal and hepatic functional reserve. Metronomic therapy is a viable palliative option for recurrent STSs and recurrent abdominal organ tumors. With metronomic therapy, we educate the client to be satisfied with achieving stable disease rather than looking for complete remission.

Andre's Case (Miraculous Shrinkage of Huge Aggressive Sarcoma)

Lena and Boris Amitin brought in Andre, their 11-year-old, 32.6 kg Shepherd mix dog, with a large $7 \times 6 \times 3cm^3$ sarcoma on his lateral left chest wall. It started to recur only 14 days postop. Andre had a history of epilepsy that was being treated with carbamazepine. Andre also had early degenerative myelopathy and a left hind limb lameness that responded to steroids. Treatment with toceranib and meloxicam failed and Andre's mass enlarged to $12 \times 12 \times 6cm^3$ one month later. The Amitins chose to discontinue toceranib. Upon my suggestion, they elected metronomic chemotherapy (mCTx) with lomustine at $4mg/m^2/day$ and continued the meloxicam. Two weeks later, the Amitins elected debulking surgery for Andre.

One month later, the sarcoma displayed a rapid recurrence over 4 days to $19.5 \times 7 \times 3cm^3$ and then stabilized for 4–5 weeks. Andre continued to swim daily and remained on lomustine and meloxicam. The meloxicam served the dual purpose being necessary for pain control and for its antiangiogenesis action. To our surprise, Andre's mass started to regress over a 4-day period at $9^1/_2$ weeks after the second surgery. What was a huge second recurrence involving the left chest wall and scapula completely regressed! We noted this as a miraculous response to mCTx. Against my advice, the Amitins decided to discontinue Andre's mCTx.

Recurrent Soft Tissue Sarcoma (STS)

STSs including feline injection site sarcomas (FISSs) are the most common locally recurrent malignancies that veterinarians and oncologists grapple with. If the geriatric oncology patient received aggressive, en block resection specialty surgery followed by radiation therapy (RTx), the tumor-free interval is generally longer. Most STS recurrences take place within 6–8 months from the first excision. If the STS patient is not a surgical cure, the mass generally appears within 6–7 months or 1 year. Andre Amitin's recurrences were much faster and more aggressive and larger than most STSs. Geriatric patients with hemangiopericytoma have the longest tumor-free intervals in the STS group.

Lady's Case (Not All Third Recurrent FISSs Are Doomed)

Lady O'Donnell, a 13-year-old F/S DSH, presented with her third recurrence of feline injection site sarcoma (FISS) in the interscapular space. The O'Donnells asked me to help them save Lady. After evaluating the history, I decided that we might be able to help, even though the literature says that further surgery at the third recurrence of FISS has no survival value. In Lady's case, her attending doctor performed her first two surgeries. Her third surgery involved a referral institution that utilized photodynamic laser therapy. However, it recurred and enlarged over several months.

When we evaluated Lady, the mass was $6 \times 6 \times 4cm^3$, lobulated but moveable. Thoracic and abdominal X-rays showed no metastases and no bone involvement. Blood work and urinalysis showed that Lady was in overall good condition for her old age. We used our multimodality protocol that combined surgery, intraoperative chemotherapy, and RTx. This was followed by external beam RTx and carboplatin chemotherapy. Lady had no recurrence of her FISS for the following 3 years. She developed hyperthyroidism, malignant mammary adenocarcinoma, and GI lymphoma that were each successfully treated. Lady died of renal failure at the age of $16^1/_2$. The O'Donnells were very grateful to have the extra years with their dear Lady.

Recurrent STS and recurrent FISS are generally more aggressive than the original tumor. Tumor-free intervals shorten with subsequent surgeries. There is a point after which surgery is no longer helpful. Epidemiological studies conducted by Dr. Phil Kass of the University of California, Davis, found that there was no significant extension of survival times for cats with FVAS after the third surgery (Kass et al. 1993). In my experience, when the original tumor and its recurrences were previously treated with routine surgery or other superficial techniques, then a more aggressive definitive surgery incorporating multimodality therapy can be successful in selected cases such as Lady's.

Each geriatric cancer patient's treatment history and current health status must be completely reevaluated for restaging the recurrence. Results from radiographs, blood work, and appropriate imaging techniques, such as ultrasound, CT, MRI, or PET scans, will aid in decision making for treatment of recurrent STS (McEntee 2004). The principles used at the first approach would also apply for the second or third approaches if a cure were still possible. Long-term survivors may develop other tumors and be clinically misdiagnosed as having recurrence (see Figure 8.2). The efficacy and safety of repeating a course of radiation therapy is very difficult to assess and requires individualized case management by the radiation oncologist.

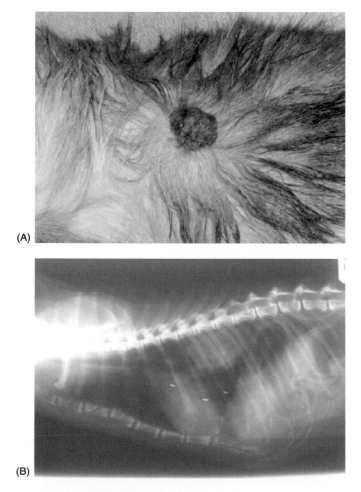

(A)

(B)

Figure 8.2.   18-year-old Hiss Clouse developed a tumor on his skin (A) suspected of being recurrent FISS, treated 4 years previously. A solitary pulmonary mass (B) was suspected to be a metastasis. The skin tumor was a hair matrix tumor and percutaneous FNA of the pulmonary mass found marked suppurative septic inflammation. This mass was also radiographically consistent with feline bronchial SCC.

Normal tissues cannot tolerate radiation therapy doses that exceed a total dose over 6.5–7 gray (Thrall 2001). In selected cases, stereotactic radiosurgery (SRS), or a high dose fraction delivered to a shrinking field, can target the most aggressive extension of a recurrent sarcoma's tentacles. Collaboration between the radiation oncologist and the surgeon is essential when considering surgery and additional radiation therapy for tumor recurrence at a previously irradiated site.

Tigger's Case (Don't Give Up if the Recurrent Tumor Volume Is Small)

Tigger, a 12-year-old M/N DSH, developed 2 recurrences of FISS in the left prescapular lymph node area. The second recurrence followed two extensive surgeries that involved multimodality treatment, which included intraoperative radiation therapy, follow-up RTx, and chemotherapy. Tigger's owner had myelogenous leukemia and underwent a bone marrow transplant while his dear Tigger received the follow-up RTx treatments. Tigger's first recurrence was within 3 months and it was treated vigorously with wide surgical excision and intraoperative RTx. The second recurrence occurred within another 2 months in the prescapular lymph node area. One of my associates told Tigger's owner that the prognosis was grim and that there was nothing else to do for Tigger.

He came to see me a month later. Tigger appeared healthy with the exception of the 3cm mass threatening his survival. I looked into his master's soulful eyes and could tell that he was brokenhearted about the thought of giving up on his best friend. I told him that I would hate to see a small lesion like that sarcoma kill his cat, and that I would not give up on Tigger if he still wanted me to fight for his life. He said that he was out of remission too and that his doctors had not given up on him and that he wanted me to try to save Tigger. The success of his decision was against the odds.

We performed a third multimodality procedure for Tigger. It involved aggressive excisional biopsy, intralesional carboplatin, and a megadose of intraoperative RTx. Tigger survived another 5 years cancer free following that gut-wrenching decision to treat his second recurrence. In fact, he outlived his master!

Recurrent Mast Cell Tumors

Mast cell tumors (MCT) are the most common potentially malignant and fatal skin tumors in dogs. They are also among the most likely to recur if not removed widely. Geriatric oncology patients with recurrent mast cell tumor (MCT) require full staging of their disease before localized therapy such as surgery or radiation therapy is elected. Staging consists of FNA of the liver and spleen and local draining lymph nodes in addition to current blood work, urine analysis, and radiographs. A subset of geriatric oncology patients with previous MCTs will grow new tumors periodically. Another subset will develop numerous MCTs in the skin. Decision making for management options are most successful when each patient is carefully evaluated and given individualized cancer care.

Katie's Case (Recurrences Every 2 to 3 years Are Treatable)

John Haddon's F/S Rhodesian Ridgeback, Katie, presented with multifocal cutaneous MCTs starting at age 3. She developed new MCTs that appeared every 2 to 3 years. Most of her MCTs were operable. When Katie was 11 years of age, she developed a rapidly growing mast cell tumor on her tail. Rather than amputate her tail, the Haddon's elected radiation therapy for Katie. Katie ultimately died of an aggressive MCT that swelled her right axillary lymph node and metastasized at the age of 12. Katie battled recurrent MCT, and I have seen other patients like her.

Jodi's Case (Cryotherapy, an Option for Mast Cell Recurrences)

The Andy Hoffman family was referred with Jodi, their very high-strung 8-year-old F/S Boxer with a history of MCTs that developed after surgical removal every 3 to 4 months over a 1-year period. Jodi was also stressed with the rigors of dealing with a large chronic corneal ulcer. The Hoffman's dreaded the thought of more surgery every time a new MCT appeared. We offered the alternative of using cryotherapy for Jodi's next MCT. She was given local anesthesia with lidocaine and we infiltrated the area surrounding the mass with Benadryl® and dexamethasone. Liquid nitrogen was applied for three freeze–thaw cycles. The lesion swelled initially and then regressed over a 3–4-week period with no complications. This option spared Jodi's family the cost and emotional trauma of putting her through yet another stressful surgical procedure.

Options for Clients Who Decline Multiple Surgeries for Recurrent Cancers

For clients who decide that they do not want further conventional surgery to manage recurrent MCTs, cutaneous hemangiosarcomas, SCCs, and other accessible tumors, we can certainly offer more options. For MCTs we can offer intralesional (intratumoral) injections of steroids. We use dexamethasone sodium phosphate, regular dexamethasone, and/or triamcinolone, or Depo-Medrol® mixed with an equal volume of patient serum. Intralesional injections may be very effective in reducing mast cell tumors without surgery and may be given into tumor beds of incompletely removed MCTs to reduce recurrence. Injections need to be repeated at intervals relevant to the duration of effect of the agent. Intralesional injections seldom require sedation, unless the patient is fractious or the procedure needs to be given in a sensitive area or if it seems painful. We can offer cryotherapy for small cutaneous cancer lesions. We can offer radiation therapy if the site is amenable and if the client can afford it and if the geriatric patient can handle it. Intralesional yttrium 90 in a polymer gel device (Y-90 IsoPet™) is another excellent option to reduce accessible tumors via pure beta radiation brachytherapy (www.isopetsolutions.com). Injecting immune stimulating agents intralesionally into tumors may help to shrink them without surgery. Immunocidin™ has been used successfully for this purpose (www.NovaVive.com).

Electrochemotherapy (Electroporation) is another excellent option that may control recurrent tumors and tumors that are difficult to resect. Clients must be advised that there will be a necrotic wound at the site. See the section on ECT/EP at the end of Chapter 6.

Recurrent Hemangiosarcoma

Waiting for recurrence of hemangiosarcoma in postsplenectomy patients is a dread-filled vigil. Many clients decline chemotherapy using the VAC protocol (vincristine, Adriamycin, Cytoxan) or single agent Adriamycin due to the potential for adverse side effects, cost, and poor response despite treatment. Explain to clients that when hemangiosarcoma recurs, the patient will generally slow down or "crash." Recurrence is generally multifocal and disseminated with vascular lesions that cause low grade DIC, hemorrhage, thromboses, blood loss anemia, weakness, and pale mucous membranes. Teach clients how to assess and be ready for their geriatric oncology pet to crash.

Unfortunately, surgical intervention has been hopeless against hemangiosarcoma recurrence due to its aggressive ability to form multifocal blood channels ("autoangiogenic") in the abdomen, chest, and bloodstream (Khanna 2004). Monitoring the patient with chest X-rays, as well as a periodic recheck ultrasound of the abdomen and heart, may occasionally detect a treatable, resectable lesion. However, without promising follow-up therapy, it would be very difficult for any oncologist to encourage a second surgery to remove one or two recurrent lesions due to the predictability of microscopic disease within a short time. The multifocal pattern of metastases with hemangiosarcoma makes treating recurrent bleeding episodes unsuccessful.

Consulting with clients at the time of recurrence and hemoabdomen should also be aimed at comforting them as they face the emotional trauma of pet loss. The family may want to take the patient home for some private last moments in Pawspice and hospice care. The patient may be very weak, anemic, and in shock. Most doctors would shun the idea of allowing a hemorrhaging cancer patient with DIC to go home in this near-death condition. However, the client certainly has the right to take their family pet home to die, despite our professional reluctance to discharge such a sick patient. Many families want to and are prepared to hold a hospice vigil for their dying pet. Our job is to make sure that the geriatric oncology patient is not in pain.

We can expect and hope for early detection, prevention, and better control for recurrence of hemangiosarcoma in splenectomized patients in the future. Jaime Modiano, VMD, PhD, and his research team at the University of Minnesota, along with scientists at ApopLogic™, have developed a novel detection test and a targeted therapy to control hemangiosarcoma using a bispecific ligand-targeted toxin from a *Pseudomonas* exotoxin (e-BAT). Studies show that it is a safe multiple-targeted therapy drug for dogs with hemangiosarcoma at picomolar concentrations (Schappa et al. 2013). The Modiano Lab and researchers at ApopLogic have developed a unique peptide dimer (Breceptin™) that induces apoptosis of cancer cells that express the bradykinin B1 and B2 receptors. They also have developed the biological immunotherapeutic agent (Fasaret™) that targets activated tumor infiltrating cells, and T-regulatory cells that express F as receptors. It can be used in the neoadjuvant or adjuvant setting to improve sarcoma survival outcomes.

It would be ideal if we could use a combination of effective gene therapy, antiangiogenesis agents, small molecule therapy, and possibly a histone deacetylase (HDAC) inhibitor like suberoylanilide hydroxamic acid (SAHA) (Cohen et al. 2004). Stay in touch with the use of other HDAC inhibitors such as valproic acid, which may enhance the effects of Adriamycin (Thamm et al. 2006). New technology has unfolded methods to detect circulating cancer progenitor cells (hemangioblasts) and enhance the safe treatment of this fatal vascular cancer with a bacterial toxin (e-BAT) that selectively kills hemangiosarcoma cancer stem cells (Modiano 2016).

Recurrent, Metastatic Osteosarcoma

Decision making to treat osteosarcoma (OSA) is difficult due to its aggressive biologic behavior. Most canine osteosarcoma (OSA) patients originally present with appendicular bone lesions. If the family is willing to treat, the lesions are most often managed with amputation and chemotherapy and potentially immunotherapy. Results of a 2016–2017 funded clinical trial for safety and efficacy of a live Listeria vector vaccine can be obtained from Dr. Laura Simon Treml at ltreml@aratana.com. Patients treated for OSA are at great risk to develop metastatic pulmonary disease.

Few viable options exist to successfully manage pulmonary metastases. Metastatic clones are generally very resistant to chemotherapy. Some oncologists use vinorelbine and T-K inhibitors. I have had short-lived regressions under 6 months rotating carboplatin with Adriamycin at 20mg/m^2 every 2 weeks, masitinib, and meloxicam. Dr. Chand Khanna benefited a small number of dogs in a study using inhaled interleukin-2 (IL-2) encapsulated liposomes. That study is closed.

Researchers are attempting to develop a clinically useful OSA tumor vaccine. A vaccine for OSA may become the favored option for future consideration. Check the Louisiana State University and the Colorado State University web sites for updates on clinical trials using this promising therapeutic modality. These sophisticated options may become more available for dealing with recurrent OSA lesions in dogs in the near future.

The overall prognosis for dogs with OSA is better for those patients with recurrent lesions that do not have a large soft tissue component or concurrent hypertrophic osteopathy. The prognosis is worse for OSA patients with elevated serum alkaline phosphatase (Dernell, Straw, and Withrow 2001), with lesions located in the proximal humerus and with lymph node involvement (Hillers et al. 2005).

Many caregivers decline amputation for their OSA dogs, especially if metastasis is present at diagnosis. Palliative IV chemotherapy using carboplatin along with IV bisphosphonates and oral piroxicam or radiopharmaceutical treatment with samarium may be of value to slow down the rate of growth and the painfulness of metastatic bone lesions (Dernell, Straw, and Withrow 2001). Pain control using a combination of analgesics as described in Chapter 7 is the most important goal for patient care.

Pulmonary Metastatectomy

Dogs that survive initial treatment for OSA are at great risk for pulmonary metastases. There are few viable options when dealing with pulmonary metastases. They are considered more resistant to chemotherapy than the primary tumor. Periodic chest X-rays or CT scans are the mainstay for monitoring and early diagnosis. CT imaging helps to evaluate the lung fields to rule out sub-clinical metastases that are not detectable on plain radiographs. Metastatectomy holds promise in selected cases. The best results from metastatectomy are for dogs that have been tumor-free for over 10 months with less than three metastatic tumors localized in one lung lobe. Although pulmonary metastatectomy is difficult and expensive, it is possible to extend the survival of selected metastatic osteosarcoma patients with a carefully planned procedure. If the patient has more than 300 days tumor-free interval, a limited number of tumors with a more than 30-day doubling time, and a negative bone scan, that dog is considered a reasonable candidate.

The surgical approach to these cases requires sternotomy or thoracoscopy. Close attention to perioperative pain control is essential. A tumor on the surface of a lung may be removed via sub-pleural enucleation. A tumor in the distal part of a lobe may be removed via partial lung lobectomy. When there are multiple tumors in one lobe or in the proximal lobe, lobectomy is required.

The median survival for 36 dogs treated with metastatectomy was 176 days ranging from 20 to 1,495 days (O'Brien et al. 1993). Pulmonary metastatectomy has been successful in controlling the painful symptoms of hypertrophic osteopathy in at least four dogs with pulmonary metastases from osteosarcoma. The surgical procedures were well tolerated and restored the quality of life for all four dogs for 50, 51, 246, and 265 days, respectively (Liptak et al. 2004). When consulting with clients about this option, we must educate them about the fact that another wave of metastatic nodules may overtake the remaining lung lobes. There is no guarantee that the lung fields will remain clear in the geriatric oncology patient's near future.

Leaf's Case (Pulmonary Metastatectomy Helped Him Live Longer)

Leaf, a 10-year-old M/N Yellow Lab mix, had a mandibulectomy followed by four treatments of cisplatin (we now use carboplatin instead of cisplatin) for OSA of the mandible. One year later, Leaf's chest X-rays showed a 2cm nodule in the right middle lung lobe. We followed the mass for another month and detected a satellite growth or a new metastatic nodule near the previous metastatic nodule. The family elected lobectomy for Leaf. He recovered uneventfully and survived another year before pulmonary metastases recurred. Although the new tumors also were amenable to a second lobectomy, the family declined the procedure.

Recurrent OSA Lesions in the Axial Skeleton

One-third of treated long-term OSA survivors may develop metastatic OSA lesions in their long bones. The patients are generally already three-legged. The new lesion is painful, but the family cannot consider a second amputation. They want and need more options to pursue. Palliative radiation therapy with several follow-up fractions or stereotactic radiosurgery (SRS) or a full course of 18 fractions has been successful in helping to palliate and treat some cases of recurrent osteosarcoma (Dernell, Straw, and Withrow 2001; Mauldin 2016). This option has the potential to extend the life for some dogs with recurrent OSA of the long bones.

Murphy's Case (Long Life after Limb Salvage for Her)

Murphy, a 5-year-old F/S Great Dane belonging to Dr. Robin Downing, DVM, was cancer-free for 3 years following a limb salvage procedure at Colorado State University for OSA of her left distal radius. Murphy received two doses of cisplatin and two doses of carboplatin. She developed a low grade beta hemolytic *Streptococcus* infection at the allograft, which was responsive to Clavamox®. Robin chronicled Murphy's treatment in her book *Pets Living with Cancer: A Pet Owner's Resource* (Downing 2000).

Three years after limb-sparing surgery, Murphy developed lameness in her right hind leg. She was diagnosed with a ruptured anterior cruciate ligament and a tibial plateau leveling osteotomy (TPLO) procedure corrected the problem. After $2^1/_2$ months of rehabilitation, Robin noticed asymmetry of the right malleolus. Radiographs demonstrated a prolific lesion at the distal right tibia at the distal pin site, consistent with osteosarcoma. The lesion was confirmed as OSA with histopathology.

It was presumed that Murphy's lesion was recurrent metastatic OSA and that it would be resistant to further chemotherapy. The lesion was not amenable to a second limb salvage. Robin decided against amputation. During her struggle with decision making, Robin called and asked me for a second opinion. My postulate was that Murphy's new lesion was too far away from her primary to be a metastasis. I felt that this lesion was a de novo osteosarcoma and that it had the same odds of being responsive to treatment and chemotherapy as her primary OSA. I advised Robin to try palliative radiation therapy and treat Murphy with at least four rounds of carboplatin chemotherapy.

Murphy entered a clinical study group of 15 patients that would receive full-course radiation therapy at CSU to their OSA lesions in 18 fractions, to spare the skin. Murphy survived another 13 months, totaling $4^1/_2$ years, with her original limb-sparing allograft. Murphy died peacefully in her sleep from dilated cardiomyopathy at $9^1/_2$ years of age. Necropsy found three small metastatic pulmonary nodules and no viable cancer cells in her tibial lesion (Downing 2005).

In the future, other novel therapeutic options for a patient like Murphy may be more available for OSA patients in your practice such as an OSA vaccine, use of a bone-seeking radioisotope called samarium, or use of stereotactic radiosurgery.

Advanced and Recurrent Mammary Cancer in Dogs

Some clients have chosen to let mammary tumors grow until they become a problem. Mammary tumors and recurrence are very common in older, intact female dogs and in dogs spayed after $2^1/_2$ years of age. In such cases, take the time to educate the family that their pet's entire mammary chain has undergone "field cancerization" resulting from hormonal influence on target mammary tissues. The patient may have metastatic disease and be developing new local tumors and/or having recurrence of old tumors simultaneously. New mammary tumors have a 50% malignancy rate. They may be unrelated to the patient's previously excised tumors and not as dangerous as a locally invasive recurrence of an incompletely removed mammary tumor. Occasionally some dogs develop inflammatory mammary adenocarcinoma, which involves cancer cells spreading into the cutaneous lymphatics and is very painful.

Radiographs that examine three views of the chest and sub-lumbar/iliac lymph nodes are essential to determine the stage of disease prior to radical mastectomy. If chest radiographs are negative for metastatic disease, surgery is the best procedure for advanced stage and/or recurrence of localized multiple mammary adenocarcinomas. Radical mastectomy with local lymph node excisional biopsy may be curative. If the mass is adhered to the body wall, include the body wall with the resection. Ovariohysterectomy of older mammary tumor patients does not inhibit recurrence, but it spares camouflaging recurrence with mammary hypertrophy (Ogilvie and Moore 1995; Rutterman, Withrow, and MacEwen 2001; Morrison 2002c).

Mammary adenocarcinoma in geriatric oncology dogs and cats can be treated more safely with mitoxantrone than with Adriamycin. Using dose escalation, start with 5mg, then 5.5mg, and do not exceed $6mg/m^2$ every 21 days for six IV treatments. My preference is to avoid cardiotoxic Adriamycin in aged patients unless their carcinomas are resistant to mitoxantrone.

For frail geriatric patients or clients with financial restraints or reluctance to continue IV chemotherapy, consider the use of metronomic (low dose) oral therapy. Oral capecitabine (Xeloda®) has proven activity against adenocarcinoma. (NEVER use Xeloda in cats because it turns into 5-FU, which KILLS cats.) For dogs, I use an empirical dose of Xeloda at $500mg/m^2$ PO 48 hours or preferably at $250mg/m^2$ PO daily and Cytoxan at $10–12.5mg/m^2$ PO daily. Piroxicam at $10mg/m^2$ PO daily can be added to this protocol as a chemoprevention agent along with famotidine and selected immunonutrition supplements. The metronomic approach is often welcomed by clients who decide that they want to address their geriatric pet's mammary cancer in a kinder and more gentle way, without surgery or IV chemotherapy. Be on the lookout for innovative anticancer products from ApopLogic™ that may kill mammary carcinoma cells using nanomolar concentrations with low toxicity (Schappa 2013).

Advanced Stage or Recurrent Mammary Cancer in Cats

Because cats are independent and self-groom, their mammary carcinomas may not be diagnosed until they are in advanced stages of disease. Cats with a history of primary mammary carcinoma are at great risk for local recurrence, regional metastases, and pulmonary metastases. Educate clients that bilateral chain mastectomy is the best-known precaution for long-term survival in cats diagnosed with primary mammary carcinoma. The patient's best opportunity for prevention of recurrence rests with your initial management strategy. By recommending bilateral radical mastectomy from the start, you may save the cat's life. Remove the tumor-bearing mammary chain first, followed by excision of the opposite chain within 4 to 5 weeks whenever possible.

When dealing with recurrence, make new radiographs that show three views of the chest and two views of the abdomen to rule out pulmonary metastases and sub-lumbar/iliac involvement. Restage the geriatric cat before attempting a second surgery or a first bilateral radical mastectomy. The second incision should include excision of the previous surgery site. If mammary nodules recur along the chain or at a previous surgery site, they may be approached surgically once again. If the mass is touching the body wall or is adhered to fascia overlying the ribs or body wall, excise at least one fascial layer below the mass or remove that section of the body wall.

If the cat received prior chemotherapy, select an agent that has not yet been used for follow-up chemotherapy. If you used mitoxantrone previously, then use Adriamycin and vice versa or use carboplatin at 21-day intervals. If the family declines IV chemotherapy, consider metronomic therapy with low dose oral Cytoxan and piroxicam, and suggest immunonutrition as an optional supportive therapy. On the horizon, there may be new peptides and biologics available that will target resistant and metastatic mammary carcinoma cells (Schappa 2013).

Anal Sac Carcinomas, Recurrence, and Metastasis

Tumors arising in the last inch of the GI tract are generally not noticed until they cause local irritation, swelling, tenesmus, cramping, straining, and abnormal passage of stool. This holds true for recurrence or metastasis from a previously excised primary mass. If the primary tumor caused malignant hypercalcemia (MH), calcium levels and water intake can be used as a tumor marker to monitor for recurrence or metastasis. Some patients do not have recurrent hypercalcemia until the recurrence reaches a certain tumor volume such as a large sub-lumbar mass obstructing the distal colon.

Some dogs are presented with deep sphincter recurrence along with enormous sub-lumbar lymphadenopathy. It was not the primary tumor that caused the clinical signs but the pressure from the lymphadenopathy pushing the colon downward and obstructing the passage of stool through the pelvic canal. The primary tumor may not recur following surgery in some cases. The patient's metastatic disease generally becomes clinically obvious around 6–9 months following the initial surgery. Chemistry and electrolyte panels may not show abnormalities in calcium levels.

A point to remember is that male dogs with anal sac adenocarcinomas were initially suspected to have benign hormone-dependent perianal tumors. Another issue confronting the clinician is that FNA offers no cytological help in differentiating the malignant anal sac gland carcinomas apart from the benign hormone-responsive hepatoid gland tumors. The basement membrane or wall of the anal sac must be submitted for biopsy for definitive diagnosis (Goldschmidt and Hendrick 2002). The Enlight Assay™ can be run on routinely collected tissue samples submitted for biopsy. This molecular biomarker profiling assay can precisely classify cancer types and subtypes in dogs. It should be able to distinguish between these tumors and assist in decision making for selection of chemotherapy drugs for follow-up treatment (www.innogenics.com). Tumor tissue may also be sent to make a personalized IFx-VET™ dendritic cell vaccine (www.morphogenesis-inc.com/veterinary-oncology).

Rosie's Case (Her Anal Sac Carcinoma Responded to Debulking)

Rosie, an F/S Australian Shepherd, shared her life with one of our profession's most treasured personalities, Dr. Robert M. Miller (RMM cartoons and "Mind Over Miller"). At 8 years of age, Rosie developed metastatic anal sac adenocarcinoma (ASC), manifested by sub-lumbar/iliac lymphadenopathy. Her chest X-rays were negative for pulmonary metastases and she had normal blood chemistries with no hypercalcemia.

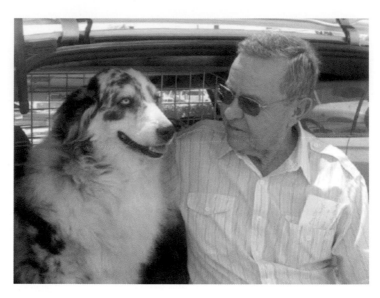

Figure 8.3. Dr. Robert M. Miller (cartoonist RMM) and Rosie celebrating her 3-year anniversary with metastatic anal sac carcinoma. A new mass was excised on the opposite anal sac after 1 year. After $2^1/_2$ years, local recurrence slowly infiltrated her anal sphincter 360 degrees. Her quality of life was good on chemoprevention and immunonutrition with piroxicam, Agaricus Bio, and IP-6®.

The Millers told me, "We were given a poor prognosis for her, so we'll let Rosie go naturally." I consulted with them about the literature and my personal experience with ASC. I recommended that they at least have the primary mass excised so that Rosie would have less discomfort, and they did. The Millers declined my suggestion for exploratory celiotomy for sub-lumbar/iliac nodectomy and chemotherapy. They elected to use piroxicam for its antitumor effects and two oral supplements selected from our immunonutrition protocol: Inositol hexaphosphate (IP-6®) and a full range of beta glucans from the Agaricus blasei mushroom.

Rosie celebrated a 1-year anniversary with a surprise: her recheck X-rays and ultrasound did not identify sub-lumbar/iliac lymphadenopathy and there was no evidence of local disease.

Two years later, Rosie developed a new mass on the opposite anal sac. The mass was excised and diagnosed as ASC. In her third year (Figure 8.3), Rosie developed tumors that slowly encircled her entire anal sphincter. She remained relatively asymptomatic. At age 12, Rosie developed tenesmus. Dr. Miller obtained several opinions regarding surgery and radiation therapy for Rosie. The consulting surgeons felt that the mass was inoperable and would create incontinence. Other options, such as radiation therapy, did not appeal to the Millers due to the fact that her iliac nodes were enlarged again. They reported that Rosie exhibited tenesmus during elimination but otherwise seemed to behave normally with an excellent quality of life. Rosie was managed with stool softeners and a soft food diet. I recommended adding an opiate pain control medication, Tramadol®, to complement the piroxicam. The Millers decided against chemotherapy.

For advanced ASC cases like this, I recommend palliative radiation therapy or palliative debulking laser surgery to shrink the local mass or localized electroporation/electrochemo-therapy. Oral chemotherapy can be helpful with metronomic oral Xeloda (capecitabine) at $250mg/m^2$ given daily or at $500mg/m^2$ BID for 10 days on and 10 days off, and metronomic Cytoxan at 10–$12.5mg/m^2$ daily or at $50mg/m^2$ Cytoxan q 48 hours (in the morning, with broth,

15–20 minutes before urination). *Always* give Cytoxan with a big bowl of broth and encourage urination afterward as this practice avoids hemorrhagic cystitis! Give famotidine first thing in the morning on an empty stomach and mix the piroxicam and other medications in with breakfast 20–30 minutes after the famotidine. If the client can afford the addition of tyrosine kinase inhibitors such as masitinib or toceranib, they may enhance the response.

Dr. Miller's goal was to maintain Rosie's well-being for as long as possible. We entered Rosie into our Pawspice program using palliative cancer medicine and she survived with a good quality of life for 3 years.

Residual or Recurrent Nasal Cancer

Decision making for treatment of nasal passage cancer is difficult due to the challenges of the recommended treatments. The radiation oncology and surgical oncology departments at North Carolina Veterinary College start out with a treatment plan for nasal tumors that intentionally addresses residual and recurrent disease. They educate clients about the shortcomings of historical radiation treatment for nasal cancer and propose a way of dealing with the expected.

Following external beam radiation therapy to the nasal cavity, patients are followed up with routine CT scans to determine and delineate residual or recurrent tumors. When detected, these are surgically removed. Patient survival times exceed those of historical controls. This multimodality approach uses a combination of radiation, imaging, and surgery to enhance survival times (Henderson 2005). Stereotactic radiation may be effective in treating nasal passage cancer in 3–5 treatments as another viable option. Chemotherapy using carboplatin has been helpful for some cases as with Rufus. T-K inhibitors (masitinib or toceranib) with carboplatin may enhance survival time.

Rufus's Case (Nasal Chondrosarcoma Responded to Chemotherapy)

Trudy Gleason was referred for consultation for Rufus, her 9-year-old M/N Black Labrador Retriever with epistaxis and stridor due to nasal passage chondrosarcoma (CSA). Trudy had previously declined definitive radiation therapy for Rufus. After our consult, Trudy elected to enter Rufus into Pawspice with aggressive palliative cancer care using carboplatin given IV every 21 days, piroxicam daily, and immunonutrition. His epistaxis and stridor regressed for $2^{1}/_{2}$ years! Rufus regained his energy and entered numerous 10 km walks with Trudy on weekends. Recurrence manifested as progressive stridor with swelling of the muzzle that enlarged steadily, causing facial deformity. His recurrent CSA was resistant to further chemotherapy. Rufus entered the hospice phase for end of life comfort care as cheerfully as he had handled his other treatments. Trudy even took him on a cross-country trip for a family reunion. Rufus survived with a surprisingly good quality of life for 4 additional months (Figure 8.4).

Multiple Primary Malignancies

What if the geriatric oncology patient develops a second, third, or fourth cancer? Aging is associated with a decline in the function of mutation repair genes and tumor suppressor genes, which reduces immunosurveillance. Some scientists propose that cancer should be considered another geriatric syndrome (Ershler 2004).

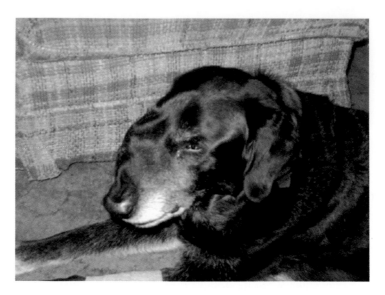

Figure 8.4. Rufus Gleason in hospice with recurrence of nasal chondrosarcoma after $2\frac{1}{2}$ years of remission with carboplatin and piroxicam chemotherapy, and immunonutrition. His recurrence caused extensive nasal deformity and was resistant to further carboplatin. Rufus went on a cross-country trip during his hospice.

Ruben's Case (He Developed 7 Types of Cancer in 4 years!)

One of my patients, a 13-year-old black Cocker Spaniel named Ruben, developed seven types of cancer over 4 years. Ruben started out with lymphoma at 9 years of age. He responded well to chemotherapy. Along the way, he developed sebaceous gland adenocarcinoma, ceruminous gland adenocarcinoma, sweat gland adenocarcinoma, bladder cancer, and malignant melanoma. Ruben responded well to treatment for these new primary neoplasms and maintained a good quality of life. Finally, he developed SCC deep in the nasal septum.

We helped the family understand that Ruben had experienced a failure of his innate immune system. His repair genes and tumor suppressor genes, which normally suppress the genetic mutations that lead to cancer, were dysregulated in the process of senescence. We also explained that chemotherapy has a negative effect on the immune system. The family understood that Ruben developed his cancers due to a decline of his normal immunosurveillance system. This explanation helped the family in their decision making. It was the challenge of the SCC that caused Ruben's family to finally surrender his battle against cancer.

The Role of Integrative Medicine in Advanced Stage and Recurrent Cancer

Many pet owners want to leave no stone unturned, especially when facing recurrence, relapse, or metastasis in their geriatric pet. They appreciate having options to pursue when conventional medical technology can no longer help their pet. Some carers observe that their pets feel better when a combination of supportive alternative therapies is provided alongside conventional protocols. Some clients with pets in chemotherapy feel that the drugs cause too many side effects and make their pet sick. They shun conventional therapy in preference to holistic and complementary and alternative medicine (CAM), hoping that it will cure their pet without the usual side effects.

According to a survey by the American Animal Hospital Association (Moore 2005b), the percentage of clients seeking CAM therapies went from 6% to 21% over one decade. When the attending clinician loses patience with the client or gives up on the case, clients often feel that they have nowhere else to turn. If carers feel that the doctor is unable to help their pet, they will often seek out CAM and integrative medicine with or without their doctor's blessings. They seek solutions to the problems with CAM therapies such as nutritional therapy, acupuncture, chiropractic, homeopathy, herbal medicine, massage therapy, magnet therapy, aromatherapy, and so forth. Many pet owners feel that blending alternative techniques along with a doctor's conventional orders could potentially benefit their pet's quality of life.

When clients ask my opinion about trying CAM for their pet's recurrence, the first thing I do is take a moment to praise their love and devotion for their pet because it is their special love bond and anticipatory grief that are motivating them to keep searching for a "cure."

Regardless of efficacy, one very important ingredient that CAM offers is hope. This is in contrast to the evidence-based paradigm of our conventional Western medicine that generates statistical data on response rates, disease-free intervals, and survival times. Western medicine shares some aspects of the herd health care system, treating large groups of patients with A or B and analyzing the results with statistics, percentages, and survival charts. Holistic medicine focuses on the patient as a whole, unique individual and is one-on-one oriented. This approach can be very comforting and nurturing for the weary family of a geriatric cancer patient.

A working definition for hope is to wish for something with expectation. CAM therapies are ministered to the patient with hope. The promise of hope is alluring and very difficult for carers to resist when their geriatric pet has recurrent cancer with comorbidities, discomfort, and a poor prognosis.

Point out that NIH researchers have examined a number of the most efficacious remedies offered in holistic and CAM and that some techniques do have merit and efficacy (https://nccih.nih.gov/health/atoz.htm). Many other remedies may have the placebo effect, which is about 30%, while most are unsubstantiated or questionable. The American Holistic Veterinary Medical Association has a journal that may have a peer reviewed article about the topic of interest (editor.jahvma@gmail.com). It is best to advise your curious clients to check the authenticity of a particular CAM treatment that they are interested in using for their pet at: www.quackwatch.com and at: http://www.fda.gov/Animal Veterinary/default.htm.

As a rule, if a treatment is used *instead* of a conventional treatment, it is considered alternative. If a treatment is used *along with* conventional therapy, it is considered complementary and by accepting it you are practicing integrative medicine. If the complimentary technique seems to alleviate pain and adverse conditions or improve the patient's well-being and survival, then it is good to continue. If there are no benefits after four visits or treatments, then it makes sense to stop the treatment unless the effect is expected to be long range, as with immunonutrition and chemoprevention.

Nutrigenomics, Immunonutrition, and Chemoprevention

Today's scientists have a greater understanding of how nutrients affect health. The new field of nutrigenomics studies the molecular alterations of gene activities after specific dietary nutrients with specific genomes are consumed. It explores the mechanisms of how nutrients affect genes by turning them on or off to benefit the patient (Moore 2005a).

Immunonutrition is the mainstay of my integrative approach toward supporting cancer patients. Clients want to provide the best possible nutritional support at all stages of their pet's cancer (see

Table 6.9). Combining immunonutrition, chemoprevention, and metronomic therapy helps to support and palliate geriatric cancer patients struggling with recurrence. At times, this is the only type of therapy that the family is interested in or will allow.

After a considerable amount of investigation, I selected a limited number of scientifically researched and trustworthy supplements from a plethora of available products for our immunonutrition protocols. We select supplements for each individual geriatric cancer patient's specific needs. In the selection process, it is imperative that the product be prepared by an ethical company. They have high standards for quality control. There are thousands of products available on the market, but approximately 38% of the products misrepresent contents with inaccurate information on the product label. This variability creates chaos, is responsible for variable results, and validates skepticism about supplements and nutraceuticals.

The highest quality supplement companies undergo rigorous self-inspection standards that parallel the regulations of the pharmaceutical companies. At times, immunonutrition and chemoprevention are the only supportive therapies that are safe and nurturing for the geriatric patient grappling with recurrence.

Summary

There is a great deal of uncertainty in decision making for geriatric pets with advanced stage, recurrent, and relapsed cancer. There are no age-based studies from which one may extrapolate helpful information. Veterinarians need to rethink their overall reluctance to working with geriatric cancer patients. Advanced stage cancer and recurrence in older dogs and cats finds the veterinarian ministering to a very heterogeneous group of complex geriatric oncology patients. These complex cases require multitasking and may help readers gather "situated knowledge" and practical wisdom for clinical judgment in the emerging area of geriatric oncology.

Every doctor has a horror story where the outcome was far from the intended purpose of therapy. Geriatric oncology patients are complicated and challenging and they can be fragile and unpredictable, or strong and durable. Dr. Patricia Olsen, PhD, when she was President/CEO of the Morris Animal Foundation, during a 2005 interview with *Veterinary Medicine*, said, "In life, we are responsible for our efforts but not the outcome. You have to expend considerable effort, but also remember that you can't always be responsible for the outcome" (Olsen 2005).

We must ponder over the most difficult emotional, ethical, economic, and medical issues inflicted upon us by cancer's recurrence, relapse, or metastasis in our geriatric oncology patients. Once we make a treatment decision that we feel is right for that patient and family, we should be able to accept and live with that bioethical decision, no matter what complications come afterward. It is good to learn from mistakes and grow with the experience. However, if we always second guess ourselves and doubt our decisions, we hurt our spirit and integrity. If we blame ourselves for all the failures that oncology will inflict upon us, we will slip into compassion fatigue, negative self-talk, and began to wither. That is not good! Our profession has surpassed dentists and the armed services in suicide rate as per a Centers for Disease Control and Prevention report on February 13, 2015 (https://www.cdc.gov/mmwr/preview/mmwrhtml/mm6405a6.htm).

We need to recognize when our thinking and self-talk has taken a low tone or has become negative. We must vigilantly practice positive self-care to remain resilient so that we can continue to minister with compassion for our clients and their beloved pets. Please read the special added chapters in this Second Edition text by Kimberly Pope Robinson, DVM, Sandra Grossman, PhD, and Ellie Friedman,

MSC, to fortify your personal wellness program so that you know your purpose and your value to society.

Paternalistic decision making must be replaced with decision-making partnerships. When facing recurrence, many of your clients will be willing to jump into the heart of battle once again to keep an elderly pet even longer. They will enter round 2, 3, or 4 as long as they are enabled by your practice team to help them maintain a good quality of life for their geriatric pet. If you cultivate an optimistic attitude toward treating recurrence in geriatric oncology, you will be prepared to freshly assess each patient's unique situation.

Reach out to help those heartbroken carers who are stumbling down the difficult road of relapse and recurrence with their aging pets. The recurrent cancer is gnashing at their pet's survival and their personal happiness. You need to know that they are suffering from anticipatory grief. Clients intuitively look to their veterinarians as healers. You have the power and knowledge to help clients negotiate the hurdles on the bumpy road during their pet's Pawspice hoping for a next remission or for stable disease. When all else fails, you can help your clients find their way at the end of the road.

Patient evaluation using the Body Condition and Muscle Condition Score Charts, the HHHHHMM Quality of Life Scale, the performance level, and frailty assessment will add up to an impression of the overall condition of the geriatric cancer patient. These factors, in addition to staging the cancer, will have a direct impact on decision making and prognosis. It requires multitasking and creating an individualized viable treatment plan to help and, most of all, not harm the geriatric cancer patient. Always look for a kinder and more gentle palliative cancer medicine approach with excellent pain management as described in Chapters 6 and 7 and above.

Be supportive, whether clients choose the high road or the low road. Help them to pass through that difficult threshold of reevaluation and decision making, when recurrence strikes their pet. Provide the client with satisfactory options for dealing with the recurrence and pain control, while maintaining a good quality of life. Consider metronomic therapy and the newer low risk targeted therapies and immunotherapies and checkpoint inhibitors as they become available, especially for geriatric patients with reduced functional reserve.

Suggest antiangiogenesis agents and chemoprevention using currently proposed agents or COX-2 inhibitors, or when appropriate and safe. Provide immune support with immunonutrition using currently proposed immune enhancement agents and anticancer supplements. These are viable options for pet owners to pursue if they feel they must decline standard therapy. Recommend improvements on the patient's diet, with mindful knowledge of popular concepts that cancer is a metabolic disease and that food can fight cancer as with the ketogenic diet. Help the family go forward with their decision, offering encouragement and validation to help them maintain their pride and confidence.

Treat recurrence in geriatric oncology patients as a geriatric syndrome that involves physiologic stress and pain. Presume that cancer and cancer-related pain cause stress and immunosuppression on the body. It is also safe to presume that the cancer was caused by the biology of aging and its related stresses with free radical damage, exposures to environmental carcinogens, and decline in immune function. Therefore, it makes sense to support the immune system and to scavenge free radicals whenever feasible using immunonutrition.

Treat the geriatric cancer patient for cancer pain by presuming that cancer hurts by its mere presence, even if overt pain is not obvious to you or the carers. When clients are using or ask about cannabis products, be open minded and help them mindfully. Let them know that many popular products on the market are not reliable. If your state will not allow you to advise your clients about cannabis, that is a difficult situation for you. I would advise that they select a reliable, legal hemp product such as HempRx™, which contains CBD and less than 0.3% THC, because it is safe and made for animals.

Use the proposed pain scoring system at: csuanimalcancercenter.org/assets/files/csu_acute_pain_scale_canine.pd. Teach clients to assess quality of life using the 7 criteria in the HHHHHMM Quality of Life Scale described in Chapter 10 to monitor and assist the patient's needs on a weekly or daily or hourly basis as the situation requires. Give your clients the working knowledge and the tools to courageously and competently assist their geriatric pet in round 2, 3, or 4 in the battle against cancer.

You can offer the major professional helping hand during decision making, treatment, or palliation by addressing critical concerns every step of the way. Pet carers will always be grateful for your kindness and helpfulness during their pets' Pawspice, especially as their geriatric pet declines and needs more intense end of life comfort care with hospice. For me, the task at hand is to pay homage, time after time and case after case, to the amazing human–animal bond, as each heartstring is plucked out one by one. This goal bestows a greater and sublime purpose to the art of practice.

References

Balducci, L., and C. Beghe. 2004. "Cancer in the elderly: Biology, prevention and treatment." In *Clinical oncology*, 3rd edn, eds M.D. Abeloff, J.O. Armitage, J.E. Neiderhuber, M.B. Kastan, and W.G. McKenna, pp. 1317–1329. Philadelphia, PA: Churchill Livingstone.

Baum, J.I., S.E. Boston, and J.B. Case. 2016. Prevalence of adrenal gland masses as incidental findings during abdominal computed tomography in dogs: 270 cases (2013–2014). *JAVMA* 249 (10):1104.

Beardsley, T.R. 2005. The role of lymphocyte T-cell immuno-modulator (LTCI) in amplification of helper CD-4 cell response, IL-2 production, and hematopoiesis, T-Cyte® Therapeutics, Bansall, CA. Personal Communication.

Clary, E. 2016a. End-of-life medical ethics: Fundamental issues and principles (Part I). *ACVS Surgical Summit Proceedings*, Seattle.

Clary, E. 2016b. End-of-life medical ethics: An ethic of "only caring" (Part II). *ACVS Surgical Summit Proceedings*, Seattle.

Cohen, L.A., B. Powers, S. Amin, and D. Desai. 2004. Treatment of canine hemangiosarcoma with suberoylanilide hydroxamic acid, a histone deacetylase inhibitor. *Veterinary and Comparative Oncology* 2 (4):243–248.

Corbin, J. 2004. A depth psychological analysis of the human–canine bond and its implications to the grief response. Dissertation proposal, Pacifica Graduate Institute, December.

Couto, G. 2005. Protocols used at OSU. Personal Communication.

Couto, G., and N.M. Moreno. 2013. "Complications that may occur in cancer patients," Chapter 3, In *Canine and feline oncology*, pp. 38–58. Servet, Spain.

Dernell, W.S., R.C. Straw, and S.J. Withrow. 2001. "Tumors of the skeletal system." In *Small animal clinical oncology*, 3rd edn, eds S.J. Withrow and E.G. MacEwen, pp. 378–417. Philadelphia, PA: Saunders.

Downing, R. 2000. *Pets living with cancer: A pet owner's resource*. Lakewood, CO: AAHA Press.

Downing, R. 2005. Personal Communication.

Ershler, W.B. 2004. "Biology of aging and cancer." In *Comprehensive geriatric oncology*, 2nd edn, eds L. Balducci, G.H. Lyman, W.B. Ershler, and M. Extermann, pp. 67–74. Oxon, UK: Taylor & Francis.

Floersch, J. 2002. *Meds, money, and manners: The case management of severe mental illness*. New York: Columbia University Press

Gawande, A. 2014. OVERKIL: An avalanche of of unnecessary medical care is harming patients physically and financially. *Annals of Health Care, The New Yorker Magazine*, October 15th.

Goldschmidt, M.H. and M.J. Hendrick. 2002. "Tumors of the skin and soft tissues." In *Tumors in domestic animals*, 4th edn, ed. D. Meuten, pp. 45–117. Ames, IA: Blackwell Publishing Professional.

Hendersen, R. 2005. Personal Communication, *VCS NL*, Spring.

Hillers, K.R., W.S. Dernell, M.K. Lafferty, S.J. Withrow, and S.E. Lana. 2005. Incidence and prognostic importance of lymph node metastases in dogs with osteosarcoma: 228 cases (1986–2003). *JAVMA* 226 (8):1364–1367.

Hua, J., S. Hoummady, C. Muller, J.L., Pouchelon, M., Blondot, C., Gilbert, and L. Desquilbet. 2016. Assessment of frailty in aged dogs. *American Journal of Veterinary Research* 77 (12):1357–1365.

Iliopoulou, M.A., B.E. Kitchell, and V. Yuzbasiyan-Gurkan. 2013. Development of a survey instrument to assess health-related quality of life in small animal cancer patients treated with chemotherapy. *JAVMA* 242 (12):1679–1687.

Jain, R.K. 2004. Vascular and interstitial biology of tumors. In *Clinical oncology*, 3rd edn, edn M.D. Abeloff, J.O. Armitage, J.E. Neiderhuber, M.B. Kastan, and W.G. McKenna, pp. 153–172. Philadelphia, PA: Churchill Livingstone.

Kass, P.H., W.G. Barnes, W.L. Spangler, et al. 1993. Epidemiologic evidence for a causal relation between vaccination and fibrosarcoma tumorigenesis in cats. *JAVMA* 203:396–405.

Kennedy, B.J. 2004. "Aging and cancer." In *Comprehensive geriatric oncology*, 2nd edn, eds L. Balducci, G.H. Lyman, W.B. Ershler, and M. Extermann, pp. 3–10. Oxon, UK: Taylor & Francis, 2004.

Khanna, C. 2004. Advances in our understanding of cancer: Explanations for your clients. *AVMA Convention Notes*.

Liptak, J.M., E. Monnet, W.S. Dernell, and S.J. Withrow. 2004. Pulmonary metastatectomy in the management of four dogs with hypertrophic osteopathy. *Veterinary and Comparative Oncology* 2 (1):1–12.

Lurie, D.M., M.D. Lucroy, S.M. Griffey, E. Simonson, and B.R. Madewell. 2004. T-cell derived malignant lymphoma in the boxer breed. *Veterinary and Comparative Oncology* 2 (3):171–175.

Mauldin. N. 2016, PetCure oncology: Treating the "untreatable" with stereotactic radiosurgery. Veterinary Cancer Society Annual Forum, Breakfast Meeting.

McDonald, M. 2003. A framework for ethical decision making. *SVME Newsletter* 9 (3):6–9.

McEntee, M. 2004. Radiation therapy: What you and your clients need to know and what your expectations should be. *AVMA Convention Notes*.

Meyers, B. 2000. "Anticipatory mourning and the human animal bond." In *Clinical dimensions of anticipatory mourning: Theory and practice in working with the dying, their loved ones, and their caregivers*, ed. T.A. Rando, pp. 537–564. Champaign, IL: Research Press.

Milani, M. 2001. Clear and present diagnosis. *Vet. Forum*, June, pp. 42–43.

Modiano, J.F. 2016. Innovations in cancer treatment and prevention. *World Veterinary Cancer Congress*, Foz do Iguassu, Brazil.

Modiano, J.F., S.C. Helfand, et al. 2005. Innovations in the diagnosis of canine hemangiosarcoma. *Personal Communication*, *VCS NL* 29 (1):4–5.

Monjazeb, A., and M. Kent. 2013. Translating combination radiotherapy/immunotherapy from dogs to humans with advanced melanoma or sarcoma, www.OncLive.com/publications.com, and UC Davis, Advance, Fall 2016, p. 3.

Moore, A. 2005a. Nutrigenomics and the food bowl. *VPN* 17 (8):17.

Moore, A. 2005b. Skepticism still greets holistic veterinary medicine. *VPN* 17 (8):1, 12–13.

Morrison, W.B. 2002a. "Clinical evaluation of cancer patients." In *Cancer in dogs and cats: Medical and surgical management*, 2nd edn, ed. W.B. Morrison, pp. 57–63. Jackson, WY: Teton New Media.

Morrison, W.B. 2002b. "Principles of treating chemotherapy complications." In *Cancer in dogs and cats: Medical and surgical management*, 2nd edn, ed. W.B. Morrison, pp. 365–374. Jackson, WY: Teton New Media.

Morrison, W.B. 2002c. "Canine and feline mammary tumors." In *Cancer in dogs and cats: Medical and surgical management*, 2nd edn, ed. W.B. Morrison, pp. 565–572. Jackson, WY: Teton New Media.

Mutsaers, J.J., S.I. Mohammed, D.B. DeNicola, P.F. Bennett, and D.W. Knapp. 2001. Metronomic chemotherapy in veterinary oncology: A pilot study. *VCS Proceedings*, p. 41.

Mutsaers, A.J. 2014. Metronomic chemotherapy: Theory and practice, state of the art presenter. *Proceedings Veterinary Cancer Society Annual Forum*, p. 56.

O'Brien, M.G., R.C. Straw, S.J. Withrow, et al. 1993. Resection of pulmonary metastases in canine osteosarcoma: 36 cases (1983–1992). *Vet Surg* 22:105–109.

Ogilvie, G., and A. Moore. 1995. *Managing the veterinary cancer patient*, eds G. Ogilvie and A. Moore. Trenton, NJ: Veterinary Learning Systems.

Oleinika, K., R.J. Nibbs, G.J. Graham, and G.J. Fraser. 2013. Suppression, subversion and escape: the role of regulatory T cells in cancer progression. *American Journal of Clinical and Experimental Immunology* 171 (1):36–45. PMC3530093.

Olsen, P.N. 2005. Personal Communication and as quoted in interview. *Vet Med* August:551–553.

Relford, R. 2016. Hyperthyroid cats: The IDEXX SDMA Test is a more reliable indicator of kidney function than creatinine, Advertorials. *JAVMA* 249 (10): 1104.

Repetto, L., A. Venturino, and W. Gianni. 2004. "Prognostic evaluation of the older cancer patient." In *Comprehensive geriatric oncology*, 2nd edn, eds L. Balducci, G.H. Lyman, W.B. Ershler, and M. Extermann, pp. 309–319. Oxon, UK: Taylor & Francis.

Rollin, B.E. 2000. Personal Communication regarding the Asclepiad Authority and Ethics at the 137th AVMA Convention, Salt Lake City.

Rollin, B.E. 2003. Ethics. Midwest and AVMA Convention Notes.

Rollin, B.E. 2004a. Ethics and the human animal bond. *NAVC Proceedings*, January 20.

Rollin, B.E. 2004b. Ethics in veterinary practice. *SVME Newsletter* 10 (2):3–5.

Rollin, B.E. 2004c. Oncology and ethics. *AVMA Proceedings*.

Rollin, B.E. 2005. "Animal happiness, a philosophical view." In *Mental health and well-being in animals*, ed. F.D. McMillan, pp. 235–242. Ames, IA: Blackwell Publishing Professional.

Rollin, B.E. 2006. Euthanasia and quality of life. Commentary, *JAVMA* 228 (7):1014–1016.

Rowe, J.M., and I. Avivi. 2004. "Clinical use of hematopoietic growth factors." In *Hematology: Basic principles and practice*, 4th edn, eds R. Hoffman, E.J. Benz, S.J. Shattil, B. Furie, H.J. Cohen, L.E. Silberstein, and P. McGlave, pp. 1029–1043. Philadelphia, PA: Churchill Livingstone.

Rutterman, G.R., S.J. Withrow, and E.G. MacEwen. 2001. "Tumors of the mammary gland." In *Small animal clinical oncology*, 3rd edn, eds S.J. Withrow and E.G. MacEwen, pp. 455–477. Philadelphia, PA: Saunders.

Schappa, J.T., A.M. Frantz, B.H. Gorden, E.B. Dikerson, D.A. Vallera, and J.F. Modiano, 2013. Hemangiosarcoma and its cancer stem cell sub-population are effectively killed by a toxin targeted through epidermal growth factor and urokinase receptors. *International Journal of Cancer* October 15, 133 (8):1936–1944.

Stanclift, R.M., and S.D. Gilson. 2004. Use of cisplatin, 5-fluorouracil, and second-look laparotomy for the management of gastrointestinal adenocarcinoma in three dogs. *JAVMA* 225 (9):1412–1417.

Temel, J.S. 2010. Early palliative care for patients with metastatic non-small cell lung cancer. *NEJM* 363 (8):733–742.

Thamm, D.H., L. Bisson, B. Rose, S. Dreitz, and L. Wittneberg. 2006. Histone deacetylase inhibition to enhance osteosarcoma chemosensitivity. Personal Communication. *Symposium of Canine Osteosarcoma Syllabus*, Veterinary Cancer Society, p. 28.

Thomason, J.D., C.A. Calvert, and C.E. Green. 2005. The pathophysiology of DIC: When the hemostatic system malfunctions; DIC: Diagnosing and treating a complex disorder. *Vet Med* September:660–678.

Thrall, D.E. 2001. "Biological principles of radiation therapy." In *Cancer in dogs and cats: Medical and surgical management*, 2nd edn, ed. W.B. Morrison, pp. 375–388. Jackson, WY: Teton New Media.

Timmons, R. 2005. Family practice. *American Association of Human Animal Bond Veterinarians Newsletter* 12.

Tobias, K. 2005. Celiotomy, complications. *NAVC Clinician's Brief*, July, pp. 13–18.

Tremayne, J., and E. Sullivan. 2005. Stem cell transplants to benefit canines with cancer at Fred Hutchinson Cancer Research Center. *DVM News* July, pp. 1-S.

Vail, D.M., E.G. MacEwen, and K.M. Young. 2001. "Canine lymphoma and lymphoid leukemias." In *Small animal clinical oncology*, 3rd edn, eds S.J. Withrow and E.G. MacEwen, pp. 558–590. Philadelphia, PA: Saunders.

Vickery, K.R., K.E. Burgess, B.S. Phillips, et al. 2016. *Veterinary Cancer Society Proceedings*, Annual Forum.

Villalobos, A. 2016a. End of life medico-ethical decision making. *ACVS Surgical Summit Proceedings*, Seattle.

Villalobos, A. 2016b. Preventing over treatment. *ACVS Surgical Summit Proceedings*, Seattle.

Villalobos, A. 2016c. Veterinary hospice care: Theory and practice. *ACVS Surgical Summit Proceedings*, Seattle.

Yeates, JW, and D.C.J. Main. 2010. The ethics of influencing clients. Views: Commentary. *JAVMA* August 1, 237 (3):263–267.

Zollers, B., J.A. Wofford, E. Heinen, M. Juebner, L. and Rhodes. 2016. A prospective, randomized, masked, placebo-controlled clinical study of Capromorelin in dogs with reduced appetite. *Journal of Veterinary Internal Medicine* 30 (6):1851–1857. doi:10.1111/jvim.14607.

Suggested Reading

Ganz, P.A. "Quality of life considerations in the older cancer patient." In *Comprehensive geriatric oncology*, 2nd edn, eds L. Balducci, G.H. Lyman, W.B. Ershler, and M. Extermann, pp. 291–300. Oxon, UK: Taylor & Francis.

Gawande, A. 2014. *Being mortal, illness, medicine and what matters in the end*. Atul Gawande, Profile Books.

Klein, M.K. 2001. "Tumors of the female reproductive system." In *Small animal clinical oncology*, 3rd edn, eds S.J. Withrow and E.G. MacEwen, pp. 445–454. Philadelphia, PA: Saunders.

McDonald, M. Ethics and conflict of interest. http://www.ethics.ubc.ca/people/mcdonald/conflict.htm and www.uptodate.com. See oncology viewers page or subscribe for current information on specialty and oncology topics in human medicine.

Web sites: at the end of the book.

Chapter 9

When and How to Decide That a Geriatric Cancer Patient Is Terminal

To be a scholar is not enough. … We must realize that we live in an imperfect world, but that we are here to make it better. We should … respect … the ethic of reverence for life.

Leo Bustad, DVM, PhD

The anguish inflicted upon pet owners when they learn that their pet is terminal is heart wrenching. When you say there is nothing further that can be done to medically help their pet, the family feels helpless. Clients rightfully want to know when you think their pet's death will occur and what conditions will lead up to the death, but they need to hear this with sensitivity and regret in your heart. Let them know that you do not want to be right about the statistical prognosis and that there can be exceptions. Let them know that every bell curve has a tail of long term survivors and that there are novel therapies on the horizon that might help or slow down the disease process. We need to respond with kind, compassionate words when our clients' hearts are breaking and let them know that we care about them and will help them with the concept of cancer palliation with Pawspice and end of life hospice care.

One of the most frustrating problems in oncology is uncertainty. Science and literature tell us which cancers are incurable and allow us to quote the published survival statistics with and without treatment. Looking at statistics, we can only estimate approximately how much time a terminal geriatric patient has to live. Our educated guess is only a supposition because the literature does not provide us with focused information about the prognosis of our geriatric oncology patients with their comorbidities.

Clarification of Terminology for Terminal

Saying that a cancer is terminal is different from saying that the pet is in the terminal stages of the disease. We must distinguish how we are using this powerful and hopeless word to help guide the family in the decision-making process. Veterinarians who use the word "terminal" when speaking to the family should be careful to explain the expected overall survival time. Terminal cancer patients are expected to survive between weeks and several months. You can say, "Terminal doesn't necessarily mean tomorrow or imminently but this cancer is mostly likely going to be what causes death. The statistics we have are an average. Some geriatric pets die sooner, especially if they have concurrent illness or if they don't tolerate or respond to treatment, while others outlive the expected survival time."

Canine and Feline Geriatric Oncology: Honoring the Human–Animal Bond, Second Edition. Alice Villalobos with Laurie Kaplan.
© 2018 John Wiley & Sons, Inc. Published 2018 by John Wiley & Sons, Inc.

Using the word "terminal" when speaking to the client makes the most sense when the geriatric patient is in the advanced stages of cancer. When a physically able pet has a cancer that will eventually be fatal, it is appropriate to enter that pet into a Pawspice program, which embraces palliative cancer management to slow down the cancer. The Pawspice concept helps carers understand that their geriatric pet is in an end of life cancer palliation program with goals to sustain quality of life for the longest time possible with kinder, gentler cancer management. When the pet enters the terminal or final symptomatic stages of cancer and declines toward death, we place them in hospice care. At *that* point, it makes sense to use the word "terminal." I generally say something like this: "Bella has entered the terminal stages of her cancer ***and her time might be short.***"

Criteria for Terminal Decision Making

The criteria most commonly used to decide if a geriatric cancer patient is in the terminal stages of cancer are based upon cancer type, stage of disease (tumor burden), histologic grade, and clinical assessment of the patient's performance and biological age by the attending doctor (Repetto et al. 2004). Stage and grade factors do not always apply across the board to all tumor types. In a retrospective study of 38 cats with lymphoma, the only factor that influenced survival was the initial response to treatment. Cats with complete remissions enjoyed median survival times of 654 days, while those with partial and no response had only 112 and 11 days, respectively (Milner et al. 2005). Treatment intensity may yield superior overall responses but causes more age-related or breed-related toxicity, such as the vulnerability of Doberman Pinschers to Adriamycin cardiotoxicity (Stone, Goldstein, and Cotter 1991).

The interactions between aging and cancer and its treatment may have a positive or negative influence on quality of life and life expectancy and how we evaluate if a geriatric oncology patient is terminal. Oncology applied on top of geriatric medicine is not an exact science. This uncertainty may lead the attending doctor and client to come to the shared decision that favors no treatment, which in itself classifies the geriatric oncology patient as terminal. Having the option to choose kinder gentler cancer treatment with the Pawspice concept may be a tremendous life saver.

Animals age with great variability and vulnerability. It is useful to refer to the comparable aging charts for species and weight. Clients need to understand how old their pet is in human years (see Table 1.3). Their geriatric oncology patient may be physiologically young when compared to other animals at the same chronologic age. Other important factors to consider would be the geriatric patient's functional performance assessment, the impact of morbidity from concurrent conditions, and quality of life issues as discussed in Chapters 8 and 10. Body condition score, assessment of core components of frailty (Hua et al. 2016), assessment of age-related sarcopenia, and cancer-related cachexia are also very important clinical factors to consider. See the WSAVA muscle condition scores that identify sarcopenia for geriatric dogs and cats. External factors that have a direct influence on the veterinary cancer patient's survival include access to specialty care and new technology, the degree of emotional attachment of the carers, and the finances allocated by the family for their geriatric pet's care.

Objective data regarding evaluation of these criteria, which are germane to veterinary geriatric oncology, are becoming available. Veterinary geriatricians are enabling pets to live longer, healthier lives with antioxidant and co-factor enriched nutrition and high-tech medical care (Roudebush et al. 2005). The Dog Aging Project is conducting a long-term large clinical study on the effect of rapamycin intervention on the delay of age related conditions. Their data may be published in 2021.

The increased frequency of tumors in aging animals is largely due to senescence of the immune system and carcinogenesis via initiation, promotion, genetic mutations, environmental exposure, and age-associated changes in susceptible tissues (Lyman 2004). Another etiologic theory is that aging tissues have a changed microenvironment that allows resident cancer cells to outcompete their normal but aged peers (DeGregori 2012).

Respect for the human–animal bond and the growing population of aging companion animals will deliver more tumor-bearing geriatric patients to our exam rooms for consultation. Veterinarians who are willing to multitask through these complex cases have the opportunity to expand the boundaries and settle the frontier of clinical geriatric oncology for companion animals.

Initial Presentation of a Terminal Case

Most veterinary patients do not exhibit obvious preliminary warning signs during the sub-clinical phase of malignancy. Senior and geriatric animals are less likely to exhibit clear warning signs of cancer due to the mingling of coexisting conditions and the physiological changes associated with aging (see Table 2.2). Obesity may camouflage cancer, be associated with certain types of cancer, and shorten the pet's overall life span (Kealy and Lawler et al. 2002; Weeth et al. 2007). Geriatric pets are often presented to their local attending clinicians when they exhibit obvious symptoms due to advanced stages of cancer. Many are rushed to emergency clinics with an oncology-related crisis, which may need surgical intervention (Salisbury 2002). Initial assessments may presume or conclude the presence of cancer or an associated paraneoplastic syndrome. This prompts the need for further evaluation to establish a definitive diagnosis. The bad news often comes as a shock to the unsuspecting family, who may then be caught up in the spirit of battle against the cancer (Butler et al. 1991).

Clients may notice that their geriatric pet has some degree of gagging, coughing, or respiratory compromise, exercise intolerance, or weakness. If the signs persist or worsen, they present their pet for examination by appointment or as an emergency. Initial X-rays may find widespread pulmonary metastatic disease, pleural effusion, or a globoid-shaped heart. This may immediately indicate the terminal nature of the patient's cancer. We can offer greater relief from the symptom burden of pulmonary cancer using olanzapine (Zyprexa™), which has provided terminal people who are dying from lung cancer with a new standard of end of life comfort care (Pal 2016).

It is important to confirm the diagnosis of cancer. Although fungal disease, anterior mediastinal lymphoma, thymoma, and lymphomatoid granulomatosis may appear as terminal cancer, these conditions may be responsive to definitive treatment. Pericardial effusion causing a globoid-shaped heart and muffled heart sounds was due to a benign or inflammatory process in 44% of 42 cases reported (Berg and Wingfield 1984). However, most dogs with globoid-shaped hearts have a distended pericardial sac due to bloody pericardial effusion from right atrial hemangiosarcoma. Occasionally, some patients maintain a tenuous but apparent well-being despite extensive pulmonary involvement.

Meeka's Case (She Was Lucky 3 Times until Metastasis)

Andrew Bergman brought Meeka, his 12-year-old Black Lab mix, for my opinion on July 27, 2016, after seeing multiple specialists who documented a $5 \times 5cm^2$ left liver lobe mass, a $7 \times 8cm^2$ splenic mass, and presumptive osteosarcoma of her proximal left humerus. Meeka's comorbidities were: osteoarthritis, disc disease, and a 2-year history of "almost fainting" during walks every day. A cardiologist ruled out heart disease as the cause of her near fainting episodes.

The decision-making process for Meeka was very challenging. Images of the abdominal tumors favored benign disease. I felt that the X-rays of the bony lesion appeared to be chondrosarcoma (CSA) with a "popcorn" pattern. Meeka's triple tumor situation and weakness episodes were very complex and most likely would wind up being terminal due to bone cancer.

Andrew wanted to remove Meeka's abdominal tumors in the hope that they were causing her near fainting spells. He felt that since she was using her left foreleg, he would forgo amputation and enter Meeka into Pawspice with palliative chemotherapy. Andrew elected splenectomy and left liver lobectomy for Meeka on August 1, 2016. Lucky for Meeka, the biopsy of her splenic mass was hematoma and her liver mass was nodular hyperplasia.

Meeka recovered well but her near fainting episodes continued. In mid-August, Meeka started limping on her left foreleg due to the presumptive OSA of her proximal humerus. Meeka did not do well on pain medications, so Andrew elected amputation on August 25, 2016. The biopsy confirmed my suspicion, CSA with an initial mitotic index of 1. We were joyful at Meeka's triple good luck.

However, an addendum to the CSA biopsy reported that the neoplasm was a high grade malignancy with a mitotic index of 8/10 high power fields, in one region.

Just after Meeka's amputation, her canine housemate, Annie, needed an emergency splenectomy and Andrew had a cardiac stent placed. Meeka recovered uneventfully from her amputation surgery but was slow to feel well enough for chemotherapy as per Andrew. She had some phantom twitching and still had her near fainting episodes.

Andrew took Meeka to a rehab center for massages and to practice with her new walking harness. Carboplatin was started on September 21, 2016, one month postamputation. It was given every 21 days × 4. On January 10, 2017, Meeka was in for her 5th carboplatin, when Andrew said, "She started coughing a little last week." Chest X-rays found multiple metastatic lesions. We decided no more IV chemo and sent Meeka home on oral metronomic lomustine and antitussives as needed. Meeka was given olanzapine (Zyprexa^{TM}) to help reduce the symptom burden of pulmonary metastases during her hospice.

Hemoabdomen

There will always be surprises and exceptions to a prognosis. A geriatric dog collapses. Initial evaluation in the emergency room finds hemoabdomen with hypovolemic shock. Hemoabdomen is most often due to ruptured splenic tumors. It has been suggested that up to 20% of ruptured splenic tumors may be due to benign disease (Salisbury, Lafond, and Morrison 2002). However, 60% of 200 splenectomy patients at the University of Minnesota were found to have benign tumors (Modiano 2016). If the acute hemoabdomen is from hemangiosarcoma, hepatocellular carcinoma, and lastly adrenal carcinoma, the prognosis is considered guarded to poor. Clinical and radiographic findings such as organomegaly, ascites, carcinomatosis, abdominal lymphadenopathy, and cardiomegaly require further imaging with abdominal and cardiac ultrasound to help determine the cause and extent of disease. Ultrasound findings may show multifocal cavitated visceral lesions in multiple organs, consistent with terminal stages of metastatic hemangiosarcoma. Splenic hematomas generally appear as solitary lesions with less cavitation. Nodular hyperplasia of the spleen may appear as multiple or singular hyperechoic nodular lesions, which may be associated with a ruptured hematoma. We need to be more optimistic and cautious with hemoabdomen patients even if we are dealing with a geriatric Golden Retriever or German Shepherd, until we can verify if the cause is from hemangiosarcoma.

We can enhance hemostasis by using Yunnan Baiyo (https://www.mskcc.org/cancer-care/integrative-medicine/herbs/yunnan-baiyao).

Manchester's Case (It's Not Over Until the "Fat Lady Sings?")

David Lyon was referred by Dr. Rachel Jones on July 3, 2013 with Manchester, his 11-year-old M/N Shepherd mix. Manchester developed recurrent multiple MCTs with one being a high grade III MCT (Patnaik system) (mitotic index 14) with narrow 1–7mm surgical margins. He also had elevated liver enzymes. Manchester responded well to vinblastine IV and intralesional injections of 15mg dexamethasone SP mixed with 2ml of his own serum (given evenly and deeply into the tumor bed) every 2 weeks × 5. We dispensed oral masitinib at 150mg SID, prednisone, Benadryl, famotidine, Agaricus, and OncoSupport. Masitinib was increased to 200mg BID after completion of the vinblastine injections. On November 19, 2014, he developed a salivary cyst, which was managed conservatively. Follow-up abdominal ultrasounds (AUSs) found splenic nodular hyperplasia. He developed hypercalcemia May 26, 2015, which has been medically managed.

On October 20, 2015, I palpated a large abdominal mass. AUS indicated that the mass was close to the spleen but may not be splenic and it was not hepatic. We could not rule out hemangiosarcoma. David elected surgery with no hesitation, given that we felt the mass did not exhibit the irregular cavitation of hemangiosarcoma on AUS and that 60–70% of splenectomy specimens examined by ANTECH Diagnostics were benign.

Postsplenectomy, the mass was diagnosed as nodular hyperplasia with hematoma. Manchester has developed osteoarthritis, sarcopenia, and degenerative myelopathy. On October 28, 2016, David called 3 times saying that Manchester had acute onset of vomiting and lethargy. His alkaline phosphatase was 27,611 (normal = 5–131 IU/l). Arsenic poisoning from household exterminator was suspected. Manchester responded quickly to supportive care. At this writing on January 31, 2017, he has been maintained on masitinib, OncoSupport, Agaricus, and supplements over 3.5 years with no recurrence of MCT.

Most clinicians suggest immediate surgery or euthanasia for all patients with hemoabdomen. Please note that it is not necessary to operate on every patient because many can be partially stabilized with a belly wrap, aggressive supportive care, and Yunnan Baiyao. Hemoabdomen is a dramatic scenario that creates lasting regret for carers, who were hastily advised that the *only* options for their pet were emergency surgery or euthanasia. This "*either/or*" proposal leaves out an important *third* option. Many pet caregivers would prefer to pursue the opportunity for stabilization along with Yunnan Baiyo. Carers want to take their pet home for end of life Pawspice care, where they can say their goodbyes during a hospice vigil. Of course, the attending clinician would ask the family to sign an informed consent release form.

Cells and/or tissue samples are needed to establish a definitive diagnosis. If the AUS findings are consistent with hemangiosarcoma, sarcoma, carcinoma, or malignant histiocytosis involving multiple organs in a susceptible breed, decision making for euthanasia may be straightforward. However, even those patients should not be denied palliative care and Yunnan Baiyo for a hospice vigil. If the family cannot afford emergency surgery for a patient that has no evidence of metastasis, the odds might be in favor of the patient if resorption is allowed to take place instead of euthanasia. It is generally best for the patient if the family can afford to have bleeding splenic masses removed to prevent future problems.

To date, systemic treatment provides only a low rate of response for aggressive multifocal visceral soft tissue sarcomas, carcinomatosis, or histiocytosis. Several clinical trials are evaluating the use of immunotherapy, antiangiogenesis therapy, small molecule therapy, and gene therapy (Helfand 2003; London 2004). These agents may prove helpful as adjuncts and permanent maintenance therapy when clinically available to bolster response rates. New detection tests and targeted therapy for hemangiosarcoma may change how we practice (Modiano 2016; Schappa et al. 2013).

Osteosarcoma

Radiographic bone lesions that appear in typical locations and exhibit Codman's triangle, bony lysis, and proliferation, characteristic of osteosarcoma, allow a working diagnosis of bone cancer for decision making. The Veterinary Cancer Society (VCS) has accepted radiographs showing bone lysis and proliferation at typical sites in large-breed dogs to be sufficient evidence for making the presumptive diagnosis to accept patients into bone cancer protocols. Some clients do not want to amputate but they want pain management and often appreciate palliative cancer care during their pet's Pawspice. It is important to educate clients about options such as: limb sparing, SRS, palliative carboplatin or metronomic chemotherapy and immunotherapy. The protocols require histopathology of the lesions following amputation or limb salvage for definitive confirmation of the diagnosis. Clinical trials for the safety and efficacy of a listeria-based vaccine may provide evidence to change how we address osteosarcoma in the future.

The attending clinician often makes an immediate decision that a patient is terminal, based upon facts and figures provided on the minimum database examination. Therein lies the problem. We need to define terminal as discussed in Chapter 8. We cannot be right all of the time, even when the prognosis is obviously poor. We can advise clients that "Cats with extreme neutrophilic leukocytosis due to cancer are 14 times as likely to die unexpectedly within 30 days than cats with leukocytosis due to other diseases" (Lucroy and Madewell 2001). Nevertheless, there are patients who defy the prognosis and outlive our expectations, especially if we compassionately alleviate distressful symptoms and provide palliative cancer care.

Advising Deeply Bonded Clients in the End Phase

How do you converse with clients who want you to try to help their terminal geriatric cancer pets against all odds? This is the time to set aside personal biases against age and cancer, which *dishonor* the human–animal bond. Avoid fatalistic thinking that puts old clichés in your mind, such as, "The fat lady has sung. Let's drop the curtain on this case." Offer flexible options to pet caregivers until they make the choice that fits their wishes.

How do you speak to clients who are clearly not comfortable with the options you suggest? Some pet owners feel that they were rushed or pressured by the attending doctor or emergency clinic doctor. They felt pressured to make a final decision, given the "either or" choices of euthanasia or definitive care at a costly estimate. The veterinarian's role in pressuring clients to agree to euthanasia before the client is ready to do so has created a generation of carers who may suffer emotionally for years, sometimes for the rest of their lives, from intense guilt and regret over the situation. We need to change this!

There is a third option that many owners accept gratefully when the other two are not acceptable. All pet caregivers should be asked if they want their pet to come home and pass away in their familiar surroundings, either by house call euthanasia or by assisted natural death under the supervision of a hospice veterinarian. Neglecting to offer this option puts our bioethics and our ability to respect the human–animal bond in question.

Dealing with deeply bonded caregivers in terminal situation decision making can be emotionally draining and difficult for the doctors and staff. This emotional trauma is called "vicarious traumatization" and appears as burnout, indifference, negativity, or depression (Norton and Cooper 2001). See the compassion fatigue section in Chapter 11.

Cecilia's Case (A Deeply Bonded Carer Wants to Share Each Step of the End of Life Journey)

Julie Corbin called me for a phone consultation regarding Cecilia, her 11-year-old F/S Golden Retriever, who recovered uneventfully following emergency splenectomy for hemoabdomen. I knew Julie, because I had reviewed her PhD dissertation on the human–animal bond the previous year.

Corbin wrote: "Cecilia's biopsy confirmed hemangiosarcoma. One or two of the tumors on her spleen were benign but the rest, including the one that ruptured, were malignant. It was also confirmed that the small masses on her liver were cancer and it looks as though the cancer has already metastasized. We are in shock at that news, as her presentation is so very normal and her athleticism remains intact. I understand the seriousness of her condition.

I want to look at all options that will honor her spirit, will to live and most importantly her quality of life."

Cecilia recovered quickly, but 10 days later, she collapsed. Corbin wrote: "Her hematocrit was 18 percent. Our doctor gave her supportive treatment. The next hour, her hematocrit went up to 20 and stabilized there. We stayed with Cecilia from 1:30 till 8:30 a.m. By morning, her hematocrit was 27 percent. We made the decision to take her home. You know how I feel about that. The hospital staff is getting a deeper understanding of the human–animal bond and the power of love and intention. The Hospital Administrator is a former pet bereavement client of mine. She gave us an exam room to stay overnight at the clinic and arranged for one of the Dr.'s to be on call. They were truly wonderful and not only tended to Cecilia but to us as well. That was such a Godsend to us."

For bonded caretakers, it is important to time the end of their pet's life properly. Simply pulling the plug because it is close to the end is not acceptable. These caretakers walk a thin line and walking that line requires vigilance and careful timing. They do not want to deprive their pet or themselves of those last days, hours, or minutes, while still ensuring that euthanasia is not delayed past the point where the pet will be in pain or suffering.

Corbin wrote: "If Cecilia recuperates from this episode, would chemo still be an option or is she just too close to the end at this point? I understand the fragile nature of her condition and know that she could appear 'perfect' one day and the next be bleeding out, but she is showing us such a strong will to live. Any thoughts? Again, thank you for 'supporting' us through this time. I wish Cecilia could meet you, but in a way, I believe she already has."

In reply, I commented that palliation with carboplatin in a split dose fashion four to seven days apart might help Cecilia (as it did Wheaty; see later in this chapter) and to stay on 24-hour vigil in case she develops DIC during her Pawspice. A few days later, Julie wrote: "Just wanted to give you an update on Cecilia. I NEVER thought I would see her acting her 'normal' self again. Less than two days after her near death experience, she is prancing around as if nothing ever happened. We are all stunned. She must be wonderdog! They really did not think she would make it – I had my doubts as well. … I sensed that our doctor thought she would not pull through (we even considered euthanasia that evening) and that she was coming home to pass on. I know that the tides could turn at anytime, but I am amazed at her ability to come back from this."

Two weeks later, Cecilia was euthanized. On that day, Julie wrote: "Yesterday I took her for a walk on the trails and today I gave her peace – she was in pain and that is where I draw the line. I will call you when I have a bit more clarity. I am not able to even walk into our home, and we are at a hotel tonight. I miss my girl so much and was with her till her last breath – she is with me now in a different way but somehow right now that brings no comfort. I have never loved anything or anybody as I do her – this will be a real tough one."

The following illustrates what I call the "woulda-coulda-shoulda" stage of grief, where many people who experience pet loss are stuck. Even when the ending is handled perfectly, caretakers will still go through the stages of grief and will often want to put blame or fault on themselves, the doctor, or the clinic. Some will obsess about the final decisions and actions and question every little decision and action. A week later, Corbin wrote: "Hello Dr. V, I was wondering if you might be available for a phone consult. I would like to get your input on a few things. Cecilia's doctor was not in on that day and the treatment protocol was much different. Cecilia's hematocrit level that morning was 36 and they did not want to keep her at the hospital. I took her back later that day because she got weak. Her hematocrit dropped down to 30 in 6 hours. Forty-five minutes later, we put her down based on the attending doctor's recommendations and comments that Cecilia was in pain, uncomfortable and not getting enough oxygen. Could that be so at 30?

I have a few other very valid explanations as to why she was panting – one being her phobia of thunderstorms and we had a huge one making its way to us. When I was told she was very uncomfortable and would only get worse, I made what I believe was the correct but too quick of a decision. I should have demanded supportive treatment. If she were bleeding a major bleed, would her hematocrit levels drop faster and more drastic? 30 is not that bad, is it?

When I asked, the Dr. said that anytime from that point on was the right time. She said it will only get worse and that she will become increasingly uncomfortable. I should have contacted you to get your opinion. … I feel that in my panic driven state I made a decision without demanding more medical facts and options. I just did not want Cecilia to be in pain. She did not appear to be in pain that day at home or in the ride there – though she did collapse.

They had her in the treatment room for 25 minutes but never began any sort of treatment to help stop the bleeding. Instead, they brought her back into the exam room where I was and she got weak and collapsed down again. Now, I wonder what were they doing with her during that 25 minutes she was back there?

I would like your medical opinion on some of my questions and would be happy to get you copies of her chart and blood work for that day. I am not looking for blame – I know of her grave condition … I am just trying to understand and gain more clarity."

In answer to haunting questions like this, it is appropriate to validate the carer's emotions over their loss and grief and point out that it is natural to sift over every moment of that final day asking, "woulda-coulda-shoulda." My validation was of great comfort to her. Julie needed validation as she struggled through the grief process.

Attend to the Carer's Needs

We need to expect a display of attachment and sorrow when a geriatric pet is terminal. We need to respect the end of life issues regarding when, where, and how the family wishes their terminal pet to pass. Understanding the human–animal bond means understanding attachment and people's reactions and behavior when that love bond is threatened with terminal cancer. End of life care has achieved a new era in our profession with veterinarians feeling compelled to help the people and pets in hospice. The International Association of Hospice and Palliative Care is a growing organization that provides training and certification (www.iaahpc.org).

With proper client education and counseling, we can and must allow deeply bonded clients who want to take their terminal pet home to die, to do just that. In the end, caregivers given this opportunity are much more satisfied with how their pet passed away. The clients that I have worked with who wanted to take their terminal pet home were sincerely grateful for the precious time and privacy that they shared with their terminal pet.

Terminal patients need a special allowance from normal hospital procedure. The attending doctor can sign off patient responsibility and arrange for that terminal cancer patient to go home to die without faulting or judging the client's wishes. This would parallel the human hospice movement. Doing the same for pets creates a new perspective on expanding the options we can offer clients for dealing with the final moments for their terminal pets as a member of their family.

In this situation, we as veterinarians have a dual loyalty and a conflict to resolve. We are taught not to discharge a sick animal that is unable to stand or unable to function. When dealing with terminal geriatric cancer cases, such as intra-abdominal bleeding from hemangiosarcoma or advanced metastatic disease, we need to rethink the situation. We must be loyal to the patient's physical needs and the client's emotional needs, we must honor the human–animal bond, and we must heed our oaths.

In end of life situations when the client wishes to bring the pet home, provide a client consent form. The form should acknowledge that the patient is terminal and is going home at the bequest of the family for end of life Pawspice care.

We also have a responsibility to spare our geriatric cancer patients in Pawspice care from pain, to keep within our personal ethics, and to honor the veterinarian's oath to avoid suffering in our patients. Attending veterinarians need to have the confidence and willingness to deliver enough pain control for all terminal cancer patients (Gaynor 2001), by alleviating cancer pain with placement of a fentanyl pain patch or by teaching the caregivers to administer subcutaneous injections of nalbuphine at 0.2–0.4mg/kg every six to eight hours as needed. If death comes peacefully and painlessly for the cancer patient, then our job has been done well.

When Do You Use the Word "Terminal"?

The word "terminal" is misunderstood, poorly defined, overused, and unintentionally abused in cancer medicine. "Terminal" in cancer medicine is defined as close to causing death from progressive advanced disease with vital organ involvement in the absence of any useful further therapy. In human medicine, terminal generally means that the person has less than six months to live. However, in veterinary medicine, terminal is used on a more arbitrary basis. When one doctor uses the word "terminal," he or she may mean the pet is dying from this disease within hours, days, or weeks. Another doctor may mean that the pet will die of this disease some day. Yet another doctor may feel that the pet is too old to treat or has too many complications, and euthanasia is the easy way out. In some hospitals, the pet's disease might be considered terminal because the hospital does not offer definitive care. What is the real meaning of "terminal"?

Hemangiosarcoma and lymphoma are considered by most veterinary clinicians to be "terminal." For dogs presenting with anemia and weakness due to intra-abdominal hemorrhage from suspected hemangiosarcoma, splenectomy is routinely elected even though the patient's mean survival time is limited to 86 days (Wood et al. 1998). While doctors readily perform splenectomy for stage I and stage II hemangiosarcoma, they abdicate or discourage combination chemotherapy for stage IIIa lymphoma patients when the survival time for treated lymphoma patients is comparable to patients with renal or cardiac disease – clearly much longer than for dogs with hemangiosarcoma.

Some doctors are more comfortable with abdominal surgery than they are with the rigors of administering chemotherapy. The problem is that the medicine and options that their clients receive is based on that doctor's personal bias instead of facts. There are doctors who urge clients to "do it now" for the hemangiosarcoma dog, yet say, "I wouldn't put him through it" for the lymphoma dog. There is a lot of variation from one practice to the next. Veterinarians unconsciously influence clients with professional persuasion (Yeates et al. 2010). There are new ethical considerations to think about in the evolving art and practice of end of life care for companion animals.

Oncologists, and a growing percentage of general practice veterinarians, feel that lymphomas are very treatable. Most commercial laboratories now have antibodies against CD3, the pan T-cell marker, and CD79a, the pan B-cell marker. The doctor can order immunohistochemical stains on submitted FNA cytology slides, to determine whether the lymphoma is a B- or T-cell immunophenotype. This information can better define a prognosis and may help with decision making. We can also submit samples for the Enlight Test at Innogenics™. Their assay technology identifies the phenotype of lymphoma in addition to other malignancies and provides suggestions as to which chemotherapy agents are likely to be effective (www.innogenics.org).

Many veterinarians are not comfortable using chemotherapy agents in their hospitals and do not encourage referrals for chemotherapy. The core of this reluctance to administer chemotherapy may be personal bias, or lack of education and fear or lack of familiarity with handling the drugs, associated hazards, and adverse events. The contemporary veterinarian seeks this education. Chemotherapy and immunotherapy for cancer patients is now being emphasized in the veterinary school curriculum as well.

Combination chemotherapy protocols create a high percentage of responses, complete remissions, and high-quality survival for B-cell lymphoma patients. First remissions, ranging from four to 14 months, are achieved in over 80% of all lymphoma patients. T-cell lymphoma patients are less responsive and have shorter remissions. Doxorubicin-based protocols provide the longest first remissions for B-cell lymphoma patients. Various rescue protocols may regain remissions and improve survival, especially for dogs with B-cell lymphoma (Rassnick et al. 2002). Tanovea™ is a new rescue drug that may yield prolonged remissions in B-cell lymphoma. A sub-group of fortunate responders will remain relapse free for the rest of their lives.

The meaning of the word "terminal" should not be conditional, yet in daily practice terminal is often a conditional state of being. A geriatric cancer patient with grade III mast cell tumors, concurrent heart disease, diabetes, hypothyroidism, Cushing's disease, and obesity may be conditionally terminal in one hospital but not in another hospital. If you carefully multitask for that patient, you may find a nice response. There is useful chemotherapy for mast cell and lymphoma patients who must avoid steroids, cardiotoxic, and nephrotoxic drugs. The tyrosine kinase inhibitors have made a huge difference in mast cell patient response and survival. The use of Tanovea™ may extend the survival time of resistant B-cell lymphoma dogs. Using monoclonal lymphoma vaccines for dogs after they have gained remission may prolong overall survival times. Age by itself should not be a contraindication for comprehensive cancer treatment.

Two new lymphoma cases presented for consultation on the same day. Each family was told that their dog was terminal by their attending doctors. One patient was an 8-year-old Boxer with painful bilateral renomegaly and hepatomegaly. The other patient was a $7^1/_2$-year-old Bernese Mountain Dog (BMD) with stridor, anorexia, and enormous peripheral and sub-lumbar/iliac lymphadenopathy. Both dogs were diagnosed by their attending doctors with high-grade lymphoma. In no way, would I, or any oncologist, overtly disagree with the attending doctors about their prognoses. Both dogs were very sick and dying from untreated lymphoma. They did appear terminal if untreated. However, if given the opportunity to undergo induction with combination chemotherapy and supportive care, they could achieve remission and enjoy a quality of life for a significant period.

After consultation with the families, they both elected induction therapy for their dogs. The Boxer did not respond to induction therapy while the BMD did. This may be because Boxers have a high rate of T-cell lymphoma, which is less responsive than B-cell lymphoma (Lurie et al. 2004; Ponce et al. 2004).

The Tumor Is Inoperable, or Is It? Can Stereotactic Radiosurgery Help?

The word "inoperable" is also conditional. If an attending doctor says the tumor is inoperable, that may be true in his or her hospital. However, the same tumor may be successfully addressed by a board certified surgeon at another hospital or referral center.

"Terminal" and "inoperable" are two very negative words, and they have the effect of quashing any hopes that a client may have of obtaining help to battle the cancer in a geriatric dog or cat. Upon hearing these words, many people now go to the Internet and may find that help is available for their geriatric cancer pet at a different animal hospital or referral center, using conventional, integrative, or alternative treatments.

A contemporary veterinary geriatrician thoroughly examines each patient's medical and functional condition, researches the options, and makes recommendations for the pet owner to consider. Individualization of the older patient's treatment plans, based on the diagnosis, staging, and comprehensive geriatric assessment, may yield a surprising benefit. We are practicing in exciting times because new technology is helping us help our "untreatable" patients. Recommend a stereotactic radiosurgery (SRS) facility if one is available and if your client can logistically and financially access it.

If the patient has an overtly terminal disease, then this bad news must be gently communicated to the pet owner. Highly bonded pet owners will take your advice and look into useful therapeutic options that may restore the pet's ability to eat and function. If you offer to provide good pain control and nursing instructions for the patient, you will be surprised. Many pet owners will gratefully pursue end of life Pawspice care with palliative cancer medicine and hospice care when their pet declines towards death, instead of opting for premature euthanasia.

The Long Problem List and Polypharmacy

The attending doctor must perform a full evaluation of the geriatric cancer patient. Veterinarians wear the hat of a geriatrician, dentist, dietician, surgeon, internist, oncologist, pharmacist, hospitalist, and consultant. We must assess the combination of the acute or terminal cancer condition and the chronic diseases and geriatric syndromes, along with the drugs the patient is receiving and any complications. The patient's problem list may be long and complex. Many age- and disease-related changes can cause multivariate effects on a drug's pharmacokinetics and pharmacodynamics (Hoskins 2004).

It requires more time to think about cases that have polypharmacy for a long problem list. It takes extra research, caution, and work to negotiate interactions with polypharmacy and design a feasible treatment plan. Most veterinarians receive patients and clients alone in the exam room, without much of a support team, yet they must think on a multidimensional level for these complex cases. It is best to have immediate access to online veterinary drug formularies such as Plumb's Veterinary Drugs and human formularies such as Epocrates™, etc. The doctor must identify the patient's problems and develop a plan to resolve the problems if possible.

When the patient is not in an emergency situation, it would be better for the attending doctor to say to the client, "I'd like to evaluate all facets of Bella's complex case and perhaps consult some specialists. Can I call you tonight/tomorrow with a plan that might help her?"

Unfortunately, geriatric cases like this are often viewed as terminal due to the complexity of concurrent conditions and their morbidities. If each comorbidity problem can be improved by at least 30–50%, the complex geriatric oncology patient may improve. Consultants from other disciplines may help provide more viable management options such as interventional radiology for stenting, etc., than those available at your facility. Geriatric oncology cases are more likely to need a multidisciplinary approach in order to have a positive outcome. A full range of options should be made available for the client to consider as you partner with the client during the decision-making process.

Healer or Executioner

An inherent problem that erodes the emotional stamina of veterinarians is that we are asked to practice at both ends of the spectrum as the healer or the executioner. Some clients do not even want basic services for an old dog or cat. Some, like Corbin, want to obtain as much time as possible with their pet but draw the line at any sign of pain or suffering. Others want us to perform heroic services beyond that line because they cannot let go of a failing pet or accept the inevitability of death. Our job is to find a balance and provide patient services for every client's comfort zone. At the same time, we must clearly but gently inform clients, in adherence to our oath, when we feel that the line has been crossed.

The key to providing Pawspice care and hospice services is to offer the best palliative cancer medicine, expert multimodal pain relief, and nursing support possible to the client's satisfaction level. Another key is to realize when and if you are personally having trouble with the emotional responsibility of caring for your terminal patients and their carers (see the section on compassion fatigue in Chapter 11 and the sections on self-care and wellness).

Luna's Case (She Wasn't Too Old to Treat at 26 Years of Age)

Luna, a 26-year-old F/S white cat, had extensive invasive squamous cell carcinoma (SCC) involving the right temporal area, and the entire full thickness of her pinna and ear canal. Her fungating lesion was large, ulcerated, and looked terrible. The family took Luna to a veterinarian for an annual exam when the lesion originally appeared at age 21. They went to different hospitals each year and asked the doctor for advice on how to best manage the growing lesion. Each year, the family received conservative advice from the various attending doctors due to their reservations regarding Luna's advanced age.

At her 26th-year exam, the fifth attending doctor recommended a consultation with our oncology service. Our geriatric evaluations found Luna to be a good candidate for surgical ablation of her right ear and surrounding temporal tissue. Luna had surgery on the same day as two other (less healthy) 18-year-old cats. Luna was discharged from the hospital before either of the 18-year-old cats and she lived cancer free until age $27\frac{1}{2}$, when she passed away from renal failure.

Marty's Case (A Collie's Hemoabdomen Was Not Terminal at 19 Years of Age)

Marty Lloyd, a 90-pound M/N Collie, was 19 years old when Gary Lloyd admitted him for acute weakness and pallor. Hemoabdomen was diagnosed and abdominal ultrasound identified two masses in the spleen. His database panel, U/A, and chest X-rays were normal. We counseled Mr. Lloyd about the increased risk of anesthesia and surgery and the prolonged recovery in the oldest geriatric patients. We advised him that 80% of dogs in this situation are diagnosed with terminal hemangiosarcoma that yields less than 4 months survival. Mr. Lloyd said, "Do you mean that you can stop the bleeding now with surgery, and maybe give him 4 months to live, and maybe a 20 percent chance he could be cancer free?" I said, "Yes, you have the picture." He said, "Dr. Alice, why would I not want to do it?"

Marty recovered uneventfully from surgery. Histopathology diagnosed the splenic lesions as nodular splenic hyperplasia. We presented Marty's case and applauded Mr. Lloyd for his decision with a card for Marty's 20th birthday at the 1999 Bustad Awards ceremony. Marty enjoyed an excellent quality of life with the help of acupuncture until he was 22 years of age.

Bear's Case (A Big, Ugly Tumor May Not Always Be Inoperable and Hopeless)

Bear Smith, a 110-pound, 12-year-old intact male Akita, developed anal sac carcinoma over a two-year period. Bear did not receive treatment due to the incarceration of his master. When help was requested, Bear's tumor was enormous, ulcerated, infected, and involved 360 degrees of the entire anal sphincter. The family reported that Bear was able to pass stool without much trouble. The Smiths asked two veterinarians to operate and both doctors felt that Bear had inoperable disease and recommended against surgery due to the extensive nature of the lesions (Figure 9.1A).

A third doctor told the family that, in his opinion, the mass was inoperable and that Bear was probably filled with cancer internally. He said that surgery would do no good. Someone at Mrs. Smith's local pet store referred her to Dr. Rachel Jones for laser surgery. Dr. Jones performed a minimum database exam, which found a normal blood panel, normal sub-lumbar/iliac lymph nodes, and normal chest films. The laser procedure was very helpful in debulking the mass (Figure 9.1B). Dr. Jones referred Bear to our service for oncology management. Bear appeared bright and alert despite his postop anal sphincter issues. He was able to defecate without straining and had a normal performance assessment and a good quality of life. Our job was to help shrink residual disease and stay within the strained family budget. We placed Bear on oral piroxicam, 10mg BID, and oral capecytabine (Xeloda®) at 500mg twice daily for 10 days. This schedule was repeated every 21 days. Bear's 360-degree anal sac adenocarcinoma mass continued to regress over a six-month period (see Figures 9.1C and 9.1D) and was lost to follow-up.

The next case helps to remind us that aggressive dogs and cats can be treated, even at the end stage of their lives. Do not decline to treat them out of hand. Aggressive geriatric oncology patients can be

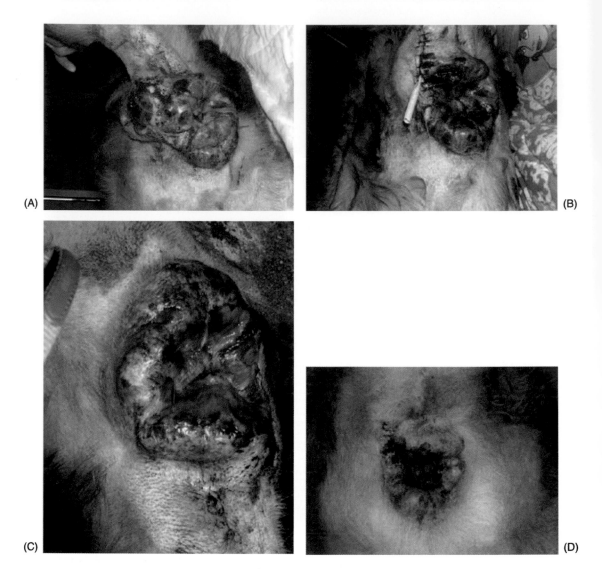

Figure 9.1. Bear, a 12-year-old male Akita with advanced anal sac carcinoma, was considered terminal according to several clinicians (A). After debulking laser surgery (B). After 3 months on oral Xeloda and piroxicam (C). After 6 months of treatment (D).

safely sedated for their treatments, although they are at greater risk for complications. A few might surprise us with a response, as in Wheaty's case.

Wheaty's Case (It's Not Over until It's Over)

Wheaty Rowe, a 12-year-old M/N Wheaton Terrier mix, was diagnosed with metastatic hemangiosarcoma involving the spleen and right ventricle of his heart. It was 4:30 p.m. on New Year's Eve when his family called me in desperation. Mr. Rowe said that they had been turned down by two different surgical specialty clinics. Each said that they could not help the family save Wheaty. The Rowes wanted my opinion ASAP because Wheaty was having trouble breathing and his abdomen was bloated.

The Rowes said their doctors recommended euthanasia, but they had faith in me since I had helped them 10 years previously. They were an hour away. I cautioned that Wheaty could expire on the way over. Wheaty presented with signs of right-sided heart failure due to a 6cm mass in his right ventricle, organomegaly, and ascites, which was a transudate from right-sided heart failure. He did not have the expected hemoabdomen from the 4cm mass in his spleen.

Wheaty had enough energy to lunge at me every time I got near him. His body condition was good but his recent performance level was compromised. The family begged me to do whatever I could for him. During the consultation, we discussed the possibility of medical management and chemotherapy and the VAC protocol for soft tissue sarcoma (STS). Adriamycin would be contraindicated and risky because of Wheaty's heart condition. I recommended carboplatin, since it has activity against some sarcomas.

Wheaty required sedation for the chemotherapy treatment due to his aggressive attitude. I thought he might die every step of the way but we all survived the procedure. One week later, Mr. Rowe returned with a seemingly different dog. Wheaty was 100% improved. The ascites was resolved; he was eupneic and more aggressive than ever. We treated him every 21 days and, to the joy of his family, old Wheaty survived with a good quality of life for 4 more months in Pawspice.

Chemotherapy for Advanced Stage Geriatric Patients

When treating advanced stage disease in geriatric patients with chemotherapy, select drugs that bypass any known compromised organ function. For instance, if the patient has kidney disease or CRF, never use a highly nephrotoxic drug such as cisplatin and modify the dose by 25–50% for drugs that rely on renal excretion. If a terminal canine patient has a heart condition or is a breed that is prone to cardiomyopathy, avoid using Adriamycin.

Management using oral and subcutaneous chemotherapy and support medications versus IV medications is preferred for advanced stage and terminal geriatric oncology patients. This approach is appreciated if the patient is fearful, stressed, or malnourished. This keeps the caregiver and patient at home and may avoid unnecessary side effects.

It is advisable to avoid using Adriamycin in very old patients because they have a greater prevalence for myocardial and renal compromise, dehydration, and malnourishment. Cisplatin should be excluded in geriatric oncology due to the high incidence of renal fibrosis and dehydration in older animals. Cisplatin is inherently nephrotoxic and using it in geriatrics creates an unjustifiable renal insult. The attending doctor needs to offer more supportive help for advanced stage and terminal cancer patients to ameliorate dehydration and malnourishment. Terminal geriatric oncology patients in Pawspice care would clearly benefit with enteral feedings and SQ fluids directed at nutritional rehabilitation and rehydration (see the Quality of Life Scale, Table 10.1). If we can improve the terminal geriatric patient's nutritional status and hydration, the pet may be able to handle palliative therapy more readily.

Metronomic (low dose) chemotherapy, chemoprevention, or conventional drugs used at the lower end of the therapeutic dose can minimize the risk of side effects. If the patient tolerates a conventional chemotherapy drug at the initial low dose range, then it is appropriate to escalate the dose on subsequent treatments (Balducci 2004). If there is no indication that the patient has received benefit from the initially selected drug, it is appropriate to try another drug using the principles of dose escalation.

When using the longer-acting chemotherapy drugs that are more toxic in geriatric cancer patients, I often split the dose. This precaution is especially important for geriatric patients with renal or hepatic compromise and obese geriatric patients. The lean body weight is determined. In addition, we reduce the traditional dose by 25% if there is renal or hepatic compromise. We then administer 50% of the dose on day 1 and day 8 of each cycle instead of giving a traditional dose on an every 21–30 day schedule. We employ the split dose method most often with Adriamycin, especially for older medium, large, and giant breed dogs. It is generally thought that the m^2 Body Surface Chart underdoses large-breed dogs and overdoses cats and small dogs weighing less than 20 pounds. By spreading the dose out over four to seven days, the patient has fewer toxicity problems.

For example, the split dose schedule that I use for Adriamycin is 20mg/m^2 on day 1 and day 8 given over 15–20 minutes for large to giant breed dogs. I use Adriamycin in this split fashion for breeds at risk for dilated cardiomyopathy, such as Doberman Pinschers. In this way, we can reduce the risk of cardiac and GI toxicity to a minimal degree while gaining a higher total dose for the geriatric patient. For geriatric dogs between 20 and 55 pounds, I use 20mg/m^2 for day 1 and 10–15mg/m^2 on day 8, depending on the size and condition of the patient. Geriatric cats and dogs under 20 pounds generally do not receive split Adriamycin doses because they experience minimal toxicity at the reduced dose of 20mg/m^2 every 21 days.

Palliative Radiation Therapy and SRS for Terminal Patients

Some terminal geriatric cancer patients may benefit from palliative radiation therapy (RTx). The normal rigorous treatment schedule that involves daily or alternate-day anesthesia is reduced to once a week for three or four weeks. The dose fraction is much higher and the tumor response time is reduced. Palliative RTx offers the patient a reasonably effective total therapeutic dose while minimizing the number and frequency of anesthetics. This schedule minimizes the stress on the compromised, terminal patient. In some cases, we maintain regression of oral masses in terminal cancer patients using monthly fractions of RTx.

If you are not sure about a case, consult a radiation oncologist to help you decide if the terminal cancer patient has a radiation-responsive mass. Many tumors that have previously been considered radio-resistant will show a response to the high fraction(s) given during 1–3 stereotactic radiosurgery (SRS) treatments. If anesthesia is deemed a reasonable risk, the client may consider either an aggressive palliative schedule or a basic palliative schedule (see the section on "The Role of Radiation Therapy in Cancer Management" in Chapter 6).

Schniffer's Case (How "Terminal" Is "Terminal"?)

Doug and Christine Gore loved Schniffer, their 13-year-old F/S German Shorthaired Pointer, who developed acute onset signs of fever, anorexia, and depression. On physical exam, the temperature was 106 degrees Fahrenheit and a 3cm mass in the left anal sac was palpated. Minimum database exam found an elevated white blood cell count and normal organ function and urine values. Chest and abdominal X-rays revealed extensive metastatic disease with nodules throughout the abdominal and chest cavities. After two days in the hospital on symptomatic treatment, Schniffer was ambulatory and regained her appetite.

The Gores wanted Schniffer to come home for Pawspice care and eventually hospice. They were sad that their infant son would never know their beloved Schniffer. They wanted to keep

Schniffer comfortable until the time came for her hospice and passing. They declined chemotherapy but accepted our suggestion for immunonutrition using Agaricus, OncoSupport, and IP-6. Schniffer amazingly survived with good quality of life for one year, befriending their son as he grew into a toddler.

Electroporation/Electrochemotherapy for Selected Terminal Patients

Megan's Case (Inoperable Oral Malignant Melanoma Responds to EP and IFx)

Dr. Christina Hutson referred Barbara Smaldino with Megan, her 10-year-old Scottish Terrier, on October 18, 2016 for consultation. Barbara was informed that Megan's oral malignant melanoma was too large to gain clean surgical margins. Megan's MRI and CT scan documented a 6cm × 4cm mass that had destroyed the right caudal hard palate and was invading the ventral right orbit. Her chest X-ray was clear and her local lymph nodes were normal. We offered to harvest tumor tissue for IFx vaccine production and perform electroporation (EP) at the tumor site, including its margins. Megan recovered uneventfully but developed an expected oral nasal fistula, which caused her to sneeze after eating. She received her IFx vaccines and remained tumor free at 6 months post-EP. For more information on EP, read the "Electrochemotherapy/Electroporation" section at the end of Chapter 6.

Client Consent Forms

Veterinarians routinely use a client consent form before anesthesia and surgery. Nevertheless, when dealing with fragile, sick, malnourished, vulnerable, and terminal geriatric cancer patients, it is reasonable to ask your clients to sign an informed consent form (Figure 9.2). This asks the client to acknowledge the severity of the pet's specific situation. Before you perform a potentially life-threatening procedure, the client must be made fully aware and acknowledge the prognosis of the geriatric pet's cancer and the increased risk for adverse events that medical therapy may entail.

The consent form should also state details regarding Advanced Directives. I ask the client this question: "In the event that Bella has cardiac or respiratory arrest, how long do you want us to resuscitate her?" I let clients know that 10 minutes is reasonable and that few patients ever recover past that critical time.

My preference is to avoid using a harshly worded legal document. I write a line or two in the medical chart regarding the poor prognosis despite treatment, including the risks associated with treatment. I also write the time lapse agreed upon to be allowed in the event that resuscitation is needed. Then, I ask the client to read the entry and sign beside it, right in the chart. This clarifying precaution is important so that everyone is on the same page and in agreement to prevent misunderstandings.

We asked Mr. Rowe to sign such a consent notation in Wheaty's medical chart before we sedated Wheaty for chemotherapy. We knew that sedation would be risky for Wheaty due to his right-sided heart failure from metastatic hemangiosarcoma. However, the family was willing to take the risk. The consent form helped the Rowe's acknowledge that Wheaty was at risk for cardiac arrest and complications. This type of personal acknowledgement of risk and prognosis is very helpful to keep the hopeful client cognizant of the reality of the situation. High-risk procedures and aggressive palliation

---

<u>INFORMED CONSENT TO FURTHER TREATMENT IN CASES WITH LITTLE OR
NO HOPE OF SUCCESSFUL TREATMENT</u>

    I understand that my pet named _____ is suffering from an incurable cancer or diseases and the treatment being rendered at _____ (practice name) is simply prolonging my pet's life by a few days to a few months. I understand that the doctors at _____ (practice name) recommend that no further surgery or treatments be performed because they are concerned that my pet may not heal or recover from such surgery or treatment, that additional medications will make my pet sicker, and/or that the tumor and complications associated with it may recur within a matter of days to weeks.

    In spite of the fact that the prognosis for my pet is poor, I am demanding that the doctors at _____ (practice name) proceed with surgery and/or all medical care that can be provided. In view of the poor prognosis, I understand that I will be required to pay in advance for all further veterinary services. Should I decide to proceed with surgery or further chemotherapeutic care, I will be expected to make satisfactory arrangements to pay for all outstanding veterinary fees totaling $ _____ as well as place $ _____ on deposit to cover the anticipated costs of surgery, medications, and possible complications from such medical or surgical care prior to the admissions of my pet to the hospital.

    In the event I am unwilling to comply with these requirements, I understand that the doctors at _____ (practice name) will be unable to provide further medical services. I understand they are, however, willing to refer my pet and me to another veterinary hospital or humanely euthanize my pet at any time at my request.

_____   _____
Signature of Owner or Agent   Date

_____   _____
Signature of Witness   Date

Figure 9.2. Client Consent Form for treatment of a terminal patient with a poor prognosis.

for advanced cancer in geriatric patients will be more commonly attempted in the future. It is prudent to clearly apprise clients of your treatment goals, despite the risks, for improving the quality of life of their geriatric cancer patients, and of your concerns as well.

Via the signed notation of informed consent in the pet's chart, the client acknowledges an understanding of the prognosis with or without treatment and the potential side effects of therapy. It is also important to convey your willingness and enthusiasm to give the patient your best effort in the event that the client elects to try to save his or her pet.

The cases selected for inclusion in this chapter are dramatic ones, involving the "oldest of the old." An essential component of practice in geriatric oncology is having finely honed decision-making skills. We need to use objective methodology to decide if a geriatric cancer patient is truly terminal or conditionally terminal. If there is a decent chance that the patient can survive a definitive or palliative surgical procedure or handle a chemotherapy protocol or palliative radiation therapy, the client may elect to proceed with treatment. If the patient's cancer has no useful therapy that can extend life, then offer pain control and support in the form of end of life palliative Pawspice and hospice care. Give the client assurance that euthanasia can and should be used to help the cancer patient pass peacefully, but only after all other approaches have been considered.

The Future is Bright

The oncology medicine of tomorrow is promising. It might change how we approach difficult, advanced, and terminal cancer in our geriatric cancer patients. We will have access to novel agents to help us battle common cancers such as Tanovea™ (rabacfosadine IV) for relapsed lymphoma in dogs and potentially in cats, and VCC-597, a dual acting tumor cell signaling inhibitor, which can be given orally for various sarcomas (www.vet-dc.com). We may have monoclonal antibody immunotherapy for lymphomas and a Listeria-based vaccine for osteosarcoma (www.aratana.com). We can submit tissue for personalized cancer vaccines for solid tumors (www.morphogenesis-inc.com/veterinary-oncology). Inoperable tumors may be treated with electroporation or stereotactic radiation, which may be well tolerated by geriatric cancer patients. Apoplogic is a biotech firm developing Breceptin™ for small cell cancers and melanomas, and Fasaret™ for Fas-resistant carcinomas, sarcomas, and lymphomas. Apoplogic is also working on an engineered biligand targeted toxin (e-BAT) that kills hemangiosarcoma progenitor cells at safe low doses (www.apoplogic.com). The Shine On Project was funded by the Golden Retriever, Portuguese Water Dog and Boxer foundations, the American. Kennel Club, and the Canine Health Foundation at the University of Minnesota, to study the detection and treatment of hemangiosarcoma. Data from the Shine On Project will provide the rationale to detect, treat, and hopefully prevent hemangiosarcoma. We may one day be able to offer our dog-owning clients a preventative cancer vaccine cocktail to offset LSA, HSA, and OSA; as mentioned in previous chapters.

Summary

When to declare a cancer patient "terminal" is not always a clear-cut clinical decision. It is best to use the word "terminal" when the patient exhibits cancer-related symptoms and distress that cannot be managed after making a good effort. Offer supportive options such as Pawspice, which embraces aggressive palliative cancer medicine along with addressing symptoms, and offer hospice, which provides an intense comfort care during the pet's decline toward death. The attending doctors should focus on palliative medicine, especially pain control, for the terminal patient until instructed otherwise by the client. Also, provide sincere respect for the human–animal bond – the deep attachment that the primary carers have for their geriatric cancer pet – during every step of the decision-making process. Some terminal geriatric cancer patients may benefit from aggressive palliation, cytoreductive (debulking or electroporation) surgery, feeding tubes, stents, and cystostomy tubes, palliative or stereotactic radiation therapy, nutritional therapy, immunotherapy, and general palliative and supportive care. Decision making should be a special partnership between you and your clients, with the terminal geriatric cancer patient's needs and quality of life prioritized as the foremost consideration.

References

Balducci, L. 2004. "Guidelines for the management of the older cancer patient." In *Comprehensive geriatric oncology*, 2nd edn, eds L. Balducci, G.H. Lyman, W.B. Ershler, and M. Extermann, pp. 525–533. Oxon, UK: Taylor & Francis.

Berg, R.J., and W. Wingfield. 1984. Pericardial effusion in the dog. A review of 42 cases. *JAAHA* 20:721–730.

Bustad, L.K. 1996. *Compassion: Our last great hope – Selected speeches of Leo K. Bustad, DVM, PhD.* Renton, WA: Delta Society.

Butler, C.L., M.S. Lagoni, K.L. Dickinson, and S.J. Withrow. 1991. "Cancer." In *Animal illness and human emotion: Problems in veterinary medicine*, eds S.P. Cohen and C.E. Fudin, Vol. 3, No. 1, pp. 21–38. Philadelphia, PA: Lippincott.

DeGregori, J., 2012. Challenging the axiom: does the occurrence of oncogenic mutations truly limit cancer development with age? *Oncogene*, 2012; doi: 10.1038/onc.2012.281.

Gaynor, J.S. 2001. "Pain management for the oncology patient." In *Small animal clinical oncology*, 3rd edn, eds S.J. Withrow and E.G. MacEwen, pp. 219–232. Philadelphia, PA: Saunders.

Helfand, S.C. 2003. "Emerging approaches for cancer therapy." In *BSAVA manual of canine and feline oncology*, 2nd edn, eds J. Dobson and D. Lascelles, pp. 115–119. Quedgeley, Gloucestershire, England: British Small Animal Veterinary Association.

Hoskins, J.D. 2004. "Pharmacologic principles." In *Geriatrics and gerontology of the dog and cat*, 2nd edn, eds J.D. Hoskins, pp. 43–58. Philadelphia, PA: Saunders/Elsevier.

Hua, J., S. Hoummady, C. Muller, J.L. Pouchelon, M. Blondot, C. Gilbert, and L. Desquilbet. 2016. Assessment of frailty in aged dogs, *American Journal of Veterinary Research* 77 (12):1357–1365.

Kealy, R.D., D.F. Lawler, J.M. Ballam, S.L. Mantz, D.N. Biery, E.H. Greeley, G. Lust, M. Segre, G.K. Smith, and H.D. Stowe. 2002. Effects of diet restriction on life span and age-related changes in dogs. *JAVMA* 220:1315–1320.

London, C. 2004. Kinase inhibitors in cancer therapy. *Veterinary and Comparative Oncology* 2 (4):177–193.

Lucroy, M.D., and B.R. Madewell. 2001. Clinical outcome and diseases associated with extreme neutrophilic leukocytosis in cats: 104 cases (1991–1999). *JAVMA* 218:736–739.

Lurie, D.M., M.D. Lucroy, S.M. Griffey, E. Simonson, and B.R. Madewell. 2004. T-cell derived malignant lymphoma in the boxer breed. *Veterinary and Comparative Oncology* 2 (3):171–175.

Lyman, G.H. 2004. "Essentials of clinical decision analysis: A new way to think about cancer and aging." In *Comprehensive geriatric oncology*, 2nd edn, eds L. Balducci, G.H. Lyman, W.B. Ershler, and M. Extermann, pp. 12–25. Oxon, UK: Taylor & Francis.

Milner, R.J., J. Peyton, K. Cooke, L.E. Fox, A. Gallagher, P. Gordon, and J. Hester. 2005. Response rates and survival times for cats with lymphoma treated with the University of Wisconsin–Madison chemotherapy protocol: 38 cases (1996–2003). *JAVMA* 227 (7):1118–1121.

Modiano, J.F. 2016. Innovations in cancer treatment and prevention, World Veterinary Cancer Congress, Foz do Iguassu, Brazil.

Norton, B.J., and S.I. Cooper. 2001. "Psychosocial issues." In *Veterinary oncology secrets*, ed. R.C. Rosenthal, pp. 15–18. Philadelphia, PA: Hanley & Belfus.

Pal, S. 2016. Psych drug helps manage lung cancer symptoms: Olanzapine eases treatment-related vomiting, nausea and disease-driven anorexia, ASCO Reading Room/MedPage Today, September 16, 2016.

Ponce, F., J.P. Magnol, D. Ledieu, et al. 2004. Prognostic significance of morphological subtypes in canine malignant lymphoma during chemotherapy. *Veterinary Journal* 167:158–166.

Rassnick, K.M., G.E. Mauldin, R. Al-Sarraf, G.N. Mauldin, A.S. Moore, and S.C. Mooney. 2002. MOPP chemotherapy for treatment of resistant lymphoma in dogs: A retrospective study of 117 cases (1998–2000). *JVIM* 16:576–580.

Repetto, L., A. Venturino, and W. Gianni. 2004. "Prognostic evaluation of the older cancer patient." In *Comprehensive geriatric oncology*, 2nd edn, eds L. Balducci, G.H. Lyman, W.B. Ershler, and M. Extermann, pp. 309–319. Oxon, UK: Taylor & Francis.

Roudebush, P., S.C. Zicker, C.W. Cotman, N.W. Milgram, B.A. Muggenburg, and E. Head. 2005. Nutritional management of brain aging in dogs. *JAVMA* 227 (5):722–728.

Salisbury, S.K. 2002. "Surgery for oncologic emergencies." In *Cancer in dogs and cats: Medical and surgical management*, 2nd edn, ed. W.B. Morrison, pp. 227–248. Jackson, WY: Teton New Media.

Salisbury, S.K., E. Lafond, and W.B. Morrison. 2002. "Blood transfusion and management of pain, infection and nutritional needs in the postoperative cancer patient." In *Cancer in dogs and cats: Medical and surgical management*, 2nd edn, ed. W.B. Morrison, pp. 303–327. Jackson, WY: Teton New Media.

Schappa, J.T., A.M. Frantz, B.H. Gorden, E.B. Dikerson, D.A. Vallera, and J.F. Modiano. 2013. Hemangiosarcoma and its cancer stem cell sub-population are effectively killed by a toxin targeted through epidermal growth factor and urokinase receptors, *International Journal of Cancer* October 15, 133 (8):1936–1944.

Stone, M.S., M.A. Goldstein, and S.M. Cotter 1991. Comparison of two protocols for induction of remission in dogs with lymphoma. *JAVMA* 27:315–321.

Weeth, L.P., A.J. Fascetti, P.H. Kass, S.E. Suter, A.M. Santos, and S.J. Delaney. 2007. Prevalence of obese dogs in a population of dogs with cancer. *American Journal of Veterinary Research* 68 (4):389–398.

Wood, C.A., A.S. Moore, J.M. Gliatto, L.A. Ablin, R.J. Berg, and W.M. Rand. 1998. Prognosis for dogs with stage I or II splenic hemangiosarcoma treated by splenectomy alone: 32 cases (1991–1993). *JAAHA* 34:417–421.

Yeates JW, Main DCJ, The ethics of influencing clients, Views: Commentary, JAVMA, Vol. 237, No. 3, August 1, 2010, pp. 263–267.

Chapter 10
Palliative Care: End of Life "Pawspice" Care

Palliative care should not be the last resort … or about giving up. It's about increased quality of life and enhanced coordination of care. It is not about dying. It is about living with cancer. It's not less care. It's more care.

Fred Meyers, MD, Davis School of Medicine, University of California

In a broad sense, most of the oncology treatments that we can offer for pets of any age that develop aggressive, recurrent, or advanced stage cancer are truly palliative in nature. Idealism and/or clinical arrogance may tempt us to characterize cancer treatment otherwise, but bad cancers continue to humble us with its millions of victories.

Defining the work of veterinary oncology as palliative, rather than cure-oriented, need not connote lower expectations. In palliation, our primary goal is to stabilize a tumor and keep it from enlarging or metastasizing. One day we may turn cancer into yet another chronic disease. In the future, we may list certain cancers as concurrent illness. It is important for practitioners and carers alike to understand that some cancers are curable, more will be controllable, and that many pets *"cancervive"* (can survive) with a reasonable quality of life on long-term palliative therapy. When the patient is expected to die, all attention should focus on comfort care to the very last days, hours, and minutes (Yaxley and Pierce 2016).

There is a true need for human and veterinary oncologists to guide colleagues and carers as to when it is time to stop the overuse of aggressive treatment and switch to palliative treatment. Some colleagues do not admit to themselves that their treatments are not effective. They are reluctant to call a time when their best efforts at further treatment have become futile. This is particularly true for cancer patients on chemotherapy. It is common to keep trying another and another and another protocol using different drugs and never stopping until the patient succumbs (Kaplan and Villalobos 2016). Most human patients less than 65 years old with incurable cancer continue to receive aggressive treatment in the last 30 days of life. By doing so, these patients often sacrificed their quality of life at the end of life. The 2012 American Society of Clinical Oncology (ASCO) "Choosing Wisely" campaign attempted to reduce futile treatments at the end of patient's lives. However, the Choosing Wisely campaign had no impact over 4 years with fewer than 20% of cancer patients receiving hospice care (Chen et al. 2016).

In veterinary medicine, the tendency to continue treating is most often in dogs with drug-resistant and relapsed lymphoma. There are many rescue protocols with variable responses. We feel obligated to try to help our patients, especially if there is a new drug available, but we must first, and foremost, preserve quality of life. Tanovea™ (rabacfosadine) is a new drug that preferentially targets lymphoma cells with a low toxicity profile. It offers invigorated hope for dogs with resistant relapsed B-cell lymphoma. When given at 1mg/kg IV over 30 minutes every 21 days, its benefit may short-cut jumping from one rescue protocol to another. It is in clinical trials for cats.

However, there comes a time when we need to be kind-heartedly frank with our clients and discuss the futility of further standard cancer treatments for their geriatric cancer pet. We need to compassionately emphasize the importance of preserving quality of life with palliative end of life home care, adopting the Pawspice and hospice philosophy. Pawspice would embrace metronomic chemotherapy, which is gentler for end of life patients, along with palliation of distressful symptoms. Hospice would provide intense comfort care as the patient declines toward death. This often requires teaching clients the basics in palliative "home care 101" all the way to the patient's last days and hours, as described in this chapter and various sections throughout this text.

I like the word "palliative" because it has the word "pal" in it. Most clients have never heard this long word before, yet they may be entering their pet into this thoughtful and supportive type of management. Palliative care can be explained to clients as finding ways to help their sick pal feel better by reducing pain and nausea, slowing down the cancer, relieving an obstruction, or improving or restoring appetite, energy, and other vital functions. Palliative care is not aimed at or expected to cure.

The primary goal of palliative care is to provide supportive care and comfort for the patient, and it may include palliative cancer care if it is desired. Pawspice embraces the simultaneous model of palliating the cancer while palliating its symptoms. Insurance companies decided that human hospice should not include cancer care, which in my opinion ruined its good intentions of relieving suffering. Human hospice became synonymous with "giving up". Sadly, most physicians refer their patients to hospice only 3 days before they die, instead of the ideal 6 months. Human hospice provides intense comfort care until death comes but it does not hasten death. In veterinary hospice, we palliate the patient and nurture the human–animal bond until we help our patients escape the final ravages of active dying with the gift of humane euthanasia. More information and certification courses are available from The International Association of Animal Hospice and Palliative Care web site (www.iaahpc.org).

What is Aggressive Palliation for Cancer?

Aggressive palliation is emerging as a very acceptable course of therapy in human medicine for geriatric cancer patients. Its goals are more optimistic than those of traditional palliation, while remaining less toxic than traditional treatment. It is used to treat advanced stage geriatric cancer patients who have a good quality of life and a reasonably high performance level. Geriatric oncology patients who can perform daily functions and still enjoy a good quality of life may be candidates for aggressive palliation.

With the Pawspice concept, you have an increasing opportunity to provide both aggressive palliative cancer care and/or palliative "comfort" care as viable treatment options for your geriatric cancer patients. The field of geriatric oncology for pets is wide open for many combinations of palliative care. Together, carers and the cancer care team can be very creative. The arena of animal hospice focuses on end of life comfort care. It requires resourceful, compassionate thinking, and imagination is the only limiting factor.

All forms of cancer therapy discussed in Chapter 6 can be modified and specifically tailored to reduce toxicity and fit into a palliative care program for an end of life geriatric cancer patient. This is the key principle of Pawspice. It is about more attentive care versus less care as it embraces the simultaneous model. The attending clinician must reassign the purpose of the treatment to be "treatment with palliative intent." Furthermore, the clinician should modify the treatment dose and schedule to deliver therapy with minimal risk to the patient, as in the split dose technique and metronomic therapy described in Chapter 6. Above all, palliative therapy must primarily be supportive. Ideally, palliative therapy would also be completely devoid of adverse events, but this is wishful thinking!

Geriatric patients are often frail and prone to reacting negatively to any type of drug or conventional treatment modality. Sedation or anesthesia is required for salvage surgery, electroporation, placement of feeding or ostomy tubes, palliative radiation therapy, stereotactic radiation (SRS), imaging, or other delicate procedures such as interventional radiology. Many sophisticated palliative and ancillary procedures may place the geriatric cancer patient at some increased risk for sedation or anesthesia-related death. The problem is magnified when the patient is fearful or uncooperative for procedures, while having concurrent illness such as heart and lung disease and other debilitating comorbidities. We should confer with the patient's carers to determine if they want resuscitation for their geriatric pet undergoing palliative care procedures. This is a request for an advance directive regarding how long they want us to continue with resuscitation efforts in the event of cardiac or respiratory arrest. I write a sentence stating the client's wishes regarding resuscitation in the medical chart and ask them to initial the statement for clarification.

One of the most dramatic areas for improved aggressive palliation has come to us from radiation oncology in the form of palliative and stereotactic radiosurgery. This may extend to the expanded use of locally delivered radioisotopes. Yttrium 90 microspheres may be safely mixed with a polymer solution, which undergoes a phase transfer into Radiogel™ after intratumor injections. Because this brachytherapy device is a short range, short duration, beta emitter, IsoPet's Y-90 RadioGel™ can be given on an outpatient basis (www.IsoPetSolutions.com). There is radiobiological rationale for accelerated fractionation of radiation therapy to treat stubborn tumors and to palliate advanced painful lesions. Old cats with CKD and ulcerative inoperable nasal planum squamous cell carcinomas were the first cases that we palliated with radiation therapy. We used four accelerated fractions given at days 0, 7, 14, and 28. Old dogs with nasal cavity tumors may also benefit from accelerated radiation protocols and combinatorial treatment. Carers may be more likely to give consent for a less time-consuming, less demanding palliative radiation protocol. They are happy to have the option to avoid the standard 16 21 fractions delivered by conventional radiation therapy. Most facilities are utilizing CT-enhanced treatment planning. Stereotactic radiosurgery delivers a targeted therapeutic dose in 1–5 treatments and avoids tissue damage to surrounding structures. It is ideal for debulking treatment of difficult to access and metastatic tumors. It can be combined with immunotherapy and sequenced with metronomic therapy that reduces regulatory T-cells, to allow the immune system to recognize and destroy cancer cells throughout the body (Monjazeb and Kent 2013).

If the family is reluctant to subject their geriatric oncology pet to a three-week radiation protocol, the next best option is to offer a palliative accelerated fraction schedule, or SRS, or Y-90, if the technology is available and affordable. In this way, the geriatric patient receives a therapeutic radiation therapy regimen with fewer treatments over a reduced period.

Today, we add piroxicam to the palliative radiation protocol. In addition, the client may be given the option of using mitoxantrone for their squamous cell carcinoma (SCC) cats and carboplatin for nasal tumor dogs. These two drugs are well tolerated as palliative chemotherapy for geriatric patients as long as we are able to keep the patients well hydrated. Metronomic chemotherapy and immunonutrition may also be applied to further palliate geriatric cats and dogs with a variety of tumor types. We can now safely add small molecule therapy using tyrosine kinase inhibitors and potentially use checkpoint inhibitors, immunotherapy, and novel products such as those from Apoplogic, Aratana

Therapeutics, VetDC, and other cancer-focused biopharmaceutical companies. In the future, we will have more treatment selections to design multimodal combinatorial palliative protocols for geriatric cancer patients that may gain welcome responses in a wide variety of tumors.

Informed Consent and Informed Refusal

Dr. James Wilson, JD, veterinarian and attorney, led a popular session at veterinary meetings titled "Paw & Order." Wilson recommends that veterinarians use improved methods and documentation to acquire client acknowledgement and compliance. Every veterinary hospital office staff is already trained to routinely have clients sign a standard consent form before anesthesia and surgery. Wilson recommends the addition of an "informed refusal" form for clients who decline the veterinarian's recommendations.

Some clients fail to recognize the benefit that their pet would gain from a certain proposed therapy. A stubborn or fearful client may be reluctant to initial the pet's chart or to sign any type of form. If this is the case, the client's lack of compliance should be noted in the medical chart. It is also important to not make the client feel guilty or bad when they make decisions that we feel are not in their pet's best interest. We do not know their extenuating and financial circumstances and the amount of stress that they are going through. Our job is to educate and inform our clients, as a partner in decision making; not to batter or judge our clients.

Informed refusal may also be used on a conceptual basis for cancer patients who will not be receiving conventional treatments. For instance, if a client declines induction therapy for a treatable cancer like lymphoma, I may ask them to sign the pet's medical chart or an ancillary note of acknowledgement but generally not an informed refusal form. The notation in the chart states the prognosis without treatment so that it qualifies for an informed refusal. Choosing a modality of aggressive palliative cancer therapy or comfort palliative therapy for a pet of any age is a very personal decision. The client should not be made to feel judged or intimidated by your request for acknowledgement and documentation of the information that you have given them during consultation.

Some clients are not likely to initial or sign the chart. I let them know, in a gentle and non-threatening way, that I am signing it in their presence for verification and documentation saying, "So that we are on the same page." This makes the client a witness to your entry into the medical record. It helps to have the facts documented in the event that there is a misunderstanding down the road. Unfortunately, some clients feel that they should only have to pay for veterinary services if the outcome is successful. Explain to clients that our work, especially in the area of palliative cancer care, has no guarantee of successful outcome. Sometimes, I tell clients that, "Cancer has cut my knees off many times." Remind clients that there is a potential for treatment-related adverse side effects. If the adverse events are fairly common with the selected treatment, it is important to describe it to them, such as, "After a few days, there will be a necrotic sore at the electroporation site for 4–6 weeks." Offer a cancer care package that provides a topical care product and medication to alleviate the common adverse events and symptoms associated with chemotherapy, especially for vomiting, diarrhea, and fever.

Taking care of the geriatric oncology patient is a partnership. You can say something like this: "The decision that you are going to make for your geriatric pet must be very difficult. We know that you love your pet. We are also aware that you may have other priorities or philosophies that may force you to decline standard or palliative therapy that we could use to treat the cancer. Some cancers respond with a certain percentage of remissions and even cures, but we cannot guarantee a remission or a cure for your pet. Remember, you can always change your mind."

For cases where the client elects no further conventional treatment, or when further treatment is considered hopeless, too toxic, or too risky, we encourage clients to enter the patient into a supportive end of life Pawspice program. Pawspice may include palliative cancer care and always includes palliation for distressful symptoms. Pawspice transitions to hospice, which provides a more intense comfort care program when the pet declines toward death. This concept, as an option, validates the family's human–animal bond for their beloved pet and restores pride and supports courage for making the difficult decision. We may ask clients to initial their pet's medical chart when entering their geriatric cancer pet into the hospice phase during their end of life Pawspice program.

When planning to administer any type of drug therapy to frail, sick, malnourished, or terminal geriatric cancer patients, discuss the concept and value of informed consent. Then ask the client to sign an informed consent form or initial the medical chart. By signing, the client actively acknowledges the severity of the pet's specific situation. Clients entering their pets into Pawspice care must be fully aware of the prognosis of their pet's cancer and of the potential adverse events that palliative and supportive medical therapy may entail. Rather than using a harshly worded legal document (see Figure 9.2), I write a line or two in the pet's medical chart regarding the poor prognosis despite treatment, including the risks associated with treatment. I read it to the client while writing and then ask the client to read the entry and sign beneath it right on the chart. This personal acknowledgement of risk and prognosis is very helpful to keep pet carers cognizant of the purpose of palliative therapy and the reality of the situation.

Aggressive Palliation and High-Risk Procedures

High-risk procedures and aggressive palliation for advanced cancer in geriatric patients will be more commonly attempted in the future. It is prudent to clearly apprise the client of your treatment goals for improving the quality of life of the pet, along with your concerns. The client needs to acknowledge and understand the prognosis with or without treatment and the potential adverse events associated with the chosen therapy. Convey your willingness and enthusiasm to give the geriatric cancer patient your best effort whenever clients elect or demand that you try to save their beloved pet.

In advanced stage cases that have a poor prognosis for successful induction or for cases that require risky anesthesia or technically complex and difficult procedures, I say something like this, "Your decision permits us to use our best medical knowledge to help your pet. We hope that we can gain a remission and that there is a favorable outcome despite the poor prognosis and risk of adverse side effects and possibly death." I always suggest to clients that they say goodbye to their pet before any procedure that requires anesthesia, in the event that the pet passes away during the procedure or in the postoperative treatment period.

Pawspice Care for Geriatric Cancer Patients

Although this book encourages veterinarians to treat cancer more effectively and innovatively, our geriatric cancer patients are at maximum risk for death. Cancer ravages over 50% of our senior and geriatric companion dogs and over 30% of our beloved cats. Our geriatric cancer patients are often preburdened with other concurrent morbidities such as dental disease, degenerative arthritis, organ failure, incontinence, and cognitive dysfunction. The level of morbidity caused by concurrent conditions confounds the decision to treat a geriatric pet's cancer. Some cancers are insidious and can be very occult in the geriatric oncology patient. Many cancers are not discovered until the companion animal is already in very advanced stages. Some cancers are discovered or suspected only after causing a seizure, collapse, or acute pain, or by causing a rapid destabilization of the compensated aged pet.

Patients needing palliative, in-home hospice care during the last phase of their end of life Pawspice program often have management issues such as: relapse, resistance, recurrence, obstructions, functional disabilities, uncontrolled pain, and reduced quality of life. There may also be other extenuating arbitrary issues with owner disillusionment, other commitments, reluctance to continue conventional aggressive or palliative cancer therapy, and budget concerns.

Most carers and their veterinarians are burdened with old wives' tales, myths, and preconceived notions about cancer and its treatment. Previous experiences may have created erroneous biases and negative ingrained emotional reactions regarding cancer. This creates a fatalistic approach toward treating cancer in younger and middle-aged pets and leaves no alternative for geriatric pets. Carers come to us with this dichotomy every day. They love their geriatric pets but they cannot rationalize treating their pet for cancer. Case by case, attending clinicians and their professional staff must overcome the defeatist attitude about the aging process, cancer therapy, palliative therapy, and end of life supportive care. We must try to dispel the old mindset and look at a new way of thinking about these issues when the family seeks our help. It is best to ask clients if they will allow you to help them examine each of their negative notions and ingrained myths or biases. Negative thinking no longer serves the human–animal bond that clients shared with their aging pet before the cancer was diagnosed.

Veterinarians must rid themselves of the old utilitarian kneejerk impulse to rank euthanasia as the second or third best option for pet carers. Instead, we can implement end of life care programs such as Pawspice, which embraces palliative cancer medicine, symptom management, and transitions to hospice care at the very end, for every client's dear pet. People come to us for advice and present their pets to us as patients; they do not expect us to prematurely terminate their pets' lives without exhausting reasonable and resourceful treatment and home care options. Our profession can, with solidarity, offer pet owners supportive, palliative options for comprehensive home care and attention to their pet's special needs when they are going down that final road toward death.

Many clients have complained to me that their initial veterinarian was too quick to recommend euthanasia if their pet's disease was incurable, if their senior pet had concurrent conditions, if treatment would be too complex, or if their pet was "too old." Refrain from suggesting or insisting on euthanasia as the next best option if the client declines the treatment plan that you recommend. Instead, say you are ready to provide pain relief for the pet and ensure the pet's comfort while the owner makes a decision regarding kinder and gentler palliative cancer therapy with the Pawspice philosophy.

Some clients complained that their veterinarian seemed to insist that the recommended procedures be done as an "all or none" policy. Some clients complained that they felt pressured to comply with procedure A or B, even though the pet's overall prognosis was poor. They complained that their attending veterinarian did not give them enough choices or offer a compromise on treatment options. They may have been told that if procedure A or B were not followed, their pet would suffer and need to be euthanized. Yet somehow the consultation ended and their pet was discharged from the clinic without being offered adequate pain control and supportive care for the ongoing condition at home. These pet carers felt abandoned, unsupported, and disappointed.

Emma's Case (It Wasn't Her Time Yet!)

Emma Moon, a 14-year-old F/S German Shepherd Dog mix, was the only pet of a childless, vibrant film-business couple. One day, a very upset man entered our busy reception room. He asked our receptionist, Jennifer, if we had time to give a second opinion. That day, two different specialists had told Mr. Moon and his wife to euthanize their beloved dog, Emma. The doctors said that Emma had two types of advanced cancer, was very old, and needed to be euthanized. Jennifer comforted him and told him that she would ask me to see if we could do anything to help. Meanwhile Mr. Moon sat on the floor with tears running down his face.

I asked him to tell me what was going on. He managed to tell me that Emma had been diagnosed with bone cancer a few months ago. Then she rapidly developed a large tumor in her groin, which was diagnosed as mast cell cancer. He said that today's X-ray of the diseased leg looked like the bone cancer would fracture. Both specialists agreed that Emma should be put to sleep that day or very soon thereafter. Mr. Moon said that he and his wife were tormented over this advice. They were not ready to let Emma go because she still wanted to eat and be with them. The clients in our waiting room and my staff empathized with his distress. I emphatically told him, "Your dog does not have to die from euthanasia today if you are not ready." I told him that we could enter Emma in a Pawspice program. I said, "If you are this conflicted and not ready yet, then it is not the right decision." I told him to bring his wife and Emma and all of her medication to me at the end of the day.

Sure enough, Mr. Moon returned at dusk with his wife. He carried Emma on a big soft pad into exam room 3. Emma's paws never touched the ground. She had pink mucous membranes and a pleasant interested look on her face. Mrs. Moon was puffy-eyed and looked at me with hope. We examined Emma. She was breathing comfortably and had no heart murmur. She had a large swelling of her left humerus that had been diagnosed as osteosarcoma. Referral X-rays showed a large osteosarcomatous lesion with lysis and erosion of cortical bone.

The lesion appeared to have a hairline fracture present but there was no displacement. A huge, bright pink soft tissue mass extended along Emma's left caudal mammary chain. The mass was $16 \times 8 \times 8 cm^3$. Fine needle aspiration cytology had diagnosed mast cell tumor earlier that day. Emma's abdomen was normal on palpation with no organomegaly. The couple said, "Look at her, she isn't ready to die yet. She still gets up to do her business and she eats and wags her tail and likes being at the center of things. We want help to keep her with us until we feel she is ready to go."

I described Emma's pain response to the Moons, saying that, "Dogs and cats don't exhibit their pain in ways that we completely understand. Dogs, by their very nature, want to stay with their pack and will fake wellness despite their pain. A pet's pain may not be recognized as such by their carers, even when they know their pet very well." I concurred with Emma's doctors and verified that Emma indeed had pain.

The sheer volume and location of the mast cell tumor warranted a poor prognosis for any dog. Emma's mast cell cancer added a negative factor to the bone cancer. The pathological fracture and the fact that she was on NSAIDs for bone cancer yet needed steroids for the mast cell tumor, compounded by her advanced age, all added up to a very poor prognosis for Emma.

I had no disagreement with her doctors' opinions yet could not disagree with the Moons, either. Emma was bright, alert, and responsive, and she seemed to be quite content. We offered palliative Pawspice care. I said, "Look at Emma with your questions and she will tell you and communicate in some way when the time is right."

We designed a special home care calendar with scheduled pre-emptive pain control for the bone tumor and palliative treatment for the mast cell cancer. We started Emma on Duragesic® fentanyl pain patches every 72 hours for osteosarcoma pain control. We administered IV dexamethasone and vinblastine for the mast cell cancer along with famotidine and Benadryl® injections, and SQ fluids with vitamins B, C, and B-12. We reviewed the calendar schedule with its specific instructions for oral prednisone, chlorambucil, Benadryl, and Pepcid A/C® along with supportive supplements from our chemoprevention and immunonutrition protocol. The Moons were instructed to discontinue all NSAIDs and recheck with us weekly for vinblastine injections and to assess Emma's quality of life.

To our amazement, Emma's mast cell tumor regressed completely, and she survived with good quality of life in her loving home for an additional eight more months in Pawspice care.

If a pet's illness cannot be treated due to financial constraints or a logistical problem, it is still a matter of good professional service to compassionately provide advice and meticulous home care instructions. When a treated pet's cancer has repeatedly recurred, metastasized, or is resistant to treatment, or if the pet is in the terminal stages of cancer, Pawspice and hospice care is a wonderful next professional service, and a helping step that keeps both pet and caregiver comfortably close to their nest. A well-conceptualized, creative Pawspice plan for pet owners may be the very best care that our profession can offer a terminal patient to support the people–pet bond.

In Pawspice, veterinarians and their staff can kindly and respectfully help carers restore and sustain a good quality life for terminal pets up to and during the very last days and hours before death. The Bond must be physically and emotionally severed. Clinic staff members can be trained in family practice skills (see Table 8.1) and be prepared to support the emotional needs of family members. This service allows the family an opportunity to enjoy the benefits of the long farewell that Pawspice offers with their beloved geriatric pet. Encourage the family to focus on enjoying the private moments with their Pawspice pet and to treasure the good parts of each day. Help worried carers realize that their Pawspice pet is still very much alive and present in the moment right there with them at home, holding court during this special end of life time.

The pet's carers – your clients – are also bonded to you and your staff. They are accustomed to the ritual and the idea of purpose and being welcome into your facility and interacting with you and your receptionists and nursing staff in an intimate fashion. All of this "social contact with purpose" ends for them abruptly with the passing of their geriatric oncology patient. Therefore, Pawspice can be more than a long farewell. It can also be a transition away from a routine that includes very meaningful connections and supportive relationships for you and your staff. Pawspice is a professional passage into the enormity of the at-home caregiving and hospice routine that they will provide for their geriatric oncology patient.

When a pet is injured, becomes ill, ages, or has arthritis, degenerative myelopathy, or cancer, the question of home care always comes up. How much care is a pet owner willing to provide for an ailing pet? After 40 plus years of experience in treating veterinary cancer patients, I can state with authority that the answer to this question is very personal. For some pet owners, the willingness to provide palliation and Pawspice care for a pet has no limit, while others are either unable or unwilling. Each owner has his or her own unique personal lifestyle considerations and tolerance levels that will support or preclude the owner's ability to provide Pawspice care for a pet.

The human–animal bond for geriatric pets may be quite fragile or very intense and occasionally not rational. This variability in the bond depends upon the pet carer's personal bias, philosophy on aging, and loyalty toward his or her elderly pet. Some pet owners have been saying their goodbyes for years before their geriatric pet has even developed any form of illness. When cancer strikes, some carers feel that their pet's time is up. They are not willing to make the personal or financial investment to challenge fate.

Other carers may feel protective or fearful of distressing or disturbing their geriatric pet. Some clients seldom or never allow their geriatric pets to have anesthesia for dental care. The periodontal disease becomes a source of infection and a roadblock in the face of palliative chemotherapy, surgery, or radiation therapy. This situation, along with other extenuating circumstances, may be why some clients elect to pursue only supportive care to alleviate pain and other distressful symptoms with Pawspice care, while declining available types of cancer palliation.

After an initial consultation regarding options for curative treatment or palliation of their geriatric pet with cancer, the family must struggle with decision making. Issues to be weighed include personal finances, the logistics of getting to and from the treatment center, and scheduling for visits and home care requirements.

Reevaluation of Attachment

Carers must face how they feel about their attachment for their pet's compromised status. They deal with feelings of guilt and remorse and they examine their sense of duty as their geriatric pet encounters problems and their disability progresses. Initial willingness to participate in a Pawspice program may wane after the pet encounters adverse side effects from treatment. Carers often find themselves reevaluating their commitment with the changing status of the Pawspice patient.

Many highly attached pet owners are overwhelmed by anticipatory grief over the impending loss of their beloved pet. They do not realize that they are cheating themselves out of the real benefit of Pawspice – months, weeks, or the final days of enjoyment with their pet. All of this good time is lost because they are so upset. Based upon the personality type, marital and financial situation, family commitments, and other personal issues that you may or may not be aware of, pet owners may respond with a wide range of emotions from panic all the way to an emotional shutdown. If, at any time, you suspect that a client is emotionally unstable, encourage that client to seek professional counseling. Always have the name and number of a counselor on hand and give that information to the client directly, with a sincere recommendation for them to seek help. I explain to my heartbroken clients that their feelings are no different than a parent who is grieving over a child stricken with cancer. In our world, the pet is like a "geriatric child" at the end of life. There is plenty of reason for clients to need pet-loss counseling.

When you outline a Pawspice plan for a geriatric patient, the owners will weigh their specific issues and then either accept the challenge to treat their pet's illness with your recommendations or decline. When a client declines an aggressive or standard treatment plan, the battle is not necessarily over. Always offer them kinder, gentler palliative cancer medicine with their Pawspice program. If you do not offer this type of help, many clients may seek a palliative cancer therapy program that is not offered at your practice. They may pursue a dietary change, and/or seek alternative or complementary treatments. They may do so without your knowledge or guidance, because they do not want to hurt your feelings. They may be embarrassed, or they may think you will be angry with them and/or disapprove of the treatment they have chosen. If their pet does well with their chosen therapy, then they will think that you misguided them or gave up too soon.

Veterinarians must refrain from being judgmental or from interpreting a client's decision not to provide a particular recommended treatment as personal rejection. Continue to educate the owner and offer options that the owner can incorporate into his or her treatment or Pawspice program. If the only contribution the owner will accept from you is comfort and support for their pet, offer that. Create a treatment calendar that shows each of the daily medications to give according to your complete protocol for supportive care. Following the treatment calendar becomes a very palatable and viable option. By showing respect for their choices, you will keep your client's professional confidence in you as their pet journeys into end of life Pawspice care.

Home Care 101 for the Pawspice Patient

When preparing carers to provide Pawspice care at home, always speak in a tender, unhurried fashion. They are most likely under a tremendous amount of personal, financial, and emotional stress. A trained nurse, technician, or doctor can make house calls to assist and coach the carers during their learning period. The family should be able to establish their own home care routine within a reasonable amount of time.

Pet carers may feel trepidation at the thought of using needles and syringes to give injections to their ailing pet. They might be upset at the thought of using a feeding tube. The use of a feeding tube may sound like heroics to one person and make perfect sense to another. Cats are more likely to need feeding tubes to provide them with proper nutrition during recovery from hepatic lipidosis, after oral surgery, or during radiation treatments to the oral cavity. Anorectic dogs may respond to Entyce™, which is a central-acting appetite stimulant. Animals with pulmonary disease and cancer in their lungs have very heavy symptom burdens, which may be alleviated with the use of Zyprexa™. This antischizophrenic drug relaxes the pet's anxiety and stimulates their appetite while reducing nausea (Pal 2016). Injections of medroxyprogesterone acetate (Depo-Provera™) may help increase appetite, well-being, and weight gain in geriatric cancer patients. Many Pawspice patients require SQ fluids to maintain hydration, especially if there is concurrent renal disease, hypercalcemia, or other electrolyte imbalances.

You and your staff can address a client's fear of needles with a cheerful approach. One technique is to ask the owner to look at a pen. The pen's function is to transfer information to the chart. Explain that the syringe and needle are like a pen; they transfer medications to the patient. Consider the syringe to be a tool, like a pen, and nothing to be afraid of. Teach carers to give mock injections with saline at the clinic and at home until they acquire the skill of handling needles and syringes. Suggest injecting teriyaki sauce into chicken or Grand Marnier into strawberries. Provide a practice needle in the gauge that will be used for their pet, and suggest they use this to inject water into an orange. Piercing the orange rind will prepare them for the sensation of piercing their pet's skin. When it comes time to give their pet an injection, carers will be more confident.

Many pet owners want to nurse their terminal cancer pet at home. They need their veterinarian and the nursing staff to teach them how to care for their pet and maintain hygiene while working within their inhibitions and concerns. Home care for a pet with incontinence or paresis is a task certain pet owners elect with the help of pet wheels, hoisting straps, harnesses, ramps, extra soft bedding, egg crate mattresses, and loads of towels and diapers.

Some pets will need frequent bandage changes. Some will need their bladders expressed. Some need diapers. Incontinent pets need frequent bathing to avoid urine scald and fecal contamination. If the pet has a resting place outdoors, the family must provide protection from flies and ants. It does not take long for maggot infestation to develop in a decubital ulcer. Some pet carers want to provide oxygen therapy for their pets with compromised respiration. Advise them to purchase portable oxygen tanks. Advise them on methods to fit their pet with an appropriate delivery mask. Teach them how to use a stethoscope, so they can routinely listen for troubled breathing and fluid sounds. Recommend a house call veterinarian who can help.

Some people get upset with a growing tumor, thinking it might rupture and cause their pet to die. We comfort them and tell them that this would be unusual and that, at worst, the wound might drain or have a discharge similar to a sliced tomato.

Some people react with a paralyzing fear or nervousness at the sight of blood or oozing wounds. They may have trouble providing wound care. They may feel squeamish looking at, touching, and treating wounds from radiation therapy mucositis or desquamation, IV slough sites, ulcerated tumors, or decubital ulcers, and so forth. We dispense an aloe vera wound cream and instruct our clients to mix $\frac{1}{4}$ teaspoon of gelatin and sugar with it just before applying it to the wound. This mixture is very helpful in caring for large wounds, especially following electrochemotherapy/electroporation.

Some clients cringe if they have to watch our nurses give injections or provide medical procedures for their pets. They cannot imagine themselves giving injections to their pet at home. We solve this problem with frequent rechecks, day hospitalization, a day care facility, or by scheduling one of our Pawspice staff to do house calls. We also refer the client to a house call veterinarian who can provide the needed in-home care, and will be on standby to help with the gift of home euthanasia at the very end of life.

Most pet owners have great fortitude and interest in learning how to administer injections and medications and nursing care to their geriatric cancer pets for Pawspice care. They truly want this level of care for their pet's convenience and they are willing to make the sacrifice. Others may be less eager but need to master technical home care procedures to save money.

Pet Aversion to the Caregiver

When a patient shows aversion to the caregiver's attempts at medication or other care, we run into a problem that may erode the human–animal bond and the home care equation. This very problem hit me broadside when Alaska, my aging Great Pyrenees in Pawspice, started to avoid me. She no longer greeted me with her usual cheer because she knew that I might have a pill, a syringe, or some SQ fluids for her. It only took one week to solve this problem. One of my assistants came to my home every day to give Alaska her injections and SQ fluids. Alaska was once again happy to see me all the time.

Sinji's Case (She Refused to Cooperate but Needed Help)

Mr. Citroen told me that he just could not torture his 12-year-old cat, Sinji, with pills or injections. Her mesenteric lymphoma responded well to the first chemotherapy treatment but he could not justify her aversion toward him when he approached her with the prednisone tablets. She would not accept any liquids or compounded medications or transdermal preparations. He called my clinic in frustration, to terminate treatment. We offered the option of visiting his local veterinarian once every two weeks for SQ injections of L-asparaginase, Cytosar-U®, and Depo-Medrol®. We also recommended that the doctor give her a 5mg capsule of lomustine on week one and week two, and repeat every six weeks following an acceptable CBC. Mr. Citroen realized that Sinji might die without the proper medication and he was grateful for a flexible modification in her palliative chemotherapy and Pawspice program.

Willingness: The Essential Ingredient on Both Sides of the Exam Table

The essential ingredient for Pawspice care is willingness. Look for willingness in yourself, in the hospital staff, and in the geriatric oncology patient's carers. When you hold staff meetings, ask the question, "Do we want to be a compassionate veterinary caregiving facility with a Pawspice program? Will our nursing and reception staff members be able to provide our clients with the necessary support?" Ask who would like to be the "Pawspice support person" for the clinic or for a special client.

Ask clients to direct phone calls and concerns to their designated nurse or to members of the clinic's cancer care support team. The nursing staff should be trained so they can handle questions regarding home care problems. The doctor evaluates Pawspice patients on a regular basis as outpatients. At those rechecks, the pet is weighed and checked for hydration and nutritional status and the quality of life score is assigned, using the HHHHHMM Quality of Life Scale (Table 10.1). The carer's questions are answered. Changes in the patient's health status and medications, as well as the patient's quality of life assessment score and adjustments for improvement, are all addressed.

The Evolution of Pawspice Philosophy

Companion animal medicine is relatively young. Our profession's founding philosophy was forged from a utilitarian stewardship of livestock and epidemiology when animals were not generally thought of as family members or pets. It is only in the last 30–40 years that companion animal medicine has emerged into the pediatrician–family practice model. The unusual situation in following this model is the baby or child is *geriatric*!

Wellness and hospice communities across the country have revolutionized how Americans care for people who are sick and dying. However, there is more work to be done to make end of life care better for people who are dying from cancer. Physicians are trained with the fight mentality to fix problems and the majority are remarkably untrained, ill-suited, and uncomfortable talking about chronic illness, the ravages of cancer and death with their human patients and their families (Gawande 2014). Unfortunately, the average terminal patient is referred into hospice care only 3 days before dying. That may be because insurance companies decline to finance cancer care for patients in hospice care. This is why palliative medicine, which includes all levels of palliative cancer care and symptom management, has evolved with wide acceptance from patients and physicians.

Our veterinary community has accepted lessons from the human hospice and palliative care movement. We realize that our highly bonded clients want us to stop delivering the euthanasia speech over every old, sick pet. Veterinarians must move away from the reflexive response of suggesting utilitarian or premature euthanasia when geriatric patients with comorbidities are diagnosed with cancer. This action greatly undervalues and diminishes the moral status of the pet owner within the human–animal bond (Tannenbaum 1985). The veterinary profession will gain more stature when practitioners learn to emulate the philosophy of the hospice and palliative medicine movement in honor of that special bond that connects people to their pets. Pawspice embraces these palliative medicine principles, and then transitions to hospice care when the pet declines toward death.

Veterinarians who offer a Pawspice program as an option instead of early euthanasia dignify the profession with a much needed and commonsense professional service. The Pawspice–hospice option resonates with pet lovers worldwide. By entering a beloved pet into end of life care, they are expressing respect for their patients and their carers honoring the human–animal bond. Bioethicists hope that companion animal professionals will be able to cultivate sensitivity and keep a courteous, caring balance with life and death, yet be vigilant against the pet owner who may blindly insist on going too far at the expense of their companion animal's quality of life (Rollin 2006; McMillan 2005).

As the veterinary community reaches out to embrace the hospice philosophy in the form of Pawspice care for pets, we must maintain a sense of balance. We must be careful not to head in the direction of the mindless machinery of medicine, insensibly keeping non-sentient patients alive who are clearly beyond hope. Our efforts to provide Pawspice care are justified in honoring the human–animal bond and attachment, as long as the patient has what we must define and defend as a good quality of life (Wojciechowska and Hewson 2005).

The Pawspice option gives pet owners more time to let go of their geriatric cancer pet slowly, lovingly, and peacefully. Many tender private moments of quiet emotion and sweet conversation are shared between the family members and their dying pet.

Education of Home Carers

In exam room consultations, attending veterinarians and staff can gracefully provide the education and support needed for efficient home care of ailing pets on a fee-for-service basis. Pet owners will gladly pay for education that alleviates pain and provides good nutritional, hydration, and medical support for their dying pet. These consultation and demonstration sessions give the family the ability to care with expertise.

The most important factors to educate home carers to confidently monitor are quality of life; minimal pain; adequate nutrition, hydration, and respiration; and detection of sepsis. When properly prepared by the veterinary staff, carers can provide end of life Pawspice care for a dying pet with all of the benefits of hospital care while allowing pets to remain in the comfort of their own home. Ask yourself, "If this pet's owners were trained to take the pet's temperature, administer subcutaneous fluids and proper pain control medications, provide food, and maintain hygiene, might this pet live more comfortably with better quality of life and perhaps live longer at home?"

A Pawspice program should include moments of pleasure or fun and joy for the pet. Owners can be overwhelmed by their pet's imminent passing and by their new tasks, such as medicating, cleaning, and providing special diets. It is important to help them avoid becoming so focused on caregiving that they forget to appreciate their pet during the additional time that Pawspice creates.

Creative carers can always find fun things to do with a pet in Pawspice care, regardless of the pet's limitations. This can be as simple as giving massages, gentle brushing and grooming, playing with toys or a laser light, or taking short walks with a dog that is able to still enjoy sniffing favorite spots. If going for walk is a dog's favorite activity, recommend short walks more often. If the pet is not able to get up or walk without assistance, instruct the owner to provide assistance with straps or harnesses or to use a pet stroller, cart, or wagon. Cats and small dogs can be carried in a pack or in a padded bicycle basket for a gentle ride. The bonded owner and Pawspice pet both benefit greatly from the continuation of happy moments and the continual creation of new happy memories to cherish later.

Benson's Case (Serum Fun Factors and Survival)

Benson Copeland, a 10-year-old M/N Newfoundland, was my first real Pawspice case. Benson belonged to Jack and Kathy Copeland of Mammoth Lakes, CA. Jack brought him down from Mammoth when his local vet, Dr. Robert Mehrhof, palpated an abdominal mass and ascites. He was treated the previous year for malignant melanoma of the buccal mucosa.

Benson was incontinent and in some mild discomfort due to abdominal distension. However, his mucous membranes were pink and he was bright and responsive. Chest X-rays were negative for metastases. Abdominal ultrasound found numerous hypoechoic lesions in his liver and large hypoechoic lesions in his spleen consistent with hemangiosarcoma or metastatic malignant melanoma. The abdominal effusion was a modified transudate, typical with non-exfoliating abdominal tumors.

We informed Jack that surgery was not an option for Benson and that his prognosis was poor. We recommended euthanasia but Jack said that his wife, Kathy, wanted Benson to come back home for one last goodbye. I had recently heard a seminar on the beneficial effect of increasing serum fun factors for women with breast cancer. Using this information, I told Jack to do all the fun things that Benson loves to do. Jack said that Benson loved to swim at Horseshoe Lake. He asked me if Benson was strong enough to go. My answer was, "Let Benson make that decision. If he stops along the way, let him rest."

Six months later, we were in Mammoth for a ski trip. The Copelands held a dinner party in honor of Dr. Mehrhof and myself and Benson. Benson had a miraculous response to serum fun factors. Old Benson was still around enjoying his swims at Horseshoe Lake! Benson looked more like a black Gordon Setter due to cancer cachexia. He still had moderate ascites, but he was cheerful and alert. The Copelands took my advice literally. They accommodated Benson's situation by getting a ramp for their trailer and parking it closer to the lake. They also took Benson swimming twice a day instead of once or twice a week. This new schedule for fun raised Benson's serum fun factors. The weightlessness of swimming twice a day seemed to have made Benson so ecstatic that he put off dying for six months. Dr. Mehrhof and I looked at each other and at Benson in amazement, wonder, and respect.

Assessing Quality of Life Using the "HHHHHMM" (H5M2) QoL Scale

The HHHHHMM (H5M2) Quality of Life Scale provides guidelines for the assessment of a pet so that pet owners can maintain a rewarding relationship that nurtures the human–animal bond, while being confident that the pet is well enough to justify prolonging life. This Quality of Life Scale will relieve guilt feelings and engender the support of the veterinary team to actively help in the care and decision making for Pawspice patients. I feel that it is ethical to prolong a life worth living. On the other hand, I feel that it is not ethical to prolong death for our patients.

There is a real need for assessing quality of life (QoL) for aging, ailing, and terminally ill pets and especially for the cancer patients under our care. Most companion animals have one or more abnormal conditions that developed in their senior years and these conditions generally worsen with time. One-third of our pet dog and cat population is overweight and/or obese. When geriatric dogs and cats become burdened with cancer and its related treatment issues, their pre-existing conditions complicate matters and limit their owner's choice of treatment options. It is always important to continually confirm and reconfirm that the patient's life is worth living.

Veterinarians are frequently asked, "When is the right time to euthanize my beloved pet? How will I know?" I may say something like this, "Ideally you will realize when it is the right time because your pet will give you a look or make a gesture or sign, or there will be a series of bad days." An easy to use QoL scale helps everyone. It especially helps those in denial about the gravity of their pet's situation. The QoL scale helps carers who feel unable to make the assessment objectively. Carers can use this itemized QoL scale to decide whether or not their pet is being humanely maintained in Pawspice. Every animal has certain needs and desires that must be recognized and respected. If we can meet these basic needs and desires at a satisfactory level for our ailing companion animals, then we are justified in preserving the life of the ill pet during the steady decline toward death.

The basic needs and desires innate to quality of life for terminal geriatric cancer patients should not and cannot, in good conscience, be ignored. It is up to the veterinary professional and the pet's family to design a supportive end of life program.

The Pawspice program needs to address each of the seven criteria that deals with quality of life openly and honestly. We can be very proactive in helping pets achieve an improved score on their

Table 10.1. **Quality of Life Scale (The HHHHHMM (H5M2) Scale)** Pet carers can use the H5M2 Quality of Life Scale to determine the success of Pawspice care. Using a scale of 0 to 10, patients can be scored. Over 5 is acceptable in each category. A total of 35 points or greater is acceptable for a good Pawspice.

H: 0–10	**HURT:** Adequate pain control, including breathing ability, is first and foremost on the scale. Is pain adequately managed? Is oxygen necessary? Nothing else matters if the pet can't breathe.
H: 0–10	**HUNGER:** Is the pet eating enough? Does hand feeding help? Does the patient require a feeding tube?
H: 0–10	**HYDRATION:** Is the patient dehydrated? For patients not drinking enough, use subcutaneous fluids once or twice daily to supplement fluid intake.
H: 0–10	**HYGIENE:** The patient should be kept brushed and cleaned, particularly after elimination, avoid pressure sores, and keep all wounds clean.
H: 0–10	**HAPPINESS:** Does the pet express joy and interest? Is he responsive to things around him (family, toys, etc.)? Is the pet depressed, lonely, anxious, bored, or afraid? Can the pet's bed be close to the family activities and not be isolated?
M: 0–10	**MOBILITY:** Can the patient get up without assistance? Does the pet need human or mechanical help (e.g., a cart)? Does he feel like going for a walk? Is he having seizures or stumbling? (Some carers feel euthanasia is preferable to amputation, yet an animal who has limited mobility but is still alert and responsive can have a good quality of life as long as his carers are committed to helping him.)
M: 0–10	**MORE GOOD DAYS THAN BAD:** When there are too many bad days in a row, quality of life is too compromised. When a healthy human–animal bond is no longer possible, the caretaker must be made aware the end is near. The decision needs to be made if the pet is suffering. If death comes peacefully and painlessly, that is okay.
TOTAL =	**35 or greater is acceptable for a good Pawspice. Over 5 is acceptable in each category.**

Dr. Villalobos created the H5M2 QoL Scale for the First Edition of this textbook based from her *Oncology Outlook* article, Quality of Life Scale helps make final call, *Veterinary Practice News* (*VPN*), September 2004.

evaluations. The H5M2 QoL scale for each factor runs from 0 to 10, where 10 is the best and highest quality rating for each factor. Since there are seven basic factors in this proposed scale, 70 would be a perfect score. If the terminal geriatric cancer patient scores at least 5 on each issue, the quality of life is considered reasonably good. We could say that a score of 35 means that the family is justified in continuing Pawspice. Each factor needs to be monitored by both the attending doctor and the family, with careful attention.

The factors in this Quality of Life assessment tool can be easily remembered as "HHHHHMM," or "five Hs and two Ms." Every Pawspice program should strive to satisfy each of the factors: Hurt, Hunger, Hydration, Hygiene, Happiness, Mobility, and More good days than bad days. A score above 5 on each factor can be considered acceptable for the decision to begin or continue a Pawspice program. A concise format is adapted for client use (Table 10.1).

Understanding the HHHHHMM Quality of Life Scale

Hurt

Adequate pain control is first and foremost on the scale. This criterion emphasizes the pet's ability to breathe properly. In human medicine, not being able to breath is ranked at the top of the pain scale. Attention to the pet's ability to breathe properly is a top priority. Cases with pulmonary effusion require thoracocentesis on an as-needed basis. Pet owners need to be trained to monitor the pet's respirations and comfort level and to identify labored breathing so they will not wait too long to provide relief. Some families are willing to provide oxygen therapy at home to help their ailing pets. The veterinarian can prescribe oxygen through a medical supply house. Zyprexa™ provides increased comfort for lung cancer patients. Pain control must be effective and should be given pre-emptively. A multimodality approach may be required to control cancer pain and may include oral, transdermal, and injectable medications.

Hunger

Malnutrition develops quickly in anorectic geriatric oncology patients, especially if they have sarcopenia and lost their lean-muscle reserve. Cancer cachexia is a negative metabolic state that may not be reversed. A new peptide that is a melanocortin (MC4/MC3) antagonist is being developed that may reverse wasting, and cachexia (www.tensivecontroles.com). Carers need to be educated about how much their pet needs to eat to maintain body weight. Help carers assess if their geriatric cancer pet is marginal or severely malnourished. A "rule of thumb" would be to start nutritional support with 250 kcal/day per 10 pounds if a pet exhibits three days of total anorexia or has lost 10% body weight (Ogilvie and Moore 2001; Remillard et al. 2000). Many Pawspice pets will live much longer if offered wholesome, flavorful foods that appeal to their dwindling appetite. Capromorelin (Entyce™) is a ghrelin receptor agonist that stimulates appetite centrally. It mimics the hunger hormone ghrelin (Aratana.com).

My own 13-year-old Great Pyrenees, Alaska, went from kibble to canned food and then to hamburger, fresh baked turkey, chicken, sausages, venison (thanks to Dr. Jack Stephens), pastrami, cheeses, and gourmet cut and marinated meats during her Pawspice for degenerative myopathy. Alaska liked smoke flavor, Alfredo sauce, and cheddar cheese soup mixed into her food along with lots of encouragement and coaxing and hand feeding. It takes patience and gentle coaxing to get some Pawspice pets to eat. It is hard not to be disappointed when such specially prepared food is rejected. Suggest to your clients that if their Pawspice pet rejects an offering, they can come back with another offering with a different flavor a little later and that meal may be more appealing to the pet.

If the pet is not taking in adequate calorie-dense nutrition willingly or by coaxing or force feeding, then placement of a feeding tube should be considered. Cats do very well with esophageal feeding tubes. Gastrostomy and jejunostomy tubes also have a role in Pawspice care. Instruct owners to use a blender or liquid diets to help their best friend maintain proper nutritional and caloric intake if they elect to use tube feeding.

Hydration

Educate the pet owner about adequate fluid intake per pound (10ml per pound per day) and to assess for hydration by the pinch method. SQ fluids are a wonderful way to supplement the fluid intake of ailing pets. Provide demonstration sessions in which the veterinarian or a staff member will teach a pet owner how to administer SQ fluids. Giving SQ fluids regularly can improve the Pawspice pet's quality of life tremendously.

Hygiene

Good hygiene is a must! Can the pet be kept brushed and cleaned? Is the coat matted? Is the pet situated properly so that it will not have to lie in its own soil after eliminations? Many Pawspice pets, especially cats with oral cancer, cannot keep themselves clean as they have done for their whole lives and they may become demoralized quickly when unclean. The odor associated with necrotic oral tumors can be offensive and cause social rejection by family members.

Prescribe antibiotics to help reduce foul-smelling infections. Also teach owners to dampen a sponge with a highly diluted solution of lemon juice and hydrogen peroxide. They should gently stroke the face, paws, and legs of the patient with the saturated sponge. This action is similar to a "mother tongue" and helps to clean the fur while soothing the unkempt cat. Dogs love this type of facial and paw grooming too!

Happiness

Happiness is important for both the caregiver and the pet. Does the patient have desires, wants, and needs? Are they being met? The Pawspice pet's bed can be moved close to the family's activities and not left in an isolated or neglected area.

Is the ailing pet willing to interact with the family and be responsive to things going on around him? Is the Pawspice cat able to purr and enjoy being on the bed or in one's lap? Is there a response to a bit of catnip? Can the cat bat at toys or look and follow a laser light? Can the ailing pet enjoy upbeat greetings from and petting by loving family members? Is the pet depressed, lonely, anxious, bored, or afraid? Do you have a routine fun time that the pet looks forward to?

Mobility

Is the pet able to get up and move around enough to satisfy normal desires? Does the pet feel like going out for a walk? Is the pet showing CNS signs, seizures, or stumbling? Can the pet be taken outdoors or helped into a litter box to eliminate with assistance? Will a harness, sling, or cart help? Is medication helping?

The answer to the mobility question has viable and variable scenarios. The scale score for mobility is acceptable anywhere from 0–10. I have met some utilitarian pet owners who are very rigid in their requirements for mobility of their pets. They may be regretful but willing to sacrifice their pet's life rather than elect amputation of a limb. Some pet owners feel that amputation is a mutilation and is not fair to the pet. Instead, they allow the pet to bear a painful limb for months before euthanasia.

More Good Days than Bad Days

Ask your clients to estimate if their pet has more good days than bad days in a week. When there are too many bad days in a row, the quality of life is compromised and Pawspice may not be appropriate. Bad days may be days filled with undesirable experiences such as vomiting, nausea, diarrhea, frustration, falling down, seizures, and so forth. Bad days could be caused by a progressive condition such as cancer cachexia, profound weakness from anemia, or the discomfort caused by gradual tumor pressure or obstruction or a large, inoperable tumor in the abdomen. If the two-way exchange needed to communicate and maintain a healthy human–animal bond is absent, then the pet owner must reconcile or be gently told that the end may be near.

Krash's Case (He Was a Very Happy Pawspice Patient)

Vickie Pancino entered Krash, her 12-year-old male 90-pound Golden Retriever, into our Pawspice program with osteosarcoma (OSA) of his left distal radius. Krash's history precluded amputation because of severe degenerative joint and disk disease, and degenerative myelopathy.

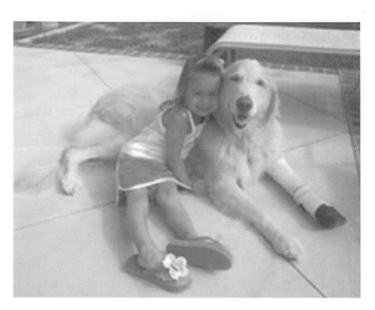

Figure 10.1. Krash Pancino at home with family. His OSA leg was splinted for visits to the dog park and at playtime to offset a potential pathological fracture. His Pawspice was full of joy and love that lasted for 3 months.

Krash had severe osteoarthritis of both his knees, along with moderate to severe degenerative joint disease from bilateral hip dysplasia. Krash's cancer leg was splinted for visits to the dog park and at playtime to offset a potential pathological fracture. His life was happy and full of joy and love for three months (Figure 10.1).

Dr. Robin Downing wrote thoughtfully about the mobility issue in her book, *Pets Living with Cancer: A Pet Owner's Resource*. Dr. Downing wrote, "Because Murphy is such a big dog – 150 pounds and very tall – her ability to get up and down and to walk under her own power are very important benchmarks in my personal 'bottom line.' She would be impossible to pick up and carry around" (Downing 2000) (Figure 10.2). "For the same reason – her size – her ability to control her urine and stool output is important."

In my opinion, the mobility scale can have a variable score from 0 to 10. The need for mobility seems dependent on the species and breed. Cats and small lap dogs can and do enjoy life with much less stress handling their mobility issues than large and giant breed dogs. If the pet is compromised and is only able to lie in bed, teach carers to create a schedule to change the position of the pet and rotate the body at least as often as every two hours.

Atelectasis and decubital ulcers must be avoided. The nursing care necessary for large immobile dogs is very demanding (burdensome care). Is the bedding material soft enough? Can an egg crate mattress be used and set up properly to avoid decubital ulcers? Is there a need for a special lifting harness, a pet mobility cart or an Evans standing cart (www.jorvet.com)? These items make a difference in the quality of life for the pet that has limited mobility, yet is still alert and responsive. Ask clients to determine if their immobile pet's life is still worth living for the pet!

Help Clients Use the QoL Scale

Sometimes carers are not sure how to assess QoL issues when the end is near. It can be made more clear to them if a standard scale for quality of life is explained and measured ahead of time and

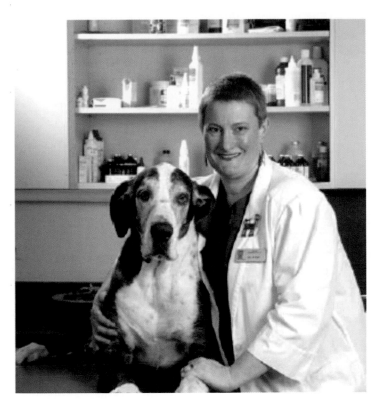

Figure 10.2. Dr. Robin Downing with Murphy, her 3-year OSA survivor. Murphy had limb-sparing surgery at Colorado State University and was featured in Downing's book, *Pets Living with Cancer*. Murphy developed another OSA lesion in her right tibia at 8 years of age.

reevaluated every couple of weeks. QoL may need to be assessed every week, every few days, or every few hours, as the situation requires. What many carers want is for their pet to pass on "naturally" at home, in their arms, in their own bed. In some cases, the veterinarian providing Pawspice care for a pet can facilitate this dream with proper pain management and sedation, as long as the pet is peacefully weakening and not suffering. As veterinarians, we need to understand that it is a very personal and natural wish when our clients request us to help their pet to die naturally at home. We are the ones they turn to for help because we took the Veterinarian's Oath: "I solemnly swear to use my scientific knowledge and skills for the benefit of society through the protection of animal health, the relief of animal suffering...."

Guarantee that the pet is pain-free during the final phase of dying. Use the most powerful preemptive pain medications and palliative sedation during the patient's last days and hours. A peaceful painless passage will help family members to cope with pet loss. Refer to the graduated scale for analgesia using the World Health Organization (WHO) pain ladder (see Figure 7.1) and review the information in Chapter 7 of this text. The WSAVA Guidelines for Recognition, Assessment and Treatment of Pain will help you manage undertreated pain (www.wsava.org/sites/default/files/jsap_0.pdf).

Suggest the helpful option of home euthanasia and, if your hospital does not offer home visits, refer the family to a house call veterinarian. The International Association of Animal Hospice and Palliative Care (www.iaahpc.org) has a list of members who are dedicated to accepting referrals at all hours.

Use the HHHHHMM (H5M2) Quality of Life Scale to facilitate the heart wrenching decision that euthanasia truly is. Your professional guidance and compassion may help to relieve the angst and regret that owners often have about their difficult decision to allow a beloved pet's death. This is a decision that too often haunts many pet owners for the rest of their lives (see Table 10.1).

Satisfaction: An Important Ingredient of Pawspice Care

Ask the pet owner if he or she is satisfied with the Pawspice arrangement. At times, there is conflict within the family about how attached the main caregiver is to the pet. Some family members feel inconvenienced with the soiling, the odors, the sacrifice, the sadness, or the diverted attention and devotion that the main caregiver is showering on the pet. This issue creates a double-edged sword for the patient's main caregiver to deal with on a daily basis. Address these issues directly with the family to help them come to a supportive consensus. If this issue goes beyond your personal counseling ability, suggest a family counselor.

One recommendation that I have found very helpful for planning ahead is suggesting to clients that they visit a pet cemetery. In this way, the pet family is introduced to all the options of afterlife services and items, before the geriatric pet passes away. They will know where to go for a memorial stone for their backyard or an urn for their pet's cremains.

You and your staff play a vital role in the Pawspice care of the geriatric oncology patient. Discuss each case to learn if the preservation of The Bond between this person and this pet will be a rewarding experience. If so, then Pawspice will be a good experience for all involved.

Veterinarians can win client loyalty by respecting and preserving the special bond that connects pet owners to their pets. If the veterinary team helps to control pain and provide nutrition in a peaceful hospice way, client-carers gain confidence. They will gain courage as the carers of their Pawspice pets and will later look back at the Pawspice experience with satisfaction.

Pawspice Programs Are Metastasizing

Many house call practitioners tell me that a significant percentage of their home visits are made to provide supportive care of companion animals in decline with end of life care needs. End of life care is being taught in many veterinary schools as an active part of patient care. The pet hospice program at Colorado State University (CSU) is staffed and run by veterinary students, and supported by faculty advisors in the College of Veterinary Medicine. Animal hospitals in the greater Fort Collins area refer terminal patients to the Veterinary Teaching Hospital Hospice Program. Every patient and caregiver is required to have a relationship with a local DVM, and that veterinarian is constantly updated about the health status of the animal and the emotional needs of their family members. The referring veterinarian also ensures that the hospice case managers understand the patient's medical needs. Many local veterinarians who work with the CSU Hospice Program will perform home euthanasia or refer their clients to the growing number of veterinarians who focus on home euthanasia.

The goal of the CSU hospice is to create the best end of life experience for both patient and family in their home, when the pet can be made comfortable at home. They teach students that when a terminal pet's medical needs can be met at home, that is where the pet should be. If the family feels that they need extra time to say goodbye or if an animal is diagnosed with a terminal illness but has good general health, hospice can help by confirming that the pet's needs are being met in that environment. When Christie C. Long was a CSU veterinary student she said, "We find ourselves in many situations providing extensive emotional support to owners, especially in helping them determine when it's time to euthanize their animals" (Long 2005).

Practical Ideas for Treating Some Specific Disease Conditions

Compliance is a huge factor in treating geriatric and end of life patients. Teaching clients the Fear-Free positive reinforcement and gentle handling techniques for home care is very helpful for gaining compliance. UC Davis, in conjunction with CABI and the International Society for Anthrozoology (www.isaz.org) organized a Compliance Symposium at UC Davis on June 27, 2017. Lynette Hart, PhD, asked me to speak on gaining compliance for end of life patients. Most carers have tremendous willingness; however, they are often burdened with a raft of emotional issues and phobias. We must train our veterinary teams to compassionately coach carers properly to help them help their pets.

Chronic Kidney Disease

Pets with chronic renal failure (CKD) that are fed special modified diets, such as Hill's k/d® and so forth, may survive longer with a better QoL, especially if they are supported with educated home care. This may include subcutaneous (SQ) fluids, Tumil-K®, famotidine, vitamins, and fatty acids (omega-3 fatty acids or fish oils), antiemetics, appetite stimulators (Entyce™), and aluminum hydroxide, and calcitriol depending on the case. Regularly scheduled recheck exams, laboratory profiles, and CBCs can monitor renal function, electrolytes, acidosis, and hematocrit. The SDMA Renal Disease Test for cats may identify CKD cases earlier. Erythropoietin (Epogen™, Procrit™) or long acting darbepoetin (Aranesp™) may be used to bring low hematocrit levels back to normal. Novel medications may help reverse or prevent sarcopenia and wasting disease associated with CKD. One CKD cat in my practice survived six happy years at home on daily subcutaneous fluids and supplements, finally passing away at the age of 22.

Senior Cats with Feline Triad Disease

Cats with concurrent inflammatory disease of the liver, pancreas, and intestines have feline triad disease. They may be palliated with fluids and oral potassium gluconate, vitamin E, prednisolone, metronidazole, ursodiol (Actigall®), pancreatic enzymes, L-carnitine, glutathione, lactulose, S-Adenosylmethionine (SAMe), and SQ vitamin K-1, according to Dr. Johnny Hoskins (2000, 2004). Cats with severe cholangiohepatitis and liver failure may be helped with Hill's liver diet l/d®, Actigall, vitamin K-1, and milk thistle. Products that contain a combination of supplements to assist hepatic function and to stimulate the appetite and to manage wasting disease are available.

Diabetic Pets

When a diabetic pet's carer is reluctant to give injections or is needle-shy, the veterinarian can offer oral hypoglycemic medication. Good clinical results can be expected with oral medication in one-third of diabetics that have no ketones in the urine. Clients feel that their veterinarian is trying to help the pet while prioritizing their own concerns. If hyperglycemia cannot be controlled by oral medication, the owner may be more inclined to then try injectable insulin as a second choice. The Cornell Feline Health Center has excellent information and instructional videos. Some carers are willing to home monitor the glucose level for their cats (www.sugarcats.net/sites/harry/bgtest.htm).

Dysrexia, Hyporexia, and Anorexia

Dysrexia is altered food preference. Hyporexia is decreased appetite. Anorexia is complete loss of appetite. Anorectic pets need to be coaxed and hand fed. Carers need instruction on the proper technique to best hand feed their ill pet. Cats generally like food warmed to body temperature. Dogs may drink broth and more aromatic wet foods. If appetite stimulators such as mirtazapine or cyproheptadine fail to help, we have a new option. Capromorelin (Entyce™) is a ghrelin receptor agonist developed for appetite stimulation via a novel mechanism of action with few side effects in dogs and cats.

Squamous cell carcinoma of the tongue in cats renders the tongue stiff, swollen, and useless and causes hyper salivation and early starvation despite efforts to eat. When a pet physically cannot eat, or will not eat, the placement of a percutaneous esophageal feeding tube may be performed under a short anesthetic with minimal risk. The procedure has been described by Rawlings (1993). After the esophagostomy feeding tube is in place, be sure to feed the pet successfully in the hospital several times before discharge. A discharge appointment must be scheduled, during which the doctor or a nurse will demonstrate feeding technique and instruct the owner about how and what to feed the pet at home. The owner should be invited to call for further instructions. The diet and supplements for feeding must be spelled out to avoid clogging the tube and to ensure that the pet is getting enough calories and liquid to maintain body weight. If the tube gets clogged, instruct the owner to use Coca-Cola® to dissolve the clog. Create a schedule that spells out morning and evening times for medications, chemotherapy, amounts of fluid, feeding volumes, and supplements on a written daily calendar. This written schedule helps to clarify the day's work order for the home caregivers.

Nasal Cancer Patients

Pets with facial deformity and night stridor, due to nasal passage cancer, may be palliated with combinations of NSAIDs such as piroxicam or carprofen, deracoxib, and so forth. Most dogs with nasal tumors have little to no trouble with stridor while they are awake and panting but have trouble sleeping at night. Most end of life nasal cancer patients will sleep more comfortably and with less stridor if given evening sedation with butorphanol or valium or a combination. Olanzapine (Zyprexa™) also enhances their quality of life.

BJ's Case (An Engineer Helped Reduce Her Stridor)

Mr. Shelton, an engineer, devised a plan to help his 12-year-old Lab, BJ, breathe more peacefully at night. BJ had trouble sleeping due to stridor and obstruction of her nasal passages. She loved to play ball and chew on bones. Mr. Shelton punched holes in a tennis ball for air passage. He taught BJ to sleep with the ball in her mouth. BJ got similar relief when she fell asleep with a large rawhide bone or any object that was big enough to keep her mouth open. This simple adjustment was a joy for Mr. Shelton as a caregiver because it provided so much palliation for BJ. Be sure to keep this concept in mind for the next case you see like BJ. Most carers can teach their dog to sleep with a toy, ball, or bone keeping the mouth open, to allow air to flow freely in and out of the trachea (Figure 10.3).

Osteosarcoma Patients

Dogs with osteosarcoma (OSA) and other types of bone cancer who do not undergo amputation are in great pain and at risk for pathological fracture. These patients can be palliated with multimodal pain

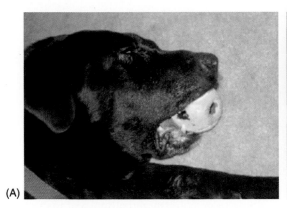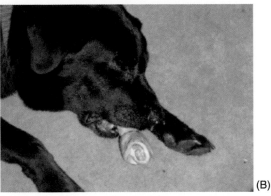

(A)   (B)

Figure 10.3. BJ Shelton, a geriatric Labrador Retriever with nasal cancer, was more comfortable when she was taught to sleep with a toy, ball, or bone to keep her mouth open. This alleviated nasal stridor.

alleviation protocols. Walking harnesses and leg braces may prevent pathological fractures during outings. QoL at home is enhanced with the use of no-slip floor mats and ramps to get in and out of the car and house and on and off the bed. If the family sleeps upstairs and the patient cannot negotiate the stairs, many carers will sleep downstairs to keep their OSA dog happy during their Pawspice days. Palliative radiation therapy or stereotactic radiation delivered to the OSA lesion may reduce pain and swelling.

The use of piroxicam at 0.3mg/kg once daily not only palliates bone cancer pain but may also actually yield a rare remission on a sporadic basis as shown by Knapp and workers at Purdue University School of Veterinary Medicine (Knapp et al. 1992). Bisphosphonates have a dual action in OSA. When given IV monthly, zoledronate or pamidronate may alleviate bone pain and slow osteoclast activity. Carprofen, deracoxib, meloxicam, firocoxib, and other selective NSAIDs may also be used, in place of piroxicam, for OSA pain palliation. All NSAIDs need to be dose adjusted and used with great caution and in combination with famotidine (long term) or omeprazole (short term) to reduce adverse events such as: vomiting, gastric ulceration, hemorrhage, nephrotoxicity, and hepatotoxicity in geriatric, frail, debilitated, or dehydrated patients. Tramadol®, a synthetic opioid, has been found to be less helpful and shorter acting than initially thought for dogs. Many clinicians still use it but in higher doses and at 8-hour intervals. When a gabapentin, amantadine, tramadol, or trazodone (GAT) are combined with NSAIDs for palliation of bone cancer pain, it can have a dramatic effect. Fentanyl (Duragesic) transdermal opioid pain patches every 72 hours or transdermal fentanyl solution (Recuvyra™) every 4–7 days can be very helpful in combination with NSAIDs for palliation of OSA pain and break-through pain in dogs. Use the GAT protocol with an NSAID at the most effective dose for multimodal pain management, as suggested by the WHO pain control ladder (see Figure 7.1) at the *initial* visit to treat bone cancer pain.

Degenerative Myelopathy or Paresis/Paralysis

These cases benefit from a wide range of resourceful home care items such as runner rugs for a slippery floor; ramps for stairs, bed, and car; slings and body harness for assistance while walking; chest and rump lifts to help larger dogs stand up; canvas suspension hammocks; wheel carts; soft bedding; and so on. Physical therapy pools, massage, acupuncture, chiropractic, and rehabilitation techniques may help to palliate these special disabled patients. Always recommend foot covers (booties) made with cloth or canvas to prevent scraping and ulceration of the metatarsals, metacarpals, and toe pads.

Decubital Ulcers

With thoughtful planning, decubital ulcers must be intentionally avoided for all recumbent animals. Instruct carers to shop for items such as soft bedding, foam rubber pads, egg crate mattresses, doughnut pads, and waterbeds, all with washable covers. Frequent inspection of pressure sites and complete cleaning of the geriatric oncology patient's coat and skin is important. If the patient is soiled with urine or feces, it is important to completely bathe the contaminated area for maximum hygiene. If the pet needs or likes to be situated outdoors, extreme caution must be taken to prevent fly strike and maggots. Patients with long hair may need to be shaved to allow more convenient bathing and inspection of the skin and orifices.

Transitional Cell Carcinoma (TCC) Patients

Older dogs, and breeds at high risk (Scottish Terriers), can now be tested for transitional cell carcinoma (TCC) using a free catch urine sample. The CADET[(SM)] test detects the BRAF mutation in urine samples that contain 10 or more cancer cells analyzed at the breenlab.org at North Carolina State University. This genetic test does not yield false positives and may detect TCC up to 4 months before clinical signs appear. Dogs and cats with TCC often survive for many months and often one year with conventional chemotherapy using oral piroxicam and IV mitoxantrone every 21 days for 4–6 treatments. It will be a tremendous help to the family if you make several simple suggestions in advance. First, suggest that they use diapers for those patients with pollakiuria and incontinence while the pet is in the house. Second, suggest frequent trips outdoors for the patient to void. Third, they can move the TCC patient's day bed close to the doggie door to help the family endure the frustrating problems associated with house soiling.

To palliate severe hematuria and avoid extreme blood loss, a weekly visit to the veterinary office for a flush can be very helpful. Mix a 1% solution of formalin with a vial of the topical ear solution Synotic®, which contains DMSO. Instill this solution into the bladder with a urinary catheter. Keep the solution in the bladder for 10–15 minutes. Then void the bladder and flush out the blood clots. This palliative procedure may reduce the hematuria for seven to 10 days and may be repeated as needed.

Some TCC cases develop tumor obstruction of urine outflow at the trigone or in the urethra. Prostatic carcinoma patients may develop obstruction of urine outflow due to extension of malignant tissue into the prostatic urethra. Some patients benefit from placement of a permanent urinary catheter. Unfortunately, the patient can easily remove these catheters, necessitating hospital visits for recatheterization.

For geriatric cancer patients with a potential for long term palliation, the surgical placement of a prepubic low-profile cystostomy tube is helpful (Stiffler et al. 2003). Carers are instructed to void the patient's bladder four times a day. The stoma provides immediate life-saving palliation by diversion of urine and bypassing the obstruction caused by the tumor. Cystostomy may reduce hydronephrosis and allow the TCC patient to maintain a good quality of life for a variable time period. Stiffler et al. reported on three dogs with TCC that lived for three, 13, and 30 weeks and one dog with uterine carcinoma that lived for four weeks following cystostomy. One elderly cat under my care lived for one year following cystostomy for prostate cancer.

Quality of life is an important objective for pet owners who want their cancer patient dogs to be able to participate in as many of their normal activities as possible. Stiffler et al. placed low-profile cystostomy tubes for TCC patients in palliation. No bandaging is required and patients have unhindered mobility with no signs of discomfort. Stiffler reports, "Owners of the dogs began their grieving process during the period of cystostomy tube placement, and their confidence in the quality of life provided by the low-profile cystostomy tube was key to their emotional comfort with their treatment decision."

Brain Tumor Patients

Brain tumor patients in palliative end of life care often experience neurologic symptoms and seizures, which may be palliated at home with confidence and with fewer emergency visits. Carers can be instructed to squirt injectable diazepam into the nasal passages or into the rectum for seizure control. Steroids, lomustine, and linolenic acid from evening primrose oil, and OM-3 fatty acids and fish oils are reasonable components of a palliative care program for pets with brain tumors. There is evidence that a ketogenic diet reduces seizures in children and it may help dogs. Hemp-derived CBD oil may also help. If seizures are not under control with medication, the pet's QoL is ruined and the family must yield to hospitalization for IV anesthesia. After two to three days with IV medications, if the patient is not stabilized, then the kindest option is to provide the patient ultimate relief with the gift of euthanasia.

Severe Refractive Vomiting

Pet owners have great anxiety and frustration when their geriatric cancer pets experience severe refractive vomiting. If the normal first line antiemetics, such as metoclopramide, fail to control vomiting, go to drugs such as maropitant (Cerenia™) that control the chemotherapy trigger zone (cereniadvm.com). Maropitant is a neurokinin-1 (NK-1) receptor antagonist, which blocks the pharmacological action of substance P in the central nervous system. It is effective in dogs and cats. Some patients may need SQ injections of maropitant several days in a row at home to control vomiting followed by the oral preparation. Some patients may need to be hospitalized and given IV maropitant or ondansetron (Zofran®) or dolasetron (Anzemet®). For home care, large dogs (60–90 pounds) may be given 8–12mg of ondansetron BID orally or one-half of a 1mg granisetron (Kytril®) tablet, crushed and dissolved in salty water. The solution can be gently dripped on the pet's lips.

On one rare occasion, I dispensed injectable atropine to help a Great Dane that had unresponsive vomiting and hypersalivation due to nausea from pressure exerted by a tumor. The tearful pet owner could not afford the costlier antiemetics and he was absolutely not ready to make the decision for euthanasia – he just wanted me to stop the vomiting on his slim budget. He was very thankful for the relief from vomiting that his dear big dog received with the inexpensive injections of atropine. Be sure to provide liquid tears for pets given atropine in this fashion, especially in breeds susceptible to keratoconjunctivitis sicca. We are constantly being asked to help end of life patients with the simultaneous challenge and ethical burden to be economically resourceful!

Severe Pain

Injectable nalbuphine is an inexpensive generic drug that offers pain control without the typical sedation effects that accompany most of the powerful analgesics. Nalbuphine doses range from 0.5 to 1mg/kg SQ every three to four hours in dogs and 0.2 to 0.5mg/kg in cats SQ every three to six hours as needed. This pain medication is not registered under the controlled substance regulations and may be of great value in pain control at home for end of life Pawspice care patients.

Managing Soft and Loose Stools

Terminal geriatric pets in Pawspice care are often plagued with soft, loose stools, and diarrhea. Abnormal stools may result from illness itself, the treatment, or an imbalance of intestinal flora, or from dysrexia, eating whatever seems palatable from one day to the next. Many Pawspice patients have a diminished appetite and will need to be hand fed. This variable appetite and food intake may cause soft or loose stools and irregular elimination times. It is difficult for some carers to manage their pet's loose eliminations. The soiling problem is magnified for recumbent patients unable to get up and use their normal toilet area.

Practical suggestions make a big difference. Instruct carers to feed the patient tasty, bland food. They can feed a prepared diet or use barley, millet, rice, potato, or pasta cooked with chicken broth, garlic, parmesan cheese, and hickory for flavor. Adding more fiber to the diet is helpful such as FirmUp, which has pumpkin and apple fiber for dogs and cats. Clients can use canned pumpkin, pectalin, metamucil, Benefiber® powder, oatmeal, oat bran, and high fiber bread as sources for fiber. Symptomatic treatment with metronidazole (Flagyl®), sulfasalazine (Azulfidine®), or Tyolsin® powder may also help. For bland protein, we recommend yogurt, egg, cottage cheese, broccoli, spinach, kale, ground chicken, or turkey cooked in broth and flavors.

Immunonutrition and Chemoprevention as Palliative Care

Carefully selected supplements play a major role in palliative care for Pawspice patients. Providing support for the "whole patient" has added more to my practice than I thought possible. Dr. Philip Bergman (1999), while at MD Anderson Memorial Cancer Center in Houston, presented an enlightening lecture on chemoprevention. This involves the use of natural or synthetic compounds that may reverse or suppress the process of carcinogenesis, metastasis, and recurrence. Nutritional advice and nutraceutical supplementation programs can be geared to play a role in cancer prevention for treated, untreated, or terminally ill companion animals. Chemoprevention and immunonutrition may be professionally and sensibly supervised at your clinic. This service creates further client confidence that the veterinarian is addressing the pet's immune system and supporting the pet's organ function as much as possible.

Most geriatric cancer patients who undergo surgery, chemotherapy, or radiation therapy are considered to be at a moderate-to-great risk for recurrence of their cancer. These older cancer patients are definite candidates for entry into a Pawspice program. The expectancy rate for recurrence and death from metastases or complications is 50–90% within four to 12 months. Dogs with osteosarcoma, hemangiosarcoma, adenocarcinoma, and lymphoma as well as cats with breast cancer, vaccine-associated sarcoma, oral tumors, and lymphoma are also at very high risk. Cats with IBD, chronic gingivitis, stomatitis, inflammatory disease, and feline triad disease are at greater risk of developing illness or cancer. Cats infected with FeLV and FIV are at risk for retroviral-associated neoplasia. Cats exposed to cigarette smoke and dogs exposed to agricultural herbicides and pesticides are also at greater risk for cancer. When these at-risk conditions are addressed with immunonutrition and chemoprevention, the pet may benefit.

Provide Emotional Support for Carers of Pawspice Pets

If carers need help to cope with pet loss issues, encourage them to join a pet loss chat room on a daily basis, such as the chat room conducted by the Association for Pet Loss and Bereavement (www.aplb.org). Carers may find it helpful to network with other people who have a geriatric pet with terminal cancer in a similar Pawspice program. With permission, you can provide telephone or e-mail contact information to promote networking between your Pawspice clients. The more experienced caregiver is often willing to share knowledge, insights, and empathy with the newcomer.

Internet support groups exist for people who have pets with specific ailments. There are chat rooms for owners with pets that have cancer in general and chat rooms for specific cancers such as: lymphoma, hemangiosarcoma, osteosarcoma, feline injection site sarcoma, feline lymphoma, and many other types of cancer. After receiving information and support at the veterinary office, many carers find it invaluable to exchange information and support with other carers. Helping clients to network brings them comfort and can be a wonderful staff time saver.

Keep several of these helpful books in your hospital lending library or for sale: *Pets Living with Cancer: A Pet Owner's Resource*, by Robin Downing, DVM (2000), is a very helpful book to orient pet carers about the ins and outs of cancer treatment for pets. Dr. Downing tells about her own dog, Murphy, and her battle against osteosarcoma with limb sparing surgery at CSU. Laurie Kaplan's insightful book, *So Easy to Love, So Hard to Lose* (2010), educates readers about pet loss, beginning with the palliative hospice care phase and through the loss and grief. It validates their thoughts and feelings, and helps them cope (www.soeasytolove.com). Kaplan's book, *Help Your Dog Fight Cancer: Empowerment for Dog Owners* (2016), provides information about canine cancer medical treatment and home care, assistance in decision making, and encouragement for carers of dogs with cancer. It also includes illustrated instructions for preparing homemade meals for cancer dogs (www.helpyourdogfightcancer.com).

Some Pawspice pets benefit from day care services provided by the primary care veterinarian's facility while the owners are at work. This service may include taking the pet's temperature and weight, bathing and brushing a soiled pet, providing SQ fluids, injections, and hand feedings. This service can be the key to sustaining a quality Pawspice for the working pet owner. Convenient monthly billing, along with drop-off and pick-up times that revolve around the owner's schedule and may be prearranged with attending staff members before and after routine receiving hours.

After orchestrating chemotherapy, radiation therapy, or any long battle with illness, the loss of a beloved pet evokes a special kind of grief in which carers feel let down, defeat, and relief. Before the pet's death, carers were dealing with anticipatory grief. We address it by encouraging them to recognize how it ruins the good days and moments that they could happily share with their pet. Whether the client made the choice for less cancer medicine or more cancer medicine, they may second-guess their decision and blame themselves for the pet's death. Relief is a natural component of grief, and we should counsel our clients not to feel guilty about experiencing relief from burdensome care after their pet dies (Villalobos 2007). Read more about counseling in Chapter 11, especially the section by Sandra Grossman, PhD, and Ellie Freeman, MFC, for more information about addressing grief after the loss of a beloved pet.

Because we are a referral practice, we make it a point to inform the referring veterinarian and their reception staff about potential problems with their client's grief. We ask the doctor to alert the staff to provide as much comfort and support as possible to the grieving pet owner during Pawspice. The attending local doctor should make an effort to contact and encourage the pet owner to seek counseling and should document this effort in the medical record.

Zorba's Case (Pawspice for Old OSA Survivors)

Zorba Tuck, a 13-year-old M/N German Shepherd Dog, had been treated for osteosarcoma two years previously but was lost to follow-up. There was a sad voice mail message from Susan Tuck, Zorba's caregiver. She was in tears. Her wilting voice thanked me for the gift of Zorba's life for the past two years. Zorba had won his battle against osteosarcoma. He had an amputation of his left hind leg followed by chemotherapy. Carboplatin and Adriamycin were given initially for two cycles, followed by five treatments with carboplatin at three- to four-week intervals over nine months. Zorba had concurrent severe arthritis and was on carprofen and injections of Legend® and Adequan® from his orthopedic surgeon. Zorba needed assistance with a support sling to get up and walk as he reached his one-year metastasis-free anniversary. He swam every day for exercise. Susan's phone message said, "It's not Zorba's cancer that is going to kill him. It's his arthritis. It pulled the rug out from under him." As Zorba approached 13 years of age, he had more difficulty with his front legs until, finally, he could no longer stand.

When I called Susan back, her phone was on call screening. She said that she wanted to speak only to her husband or to me. She did not want to take calls from her friends because they did not understand and would say hurtful things like, "Well, Zorba has had a long life" and "When will you come to your senses and let him go?" In response to this type of complaint, I generally say, "Forgive your friends. They mean well and they are sad to see your heart breaking. They don't understand how much Zorba means to you. They don't understand the depth of the human–animal bond that you share with Zorba."

When I asked Susan about Zorba's quality of life, she said enthusiastically, "He is fine, Dr. Alice, he just can't stand. He plays, he eats, he barks, he is happy. He has always been just fine lying around because of his arthritis." I asked her if she was able to keep him clean and she said, "Oh, it's not a problem and I don't mind that at all. We have a routine. Of course, I quit my job to be home with him 24/7. My husband is very supportive." Her voice cracked with grief and sorrow. I said, "If Zorba is happy, he must sense your sadness and wonder what he has done wrong." I pointed out that she seemed too sad right now for the Pawspice that she and Zorba were sharing and that she was ruining their precious moments together with anticipatory grief. She said, "That's it, Dr. Alice, I knew you would understand!" I said something like this: "Susan, you need to reconfigure your emotions. Enjoy the precious days that Zorba is giving you. He is still very much alive and with you! When you smell a rose, the fragrance gives you pleasure for that instant even though you know the rose will wilt in a few days. Zorba is like a flower. You need to inhale Zorba's fragrance and his presence today even though he will wilt tomorrow. Zorba is there with you right now. He is not dead yet. You need to focus on the moments of joy and share the happiness of your bond."

Susan thanked me for helping her to think more clearly and stay in the moment and to "Think the way Zorba did." I told her, "Look into his eyes and focus on the wellness that is right there in front of you and count your blessings about how well he is today. When more functions get subtracted from Zorba, he will tell you when the time would be right to give him back." Susan told me that she felt better and thanked me again for being so supportive.

Susan clearly needed to use a Quality of Life Scale as a guideline for future decision making. At the end of our conversation, I promised to send her articles about Pawspice, the H5M2 Quality of Life Scale, and anticipatory grief as well as the phone number for a Pet Loss Hotline. Susan left a message the next day. She said, "Thank you Dr. V. After reading the mobility section in the quality of life article, I knew that I was doing the right thing for Zorba. He is happy and playful."

Susan felt validated with her choice for Pawspice care for Zorba. Susan hoped that Zorba would celebrate his 14th birthday and a three-year anniversary with osteosarcoma, and he did!

Tips for Pawspice/Hospice Patients in Decline

Technician house calls may be set up for carers who are unable to administer injections and fluids to the Pawspice pet. The reception staff can be made aware of which pets are on Pawspice programs so they can be sensitive when family members call in for information, updates, appointments, or emotional support.

If the patient has hyporexia, anorexia or cancer cachexia or has a feeding tube, supplement the diet with high-quality glutamine and whey protein powders. Glutamine supports intestinal health, helps prevent muscle breakdown, promotes healing, and is a precursor in the synthesis of glutathione. Whey proteins such as lactoferrin, immunoglobulins, and active peptides provide the gut with highly digestible nutrients. Primal Dose™ contains bovine colostrum and is considered a superfood that improves gut health and immunity. Novel products will become available that will reduce wasting.

You and your veterinary staff should give carers all the emotional comfort and encouragement they need. Offer them a supply of hospital towels or introduce them to puppy pads for easy, frequent bed changes. Help carers establish good hygiene for the patient and encourage frequent rear end bathing. If each one of the patient's problems can be addressed and improved by at least 30 to 50%, the Pawspice patient's QoL may improve dramatically despite their prognosis.

Remind the family to use the H5M2 QoL Scale. Ask them to review each of the seven criteria and give a score every week. If the hospice patient is declining towards death by the day, ask for a daily score, or a morning and evening score, or an hourly score if the patient is entering the first of the three phases of active dying. The family may make the final call to ask for help in transitioning their beloved pet with a home euthanasia or they may prefer to bring their pet to your clinic for help to avoid the rigors of dying.

Summary

The human–animal bond between pets and their human carers is a celebrated and cherished attachment relationship (Voith 1985). When it is time for the physical departure of the pet, The Bond grows even stronger. The pet's death is heartbreaking for the entire family and each family member suffers differently. We need to address grief with more expertise, especially when dealing with children. Pet owners may express emotions that are uncomfortable for the doctor and staff to witness and deal with (Cohen and Fudin 1991). Many pet carers suffer from severe anticipatory grief, which should be addressed. Family members often want to spend as many last days and hours as possible in the hospice setting to spend precious moments with their pet at home before their inevitable loss. Veterinarians, especially emergency room clinicians, should make every effort to accommodate their clients for the hospice vigil for end of life patients. Whenever possible, offer clients the option to make arrangements for their dying pet and to go home with palliative comfort care and palliative sedation for the hospice vigil.

Being old, having more than one concurrent disorder, having two signs of frailty (Hua et al. 2016), and having cancer are associated with shortened survival times. Keeping all of this in mind, it is time for contemporary veterinarians to rethink how our profession can improve the attitude, expertise, and delivery of end of life services. We can expand services to include routine hospice care for terminal patients or consider referring to a hospice care provider. We can improve our willingness and demeanor when discussing options for palliative care and turn up the level of supportive care that we offer. We can very professionally help pet owners face the final days with their best friend at end of life. We can better equip our clients with the knowledge, support, and resources they need to successfully forge ahead into the final phase of their beloved pet's life.

References

Bergman, P. 1999. Chemoprevention. *Proceedings of the 1999 ACVIM Forum in Chicago*.

Chen, R.C., A.D. Falchook, F. Tian, R. Basak, L. Hanson, N. Selvam, and S. Dusetzina. 2016. Aggressive care at the end-of-life for younger patients with cancer: Impact of ASCO's Choosing Wisely campaign. *Journal of Clinical Oncology* 34, abstract LBA10033.

Cohen, S.P., and C.E. Fudin (eds). 1991. *Animal illness and human emotion: Problems in veterinary medicine*, Vol. 3, No. 1. Philadelphia, PA: Lippincott.

Downing, R. 2000. *Pets living with cancer: A pet owner's resource*. Lakewood, CO: AAHA Press.

Gawande, A. 2014. *Being mortal: Medicine and what matters in the end*. New York: Metropolitan Books, Henry Holt and Company.

Hoskins, J.D. 2000. Feline "triad disease" poses triple threat. DVM *Newsmagazine*, February, pp. 4S–7S.

Hoskins, J.D. 2004. *Geriatrics and gerontology of the dog and cat*, 2nd edn. Philadelphia, PA: Saunders.

Hua, J., S. Hommady, C. Muller, J.L. Pouchelon, M. Blondot, C. Gilbert, and L. Desquilbet. 2016. Assessment of frailty in aged dogs. *American Journal of Veterinary Research* 77 (12):1357–1365.

Kaplan, L. 2010. *So easy to love, so hard to lose: A bridge to healing before and after the loss of a pet*. Briarcliff Manor, NY: JanGen Press.

Kaplan, L., and A. Villalobos. 2016. *Help your dog fight cancer: Empowerment for dog owners*, 3rd edn. Briarcliff Manor, NY: JanGen Press.

Knapp, D.W., R.C. Richardson, G.D. Bottoms, et al. 1992. Phase 1 trial of piroxicam in 62 dogs bearing naturally occurring tumors. *Cancer Chemotherapy and Pharmacology* 29:214.

Long, C.C. 2005. Personal Communication as student representative of CSU Pet Hospice Program, October.

McMillan, F.D. 2005. "The concept of quality of life in animals." In *Mental health and well-being in animals*, ed. F.D. McMillan, pp. 183–200. Ames, IA: Blackwell Publishing Professional.

Meyers, F.C., as quoted by C. Morain. 2005. It's about living. *UC Davis Magazine*, Fall.

Monjazeb, A., and M. Kent. 2013. Translating combination radiotherapy/immunotherapy from dogs to humans with advanced melanoma or sarcoma, www.OncLive.com/publications.com and UC Davis. *Advance*, Fall 2016, p. 3.

Ogilvie, G.K., and A.S. Moore. 2001. "Nutritional support." In *Feline oncology*, eds G. Ogilvie and A. Moore, pp. 113–125. Trenton, NJ: Veterinary Learning Systems, 2001.

Pal, S. 2016. Psych drug helps manage lung cancer symptoms, side effects: Olanzapine eases treatment-related vomiting, nausea and disease-driven anorexia. ASCO Reading Room/MedPageToday. September 16, 2016.

Rawlings, C.A. 1993. Percutaneous placement of a midcervical esophagostomy tube: New technique and representative cases. *JAAHA* 29:526–530.

Remillard, R., W. Burkholder, S. Abood, and K. Michel. 2000. In dire need of food. Roundtable on Nutritional Support, *Veterinary Forum*, September, pp. 51–61.

Rollin, B.E. 2006. Euthanasia and quality of life. *Commentary. JAVMA* 228 (7):1014–1016.

Stiffler, K.S., M.A. McCrackin Stevenson, K.K. Cornell, L.E. Glerum, J.D. Smith, N.A. Miller, and C.A. Rawlings. 2003. Clinical use of low-profile cystostomy tubes in four dogs and a cat. *JAVMA* 223 (3):325–329.

Tannenbaum, J. 1985. Ethics and human–companion animal interaction, a plea for a veterinary ethics of the human–companion animal bond. *Veterinary Clinics of North America*, March, pp. 431–447.

Villalobos, A. 2007. Relief is a natural component of grief, The Bond and beyond. *Vet Practice News*, November, pp. 24–25 (www.pawspice.com/clients/17611/documents/ReliefArticle.pdf).

Voith, V.L. 1985. "Attachment of people to companion animals." In *Symposium on the Human–Companion Animal Bond,* Veterinary Clinics of North America, pp. 289–296. Philadelphia, PA: Saunders.

Wojciechowska, J.I., and C.J. Hewson. 2005. Quality of life assessment in pet dogs. Vet Med Today: reference point. *JAVMA* 226 (5):722–728.

Yaxley, P., and J. Pierce. 2016. Hospice care and palliative sedation. *Veterinary Team Brief* 4 (10):35–40.

Suggested Reading

Dobson, J., and D. Lascelles (eds). 2003. *BSAVA manual of canine and feline oncology*, 2nd edn. *Quedgeley, Gloucestershire*, England: British Small Animal Veterinary Association.

Hunt, L.E. 1998. *Angel pawprints: Reflections on loving and losing a canine companion.* Pasadena, CA: Darrowby Press.

Lagoni, L., D. Morehead, and C. Butler. 1999. The bond-centered practice: The future of veterinary care. *Proceedings of the 1999 ACVIM Forum in Chicago.*

Mauldin, G.E. 2001. "Nutritional considerations." In *Veterinary oncology secrets*, ed. R.C. Rosenthal, pp. 101–108. Philadelphia, PA: Hanley & Belfus.

Meier, D.E., S.L. Issacs, and R.G. Hughes (eds). 2010. *Palliative care: Transforming the care of serious illness*, 452 pp. San Francisco, CA: Jossey-Bass, A Wiley Imprint.

Morrison, W.B. 2002. *Cancer in dogs and cats: Medical and surgical management*, 2nd edn. Jackson, WY: Teton New Media.

Mutsaers, A.J. 2014. Metronomic Chemotherapy: Theory and Practice, State of the Art Presenter, *Proceedings Veterinary Cancer Society Annual Forum*, p. 56.

Ogilvie, G.K. 1999. Hospice and bond centered practice: The future of veterinary care. *Proceedings of the 1999 ACVIM Forum in Chicago.*

Ogilvie, G.K., and A.S. Moore. 1995. *Managing the veterinary cancer patient.* Trenton, NJ: Veterinary Learning Systems.

Veterinary Learning Systems Co., Inc. 1995. *Managing the veterinary cancer patient: A practice manual.*

Villalobos, A.E. 2000. Conceptualized end of life care: "Pawspice" program for pets. *AVMA Proceedings*, pp. 322–327.

Chapter 11
Euthanasia for the Geriatric Cancer Patient

Euthanasia is a time when you can do more for the family than at any other time in the pet's life. That is why veterinarians must sensitively respect the bond that exists between the pet and caregiver.

Cathy Adams, DVM

A Philosophy and Principles

Pet caregivers wish that their beloved pets would pass away peacefully at a ripe old age during sleep in the privacy of their homes. However, that wishful ideal is seldom the case. The slow decline of a sick geriatric cancer patient can be a bumpy and exhausting road. Some pet carers say they want their old pal to have a "natural" death without understanding that they may be prolonging death and that their pet may suffer unnecessarily (Feldman 2004).

In keeping with the Pawspice philosophy, the pet's quality of life (QoL) and freedom from pain must be regarded as the most important priority. Cancer is a merciless and relentless disease. Our geriatric oncology patients are stoic as they suffer and unable to comprehend the human concept of sacrifice for extra life. These factors lead to unrecognized pain and frustration, and untreated suffering at the end of life. The attending doctor, as the pet's advocate, should help carers understand these factors and assist them in every way possible to be vigilant to ensure that their pet will have a peaceful and painless death (Rollin 2006). We must initiate that difficult conversation with our clients to gain insight about their diverse beliefs and feelings about euthanasia. It is difficult and morally stressful for us to understand clients who refuse to consider euthanasia or properly manage a terminal geriatric pet that is suffering needlessly. The courageous conversation approach is to shift your internal stance from "*I understand*" to "*Help me understand*" (Bateman 2016). However, with professional hospice help, we can provide carers with emotional support and provide our dying patients with palliative sedation to ease anxiety during their last days and hours (Yaxley and Pierce 2016).

For some carers, it may be too difficult to accompany or witness their dying pet all the way to the end. We need to prepare our clients about what to expect during their pet's final decline toward death and give them the tools to make end of life decisions. We need to help carers accept the inevitability of death and understand the experience and the value of a good death and the process of euthanasia. We should always let carers know the meaning of the word euthanasia is "well death" and that it is our honor and privilege to help their pets pass peacefully. Thanatologists know that veterinarians have a lot to contribute to the Death with Dignity movement in the US and beyond. Thanatologists asked me

---

Canine and Feline Geriatric Oncology: Honoring the Human–Animal Bond, Second Edition. Alice Villalobos with Laurie Kaplan.
© 2018 John Wiley & Sons, Inc. Published 2018 by John Wiley & Sons, Inc.

to contribute to their literature. The title of my commentary is a question, *Are Veterinarians Kinder to Their End of Life Patients than Physicians?* and it was the most downloaded article in that issue of *International Journal of Ethics* (Villalobos 2014).

Emergency-Related Euthanasia

Unfortunately, many geriatric pets develop cancer quietly without notice and they wind up in an unfamiliar emergency clinic due to acute onset issues instead of your hospital, among the doctors and staff that they have known their whole lives. Occult cancer often reaches a threshold that precipitates an acute symptom or paraneoplastic syndrome. Geriatric dogs are commonly presented to emergency rooms for cancer-related disorders such as hemoabdomen, weakness, epistaxis, seizures, pathological fractures, syncope, dehydration, vomiting, diarrhea, anorexia, pain, metabolic problems, labored breathing, and so forth. Geriatric cats with occult cancer commonly present with dyspnea, dysphagia, vomiting, diarrhea, weight loss, obstruction, dehydration, cachexia, anorexia, etc. The emergency room clinician may be the first to diagnose cancer in the geriatric patient. Many are euthanized within hours of the emergency visit, while others undergo emergency treatment and surgery. There is an increasing demand to arrange a hospice vigil for terminally ill patients so that family members can have more time to say their goodbyes. The hospice vigil allows beloved pets to go home, after their crisis and emergency clinic visit, with the option to have a house call veterinarian help them transition in the presence of friends, family, and other household pets.

Kathryn D. Marocchino, PhD., Professor of Thanatology at California State University in Vallejo, started the Nikki Hospice Foundation for Pets in 1996. She felt that the end of life hospice movement for pets addressed a "sense of coercion" faced by owners of sick pets who were forced to decide between aggressive treatment or euthanasia. She objected to what I call "either–or" medicine, which can be devoid of compassion. I feel that our entire profession must provide carers with the third option for the hospice vigil and home or clinic euthanasia when appropriate. People thanked her, with comments like: "Where were you 30 years ago? They made me kill my dog."

Geriatric patients with comorbidities are at greater risk for death and complications from diagnostic, surgical, and therapeutic procedures. Aging causes increased susceptibility to sepsis, poor organ system functional reserve, and a decreased ability to cope with the physiological stress of anesthesia, surgery, tissue damage, and pain. The risk for complications and adverse events to cancer therapy increases for the oldest of the old, especially if they are obese or have concurrent disease and chronic debilitating conditions (Balducci et al. 2004).

Geriatric oncology patients are at risk for more oncologic emergencies than younger cancer patients receiving similar therapy. Oncologic emergencies related to treatment toxicity commonly involve vomiting, diarrhea, leukopenia, sepsis, thrombocytopenia, renal failure, heart failure, hepatic toxicity, tumor lysis syndrome, drug and radiation therapy-related reactions, and so forth (Ogilvie and Moore 1995). Carers of geriatric oncology patients receiving therapy may feel they must give up if their pet becomes extremely ill. They may feel guilty about stressing their old pet and for making the decision to treat the cancer in the first place.

When consulting with clients who cannot emotionally face death, we should discuss the bioethics of prolonging death for a suffering animal and discuss futile medicine at the end of life. They may be asking you to continue futile treatment or to help them seek clinical trials, or complementary and alternative medicine for their terminal pets. The first thing to do is take a moment to be supportive and empathetic. Praise their love and devotion for their pet. Acknowledge their special human–animal bond and their struggles with anticipatory grief, which is driving their search for "a cure." More often, carers are looking for hope and a nurturing, palliative hospice care program that your practice is not offering them.

Cabo's Case (Love Blindfolds Some to Hope Against Hope)

During one of many phone consultations with Elaine, I said, "I know that you love Cabo very much and that she means everything to you. I know that you would do anything if it would help make the renal cell carcinoma in her abdomen and the lesions in her lungs go away. Her tumor burden is too high to expect that any more chemotherapy would be able to help her. At this point, chemotherapy would most likely burden her one functional kidney and make her very sick. Furthermore, chemotherapy in the face of the huge tumor burden that she has would offer little or no benefit. There are some experimental small molecule therapies being developed but we don't have access to them yet. My job as Cabo's doctor is to make sure that we do no harm to her in these final days. Just slow down your quest for a cure, and stay home with Cabo and try to enjoy her final days of wellness until she crashes."

When deeply bonded clients like Elaine keep asking if there is anything else you can suggest to help Cabo and make the tumors shrink, they need to know what you know about the cancer and its impact on the patient's body and what to expect. They also need to know what you do not know. They need all the emotional support you can give them, along with the best palliative care that you can recommend for their terminal patient. Today, I would give Cabo: metronomic chemotherapy, antiangiogenesis therapy, small molecule therapy, and Zyprexa™ to ease the stress of pulmonary metastasis.

If carers feel you are a dead end for their pet, they will often seek out complementary and alternative medicine, and integrative medicine with or without your blessings. I point out that researchers have examined many the most efficacious remedies offered in holistic and alternative medicine and that some techniques do have merit, while others are unsubstantiated, unproven, and even questionable.

The one high touch ingredient that complementary and alternative medicine offers carers and patients is hope. This is in contrast with the evidence-based paradigm that our conventional Western medicine generates with statistics on response rates, disease-free intervals, and survival times. A working definition for hope is to wish for something with expectation. Alternative therapies generally require one prerequisite, and that is to be ministered to the patient with hope.

As a general rule, if an integrative technique seems to alleviate pain or adverse conditions or improves the recurrent geriatric oncology patient's well-being, then it is good to continue and incorporate it as complementary to your treatment. If there are no benefits after four visits, then it makes sense to stop the treatment. Many of my clients take their geriatric pets to holistic doctors for detoxification, herbal therapy, acupuncture, and massage after receiving chemotherapy at our office. We record the Rx's in the chart.

Elaine's bond for Cabo was very deep. She consulted with our service, another oncologist, a holistic practitioner, and a health foods store from the start. She acquired some last-minute supplements at her health food store and opted to try interferon therapy under the direction of her other oncologist in a last-ditch effort to help Cabo. Elaine told me that she knew that she was hoping against hope. She felt that it was all she could do. This happens to pet owners who cannot face the fact that their pet is terminal. They still prefer hope against hope, to hope with little reason or justification.

When Cabo went into respiratory failure, Elaine wanted the emergency room doctors to resuscitate her. After 20 minutes, she finally let Cabo go. Afterward, Elaine second-guessed herself at every step of the way. She asked me about harmful side effects from interferon. She was moving through the typical stages of grief. I comforted Elaine by helping her recognize that she was going through the "woulda-coulda-shoulda" phase of grief. She told me that she felt compelled to do all that she could for Cabo and that she would miss her forever.

Emergency-associated euthanasia is generally an emotional shock to the pet's family. They have had no time to prepare emotionally for the loss and to make matters worse are required – sometimes pressured – to make the decision to euthanize. Understandably, carers may have intense guilt. They may blame themselves for not knowing or for procrastination – for letting some small innuendo or symptom slide. Some pet owners feel that they abandoned or gave up on their best friend. Self-doubt haunts some carers, causing angst, sleep disturbances, weight loss, and depression. They sift over every moment of the visit asking "woulda-coulda-shoulda" about each step, each action, and every decision. Their feelings of guilt may persist for a long time. Some carers feel that no one understands their sorrow and that they have no one to talk to about their feelings of loss. Elaine needed a referral to the Association of Pet Loss and Bereavement to help her process her profound grief.

Cecilia's Case (Self-Doubt Follows Even Good Decisions)

Many clients need emotional support following their decision. You may recall Cecilia, the Golden Retriever with hemangiosarcoma in Chapter 9. Corbin (2004) wrote the following letter seven days after Cecilia was euthanized:

"When I was told she [Cecilia] was very uncomfortable and would only get worse, I made what I believe was the correct but too quick of a decision. I should have demanded supportive treatment. If she were bleeding a major bleed, would her hematocrit levels drop faster and more drastic? 30 is not that bad, is it?

When I asked, the Dr. said that anytime from that point on was the right time. She said it will only get worse and that she will become increasingly uncomfortable. I should have contacted you to get your opinion. … I feel that in my panic driven state, I made a decision without demanding more medical facts and options. I just did not want Cecilia to be in pain."

Planning for Death

Carers who have a geriatric pet with terminal cancer in Pawspice care may have many questions and great fears about death and euthanasia. "How will I know when the time comes? What do I do? I can't go through this." The answer to the first question should rest with the pet. Advise the family that their old pal will give them a clear sign. The signs may be physical, such as unresponsive vomiting, uncontrollable diarrhea, dyspnea, crying, and loss of mentation or slipping into a moribund state. Some geriatric cancer pets decline to the point where the carer notes that they are having more bad days than good days. Use the HHHHHMM (H5M2) Quality of Life Scale (Table 10.1) as a guide to help in decision making about euthanasia. When counseling carers, you might say, "Look into Stormy's eyes and he will tell you when it's the right time for him to go. The message will be clear and you will know." The eyes usually tell the story: pupils are dilated, the cornea appears glossy, the third eyelid may be prolapsed, and the pet may be squinting (Cohen and Sawyer 1991).

The answer to the second question, "What do I do?" is more logistical. When the time approaches for the pet to be humanely euthanized, the emotional pain for the family may be softened if they know that euthanasia can be performed at any time of the day or night. Arrangements must be made in advance to cover the patient's needs 24 hours a day. Referrals to a house call doctor or an after-hours emergency room facility need to be set up so that the decision about the right time for euthanasia is made on behalf of the pet, not the doctor's office hours.

When the time comes for the emotional pain that is unavoidable with the euthanasia of a companion pet, carers whose pets are in Pawspice care are empowered to make the best decision for the pet. Advise the client to have several plans in mind. Plan A may be their ideal wish, for their terminal pet to pass away peacefully at home. Plan B may be with a house call doctor who will perform home euthanasia. Plan C may be euthanasia at your hospital during regular office hours. Plan D may be euthanasia at a specified emergency clinic in the event the need comes after hours. Also, ask the family if they have planned ahead or if they need help making arrangements for cremation or burial.

Pye's Case (Leave Room for Every Carer's Plan A)

Dearest Dr. Alice:

My beloved Pye passed away Friday evening. I write this note of thanks to acknowledge that it is by cause of your good work and guidance of Pawspice that we were afforded a long, peaceful goodbye. I had the time to say all the things that I wanted to say to him and also tell him that I know how much he loved me, too. Pye was home with his brother Joie and I when he passed. I am confident that he was exactly where he would have chosen to be.

As I was armed with your knowledgeable counsel regarding Pye's particular type of cancer (hemangiosarcoma), I was able to see him through his several 'incidents,' and rather than have him euthanized prematurely (as I had contemplated more than once prior to learning of 'Pawspice'), I was able to provide Pawspice care at home for him and we were afforded the most loving of farewells. I could not have designed a more beautiful end of life for him and I pray that when his brother's time comes, he too, will be able to remain at home with me caring for his end of life (Pawspice) and a safe, loving, slow return to his brother. Fifteen years has been far too short a time together and I selfishly wish my beloved pets could live with me forever. But I remind myself that the death of an OLD and BELOVED man (pet) can NOT in any manner of honesty, be called a tragedy.

In loving thoughts, Ginger Atkynes

Euthanasia Always a Two-Step Process at the Hospital

Many pet carers make the statement, "I can't go through this." We should not ignore this cry for help. We can be supportive and say something like, "You are doing a wonderful job caring for Bella right now. She is depending on you to do the right thing when her life is no longer worth living. When that time comes, it will be as if you have a curtain call. You must go out on stage, like an actor, and go through the motions. You may not feel that it is real, but you know your role and what you have to do and say, as a farewell to Scooter. When you get back home, you can have your breakdown and cry."

Many families plan to bring their geriatric oncology pet to your facility for euthanasia. This is a sad and very difficult occasion for carers but with just a little effort, you and your staff can make the moment as pleasant as possible. Comfort your clients. Encourage them to bring their pet's favorite blanket, toys, candles, and music. Let them know that they can bring their children, other pets, and close friends as well. Alert your staff that there is a euthanasia service going on and that they should keep their voices down to show respect for the grieving family.

Many new and remodeled hospitals have added a comfort room or rainbow room furnished with a couch and carpeting for a warmer atmosphere. If your facility lacks a comfort room, it helps to create a gentle atmosphere in one of your exam rooms. Turn off or dim bright overhead lights or use a small room lamp.

At our clinics, we shut off the overhead lights in the exam room, turn on a soft light and light candles, and bring in blankets. This subtle change in lighting works well to soften the harshness of the room. We light candles for ambiance and symbolism, and to show reverence and respect at this sad time. We place flowers and leafy greens nearby on the pet's blanket.

Next, we explain to the family that you have a two-step process for euthanasia. The first step is to give a sedative to the cancer patient and the second is to give the final injection. Now we ask if the family is ready for the first step.

Giving the patient a deep sedative allows the stressed caregivers to relax while their beloved pet gently falls into a relaxed state and loses consciousness. We always keep the terminal pet in the presence of the owner. I use a 27-gauge needle and give a deep intramuscular injection of dexmedetomidine (Dexdomitor®) with butorphanol to prevent nausea. For deep sedation dose go to: dexdomitorcalculator.com. The patient seldom feels the injection, but if the patient objects or struggles, apologize immediately.

Some doctors prefer to use Telazol®, SQ, or IM injections of butorphanol-acepromazine. It helps family members to know that Dexdomitor is reversible in case they change their mind. To avoid emesis, we give an SQ injection of butorphanol as a pretreatment 5 to 10 minutes before the sedative if the pet had eaten recently. Otherwise give the combination IM. The presedation allows that first big step of physical separation and loss of consciousness to be an easy step for the family to witness. Gently instruct family members to say their last goodbyes as they watch their beloved pet slowly falling into a relaxed sleep. Caregivers often comment that they sensed that their pet seemed very peaceful with the sedative. Let the family know that the heavy sedative provides powerful control against cancer pain (De Lorimier and Fan 2005).

Give the family privacy by leaving the room. Place a marker on the door so that staff will not mistakenly enter. Return in 5 or 10 minutes. At this time, ask if each person in the room wants to stay for the final injection. Some family members feel that they cannot be present for the "final" procedure. They are content to leave their beloved pet in the sedated state because they are uncomfortable with witnessing the death and they trust us. Many carers want to be present for the final injection and be holding their pet during the last breath. This is the time to assure the family that the next step will be the painless euthanasia injection, and that it will cause the heart to slow down until it stops beating.

The next step is to place a towel over the pet's body and cover the chest area up to the neck. Let carers stroke the pet's face and paws. At this time, it is best to explain that the final injection is an overdose of a barbiturate. It can be given into any vein, the heart (IC), any organ, or into the abdomen (IP). Depending on the route of delivery, the drug will cause the heart to stop beating fast if given IV or IC or slower if given into an organ and more slowly over 20 minutes or so, if given IP. We must advise attending family members that reflexes are powerful and that their pet may gasp or sigh even several minutes after death.

For IC injection, gently lift the towel for access to the chest. Listen for heartbeats with your stethoscope or palpate using your fingers, and give the euthanasia solution directly into the heart while directing the family to lovingly stroke their pet's head. Some house call doctors prefer to give the final injection IP or into a kidney or into the liver. The patient takes longer to pass but the passing is peaceful. Family members may want reassurance that their pet is truly gone. Offer them the use of your stethoscope to be rest assured that their old pet's heart has stopped beating.

Since we started using these procedures, we found that it eliminates pressure on our technical staff. The nursing staff does not have the stress, worry, and struggle of trying to place an IV catheter into a hypovolemic, dying patient. I believe that this technique reduces moral stress and compassion fatigue.

Most house call and hospice veterinarians have found this two-step method of sedation and euthanasia to be of great relief to them. No more tension and anxiety trying to place a catheter. A house call doctor is often the provider of Pawspice and hospice care services and develops a relationship with the expectation of being the one who will be performing the final home euthanasia visit. The chore of placing an IV catheter in the home environment can be overwhelming. One doctor told me horror stories of trying to get an IV catheter into a hypotensive cat. Another colleague told me about a disaster house call trying to put an IV catheter into an obese dehydrated nasty dog that urinated and defecated on the living room carpet. Afterward, she and her assistant had to carry the pet's body to her car for a cremation service pickup at her home office. All these unpleasant scenarios can be avoided using the two-step euthanasia protocol.

At the AVMA Human–Animal Bond Session in 2000, Bonnie McKinley, my long-time oncology nurse, co-presented a lecture with me on Pawspice (Villalobos 2000). We ended the lecture with this two-step method of letting pets go. General practice and house call doctors were relieved to learn that they could bypass the ritual of placing IV catheters into stressed, fearful, near-death pets. They welcomed our protocol of presedation and delivery of euthanasia by IV, IC, IR, IH, or IP injection according to preference. House call doctors can inform clients that they will leave large deceased pets in the home. This gives the family the opportunity to hold a wake for their deceased pet. Provide a list of private cremation services that will pick up the pet's body for specified cremation or burial.

Some of my clients will invite friends and family to come to the clinic for the euthanasia service. Some invite friends and family to their house to visit their pet to say their final goodbyes before the house call doctor arrives. I always encourage clients to hold a wake for a few hours either a day or two before the euthanasia or on the day of euthanasia to allow friends to say their goodbyes. See the section on holding a wake below.

Do Not Betray the Human–Animal Bond Before Euthanasia!

If euthanasia is to be performed at the hospital, the very last thing that we want to do is to take near-death geriatric pets away from their grief-stricken carers, even for one minute. Many institutions teach that the euthanasia solution must be given as an IV injection through an indwelling IV catheter. Often, the pet is taken out of the exam or comfort room and away from the family, into a treatment room where the IV catheter is placed into the patient's vein as the first preparatory step before euthanasia. This runs counter to the definition of a sensitive and caring enactment of euthanasia. Catheter placement can be traumatic for a dying, dehydrated, hypotensive geriatric oncology patient and the patient might struggle. Near-death pets may be in extreme discomfort. They may have pulmonary or abdominal effusions, dyspnea, dehydration, anemia, and/or cachexia. That struggle would be too difficult of a scene for the pet owner to witness.

Taking a pet that is about to be euthanatized away from their pack, the tearful family, dismisses and violates qualities of their special attachment (Voith 1985). I feel that placement of an indwelling catheter in a back room is done purely for the doctor's convenience and is disrespectful to the pet and the family. If we want to be the geriatric oncology patient's advocate, ideally, this scenario would never happen. If we honor the human–animal bond, separation of the geriatric cancer pet from family for catheter placement is avoided at all costs. Nurses get frustrated, even though the pet owner is not present. They feel that placing the euthanasia catheter is a behind-the-scenes unpleasant chore and a betrayal to the pet and to the client. Clearly, separating the pet from the family breaks the human–animal bond by disconnecting them at a critical moment before death. For all these reasons, contemporary bond-centered veterinarians should redesign their old standard euthanasia protocol. This will help their patients receive the highest quality death and their families receive much needed emotional support, as described in this chapter.

Think only about making the very last moments of life easiest for the patient and family. Use SQ or IM heavy sedation as step 1. While the sedation takes effect, allow private time for the pet to fall asleep comfortably on familiar bedding, surrounded by the loving faces and soothing voices of their family. Then give the final injection IV, IC, IP, IR, or IH. This ends the patient's life but it opens the need for thoughtful after-life services.

Suggest a Wake

There is not enough reverence, service, ceremony, or emotional support offered by our profession and society to grieving families on the occasion of a dear pet's death (Villalobos 2002; Corbin 2004). One very special way to validate and enrich the experience of a beloved pet's passing is to encourage the family to have a wake with flowers, candles, soft lighting, and poetry. Invite the family to hold a wake and stay for as long as they want to view, grieve, and reflect beside the body of their deceased pet (Figure 11.1). This is precious time! The special bond that connects clients to their veterinarian is severed when the patient dies. Clinicians, who make the euthanasia experience an enriched occasion, will not lose their veterinarian–client bond with the family. Instead, they will be showered with gratitude.

The wake is a special time for the pet's family and close friends to grieve and comfort one another. During the wake, I like to read poems, and talk about how important and sweet and special their beloved pet was. Suggest writing a poem or a story about who this pet was to the primary carer, their family and friends, and what made their relationship so special.

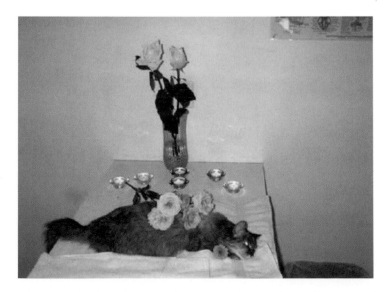

Figure 11.1.   Create reverence at the time of euthanasia by suggesting a wake with flowers, candles, and soft lights. Console the family and encourage them to stay for a while to view and reflect beside their deceased pet.

Offer the family a lock of fur. Gently clip the fur from a familiar site and place it in a windowed envelope with the date and the pet's name on it as a remembrance. This is also a good time to make a plaster imprint of the pet's paw as a memorial. Take pictures.

As part of the wake, you or one of your staff can sit on the floor next to the pet and read the special poem "Rainbow Bridge." If time permits, select a few short poems from *Angel Pawprints* (for dogs) or *Angel Whiskers* (for cats). These two books are wonderful anthologies of poetic reflections on loving and losing a canine or feline companion edited by Laurel E. Hunt (1998, 2001). My favorite reflection from *Angel Whiskers*, titled "The Last Will and Testament of Silverdene Emblem O'Neill," is written by Eugene O'Neill (Hunt 2001). It has thoughtful humor and helps one to think of forming new attachments in the near future. Give handouts and booklets that will help carers to weather the difficult days of pet loss that lie ahead of them and write a message to the family on the inside cover.

The grieving family should feel welcome to stay in the comfort room as long as they need to. Give them private time to cry and grieve alone with their deceased pet. Every 5 or 10 minutes, check in on the family and see if they need a cup of water, new tissues, or any other assistance.

After the wake is over, ask who is driving home and confirm that, in your judgment, the person is competent to drive. After such an emotional experience, it can be difficult to focus. If you have any doubts, recommend that the family sit for a while or take a walk outside the clinic for a few minutes to get fresh air and regain their composure before leaving in the car.

Encourage carers to create a little shrine for their pet at home, with pictures, their pet's favorite toys, collar, other keepsakes, and candles. I tell them to light a candle every night for the first couple of weeks and every time that they feel sad. I also let them know that every Monday night worldwide, people light a candle in honor of the human–animal bond that they shared with a belated pet at 7:00 p.m. PST.

When bidding farewell to the family, mention once again that you would like them to write a story or a few paragraphs about their dear pet to help in the grieving and closure processes. Ask them to email or send you a copy of this tribute to so that you can share it with your staff. Many carers post their pet's eulogy on Facebook or on the website of an animal charity to which they or their veterinarian made a donation in honor of the pet's memory.

Compassion and After-Life Services

When a geriatric cancer patient dies in the hospital or at home or is euthanatized under a veterinarian's medical care, the family may ask about after-life services. The family may expect the hospital staff to provide information and guidance about what to do and where to go. Veterinarians can improve and update procedures and protocols concerning how the hospital staff offers the bereaved family this sensitive information. The staff should conduct conversations of this nature in a private room – not at the front desk. They should offer condolences and hugs, and they should compassionately offer comfort and console the family during this emotional time.

Veterinarians play a complex role at death time. We wear many hats when a geriatric cancer patient is in the process of dying and after the pet has passed. Clients frequently ask, "How do you do it, Dr. Alice?" I say, "I know that I am helping you step over a very difficult puddle and I'm holding your hand. It is my honor to help you say goodbye to Bella. I can help you go through the cycle of life, which is also accepting death with natural grief and love. In time, your feelings of grief and sadness will evolve into gratitude and joy that you were blessed with Bella."

Veterinarians wear many hats! We provide the services of the attending doctor, the grief counselor, and the funeral director. Physicians in human medicine routinely disconnect with the family upon the death of a patient. They may not ever see that family again. A human body is quickly transferred to a cremation service or funeral home. Funeral home personnel are trained to help with arrangements and prepare the deceased for either cremation or burial. After a person dies, the family spends a great deal of time at the funeral home making the arrangements, picking out memory cards and poems and writing an obituary for their loved one, deciding what clothes to bring back for the service, and many other related activities. There are wakes and rosaries and church services and the funeral, burial, or interring of cremains at a mausoleum. These activities help with closure, but pet caregivers have very little ritual to help them deal with their profound loss. Society seldom understands the depth of the human–animal bond at death.

We accept that there is a need to grieve the loss of a companion animal but provide no formal outlet service. Regardless of the circumstances surrounding a pet's death, the carers are always in a time of need. Any support offered by the veterinarian at this sad time deepens the doctor–client relationship. The attending veterinarian, if willing, can become the provider of supportive care for the client's emotional crisis. Do not recoil from this responsibility; do not neglect to offer solace.

A well-trained, compassionate staff will also play an important role in consoling bereft carers. Staff can comfort grieving clients by offering hugs and consolation and providing information for pet loss counselors who offer professional emotional support. It takes caring, planning, teamwork, and coordination to enrich the euthanasia experience to be as pleasant and sensitive as possible for the geriatric oncology patient's family. Half of clients who elect euthanasia question themselves after the pet has died and feel extreme guilt (Adams and Shaw 2006). "Humane euthanasia is a time when you can do more for the family than at any other time in the pet's life. That is why veterinarians must sensitively respect the bond that exists between animals and their caregivers" (Adams 2005).

Dealing with the Pet's Body for High-Need Clients

When a geriatric cancer pet dies, the human–animal bond remains precious to the caregivers and it is often carried over and symbolized by loyalty and respect for the pet's body. The family is generally unprepared for handling a deceased pet's body. They depend on their attending veterinarian's kindness for counseling and recommendations to pet cremation services or cemeteries. Some clients elect the traditional in-house group "disposal" service if they cannot afford or do not want specialized private arrangements. Most clients will be grateful for information about their options. NEVER use the word "Dispose" or "Disposal"! It is part of everyday practice for the attending veterinarian's staff to gently and compassionately advise and make arrangements. NEVER use the word "Disposal." Ask, "What arrangements would you like us to make for your deceased pet?"

The human–animal bond may have been very intense due to the pet's special training. The pet may have been a service dog, a show dog, or an unconditional loving companion to a "high-need" person or a person who lives alone and has no other pets. The sense of loss can be overwhelming for some pet caregivers. They may feel emotionally drained, vulnerable, and unable to make any after-life decisions without your help.

The family may expect that your hospital will cremate their pet's body. They may not know that options for private cremation, aquamation, or private burial are available. They may ask you what they should do. Instead of saying what they should do, you might share with them what you have chosen to do. I tell clients who ask, "My pets are all cremated. Their ashes are in containers behind an angel statue on top of a cabinet at my house. It is in my will that their ashes go with me, wherever I go, up or down, whenever the time comes."

I served as a board member for the Los Angeles Pet Memorial Park for a decade. The park itself is beautiful, with lovely memorial benches under large trees for people to sit and look at hundreds of headstones. The park offers viewing services, private cremation services on site, burial services, and a pet mausoleum for those who cannot afford a full burial due to land fees. There is a little Rainbow Bridge section on the grounds. This park is a wonderful place for people to visit before and after their pet has passed. Members get a newsletter and a yearly invitation to a fundraiser at the park and some stay connected this way. Pet owners have an open invitation to visit their pet's gravesite 7 days a week. The staff at the park is very sympathetic to bereaved pet owners.

Only a small percentage of pet owners request burial and a memorial headstone in remembrance of their beloved pet. Some carers take their deceased pets home for private burial on personal property. Most veterinary clients choose to have cremation for their deceased pets on an individual basis. As aquamation becomes more available, this will be an additional option. They want their pet's body handled with respect and the cremains to be returned to them. This service generally goes through the hospital's chosen cremation service providers. Most pet owners accept their veterinary hospital's contracted cremation service provider. The deceased pets are picked up and the cremains returned to the clinic for the family to pick up.

I try to be present when a beloved pet's cremains are given to the carers because that is an emotional moment. We give hugs and take a few minutes to see how they are coping with pet loss. Make it a policy to greet the family privately when they come to pick up their pet's cremains from your hospital. This is an opportunity to give the grieving carers a hug and see how they are getting along. Take this second chance moment to encourage carers to write about their pet and send an e-mail tribute to friends and family and to copy you in if they have not already done so. These after-life encounters may be fading away from veterinary practice. There is a growing new service that will pick up deceased pets and hold them for a few days until they can deliver several to a cremation facility. Afterward, they return the cremains to the family with a kind visit mixed with pet loss counseling and sympathy. Some house call veterinarians take the pet's body for cremation and will follow up to return the cremains. Others refer to one of these compassionate pickup and delivery service providers or to a contracted cremation facility that will pick up the body, especially for large and giant breed dogs. The entire branch of after-life pet care services has expanded tremendously in the last 2 decades.

When your hospital refers clients to facilities for cremation or burial, those facilities become an extension of your hospital. Evaluate any facility that you recommend to clients for after-life services. Make sure that they are professional, thoughtful, and respectful. Distressed clients are amenable to trusting their doctor's choice for a good and reputable cremation or burial service for their pet's body once they make the decision.

Cecilia's Case (Respect the Client's Spiritual Belief System)

One more important aspect about Cecilia, our Golden Retriever with hemangiosarcoma, involved her after-life care. Julie Corbin wrote this email to me:

Dr. V,

I am glad that you agree about post-euthanasia/follow-up care. I never gave that a second thought until now and how that is such a powerful bridge to one's grieving process. Another issue is the handling of the body.

While the life force may have left the body, should we not honor the body with dignity and respect – especially if that is part of one's spiritual belief system? We would never just throw a human body on the ground of some cold warehouse wrapped in a garbage bag (yes, that is where I found Cecilia's body, 100 miles away from the clinic, and I know this is common practice). Why do we not extend the same dignity and respect for the body of our companion animals that we do humans?

… Seeing Cecilia's body stuffed in a trash bag laying on the ground like a heaping pile of garbage with the "Pet Memorial" staff just staring at me with these blank looks was more than I could take. Ever hear of a gurney or a table to transport her into my car or something a bit more dignified? My girl was better than that, and I am glad that I heard her call for me to pick up her body and take it to a place that would treat it with dignity and respect. It was quite odd how all that happened. … Through this experience, I see so many areas that need to be addressed if we are to truly honor the human–animal bond. I know my thoughts and ideas may not be readily embraced by all veterinarians but those are the ones that need to hear it the most!

Thanks for your encouragement. J.

Also, suggest a memorial service. Carers may find that holding a memorial service for their pet provides great emotional support. In the matter of a wake, invite friends and family to gather together in honor of the deceased pet. The carer may want to prepare a eulogy to present during the service. The following eulogy, written for 14-year-old Bullet by his carer, Laurie Kaplan, might help your clients in writing their own eulogy. Bullet survived more than four years with lymphoma and two years with dilated cardiomyopathy before passing from renal failure. Kaplan is also the author of the book, *Help Your Dog Fight Cancer*, which she wrote to help others with cancer dogs through the journey (Kaplan 2008; Kaplan and Villalobos 2016). Kaplan also wrote *So Easy to Love, So Hard to Lose*, which is a workbook that helps carers step by step through the grieving process (Kaplan 2010).

Bullet's Eulogy (by Laurie Kaplan)

"Thank you all for coming today to share some memories of Bullet, to help me celebrate his life and to say a loving farewell.

Bullet and I walked these trails thousands of times in the 12 years, 2 months, and 1 day that he was with me. I calculated that we crossed these very stepping stones more than 2,000 times. I can almost see him now, prancing regally, wearing that wonderful husky smile and lifting each paw high with every step … moving from stone to stone with the pure, natural grace that can be seen only in a wild creature completely unaware of and unimpressed by his own beauty.

Rarely did anyone pass by us without stopping to admire Bullet. But he also had a great inner strength, a strength and temerity that enabled him to survive lymphoma. That same indomitable spirit enabled him to survive a heart disease expected to kill him within 6 months. That was 2 years ago.

But there's one thing that Bullet was NOT – he was not an easy dog. (I have a funny feeling we might hear a story or two today reflecting that.) But to me, his willfulness, his wildness and his "growliness" were all just part of his charm.

Bullet stole my heart in a split second in September 1992 and Bullet will always have my heart. He is my heartdog, the love of my life and the dog of my dreams. Thank you all for coming today. Thank you for listening. It means a great deal to me that Bullet's favorite people – and mine –are here to share this moment. Now Ru is going to say a prayer and then whoever wishes to will share a special memory about Bullet."

Invite your clients to come back into the human–animal bond and embrace the cycle of life with a fresh set of paw prints by their side. "Doctor's advice" for bereaved caregivers should be, "Don't remain '*petless*' for long. Stay in touch by stopping by to visit us, and bring us cookies."

Home Euthanasia and Hospice: A Movement in Response to a Need

Annie Forslund, DVM

Pet owners yearn for personal touch and intimacy with the professionals who step in to help them in their pet's End of Life (EoL) care. A pet's imminent EoL can be one of the most emotionally impacting events of a person's life. Many pet owners state emphatically that the loss of their pet was harder than the loss of a parent. With the advent of corporate and multiple-doctor practices, the old "James Herriot" model is dying out. The need for a return to this model is most desperately felt in the EoL phase, when pet owners are in desperate need of guidance through the surge of emotions and the ups and downs that the good days and bad days bring about. EoL is a unique and often demanding phase of life where veterinary care involves much more than just caring for the physical body of the pet. In the EoL phase, a veterinarian who is grounded in the Pawspice philosophy, in addition to being a competent professional, is also able to counsel the family through the many vicissitudes they encounter caring for their pet during the final decline.

Pet owners often feel lost and are afraid that they may make the wrong decision. In the prime of life of a pet, when illness hits, the "right decision" is often cut and dry, but in the EoL phase, there may be a fine line of fear and doubt with decision making. A decision for definitive diagnostics and standard treatment can be just as wrong for a geriatric pet as a decision against it because there is no right or wrong answer. The decision must be reasonable for the patient and acceptable to all family members involved. A skilled EoL and Home Euthanasia (HE) veterinarian can help the pet's family navigate through the difficult decision-making process. They can counsel the family on what the best choices are for their pet, considering not only the pet's medical condition and personality but also the family's situation in regards to finances, time, lifestyle, religious and spiritual beliefs, emotional condition, physical condition, mental condition, the presence of children, other pets, logistics, and so forth.

An EoL Pawspice veterinarian has developed skills that are not taught in veterinary school. I attended several lectures on the human hospice model. I was enthralled to learn about the resources that are available to the hospice doctor. The human hospice patient benefits from a multitude of resources: the primary physician, oncologist, cardiologist and other specialists, the physiotherapist, an array of nurses, PAs, ministers, chaplains, and the psychiatrist. In the veterinary field, the services and benefits provided by these ten specialties are generally provided by one person: the attending veterinarian, who is caring for the EoL pet and their family members. No matter how much we dream that one day we will be able to apply a similar model to veterinary medicine, it would never be financially feasible.

When I first started my HE practice, it was practically unheard of to have a service solely dedicated to HE. Most mobile veterinarians perform HE by default. It is not their vocation, but because they perform home visits, they are called upon to euthanize pets at home for their established clients. Many general practice mobile veterinarians decline to perform this service for families with whom they do not have an established relationship. Because there is such a need for this service, they feel like their practice will become a morbid drudge of one euthanasia after another rather than the upbeat mobile practice they had initially envisioned.

When I started my practice in February 2009, other HE practices started all over the country and some practices have expanded with franchise management such as lapoflove.com, which is nationwide. Most HE practitioners found themselves also tending to pet hospice as part of their practice, in response to a need. In a dedicated HE practice, the veterinarian sometimes makes a house call only to find that the pet and/or their family are "not quite ready." They might find that QoL issues can be improved for some time using supportive approaches such as improved pain management, wound care, nutrition counseling, environmental modifications, home care education, etc. Therefore, HE veterinarians found themselves embracing pet hospice or, as Dr. Villalobos brilliantly coined it in 1999, "Pawspice."

Practices solely dedicated to HE and hospice have now been established around the US and across the world. Dr. Villalobos heralded the movement with her writings, lectures, and seminars. She introduced the Pawspice concept in 2000 at the AVMA Convention. She gave our profession the philosophy and format for pet hospice with the First Edition of this textbook in 2007. Prior to 2000, pet hospice was practically unheard of except for the services offered at Dr. Villalobos's practices. Veterinarians have always been involved with house call practices, and cared for dying pets, and they dutifully provided euthanasia at home as part of a more diversified general mobile practice. Veterinarians very rarely had a dedicated EoL Pawspice practice. It has been over 20 years since Dr. Villalobos started promoting improved expertise in EoL care, but in the last decade there has been a definite growth of the home care hospice movement to better serve society's companion animals at EoL.

In March of 2008, the First International Symposium on Pet Hospice was held at UC Davis, which revealed the need for veterinary leadership in the animal hospice field. In 2010, the International Association of Animal Hospice and Palliative Care (IAAHPC) was founded by Dr. Amir Shanan, an attendee of the 2008 meeting. The first IAAHPC Conference was held in 2011 with 35 attendees. The following year, 150 attended and, since then, the attendance has grown by about 15% per year. The 2016 Conference had an attendance of 225 and the association's membership stands at about 400. Other hospice-related associations are also in existence and their number and importance across the world will undoubtedly continue to grow.

While academic attention to specialized education in hospice remains low, increasingly more universities are offering pet hospice classes such as: UC Davis, Colorado State University, Cornell University, University of Florida, Missouri State University, Ohio State University, Tufts, and more will follow. In 2016, the American Animal Hospital Association, in conjunction with the IAAHPC, officially published End-of-Life Care Guidelines in the organization's November/December journal, *JAAHA* (Bishop et al. 2016). Veterinary Information Network (VIN) launched the Hospice and Palliative Care folder in October 2015. The IAAHPC has developed a certification program timeline that is offered in modules for Veterinary Hospice and Palliative Care (www.iaahpc.org/certification.html).

During the End of Life phase of a beloved geriatric cancer patient's life, many pet owners prefer to avoid an aggressive treatment approach. They feel as if they need to protect their pet from treatment-related adverse events. Some families want to avoid spending money on expensive diagnostics and definitive standard cancer treatments, especially if their pet is old and frail. They are reluctant to elect a pathway of prolonging their pet's life if there will be suffering. What these owners want is for their geriatric pet to live out their old age peacefully and comfortably, without pain, until they are "ready." The HHHHHMM (H5M2) Quality of Life Scale that Dr. Villalobos published has been a mainstay decision-making tool in my practice brochure for helping families know when to make the final call for help with euthanasia at home. Dr. Villalobos is regarded as the mother of veterinary hospice and the queen of QoL for her pioneering work and contributions in creating the new field of veterinary hospice.

When the primary veterinarian makes the diagnosis of cancer, or uses words such as: geriatric, organ failure, suffering, advanced arthritis, etc., the client may feel that the red flags are raised over their pet. Combined with fear and anticipatory grief, the red flag diagnosis and words may get processed as "no hope and no more vet visits." If the family hears "there is nothing more we can do" from their veterinarian, it confirms what they may already feel or know. They may not have been referred to an oncologist or encouraged to seek a second opinion. The ailing pet may be brought back home to decline without help, even though, unbeknownst to the family, there is always something more that can be done to comfort the dying pet using the palliative Pawspice philosophy. The ground-breaking End of Life Care Guidelines recommends that primary care practices should establish a dedicated team to implement palliative and hospice care for EoL patients or refer them to a hospice care provider. The only time when nothing more can be done is after death. This is what pet hospice provides: it bridges the gap between "no hope" by providing professional help during the months, days, and hours before a beloved pet passes away and/or helps transition the pet from life by providing the gift of a peaceful euthanasia.

Note: I have known Dr. Annie Forslund since before she started her HE practice in Orange County in 2009. She has devoted her career to helping companion animals at EoL and working with the IAAHPC. Her very insightful web site has sections on pain detection, QOL assessment, and decision making. Pet owners can learn important details at EoL: www.homepeteuthanasia.com. *(AV)*

Compassion Fatigue and Ethics Fatigue

Our profession is keenly aware that veterinarians may experience feelings related to burnout. It comes from stressors and pressures encountered in veterinary life with euthanasia, medicoethical decision making, student debt, staff and employment issues, social media, in addition to personal life issues, and so forth. Euthanasia is sad and sadly it triggers undue stress on some veterinarians who feel morally stressed with it.

Practicing oncology plays tug-of-war with our emotions, values, and dictates of conscience. One minute we are struggling with medicoethical decisions to save a pet's life and the next minute we are asked to euthanize that same pet. One minute, we are responsible for the medical care and management of the patient and the next minute we are acting as the executioner and the mortician. The loss is felt by the nursing staff, receptionists, and everyone else involved in the case. It is especially hard to lose our long-term geriatric oncology patients and their loving caregivers. It is easy to get attached to clients and pets in geriatric cancer care.

The veterinarian must jump back and forth from one exam room obligation to the next. In general practice, one exam room may be filled with grief while the next exam room client has a new pup or kitten. These extremes in professional task performance represent the rich dichotomy in our practice lives. Every chance we get to hold puppies and kittens allows us to bear witness to new beginnings. Every time we are there to help a client celebrate the adoption of a homeless pet, it brings us back from an ending to a new beginning. Sometimes, I bring grieving clients into the homeless ward at our clinic and place a kitten or a puppy in their arms to cheer them up. If a grieving client is clearly not ready to take a new pet into his or her heart, suggest that the client foster a pet from the local shelter or join a volunteer club or an animal shelter to help socialize kittens and care for homeless animals. Our oncology team finds that feeding kittens in the homeless ward gives us cheer when our losses are piling up. Be sure to find time to eat lunch together and develop pleasurable outlets for your staff during the tough times, to avoid compassion fatigue.

Compassion means: "Suffer together, deep sympathy." Unfortunately, the dictionary includes the word "pity" as a synonym for compassion. Fatigue: "Exhaustion or weariness, to tire out." Weariness: "Worn out, without patience or zeal." Exhaust: "To use up, to empty completely to drain." The phenomenon of compassion fatigue is complex. Overall the syndrome refers to the negative effects on people in the helping professions who are working in a job that requires compassion. Burnout applies to job frustration or weariness, apathy, and depersonalization.

The moral and emotional stress surrounding euthanasia can be enormous. In fact, this stress was found to be the single largest source of job dissatisfaction for companion animal veterinarians (Rollin 2003). Most veterinarians experience some of these feelings and emotions daily. I want to change how veterinarians view euthanasia. Instead of feeling bad about it, we can rethink and feel ***honored*** to be the one that peacefully escorts beloved pets over the Rainbow Bridge. This attitude change can lighten the negative emotional load of euthanasia that triggers stress. As you will read in Dr. Kimberly Pope-Robinson's wellness care section, thinking differently can be a balloon that lifts the heavy sinkers off your shoulders.

In his book, *Compassion: Our Last Great Hope* (1996), the late Dr. Leo Bustad tells us what compassion is not. "It is not pity, which is feeling sorry for someone. With pity, there is condescension and separateness; one does not celebrate with a person one pities. Compassion is suffering with, having empathy with, or feeling for. It includes joy as well as grief. It is the feeling of togetherness. … Compassion is not only feeling or sentiment, but also actively helping to relieve pain and suffering in others."

Compassion fatigue is internal emotional depletion. It is different from burnout, which comes from organizational bureaucracy or policies and procedures. Compassion fatigue comes from caring and feeling responsible for patients and sharing the burdens and sorrows of their caregivers without relief.

Ethics fatigue is an underrecognized issue in veterinary medicine. Some of us are bottomless pits of compassion, and we will never run out. However, if we feel bad, it may get labeled as compassion fatigue, when it just is not so. This can make us feel even more frustrated. Around 5 years ago, I pinpointed my concept of ethics fatigue on Dr. Dani McVety, cofounder of lapoflove.com. I asked her if she had compassion fatigue and she said, "No." Then she told me that she felt drained from making so many ethical decisions in emergency work. That is when I pointed out that she was suffering from ethics fatigue. Dr. McVety wrote eloquently about ethics fatigue in DVM360.com on January 17, 2017. "My fatigue stemmed from making ethical decisions within the boundaries of someone else's (often) illogical values or unreasonable budget" (McVety 2017)

Veterinarians and their teams deal with morally stressful medicoethical decisions every day, depending on their line of work. Shelter veterinarians face the tragedy of euthanizing unwanted animals. Emergency veterinarians face the fluctuations of pet owner issues that span from neglect of the human–animal bond all the way to heart-wrenching scenarios. Oncologists, cardiologists, neurologists, and most specialists often deal with medicoethical dilemmas of end stage disease and pressure from clients that may strain and fatigue their moral principles.

The physical and mental symptoms of compassion fatigue and/or ethics fatigue are varied. They are similar to the feelings of regular burnout: GI symptoms, headaches, sweating, blurred vision, along with mental indifference, frustration, anxiety, negative thinking, and depression, to name a few. If you experience these physical or mental symptoms, be sure to recognize that it is natural and understandable. Give yourself a break, change your routine, be kind to yourself, and exercise. Pamper yourself and get your cognitive spirit reenergized. Hug some kittens and puppies. Do not allow your internal emotional resources to become depleted. Never quit caring about each and every human–animal bond that you encounter and the unique people who entrust you with their companion animals. Our highly attached clients need and expect us to keep caring (Mitchener 2005).

Compassion versus Cure without Care

Dr. Leo Bustad, the father of the term "Human–Animal Bond," quoted the spiritual theologian, Matthew Fox, who wrote extensively about compassion. "Compassion is the world's richest energy source and compassion is our last great hope." I personally feel that veterinarians are among the best people and most compassionate healers on the planet. We are the energy source for great compassion and for honoring the human–animal bond. When people ask how you can go on, tell them your spirit is like a candle, no less bright for lighting another candle.

Bustad lamented the exile of compassion from medicine and the mechanization of medicine and the hazards of "cure without care." I call it the "mindless machinery of medicine." Bustad wrote, "Cure without care makes us preoccupied with quick fixes and makes us impatient, and also unwilling to share one another's burdens, unable to experience compassion. Care is more important than cure. In fact, cure without care may be, in the long run, more harmful than helpful." Bustad wrote that compassionate people have a keener awareness of the interdependence of all living things: "We feel a kinship with animals and are stewards of the earth and all within it."

Posteuthanasia Follow-Up

When a long-term geriatric cancer patient dies, a little part of your practice goes with them. Your staff will miss seeing the pet and the family. Send one or two sympathy cards with staff notes and signatures. Ask the pet owner to visit and bring pictures of their deceased pet. Put the owner's e-mail address on your hospital list of dog or cat lovers so you can contact them with pet-related issues, news, and pictures. Let clients know that you believe that they should remain within the human–animal bond because it will benefit and enrich their lives and encourage them to get back into the love cycle again by adopting a homeless pet. Let them know that you would be honored if they considered adopting one of your hospital's rescue pets. Ask them to call when they feel the time is right for them to adopt. We say, "It would be hard to imagine you walking around this planet without a set of paw prints at your side." Offer a genuine invitation for your pet-loss clients to come back and visit the hospital at their old appointment times or during lunchtime with cookies and pictures.

Give the family a phone call anywhere from one day to several weeks after their pet has passed to ask how things are going. This is often the toughest call to make because now we are not talking medicine or a protocol. You can start by asking a question, "How are your heart and soul doing? I know you must be missing Bullet very much. These days of pet loss are difficult and we all want you to know that we are thinking of you." Talking about a deceased pet often helps the grieving family. If the carer is having trouble processing grief or if you suspect maladaptive grief, offer emotional support, and a referral to a pet-loss counselor. Other great sources for help and comfort are the pet-loss hotlines and the www.aplb.org, which offers chat rooms every day conducted by people trained to handle pet-loss issues.

A very helpful piece of advice that you can offer grieving carers is to set aside special times for tears and feelings of grief. Instruct clients to limit their sad feelings, perhaps to 30 minutes a day, preferably in the morning or the evening. This encourages carers to continue working through the grieving process while helping them face their workaday world with more clarity. If the client needs pet-loss counseling, make sure to initiate a pet-loss counseling referral or have them contact a pet-loss hotline.

The family may also draw closure by conducting a memorial service or donating to animal charities (Butler et al. 1991). If clients ask for your direction, you can suggest that they donate to your alma mater's cancer center, the Veterinary Cancer Society, the Morris Animal Foundation, Animal Cancer Foundation, AVMF, the Magic Bullet Fund, or the Veterinary Cancer Foundation. These last two raise funds to help pay for cancer treatments for privately owned dogs. Suggest other innovative ways that will help your clients and their children (ages 0–6, 6–14, and 14–21) honor their deceased pets with art, jewelry, poetry, books, ceremonies, and so forth (McVety 2016). Tell clients that you and your staff miss them and then encourage them to make the full cycle back into the wonderful world of the human–animal bond with another loveable pet and to come and visit you (with cookies) as soon as they feel up to it.

Sending an After-Life Gift

Sending flowers, a potted plant, a bronze paw print, or a memory gift to a favorite charity honors the human–animal bond that the family shared with their pet. A gift symbolizes that you care about the family's emotional pain and loss (Butler et al. 1991). As an after-life gift, we sent the grieving family a six-inch bronze memorial paw print with an engraved plaque that reads, "In Loving Memory of Bella." We call our engraver with the pet's name and they send the plaque to our office. We attached the plaque on to the base of the bronze paw print and ship it a few days after the sympathy card.

When the family receives the gift, their emotions may be settling down but their hearts are still heavy. We receive very touching letters of gratitude. Carers truly appreciate these remembrances that honor the human–animal bond, which they allowed us the privilege of sharing during EoL Pawspice care for their beloved geriatric pet.

Sir Walter Scott on the Human–Animal Bond

There is a quote by Sir Walter Scott that helps caregivers when they are dealing with pet loss. The quote is featured in *Angel Pawprints*, by Laurel Hunt (1998). With one changed word (dog to pet), his words can be expanded to include cats and other species of pets.

> I have sometimes thought of the final cause of dogs [pets] having such short lives, and I am quite satisfied it is in compassion to the human race; for if we suffer so much in loving a dog [pet] after an acquaintance of ten or twelve years, what would it be if they were to live double that time?
>
> *Sir Walter Scott*

References

Adams, C. 2005. Personal Communication. Rothesay, New Brunswick, Canada.
Adams, C., and J.R. Shaw (eds). 2006. *Console pet loss support system clinic training guide*, pp. 3–24. Bogart, GA: Bioniche Animal Health USA, Inc.

Balducci, L., G.H. Lyman, W.B. Ershler, and M. Extermann. 2004. "Prognostic evaluation of the older cancer patient." In *Comprehensive geriatric oncology*, 2nd edn, eds L. Balducci, G.H. Lyman, W.B. Ershler, and M. Extermann, pp. 309–319. Oxon, UK: Taylor & Francis.

Bateman, S. 2016. Addressing diverse beliefs with courageous conversations: A courageous conversation about euthanasia, *VetTeam Brief*, Vol. 4, Issue 10.

Bishop, G., K. Cooney, S. Cox, et al. 2016. 2016 AAHA/IAAHPC End-of-Life Care Guidelines. *Journal of the American Animal Hospital Association* 52 (6):341–356 (https://doi.org/10.5326/JAAHA-MS-6637).

Bustad, L.K. 1996. *Compassion: Our last great hope – Selected speeches of Leo K. Bustad, DVM, PhD*, 2nd edn. Renton, WA: Delta Society.

Butler, C.L., M.S. Lagoni, K.L. Dickinson, and S.J. Withrow. 1991. "Cancer." In *Animal illness and human emotion: Problems in veterinary medicine*, eds S.P. Cohen and C.E. Fudin, Vol. 3, No. 1, pp. 21–38. Philadelphia, PA: Lippincott.

Cohen, S.P., and D.C. Sawyer. 1991. "Suffering and euthanasia." In *Animal illness and human emotion: Problems in veterinary medicine*, eds S.P. Cohen and C.E. Fudin, Vol. 3, No. 1, pp. 101–109. Philadelphia, PA: Lippincott.

Corbin, J. 2004. Personal Communication as an external reader. Dissertation Proposal, "A depth psychological analysis of the Human–Canine Bond and its implications to the grief response: A phenomenological study." Pacifica Graduate Institute, Carpenteria, CA, December.

De Lorimier, L.P., and T.M. Fan. 2005. Understanding and recognizing cancer pain in dogs and cats, treating cancer pain in dogs and cats. *Veterinary Medicine*, May, pp. 352–377.

Feldman, B.R. 2004. On dying a "natural" death. Clinical Ethics, Veterinary Forum, June, pp. 41–45.

Hunt, L.E. 1998. *Angel pawprints: Reflections on loving and losing a canine companion*. Pasadena, CA: Darrowby Press.

Hunt, L.E. 2001. *Angel whiskers: Reflections on loving and losing a feline companion*. New York: Hyperion Press.

Kaplan, L. 2008. *Help your dog fight cancer: What every caretaker should know about canine cancer*. Briarcliff Manor, NY: JanGen Press.

Kaplan, L. 2010, *So easy to love, so hard to lose; A bridge to healing before and after the loss of a pet*. Briarcliff Manor, NY: JanGen Press.

Kaplan, L., and A. Villalobos. 2016. *Help your dog fight cancer: Empowerment for dog owners*. Briarcliff Manor, NY: JanGen Press.

McVety, D. 2016. Top 5 ways to honor deceased pets. *VetTeam Brief*, Vol.4, Issue 10, pp. 22–27.

McVety, D. 2017. The myth of compassion fatigue in veterinary medicine, DVM360MAGAZINE.com.

Mitchener, K.L. 2005. Oncology professionals at risk: Compassion fatigue. *Veterinary Practice News*, March, pp. 28–29.

Ogilvie, G.K., and A.S. Moore. 1995. "Oncologic emergencies, section III." In *Managing the veterinary cancer patient*, eds G. Ogilvie and A. Moore, pp. 149–189. Trenton, NJ: Veterinary Learning Systems.

Rollin, B.E., as quoted by Verdon, D.R. and J. Fleisher. 2003. *DVM Magazine*, p. 34.

Rollin, B.E. 2006. Euthanasia and quality of life. Commentary, *JAVMA* 228 (7):1014–1016.

Villalobos, A.E. 2000. Conceptualized end of life care: "Pawspice" program for pets. *AVMA Proceedings*, pp. 322–327.

Villalobos, A.E. 2002. Cancer pain: Understated shouldn't mean underestimated. *Oncology Outlook, VPN*, July.

Villalobos, A. 2014. "Are veterinarians kinder than physicians at end of life?" In *International Journal of Ethics*, Vol. 9, No. 4, pp. 223–235. Nova Science Publishers, Inc. ISSN: 1535-4776.

Voith, V.L. 1985. "Attachment of people to companion animals." In *Symposium on the Human–Companion Animal Bond*, Veterinary Clinics of North America, pp. 289–296. Philadelphia, PA: Saunders.

Yaxley, P., and J. Pierce. 2016. Hospice care and palliative sedation. *Veterinary Team Brief*, Vol. 4, Issue 10, pp. 35–40.

Suggested Reading

Downing, R. 2000. *Pets living with cancer: A pet owner's resource*. Lakewood, CO: AAHA Press.

Gawande, A. 2014. *Being mortal: Medicine and what matters in the end*. New York: Metropolitan Books, Henry Holt and Company.

Lagoni, L., D. Morehead, and C. Butler. 1999. The bond-centered practice: The future of veterinary care. *Proceedings of the 1999 ACVIM Forum in Chicago*.

Ogilvie, G.K. 1999. Hospice and bond centered practice: The future of veterinary care. *Proceedings of the 1999 ACVIM Forum in Chicago*.

Villalobos, A.E. 1999. Pet hospice nurses the bond. Oncology Outlook, *VPN*, September.

Villalobos, A.E. 2001. Comprehensive pain management vital to oncology patients. Oncology Outlook, *VPN*, July.

Villalobos, A.E. 2003. Cancer causes cachexia, an insidious weight loss. *VPN*, December.

Villalobos, A.E. 2004. Quality of life scale helps make final call. Oncology Outlook, *VPN*, September, p. 38.

Withrow, S.J., and E.G. MacEwen. 2001. *Small animal clinical oncology*, 3rd edn. Philadelphia, PA: Saunders.

Chapter 12

The Veterinary Professional/Client Relationship: Supporting Your Clients – Supporting Yourselves

Sandra Grossman, PhD and Ellie Freedman, MFT

> There's more to being an expert vet than just offering professional medical advice. The most successful vets are those who care for the pet and for the family.

Anonymous from EOL Survey

Pet Loss Partners is a group practice comprised of certified Pet Loss counselors and certified Compassion Fatigue educators. Pet Loss Partners members have the unique perspective of seeing both sides of the veterinary care experience (www.petlosspartners.com).

In 2015 Pet Loss Partners conducted an online End of Life Care/Pet Loss Study©. The objective of the study was to find ways to bridge the communication gap that often exists between veterinary team and client. The study was copyrighted on March 15, 2015 and results provide information that will help clinicians create an environment in which both clients and veterinary professionals feel understood and appreciated. The results reveal how you and your practice might better deal with and support grieving clients, and how veterinary professionals can use self-care strategies to manage and combat Compassion Fatigue.

According to the study result, grieving pet parents do not share their feelings about their pet's end of life experience with their veterinary teams. This information is very valuable to veterinary professionals. It may teach veterinarians to provide better care to their patients and to their clients, and ultimately may help veterinary professionals care better for themselves.

Compassion, understanding and good communication with pet owners are all important pieces in managing some of the challenges and stressors you face when dealing with pet parents under very difficult and stressful circumstances.

> "I can't say how grateful I am to this vet. He did all he could for both me and my dog and he always kept me in the loop. He was amazing and is my forever vet."

> "The vet I used at the time was a cold fish. I never went back to this practice after my pet passed away."

A successful Veterinary Practice is one that takes into account the needs of its patients, clients, and staff. The relationship between all three entities is at the heart of a thriving practice.

Canine and Feline Geriatric Oncology: Honoring the Human–Animal Bond, Second Edition. Alice Villalobos with Laurie Kaplan.
© 2018 John Wiley & Sons, Inc. Published 2018 by John Wiley & Sons, Inc.

Creating a Compassionate Practice for both Clients and Veterinary Professionals is a copyrighted book and workshop belonging to Dr. Grossman.

Background of the End of Life Care/Pet Loss Study

At the outset, it was extremely important to us that the information in the study be relevant to what clients experienced. We decided to get input from our clients and other pet parents who had lost a beloved pet in order to create the topics and questions in our study. All the questions and sections were developed from our conversations with them about what they felt they expected and needed during this time and what their actual end of life care experience was like.

The study was conducted online. The only requirement for completion was that respondents were at least 18 years of age and had lost a pet. The study was promoted through Social Media outlets including Facebook, LinkedIn, and Yahoo groups. It was posted on web sites such as www.petloss partners.com and www.pet-loss.net. We also asked members of The Association for Pet Loss and Bereavement (www.aplb.org) to complete the survey.

In 3 months, 461 respondents completed the survey representing 45 states and 9 different countries. The survey was taken by pet parents who had visited all different types of practices (primary, specialty, emergency hospitals) as well as in-home veterinarians. In order to get a complete picture of the end of life care experience, we included questions about the client's expectations, ratings of the different types of practices, their satisfaction and retention, and their experience during their pet's euthanasia, pet loss, and follow-up. A combination of quantitative and qualitative questions was used.

Supporting Your Clients Through the End of Life Care Experience

"Our vet did her best to be sure I understood the disease, the effect on my dog, and how to know when it was time to put her down"

"My doctor was knowledgeable and compassionate when diagnosing my pet with a brain tumor. She talked to me honestly about what to expect with this diagnosis."

According to this study, the vast majority of pet parents understand that your primary role is to provide the best medical care possible for their beloved pets. They acknowledge and appreciate what their veterinary teams have done for their pets and for themselves. They also understand that their vet is not trained as a mental health counselor.

That said, the relationship between pet parents and their pets is a complex one, with the pet being considered a "family member" more than ever before. It is beneficial for all parties when a veterinary team acknowledges the relationship between their patients and clients, considers them as a family unit, and applies that awareness to the implementation of a treatment plan.

Clients look to their veterinary team to provide medical care for their pets, but more is needed. The compassion provided by the veterinary team is a key driver in the end of life care experience. In fact, 76% of pet parents agreed strongly that the compassionate care they and their beloved pets received was *just as important* as the veterinarian's knowledge and ability to treat their pet's disease or condition.

There are three distinct benefits of a veterinary team understanding this. First, it provides insight and understanding into why pet parents react as they do. Second, it provides insight into how to communicate with clients to minimize stress levels. Finally, it highlights the importance of the fact that the end of life care experience leaves a lasting impression on clients. The experience very often will influence their decision to stay with the practice and/or return with another pet in the future.

In a successful veterinary practice, the team takes the time to understand the bond between the clients and their pets, and makes caring for both a priority. This practice will win overall client satisfaction and, ultimately, client retention.

So how do you offer support to your clients while still keeping your focus on your patients? The good news is that there are simple steps that can be taken that can make a big difference in helping your clients. Let us first focus on the end of life care experience before discussing supporting your clients through the loss of a pet.

Support starts with a basic understanding of what these clients need. Pet parents going through end of life care with a pet have four important needs:

- Information
- Resources
- Choices
- Support

Information

Your clients will feel well informed if you provide them with the opportunity to speak freely about their questions and concerns. They will feel that you are working together as a team for the best interests of their pet. Make sure clients get their questions answered during each appointment. Ask clients to bring a list of questions with them, and before the appointment is over make sure all their questions have been answered. Based on how emotional your client is, you may also want to suggest they bring a friend or family member with them, both for support and to be sure all issues have been addressed. We also recommend letting your client know early on the best way to reach you (phone, email, text) and the best time to call you should they need to. If there is an associate you work with who can also answer questions when you are not available, let them know who that is, and how to contact them. If possible, arrange an introduction.

In this way, you can lower your client's anxiety and make them feel that they are being heard. There are also benefits for you as well. Providing the time for clients to have their questions answered during the appointment and lessening their anxiety will lessen the chances they will call you as often, and if they do, it will be at times and in a manner more convenient for you.

Resources

Providing resources means providing pet parents with the information they need to feel comfortable about their pet's condition, treatment, and prognosis. Often, clients will turn to "Dr. Google" or to online pet support groups for information, like many of us do when we are sick. This can often lead to misinformation that may not apply to their particular situation and can cause them even more stress.

In order to compete with these resources make sure your client has enough information from you. Provide good printed information sheets and provide online resources where they can find accurate information. The benefit for your clients is they will have accurate information to reduce their stress and worry. The benefit for you is that your clients will not be misinformed and come to you with inaccurate information, which may necessitate stressful, defensive conversations that are stressful and cumbersome for you and for your client.

Choices

A client dealing with end of life with their beloved pet is also dealing with high levels of anxiety, stress, and worry, all of which can make information processing and decision making that much harder. Providing clients with both verbal and written information about treatment options will help them make better choices.

Provide your clients with a written "take-away" outlining their options, along with explanations of how the procedure will help their pet, the possible negative consequences, and the costs involved. This will benefit your clients, by giving them something to refer to when they have questions or cannot remember what you said. It will benefit you because in the printed or written confirmation you have laid out all the options, and chances are good that they will later have less questions, saving you time and stress as well.

Support

> *"Clients don't care about how much you know until they know about how much you care."*

When clients are coming to terms with the fact that the time they have left is limited with their beloved pet, the compassion they receive from you becomes much more important. Let them know through your words and actions that you truly care and that you understand how important their pet is to them. You can make sure they feel supported by connecting with them through active listening techniques. Make direct eye contact. Acknowledge their concerns and reassure them that you are doing all you can to help their beloved pet. This support will go a long way to give them the support they need and it will help you solidify your relationship with the client.

Going through this end of life care experience with their beloved pet is traumatic and emotionally exhausting for your client. The experience will often stay with them for quite some time. *The compassion that you and your staff provide or withhold will have a major impact on how clients experience and how they will remember the end of life care experience.* With some careful planning and thought, offer your clients the information, resources, choices, and support they need. This will prove invaluable to making sure the experience is one that satisfies and benefits everyone involved.

Pet Loss: Supporting Your Clients – Supporting Your Practice

> *"I was not prepared for the extreme emotional grief my family and I have experienced. I feel guilty for feeling so lost, and inconsolable regarding our pet's death. How do we handle this?"*

> *"I wish someone had told me about pet loss support. It was devastating, and I had to go through it alone."*

These statements demonstrate the impact that the loss of a beloved pet has on pet carers. The loss of a pet is difficult for everyone involved. You are also affected by the loss of a patient, with whom you have grown close and have done all you can to help. Even though veterinary professionals are not mental health professionals, it is important to realize that when there is no longer anything you can do medically to help your animal patient, there is still a great deal you can do to help your human client.

The results of our study and our conversations with grieving pet parents both clearly indicate the gap between what is needed by pet carers at this difficult time and what they are offered by their

Table 12.1.   Support Options Offered

Type of Support	Percentage
Brochures/pamphlets on pet loss or resources	12%
Information on online resources/chat rooms	4%
Books on pet loss	3%
On-site pet loss counseling services	3%
Outside pet loss counseling services	4%
No resources offered	83%

veterinary teams in terms of pet loss support. As can be seen in Table 12.1 and Figure 12.1, 83% of pet parents reported that they received no support from their clinic (in person, online, or brochures) upon losing their beloved pets. Of those same pet carers, 87% rated receiving some type of support to be either very or somewhat important. Furthermore, for those pet owners in our study who did receive some type of pet loss support, 55% rated that support as poor, as shown in Figure 12.2.

Most veterinary professionals and their staffs have received little to no proper training in how to offer support to their clients. Subjects like pet loss support receive very little attention in veterinary schools. In fact, although pet loss support has been available to pet parents as early as the late 1980s through organizations such as the Association for Pet Loss and Bereavement (www.aplb.org), it has been only in the last 10 years that pet loss support has begun to receive the attention it deserves. The good news is that today, more than ever, there are resources available for veterinary professionals to use that can help them provide adequate support for their clients.

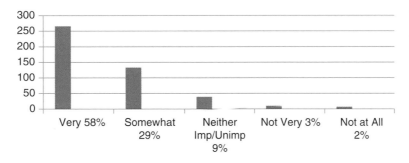

Figure 12.1.   The importance of offering pet loss support.

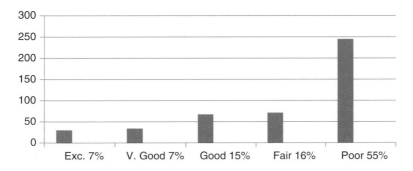

Figure 12.2.   Rating of pet loss support offered by veterinary practices.

Table 12.2. Common Reactions to Grief

Category	Reactions
Physical	Changes in eating habits, changes in sleeping patterns, aches and pains, extreme exhaustion and fatigue
Emotional	Sadness, guilt, anger, shock, numbness, irritability, depression, disbelief, feeling overwhelmed, vulnerability
Behavioral	Difficulties in communicating, difficulties in relationships, difficulties in socializing and rationalizing, easily distracted, confusion
Spiritual	Anger/bargaining with God, loss of faith, renewed s pirituality

In our conversations with veterinary professionals and their staff, we learned that part of their reluctance in attempting to support their clients through pet loss is their lack of knowledge and their uncertainty about what support is needed. Some basic knowledge and understanding can go a long way in supporting grieving clients. While there are some commonalities in what grieving pet parents go through, no two people who will go through the grieving process react in the exact same way. Table 12.2 provides examples of various ways clients experience this grief.

We have dealt with many couples grieving the loss of a beloved pet, and found that the grief each feels is somewhat different from the other, as is the time it takes them to begin to heal. In fact, one of the most important things to understand about grief is that it has no time-line. Grief is an individual journey for each person. How grief is experienced is based largely on four factors:

- **Life circumstances**. Has your client lost a job, or gone through a divorce? Are they dealing with family problems, etc.?
- **Support system**. Does your client have a good support system at home or at work or are they isolated with no one to turn to in challenging times?
- **Relationship with pet**. Does your client consider their pet to be "fur-kids" or pets? How close is the relationship between them?
- **Grief history**. Has your client experienced a lot of loss in the past? How long ago were these losses? Is this the first major loss they have experienced?

Having this information about a client's situation will greatly assist the practice's ability to evaluate the client's need for emotional support. You have the opportunity to learn more about your clients and their lifestyles during the time that they come to your practice with their pets. Create a special section of a client's folder for notes regarding who the client is as it relates to these four areas. By having it written in the folder, it gives everyone access to this information so that they know with whom they are dealing. Here are some suggestions for easy and appropriate ways to offer support to your clients.

Do: Allow your clients to talk about their feelings and concerns after a loss. Let them tell "their story" as many times as they need to. For a grieving person, telling their story can begin to make the sad and painful feelings lose power over them.

Don't: Schedule a time to talk to your client when you are too busy or don't have the time. Not focusing on the client and their needs can make the client feel unimportant and can worsen their grief.

Do: Use words of condolences from the heart. Even saying something as simple as "I'm so sorry," followed by a pause, is sincere and speaks for itself.

Don't: Try and use logic to help a grieving client. Expressions like, "They aren't suffering anymore," or "Time heals" can be seen as insensitive canned responses.

Do: Listen more than you talk. Listen in a non-judgmental manner and allow periods of silence.

Don't: Invalidate your client's loss by not responding at the appropriate times. A simple nod of the head or touch on the arm can go a long way in letting them know you're paying attention.

Do: Share and reminisce about your memories of the pet. Tell a story about something you remember about their pet, and what made him/her special to you.

Don't: Avoid using the term "I know how you feel." Everyone experiences loss in their own way. Instead, try some self-disclosure by saying something like, "I felt a similar pain when I lost my dog/cat last year."

Do: Always provide the client with grief counseling resources and information. Let clients know you are there by following up with them.

Don't: Act as a psychologist or counselor. Know your limits. Your role is as an educator, supporter, and referral source. Trying to do more than you are able to do or trained to do can hurt your grieving client and can also put you at risk.

The last suggestion above is extremely important. Veterinary professionals often tell us that they struggle with the decision about whether or not a client needs pet loss counseling from a professional counselor. Our answer is simple. Make it a practice to offer resources to every one of your clients who loses a pet. No matter what the circumstances of the death, one thing is certain: there is always a sense of shock or disbelief that their pet is no longer with them. Most often, for the first day or two after the loss, your client will be filled with emotion and trying to make sense of what has happened. As the reality of the loss sets in, a client may or may not realize they need counseling or therapy. Some may benefit from a pet loss book, or an online chat at a pet loss support group, or a local counselor for private or group therapy.

Since you are not a psychotherapy diagnostician, provide every client with a grief folder with coping suggestions, a pet loss bibliography, and a list of pet loss support groups and counselors. By providing each client with a grief folder with resources, it allows them to decide for themselves how much support they may need. It also demonstrates how much you care not only about their pet but also about them.

Another way to provide support for your clients at this difficult time is to have a staff member become trained as a pet loss counselor. Perhaps the best online training program is offered by the Association for Pet Loss and Bereavement (www.aplb.org). If training a member of your staff is not an option, consider working with a certified pet loss counselor who can run a support group at your practice once a week or once a month. Implementing these suggestions takes pressure off of the veterinary professionals who want to keep their main focus on the medical care of the pets. It is also a way of honoring the pet that you cared for by helping their family begin to heal.

Red Flag Signs

In our pet loss consulting with various veterinary practices, we are often asked how to determine if a client is experiencing "normal" grief or if there may be something more to be concerned about.

Below are some of what we call "Red Flag Signs" to watch out for that may indicate that a client is in need of additional support.

- Clients who live alone and cannot identify other sources of emotional support
- Clients who you believe may be clinically depressed or those who make references to suicide, homicide, or violence
- Clients who exhibit obsessive guilt, remorse, or blame after the death
- Clients who have exhibited extreme emotionality in general during their relationship with you
- Clients who have recently experienced other significant losses or stressors (the death of another family member, loss of a home or job, divorce, etc.)

Suicidal Ideation

Many pet owners, especially immediately following the loss of a beloved pet, find it difficult to imagine their lives without their pets. A remark about not wanting to go on may be a normal reaction, as losing such a significant relationship can feel overwhelming. On rare occasions, however, there may be suicidal intent underlying the client's comment. It is therefore important for you to have a professional counselor or therapist available, to assist you in determining if this is a credible threat or a normal grief reaction. When a client's well-being is at stake, better safe than sorry.

In this situation, it is very helpful to have a client information folder as mentioned above (a record of their life circumstances, grief history, relationship with pet, and support system). If you have a client who exhibits any of these signs, we strongly recommend that you urge them to seek outside support. If there is a trained professional working with your practice, consult with them about the case.

The Importance of Follow-up

> *"I know we weren't technically their clients anymore, but it was like when our dog died, we died too. I guess I thought they cared more than they did."*

Another really important piece to supporting your client through the loss of their beloved pet is the area of client follow-up. Along with offering pet loss support resources, veterinary practices have another opportunity to show pet parents they care about their beloved pets and the families they leave behind. It is important to remember not only do your clients lose a beloved family member but they also lose their connection with the veterinary team who very often have become a significant part of their lives. Letting the families left behind know you care about their welfare goes a long way in helping them to heal and impacts the impression they have of the practice.

In an effort to see how pet's family members felt about the importance of follow-up and whether or not follow-up was offered to them, we included the following questions in our study:

- Did your practice follow up with you to see how you were doing after the loss of your beloved pet?
- How important do you think it is that your practice follows up to see how you and your family are doing after your loss?

In our study, pet owners reported that only 28% of veterinary practices had followed up with them after the loss of their pet. Yet, as the results in Figure 12.3 demonstrate, another gap clearly exists

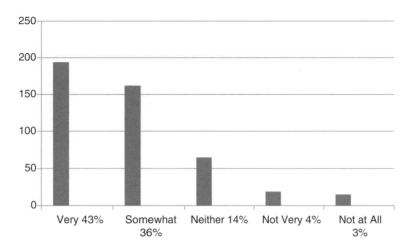

Figure 12.3.   The importance of following up with clients.

between what clients want and what they receive when it comes to their veterinary team following up with them. Taking note of this and acting upon it provides another opportunity for veterinary practices to leave their clients with a positive feeling.

Dr. Villalobos and her Pawspice practice are at the forefront in providing follow-up support. Often, after their clients lose a beloved pet, they are told to "come back and visit with cookies." In counseling her clients, many have mentioned this as being so helpful in their healing and their belief that Dr. Villalobos truly cared not only about their beloved pets but about them as well.

Certainly, not every practice is able to go as far as Pawspice, but there are ways to follow-up with your clients that will make a difference. If your clients come to the practice with their pet for euthanasia, make sure to let them know afterwards you are there to support them and they can call you with any concerns. Designate a front office staff member to make a call to them a few days later and let them know you are calling to "check in" and see how they are doing. Let them know you are there if there is anything they need. Many practices will send a condolence card after the pet's passing. This can really make a difference as well, but *the important thing to remember* is the card should be personalized with written messages from those who treated the pet rather than having a "canned saying" that goes into every card. If the client comes to the practice to pick up the cremains, be sure and take a few minutes to see how they are doing. You may want to remind them that support is available if they are having a hard time. All of the above suggestions can go a long way in both honoring the memory of the beloved pet and helping to sustain a long-term relationship with satisfied clients.

Pet Loss and the Impact on Veterinary Professionals

Up until this point, we have been focusing on supporting clients dealing with the loss of a beloved pet. Now we will bring our focus to Compassion Fatigue/Self-Care Strategies for Veterinary Professionals. However, we do feel it is appropriate to end this section by addressing pet loss and the impact it has on veterinary professionals. When we conduct some of our Compassion Fatigue support groups, it is not unusual for someone to bring up how the loss of a patient has affected them. They will often bring up their level of discomfort when it comes to sharing their sadness with both their clients and their colleagues. Unless you are working in an Emergency/Specialty Hospital setting, it is normal and understandable that you would often develop special relationships with your patients whom you have cared for, sometimes from puppyhood to adulthood/old age. Even those professionals working in specialty settings can get close to patients who they are caring for during a specific illness. It is completely normal and understandable to feel sad and upset upon the pet's death.

We understand, too, that you are put in a difficult position. As a professional, especially if you are performing the euthanasia, you are limited as to how much emotion you can display. Yet, in conversations with almost all of our pet loss clients, they told us how much it meant to them that their veterinarian and staff did show emotion and let them know how much their beloved pets meant to them. We strongly believe that it is vital for everyone involved to have the opportunity to grieve for the loss of pets who have touched your heart in some way. We also understand the difficulty in doing this when, during the course of a given hour, you may have to go from euthanizing a favorite patient to caring for a young puppy that is full of youthful energy.

So how do you honor your own feelings of loss of a special patient? We believe it starts with you first acknowledging that your own feelings are real and valid and should not be ignored. Allowing yourself to care about and feel for your patients is what helps you do your job well.

When you are at the practice, if you are able, see if you can arrange your schedule so that you can take even a little time off to allow for your own feelings. Take 15 minutes to go for a walk or sit quietly in a room or your car by yourself. After the client leaves, if it is possible, take some alone time with the beloved pet and let him/her know how much they meant to you. We recommend setting up a place in a break or conference room where you can honor special pets who the staff has treated. Think about putting up an "In Memoriam" corkboard, with a picture of the pet or perhaps some electric candles. If possible, schedule some time during staff meetings to honor pets who made an impact on different members of the staff.

On a personal level, do what you need to do to honor your own grief. When signing the condolence card for clients, make sure to let them know how much their pet meant to you. Think about memorializing him/her by making a donation in their name. Take the time to share with a friend, family member, or co-worker about how much the pet meant to you. Take some time to remember all you did to help the pet in the time you cared for them. Again, the main thing is to take the time to honor the relationship you shared with them and the grief you feel. Taking this time not only honors the relationship you had with the pet but also helps you to provide the best care for pets in your practice now and in the future.

Compassion Fatigue and Self-Care

Up until now, the focus of this information has been on helping you help your clients during the difficult end of life/pet loss experience. As we believe, and what is the focus of our "Compassionate Practice" concept, caring for clients and caring for yourself are intricately bound, with compassion and communication being two of the core elements.

The goal for this section is to provide you with information and strategies on how to care for yourself and your practice. Before getting into self-care though, it is important to have at least a basic understanding of what causes some of the underlying stress that is a part of veterinary work.

When we go into veterinary practices to do workshops on Compassion Fatigue and Self-Care, we will often start out by asking how many people have heard of Compassion Fatigue, how many feel they have a good understanding of what it is or have previously been to a workshop? Almost everyone will raise their hand when it comes to having heard of Compassion Fatigue, but not as many hands go up when it comes to understanding what Compassion Fatigue is, its causes, or how to manage and combat it.

We have all heard of the tragic incidences of talented and caring veterinarians who have taken their own lives, so it is not surprising that many have heard of Compassion Fatigue. Some may know colleagues who have just had enough and walked away from a profession that they once loved. It is not uncommon to find people with the best intentions coming in to the veterinary field and then losing the joy or becoming disillusioned because of situations at work that may be beyond their control. This is sad on many levels. First, not everybody gets to find work that brings them joy, and when they do, they are a true gift to those they help. Second, we can tell you that as pet parents and as pet professionals representing pet parents, we really need good people to care for the pets we love so much. The fact is with some knowledge and strategies in place all of this heartache and distress can be managed.

We are firm believers that knowledge is power, and we feel that really understanding what you are up against gives you the best chance to put a working individualized self-care plan in place to combat Compassion Fatigue. It is our hope to provide you with some basic information on Compassion Fatigue and then to focus on helping you develop a self-care plan so that you can continue to help the animals you care about and do the work that brings you joy. There are many books and resources written on the topic of Compassion Fatigue. We have found the best out there to be *Compassion Fatigue in the Animal Care Community* written by Charles Figley and Robert Roop. (Figley and Roop 2006). Charles Figley has researched and written on the area of Compassion Fatigue for many years and is considered an expert in the field. Figley defines Compassion Fatigue as:

> The inner exhaustion caused by the stress of caring for and helping others who are traumatized or suffering.

While Compassion Fatigue can be found in all the helping industries, some studies have found it to be most prevalent in the veterinary profession. The important thing to realize is that no matter how skilled or experienced an animal care professional you are, you cannot help but be impacted by the traumas you see each day. Compassion Fatigue is not a diagnosis or a mental illness, but a normal consequence of working in a helping field.

We have often heard the terms "Compassion Fatigue" and "Burnout" used interchangeably. However, they are not the same, and the distinction needs to be made. Burnout can be defined as "the physical, mental and emotional exhaustion related to long-term, cumulative stress of emotionally difficult work and lack of job satisfaction" (Figley in Figley and Roop 2006). Burnout is what happens when you feel the effects of work-related stress over a longer time period and do nothing to take care of yourself. You have lost your energy and passion for your work. You have reached the point of no return. Compassion Fatigue allows that there is still hope as long as steps have been taken for self-care. This distinction clearly highlights the importance for awareness and the willingness to take action so that the situation does not get to the Burnout point.

Causes and Symptoms of Compassion Fatigue

Struggling with the symptoms of Compassion Fatigue does not mean something is intrinsically wrong with you, but rather it is a very normal consequence of working in the helping industries. Compassion Fatigue is caused by both external and internal causes.

External Causes

On the external side, one of the main causes is the fact that in the veterinary profession you are faced with dealing with, and trying to help, traumatized pets and their families on a daily basis. The other main external cause has to do with your work environment (culture of the practice, personnel policies and reward structure, work ethics, etc.) and how you are able to work within it. While there is not much that can be done about working with traumatized animals and people, as it is just an inherent part of being in veterinary work, the work environment is something that you do have some control over.

We always recommend to veterinary professionals that they think about the type of environment in which they feel most comfortable working. Take a few minutes to ask yourself these questions:

- Are you more comfortable working in a fast-paced, "workaholic" type of atmosphere where you are always on the run or do you need more of a slower paced environment within which self-care is promoted?
- Are you the type of person who needs feedback on the work you are doing and likes working as part of a team or do you prefer to work more independently with no supervision?
- Now ask yourself how your work environment matches the environment in which you are most comfortable working?

The closer your ideal work situation matches the work environment in which you currently find yourself, the less stress you will have. The further away your ideal work environment is from where you are working, the more work-related stress you will feel. If you are feeling a lot of stress in this area, think about whether or not anything can be done to resolve these issues. While everyone, no matter what their occupation, should try and work in the most comfortable environment possible, those working in helping/veterinary professions need to pay more attention to this factor. Awareness is an important piece of being able to handle the effects of Compassion Fatigue.

Internal Causes

Internal stress factors have to do with the traits that make you who you are. The majority of us working in the helping industries are very empathetic and committed to helping others. That makes us special in many regards, but it can also be a detriment if we forget to take care of ourselves. Sometimes we may have unresolved issues and traumatic memories that may surface in doing this work. These issues should be worked on and resolved so that they do not interfere with your work and well-being. It is also not uncommon to find many in the veterinary field to be over-achieving or over-pleasing, highly sensitive and prone to perfectionism. Again, awareness is an important first step in taking care of ourselves. Take a moment and reflect on which of these traits you may have and how they may be making you more vulnerable to the effects of Compassion Fatigue.

If you rate yourself high in any of these areas, think about what you can do to keep them in check when dealing with some of the more stressful situations during the day. Carmen Berry writes about a phenomenon she calls "The Messiah Trap" (Berry 1989). This is where people have a strong tendency to put everyone's needs first and ignore their own. They tend not to accept help even when it is offered because they believe, "I, and only I, can make things right." Those working in the helping professions often tend to be more this way. Again, the awareness of who we are and how it may affect our susceptibility to the effects of Compassion Fatigue are important factors to pay attention to.

Symptoms of Compassion Fatigue

Along with knowing what causes Compassion Fatigue, it is also important to understand what Compassion Fatigue looks and feels like. Because the idea of Compassion Fatigue has become somewhat of a "buzzword" in the profession, it is often mistakenly used to describe people in the profession who are feeling burned out. People who have been affected by Compassion Fatigue have symptoms or behavioral changes that require a more comprehensive definition. A breakdown of these symptoms with examples is below. Contemplate the following symptoms. How many have you been feeling? Are they out of the ordinary from your natural state of being? Have you noticed an increase in any of them?

- **Physical Symptoms include** extreme fatigue/recurrent illnesses/weight gain or loss.
- **Psychological Symptoms include** increased negativity or irritability/numbness or apathy/ increased anger.
- **Social Symptoms include** isolation/disengagement/complaining.
- **Spiritual Symptoms include** a loss of faith/loss of purpose or meaning.

Once again, the importance of awareness becomes apparent. It is most important to notice when you are feeling symptoms you have not experienced in the past or if any of the symptoms that you have experienced have increased significantly. If so, it is likely you are struggling with Compassion Fatigue. Once you become aware that you are feeling the effects of Compassion Fatigue, the next step is to develop a self-care plan to manage and combat them. Before we begin to discuss the steps necessary to develop a self-care plan, let's take a brief look at how Compassion Fatigue can affect a veterinary practice as a whole.

Compassion Fatigue and the Veterinary Practice

It is often said that an organization is only as good as the people in it, but what happens when a part of, or the majority of, the staff within a veterinary practice is struggling with Compassion Fatigue? The practice would not be able to run effectively when everyone working within the organization is affected by Compassion Fatigue symptoms. It is as though the practice has a widespread Compassion Fatigue "staff" infection.

What causes Compassion Fatigue to occur within an organization? Occasionally, a new person struggling with Compassion Fatigue will join a practice and can "infect" others working there, but more often than not it happens the other way around. As stated earlier, the very nature of the work done in a veterinary practice makes the people in it more susceptible to Compassion Fatigue. Add to that an environment in which the well-being and needs of the staff working in the practice are not taken into account, and chances are high that some, if not all, of the staff are likely to struggle with at least some symptoms of Compassion Fatigue. It is understandable, too, that new staff entering the practice will not be immune to the environment and will also begin to feel the effects.

So, what does a practice suffering from a Compassion Fatigue "staff" infection look like? Think about the practice you work in now. How many of these symptoms of Compassion Fatigue can you identify?

- Negative attitude or low morale
- High rates of absenteeism/tardiness and/or staff turnover

- Lack of communication or miscommunication
- Increase in interpersonal conflicts
- Poor level of service provided to clients

Workplace settings in which these symptoms are prevalent are more likely to have employees struggling with symptoms of Compassion Fatigue. Knowing this, it becomes incumbent upon management in veterinary practices to take steps in order to avoid a "staff" infection and to create a work environment with personnel policies and rewards that take into account the needs of the staff. Doing so will help to ensure a well-run practice that benefits everyone.

More information on this topic is included in the "Creating a Compassionate Practice" section.

A Self-Care Plan – Managing the Effects of Compassion Fatigue

> In dealing with those who are undergoing great suffering, if you feel burnout setting in, if you feel demoralized and exhausted, it is best for the sake of everyone, to withdraw and restore yourself. The point is to have a long-term perspective.

The Dalia Lama

This quote provides such an important message. In order to enjoy a long and enjoyable career, it is crucial that you take the time to care for yourself. Interestingly enough, when we conduct workshops on Self-Care or even during our Compassion Fatigue support groups, when the topic of self-care comes up, we can feel an underlying reluctance on the part of participants. Some veterinarians and their staff tell us that they just do not have time for self-care. They tell us on a busy day there is barely time to go to the restroom, let alone take a break. There are patients who need their help. When they leave for the day, there are errands to run and families to help and care for. How can they possibly take time to go to the gym or read a book?

However, who are you going to be able to help if you are unable to help yourself? How many times have you walked out of the practice at the end of a day saying, "I just can't take any more sadness and stress today," only to have to go home and deal with family or personal issues? How much are you able to give to anyone else on those days?

Think back to a really hard day at work, knowing you have to go in the next day and do it all over again. Were you able to give everything that you wanted to give? Or were you physically and/or mentally exhausted just giving enough to get by? Who did that benefit?

It is critical for those in the helping professions to find time for self-care. It is crucial if you want to be able to make a difference in the lives of pets and their families, and it is crucial for your own well-being. Implementing self-care into your life does not have to be time consuming, nor does it have to be done all at once. You might be surprised by the effect that a few simple changes can have on how you feel about yourself, your work, and your home life.

Charles Figley (in Figley and Roop 2006) talks about self-care as a way to move from Compassion Fatigue to Compassion Satisfaction. He defines Compassion Satisfaction as the following:

> Compassion Satisfaction is the pleasure you get from being able to do your job well and the pleasure you derive from feeling positive about your colleagues or your ability to contribute to the work setting or even the greater good of society.

The Basics of Self-Care

This section will provide you with information about developing a self-care plan that works for you, including easy-to-implement self-care suggestions, strategies and exercises that you can use to develop a personalized self-care plan.

First, it is important to realize that there is something inherent in all of us that can help us stave off the effects of Compassion Fatigue. Charles Figley talks about how we can build our levels of resiliency to help us be less affected by Compassion Fatigue. He defines Caregiver Resilience as:

> … the tendency to cope with the work-related stress naturally or through the help of others (organizations, colleagues, friends, or family) and to be able to avoid the negative consequences and savor the satisfactions of the work.

Increase your Level of Caregiver Resilience

- Make Connections.
- Keep things in perspective.
- Avoid seeing problems as insurmountable and avoid taking decisive action.
- Look for opportunities for self-discovery.
- Nurture a positive view of yourself and maintain a hopeful attitude.
- Take the time to care for yourself.

Think about your level of resiliency before you entered the veterinary profession. Do you think it has increased, decreased, or stayed the same? Which of the steps above do you think you can use to build your resilience level?

Awareness

Taking the time for awareness is an important part of self-care and developing a self-care plan. Several times in this chapter we have mentioned the need to become more aware of how you are feeling or of your surroundings. Awareness is the first step towards developing a self-care plan, along with Assessment, and Planning (Figley).

Those who are lucky enough to work around animals understand that when it comes to being aware, staying mindful, and living in the moment, pets are truly the experts. Our society judges us on how much we can do and how fast we can do it. We strive to be excellent multitaskers. All of this helps us to lose touch with what or how we are feeling. By staying in the moment and becoming more aware of how and what we are feeling, as well as how our environment is impacting us, we can become better able to handle the stressors we are facing and find solutions for them.

Stress Awareness Exercise

Our bodies guide us to recognize how much stress we are holding inside. They can be barometers to help us realize what our triggers are and which things will get under our skin and make our stress rise. Unfortunately, we often do not pay attention to the signals our bodies are sending us.

The following exercise can help you get into the habit of listening to your body so that you can realize what your stress triggers are and how they affect you. If you are able to recognize this, then you will be better able to defuse stress when you feel it.

Can you identify where in your body you feel stress? Start by taking a moment to relax and take some deep breaths. Now think about the last several times you felt stressed. Where in your body did you feel it? Is it your neck, your back, your stomach? Take a moment and write down all the places in your body where you felt the stress. Also, write down the things that caused your body to feel that way. Those are your trigger points.

By paying attention to which stressors affect your body in what ways, you can be better prepared to handle them. It can also give you the opportunity to have solutions readily at hand. For instance, if you know that your stomach bothers you when you are stressed, you can keep some antacids on hand at work. If it is your neck/head that bothers you when you are stressed, do some stretches, use a hand-held massager where you hurt, and keep some Tylenol at the ready.

This exercise can be an eye-opening experience to how much your body is affected by the stress you feel on a daily basis.

Creating a Well-Rounded Self-Care Plan

Ideally, the goal is to work toward a well-rounded life, in which all of these dimensions are balanced. A good self-care plan includes strategies for taking care of all dimensions of our lives, including:

- Physical health: strategies to sleep/eat/exercise properly
- Mental health/personal growth: honoring your emotional needs and make time for the things that lead to personal growth
- Spiritual: finding a place to worship or just having meditation exercises or prayer time alone or with a group
- Interpersonal: taking care of relationships both inside and outside of work
- Pleasure: pursuing hobbies or anything that gives you pleasure
- Work: doing work that makes you feel good/satisfied

An Exercise in Balancing Your Life

When we introduce this exercise to veterinary practices, we always get some "eye rolls" and spoken or unspoken comments of, "A balanced life? Who is able to have *that* these days?" We are not under the delusion that any exercise can make your life more balanced. However, we have done this exercise with many veterinary practices with whom we consult. It does offer a chance to raise awareness of how balanced or unbalanced our lives may be, and it does offer a chance to assess how we are doing in our quest for a balanced life. Our clients who have taken the time to do this exercise have found it to be enlightening, as well as an inspiration to make a change or two.

See the two pie charts in Figure 12.4 with the six areas/dimensions mentioned above. Divide the pie into slices that represent how much time you spend on each of the dimensions. When you are finished, take a look at your pie chart. Work will likely be the biggest slice of the pie. Is it between 40% and 60% of the pie? Answer the following questions about your pie chart:

- Were you able to fill all six dimensions in your pie?
- What surprised you most about reviewing your completed pie chart?
- What area do you most want to increase/decrease?

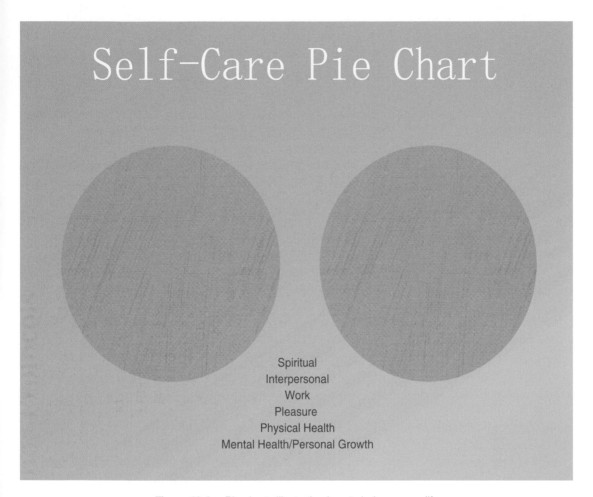

Self-Care Pie Chart

Spiritual
Interpersonal
Work
Pleasure
Physical Health
Mental Health/Personal Growth

Figure 12.4. Pie charts illustrating how to balance your life.

There is a second pie chart in the figure. Use your first pie chart to evaluate where you currently are and formulate a plan of change. Then wait a month or two and use the second pie chart to see if you have made any positive changes.

One Step Further

As we stated earlier, a good well-rounded self-care plan should include strategies for all aspects of life. Thinking about the pie chart that you completed, look at the areas you wish were larger. What one step can you take in each of the areas you want to improve upon that will bring things more into balance?

Taking Care of Your "Self"

Up until now we have been focusing on the importance of becoming aware, of assessing how you are doing, and of creating a self-care plan. However, any good self-care plan should also include care-taking basics such as eating well, sleeping well, exercising, and other fundamentals. The reason we

CARING FOR YOURSELF IN THE FACE OF DIFFICULT WORK
Our work can be overwhelming. Our challenge is to maintain our resilience so that we can keep doing the work with care, energy and compassion.

10 Things To Do For Each Day

1. Get Enough Sleep

6. Focus On What You Do Well

2. Get Enough to Eat

7. Learn From Your Mistakes

3. Do Some Light Exercise

8. Share A Private Joke

4. Vary The Work That You Do

9. Pray, Meditate Or Relax

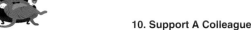

5. Do Something Pleasurable

10. Support A Colleague

From Sandi & Ellie - Your Friends at "PetLoss Partners"

Beth Hudnali Stamm, Ph.D – ProQOL.org & Idaho Sate University/Craig Higson-Smith, M.A. South Institute of Traumatic Stress/Amy C. Hudnali, M.A.ProQol.org & Appalachian State University/Henry E. Stamm, Ph.D ProQOL.org

Figure 12.5.   Chart of caring for yourself in the face of difficult work.

need to include them is simple. As caregivers, we are experts at making sure our patients, clients, family, and even colleagues take good care of themselves. When it comes to our own self-care, we may come up with a million excuses as to why we do not have time. However, making time to enact a good self-care plan is what will allow us to perform well and enjoy what we do.

The "Caring for Yourself in the Face of Difficult Work" chart (Figure 12.5) is a good and fun reminder of basic self-care tasks that we need to take into account. Print it out and keep a copy on your bathroom mirror, at your desk, in the break-room, in your car, or wherever it may serve as a good reminder.

The Gift of Saying "No"

Volumes have been written about the importance of setting boundaries, especially when it comes to those in the care-giving profession. A big part of boundary setting is the ability to say no to others when necessary. Whenever we discuss "The Gift of Saying No" with our veterinary practice clients, we almost always encounter resistance at first. It is not a surprise. People who are caregivers feel uncomfortable about saying "no" to others, especially to people they care about and for.

We often hear, "If we don't work the extra hours, then the pets won't get taken care of" or "But the work has to get done." Perhaps the questions should be, "If you do work the extra hours, then what about you? Does that mean you lose the time you needed to rest, spend time with family, and take care of yourself? How effective will you be when you work those extra hours? What consequences have you paid for not being able to say 'No' at work or at home?"

What if you could reframe saying "No" to others as saying "Yes" to yourself and your own needs? Just like anything new, this may feel uncomfortable at first, but the more comfortable you become saying "yes" to you, you will realize that you are really saying "yes" to everyone. Taking the time for self-care allows you to give your best to others as well.

Self-Care in the Veterinary Practice

The information, suggestions and exercises we have offered are intended to help you become more aware of yourself and better able to assess how you are doing, with the ultimate goal of implementing self-care strategies that work for you. Bear in mind that although it is important to have strategies and tools in place that can be used to support you in the important work you do, it is just as important in supporting the practice as a whole.

Helping the Helpers

Caregivers are experts at helping others, but when it comes to asking for help, it can be very difficult and sometimes uncomfortable. However, your ability to be able to ask for help when necessary is critical in order to continue to do the work and help the pets you care for so much. It is important to take the time to realize or acknowledge that the colleagues working with you can and should be thought of as resources when you have questions or need help in your work. All of you have individual knowledge and experiences that can be used to help each other. Part of the success of a practice as a whole depends on the ability of the staff to pool its resources for the good of everyone involved. It is important and necessary for everyone to become comfortable leaning on others.

When we go into veterinary practice, we encourage the staff to take that chance and rely on each other for support by doing two things:

- Have each person in the practice create a "crisis plan" with the names, e-mail addresses, and telephone numbers of their colleagues on whom they can rely and to whom they can delegate responsibility in case they have a personal emergency or need help with their work.

- Have each person in the practice designate a co-worker as their "self-care buddy." This is a friendly colleague from whom they can find support and encouragement to take care of them when needed. Chances are good each staff member already has at least one colleague with whom they have developed a good working relationship. Why not agree to be each other's "self-care buddy?"

In the beginning, asking for help or relying on others can feel awkward and uncomfortable. However, we ask you to take a chance and try it. The benefits for each staff member can be huge and will bring the staff closer as a team.

Get Inspired

As Pet Loss counselors and Compassion Fatigue educators, we know and admire the work you do. The help you give to so many pets is very much appreciated by your clients. We also know that your work is very rewarding and very challenging on a daily basis. This can make it difficult to feel appreciated and cause you to wonder if your work makes a difference.

Feeling a lack of appreciation is only made worse by the reach of today's social media that allows those with grievances an immediate opportunity to voice their feelings and the ability to instantly reach so many. If you are not taking the time to care for yourself, you will easily be affected by a bad "review" or begin to pay more attention to what you did "wrong" rather than all you did "right." How do you keep your spirits up and stay focused on all you do well in light of these challenging situations?

The "Get Inspired" exercise below will help you focus on how much of a difference your work makes to so many. We call it the "Anti-Yelp" exercise. Take some quiet time to write down the answers to the following questions. When you are done, read what you have written. How does it make you feel? Post a copy on your bathroom mirror, at your desk, in your car, or wherever you can see it when you need a reminder.

- What was the most rewarding moment you had at work last week?
- What are 3–5 things that you love about your job?
- Name 3–5 co-workers, clients, or patients whose lives you have touched in a positive way this week or this month.
- Why did you take the job you currently have?
- What are 3 things you did well this week or this month?
- What are 3 compliments you received in the last week? In the last month?

Knowing that there are others at work on whom you can rely, and taking the time to keep your focus on your positives, will help you during challenging times and will help you manage and combat the effects of Compassion Fatigue.

Self-Care Suggestions for Veterinary Management

Individual self-care, as well as having self-care strategies in place for the practice, is crucial for veterinary professionals and staff. Management's role is just as crucial and can have a major impact on the success or failure of self-care in the practice environment. Providing education and support for those working within the practice can make the difference between having a staff that works as a team and is prepared to deal with the challenges that arise or a staff left to their own devices that is ill-prepared to work as a team and fails to meet challenges.

How does management support self-care within the practice? We recommend the following strategies:

- Promote staff input. This can be done either through the use of an inconspicuous suggestion box or an anonymous survey. Think about forming a Staff Task Force that is run by staff and acts as a liaison between staff and management. Promote an "open door" policy where members of staff are encouraged to speak freely with management.
- Regular staff meetings. We cannot emphasize enough the importance of making time for regular staff meetings. While we understand that this may be difficult in larger or 24-hour/emergency facilities, the benefits far outweigh the effort and time it takes to plan and coordinate these meetings. When well planned, meetings will offer everyone a chance to brainstorm solutions for key practice-wide stressors, come together as a team (team building exercises), and catch up on practice news.
- Promote a self-care environment. Take the time to encourage and promote both individual and practice-wide self-care. Providing healthy snacks or offering discounts on gym memberships can go a long way to letting the staff know you care about their well-being. Celebrate

practice-wide successes during staff meetings. Institute self-care practices and encourage individual self-care to benefit the practice as a whole, as well as the individual staff members and, ultimately, the clients and patients.

- Bring in outside expertise. We recommend finding an outside certified Compassion Fatigue educator/consultant to provide support and education for you and your staff. A trained professional from outside of the practice is more likely to see things clearly and objectively, and be able to offer solutions and opportunities for growth that someone working within the practice would not be able to do.

Making the Commitment

Throughout this section, we have provided information demonstrating reasons why both individual and practice-wide self-care is so important. We understand that finding time for self-care can be challenging, but we encourage you to ask yourself this question: How much more challenging will it be for me and everyone around me if I don't take the time for self-care?

We also understand that implementing a self-care plan can be overwhelming. For that reason, we encourage you to take the commitment walk with us. Instead of thinking of all you would have to do to implement a self-care plan, think of one easy and manageable step that you can implement this week that would serve you well. Write it below:

My first step towards self-care is:

_____

_____

_____

_____

Write it down on a separate piece of paper and hang it on your bathroom mirror, your car dashboard, your desk, or wherever it will serve as a reminder for you. Remember, taking the time to care for yourself will allow you to take better care of the patients and clients you serve and to continue working in a profession that you enjoy.

Creating a Compassionate Practice for Clients and Veterinary Professionals©

We believe that veterinary medicine is one of the most rewarding and challenging careers. So we have a book and course with the May 5, 2016 copyrighted title, *Creating a Compassionate Practice for Clients and Veterinary Professionals* (Grossman 2016). Those who choose to work in the field do so because of their love of animals and their desire to help them. Some choose the field because of a special relationship with pets they had growing up. They may even have wished more could have been done to save their pet. Some have a more global view and, because of their love of animals, they want to find a way to help them live long and healthy lives. The common thread is the love of animals.

Whether or not you realize it, this is also the common bond you share with the majority of clients whose pets you treat. It is their love for their pets and desire to make their lives happy and healthy that has them reaching out to you and entrusting their pets to your care. Speaking as current pet parents and ones who have also grieved intensely for very special pets, we appreciate and admire all you do for the pets we love so very much. We believe that it is so important for you to realize this because we also know that pet parents, especially when dealing with critical care or end of life situations, can be challenging to work with. These challenges are mostly due to the fact that they love their pets, are worried about them and want desperately to make the right treatment decisions. Their anxiety and distress can affect everyone involved.

As we have discussed in previous sections, these challenges, and many others that you face in your work can begin to take a toll on your joy in the work you do and on your ability to practice effectively. That is why we stress the need for self-care. Looking holistically at the relationship between clients and their veterinary team, we can see two sets of people who care very deeply for animals and face their own set of challenges in trying to do what is best for them.

This point was the impetus for the idea of a "Compassionate Practice." We began to think about how effective and successful a veterinary practice could be if it were to take everyone's needs (the patients, the clients, and the staff) into equal consideration. We define a Compassionate Practice this way:

> *A Compassionate Practice promotes a healthy work environment in which caring for staff, clients, and patients is valued as highly as the curing component.*
>
> *Protocols for staff wellness are identified and monitored to keep stress levels at a minimum.*
>
> *Relationships between staff members and staff and clients are based upon open and supportive communication that meets the needs of everyone involved. All feel seen, heard, and respected.*

A healthy, happy staff leads to a healthy, flourishing practice, which, in turn, leads to satisfied clients.

Satisfied Clients Lead to Higher Client Satisfaction and Retention

In a compassionate practice, there are benefits for everyone:

- Staff benefits. Staff feels good about themselves, their co-workers, and their work. They experience less stress, more client appreciation. They feel less effects of Compassion Fatigue and more benefits of Compassion Satisfaction and self-care.
- Client benefits. Clients feel more confident and satisfied with the care the pet is receiving. They feel more supported by their veterinary team. They have a stronger desire to remain as clients of the practice with current and future pets.
- Patient benefits. Pets receive the best care from their veterinary team and family and experience less stress.
- Practice benefits. Doctors and staff feel appreciated. Clients feel confident, satisfied, and appreciated. Patients are well cared for. There are lower rates of practice-wide Compassion Fatigue and higher rates of client satisfaction and retention.

At first glance, you might ask, "That looks great on paper, but how could something like this ever be achieved?" By having easy-to-implement actionable steps using some CORE principles, a Compassionate Practice is possible. In the book *Creating a Compassionate Practice for Clients and Veterinary Professionals* (Grossman 2016), we provide specific information, strategies, and exercises on how to turn an existing practice into a Compassionate Practice using the CORE principles. CORE stands for the four areas that need to be addressed in order to create a Compassionate Practice. They are:

- Compassion. Practices are designed to promote more compassion for the veterinary team individually and as a whole (mental health/self-help), the clients (education and support), and the patients (best-care practices).
- Open communication. Practices are designed to promote better communication between the veterinary team, management, and clients. This includes education and support in the areas of teamwork, conflict resolution, and client communication.
- Resiliency. Practices are designed to manage and combat the effects of Compassion Fatigue by developing resiliency and self-care strategies (education and support).
- Expectations/client experience. Practices are designed to understand and fulfill the client's expectations, enhance the client's experience through surveys and oral communication with clients, and turn the results of that information into actionable steps.

The key to creating a successful "compassionate practice" is to start by coming up with a few small actionable and measurable steps. This process does not have to be completed all at once. We believe you will begin to see improvements by completing the first steps you choose. Then you will review how things are going and build on that, making adjustments as needed. We also recommend that you get assistance from an outside consultant to help with the process. Often, it is easier for someone on the outside to see things objectively than it is for people in the middle of the situation. By taking the time to do the work, we know that you will begin to see the benefits of creating a practice environment in which the doctors, staff, and clients all feel appreciated and satisfied, and the patients get the best care possible. This benefits your practice as a whole, by helping to achieve high client satisfaction and retention.

References

American Psychological Association/Discovery Health – The Road to Resilience.

Berry, B.R. 1989. *When helping you is hurting me*. Harper Collins.

Figley, C.R., and R. Roop. 2006. *Compassion fatigue in the animal care community*. Washington, DC: Humane Society Press.

Figley Institute/Green Cross Academy of Traumatology, Charles and Kathleen Figley, Certification for Compassion Fatigue Educators.

Freedman, E., and Grossman, S. (2015) *End of life care/pet loss study*.

Grossman, S. 2016. *Creating a compassionate practice for clients and veterinary professionals*.

Beth Hudnali Stamm, PhD, ProQOL.org and Idaho State University/Craig Higson-Smith, MA, South Institute of Traumatic Stress/Amy C. Hudnali, MA, ProQOL.org and Appalachian State University/Henry E. Stamm, PhD, ProQOL.org.

"What about you, a workbook for those who work with others." The National Center of Family Homelessness.

Chapter 13
Professional Support: The Well-Being of the Veterinarian and the Team

Kimberly Pope-Robinson, DVM

> Shame is the intensely painful feeling or experience of believing we are flawed and therefore unworthy of acceptance and belonging.

Brene Brown, from her book "Daring Greatly" (2015, Penguin Books Ltd)

If we choose to help geriatric cancer patients and end of life patients, we need more skills. When visiting the space of emotional well-being in the veterinary profession, compassion fatigue is often discussed as a focal point. However, I have found that there is much more at play in this space. To ensure the emotional well-being of the veterinarian and the veterinary team, I feel that we must begin with a discussion about shame.

In managing the day-to-day actions of working in this profession, we sit floating on what I call the *"Ocean of Shame."* Brene Brown's definition of shame, above, well describes the feeling experienced by many practitioners when making life and death decisions for their patients, particularly when they are involved with end of life decisions.

Picture yourself floating on this ocean, and now picture all of the factors that are working to pull you under the water line. These factors, which I call *"sinkers,"* can show up in many forms: client pressures, patient pressures, practice pressures, financial pressures, career pressures, societal pressures, etc. Sinkers are not just related to death and dying situations. For example, one important sinker is the pressure you may feel to stay current and always have the complete knowledge and information needed for the decisions you make each day. We blink, and there is a new flea/tick product out. How can we keep up?

Sinkers pull us down into the Ocean of Shame. We may start to sink into the ocean and begin to go under the surface gasping for air. It may be a natural reaction to fight the downward pull by turning to fear and blame. In this place, we resort to *naming, blaming, and judging*. This can drive us into a place of negativity, cynicism, and anger, which feels comfortable and safe and can even give us buoyancy for a bit, although it is only a temporary fix. Ultimately, it will just make the sinkers stronger as we begin to disconnect from our passion and life. The next time the sinkers come along, we sink faster and deeper.

In the processes of working to tread the ocean water as the sinkers become heavier and heavier, we can instead fight the downward pull by focusing on our mental, spiritual, physical, and emotional

---

Canine and Feline Geriatric Oncology: Honoring the Human–Animal Bond, Second Edition. Alice Villalobos with Laurie Kaplan.
© 2018 John Wiley & Sons, Inc. Published 2018 by John Wiley & Sons, Inc.

well-being. I call this *"filling our well-being balloons."* The well-being balloons are balloons that only we know how to fill. We hold these balloons in our hands and they keep us from sinking into our Ocean of Shame. These wellness balloons can counteract the sinkers. They keep us afloat and allow us to turn to *recognizing, embracing, and connecting* instead of naming, blaming, and judging.

In this chapter, we will go on a journey, to paint the picture of how we can be most helpful to our clients and make the very best recommendations for the care of their geriatric cancer pet, without feeling shame regardless of the outcome. We must be able to make recommendations and, when the outcome is not what we anticipated, it can be a sinker, but we need to accept that we cannot save them all.

When a negative situation presents itself, we can allow it to sink us into our Ocean of Shame, where we then look for someone to blame. Once we blame, then judgement shows up. This negative thinking could be externally focused or it could be internally focused. An example would be something like this: I was walking my dog, Iz, the other day. She was super excited to be out. I was having a difficult day with my hands due to a chronic inflammatory disease, and I was frustrated and angry and just plain painful. Iz kept pulling and hurting me. Name: My hands are so weak and painful, this sucks. Blame: It is Iz's fault. She is pulling so much. Judge: She is such a badlybehaved dog. In fact, all Frenchie's are not well behaved. Name, Blame, Judge.

We can allow the sinkers to take us to Name, Blame, Judge, or we can fill our balloons to lift our spirits and go instead to Recognize, Embrace, Connect. This chapter will show you how to find and maintain the path to Recognize, Embrace, Connect.

A few years out of school, I was practicing as a lead veterinarian in a multiple-doctor general focus practice. At that stage in my career, my confidence was good, but I recognized that there was much I still had to learn and become comfortable with. I prided myself in the connection I made with clients, and found peace in empathy and in helping to guide each owner through the journey of caring for their pet. I was content, but still in the honeymoon stage of my veterinary career. I had not yet spiraled down into the negative world that was to come in the not so distant future.

Then I met a client and patient I will never forget – the client and patient that made me start to question myself, the profession, and the world. This was my introduction to the Ocean of Shame, sinkers, and wellness balloons.

To help understand the dynamics of managing these emotions, let us look at a case. This is a real case, however details have been altered to provide privacy to the client and pet.

George's Case

The patient was a 12-year-old male orange domestic shorthair tabby cat who presented for on/off inappetence and weight loss, which progressed quickly into not eating at all and vomiting. We will call him "George." George's owner was a woman who was in her mid-30s, living alone with no significant other, kids, or direct family nearby. Her job and George were her life. We will call her "Sarah." Sarah came in sick with worry for George. She had wanted to bring him in earlier, but she was busy with her job. With the current immediate change, she finally made it a priority.

I went in to work up a vomiting and anorectic middle age DSH cat. Through history and physical exam, I made the decision to start with blood work and radiographs. At the time, an ultrasound was not a readily available diagnostic tool in a GP setting; it would have required a referral. Blood work was fairly unremarkable, with the exception of evidence of a little dehydration. Unfortunately, this was not a case to review the medicine; this was a case to look at the emotions involved.

The radiographs showed clear evidence of a density in the intestine, suggestive of a foreign body or mass. When I discussed these results with Sarah, she clearly remembered that one of his toys was missing. With this news, there was a high chance that the toy was what we were seeing. Maybe he had eaten it and it remained in the stomach, causing minimal clinical signs and recently moved into the intestine to cause more of an issue. It was a good theory, however my veterinary "gut feeling" sensed it was more than that. We all know that "gut feeling" where we cannot quite explain it, it makes really no sense, has no analytical evidence to support, but yet we feel it, deep in our gut. This was not going to be a foreign body.

Sarah and I made the decision to do an exploratory surgery and then move forward from there as indicated. The first place of the "what ifs" presents themselves. Some would question why I did not push to refer for an abdominal ultrasound before surgery? Enter a sinker of the unknown; did I make the right recommendation type? When I discussed it with the Sarah, an ultrasound would not have changed going forward to surgery. Therefore, an estimate was presented based on suspected foreign body removal and after care. George otherwise was rather stable and so appeared to have a positive prognosis at that time. We adjusted our day to squeeze George in and moved forward. George stabilizes into anesthesia beautifully and we prep him for the exploratory procedure. During the exploratory surgery, I start to palpate George's bowel and immediately find the "density" we saw on radiographs. My heart drops; it is not a foreign body, but a mass. My gut feeling was right and now I have the sinking feeling this is more than "just an isolated easy to remove mass." A mass can always be one of three things: inflammatory, infection, or cancer, and my gut was leaning on cancer. I examined the entire bowel and found no other lesions, not one. In addition, the lymph nodes all appeared normal. I knew these findings did not rule out microscopic disease, although the lungs were also clear on the radiographs we had taken earlier.

Now I have that call to make. "Hello, I am in surgery and I found more than what we thought." That dreaded "your pet may have cancer" talk, while the pet is under anesthesia and we need to make a decision now with limited information. I have my team dial the owner on the phone and put it on speaker so that I do not have to scrub out. Thankfully Sarah answered on the second ring.

How do you start that conversation? Well there is no easy way to break the news; "I found something, and it is bad." I shared what I found and the decision we were in. I discussed the types of cancer it could be, how it is an isolated lesion and so could be an inflammatory response to something, although infection was low on my list. Again, my gut feeling said to me – this is lymphoma, but that was a "gut" feeling and I had nothing to confirm that and I very well could be wrong. Sarah was obviously upset and we discussed all outcomes but, again, George is under anesthesia and so we have a bit of urgency to make a decision. She then asks me the question I dread: "What would you do?" Why do I hate that question? Because I do not want that pressure. I am doing my best to give her what I know, but I cannot make that decision for her to stop or move forward. I get why people ask us. Asking us this, I recognize, shows such a value in our opinion and a trust in us, but personally, I hate it. I hate having this cat's future in my next few words. Will I tell her the right thing? What if I am wrong and it isn't cancer? What if I am right and we do surgery only to have him crash 10 days later? I think you can each go through the "what ifs" that circled in that 15 seconds as she waited for my answer.

I told her that I would remove the mass and submit it for histopathology and then decide from there. I explained that without knowing what it was I did not know if she would have a fully recovered pet or if we would be still making hard decisions in the future. Oh, and did I mention she did have a limit of funds, enough for the surgery, but that was about it? If it was cancer, oncology therapy would be very limited. This was a time before the amazing financial supports we now have available and she did not have insurance on George. Therefore, I had all that on my mind as well. She agrees to remove the mass, find out what it is, then cross the next bridge.

With George's blood work and other parameters looking well, seeing no evidence of disease in the lungs or lymph nodes or anywhere else in the bowel, I hung on to the hope that maybe this was a local smooth cell tumor and we caught it. It was a stretch, but I was holding on to it. I excised a large section to manage the possibility for local infiltration, closed him up and woke him up. He recovered beautifully, we designed a recovery plan for him postop and he was textbook in his recovery. We sent the mass out to histopathology, but knew it would take 5–7 days to have full results, as it was a large sample.

George's postop week was amazing. He was right on track in his recovery. Sarah shared that he was back to himself, begging for food, and greeting her at the door. I was starting to believe that my gut feeling had been wrong. In the end, I think you know where this is going. I was not wrong. The histopathology came back as lymphoma. Again, my heart sank and I would have to have another difficult conversation with Sarah. George was scheduled for a recheck in the next 48 hours, and I elected to wait until then to discuss the results in person. I knew that calling Sarah would worry her, and since George was still recovering from surgery, nothing was going to change in his therapy for a least another 5 days. Maybe that was the wrong decision. Enter yet another sinker for the case.

When I walked into the exam room, Sarah knew that the results in my hand were bad news. This is when she truly broke down. I knew that Sarah did not have the means to move forward with aggressive therapy, but I encouraged her to go to an oncologist for a consult and hear the options and prognosis. She made an appointment with the local Vet School for the following week. As for George, he was doing surprisingly well. We made a recheck appointment for the day after her appointment with the oncology department so that we could discuss the next steps.

At that appointment, she confirmed she was at limited resources and just wanted to support George to be comfortable. We made a plan and moved forward. For 4 months, he did more than fabulous, he thrived. Sarah was very happy, but in my heart I knew that the moment would come when George would start to decline. I hoped it would be many months away, but my hope was short lived. Five months postop, clinical signs started to return. Six months postop, I could feel thickening in the bowel on external palpation. We entered the stage of managing his clinical signs for comfort. We were able to help him for a couple of months as he continued to move toward his final weeks and days. The day finally came when Sarah made the decision to stop.

Euthanasia is always a very difficult decision. Did we wait too long, did we jump too soon? When clients asked for guidance, we used to say "When there are more bad than good moments" or "You know your pet, you will know, they will tell you." Today we have great tools to provide to clients, to help them determine their pet's quality of life.

After more than 10 years why do I remember this case so well? I remember it because I question every decision that I made. I went to a place of failure and shame, not because I didn't do a good job, but because I did not know if it was the "right" path. The sinkers came at me and, at the time, I did not know how to offset those sinkers with wellness balloons. George and Sarah had a profound effect on me as an individual and as a veterinarian.

After we supported George to his final resting place, I questioned so much of what I had done. Did I check for this? Did I check for that? Why did I move forward when I felt it was bad? Why did I refer her to an oncologist when you knew she couldn't afford it? Why did I…? Today I can see I did the best that I could and easily there were many ways the case could have gone, but I feel truly confident that it took the path it was meant to take for George, Sarah, and myself. I was vested in George the minute the owner asked me, "What would you do?"

To be sustainable in our chosen veterinary career, it is not just about the client and the pet. We need to look at what the veterinarian and the team need to understand in order to manage the sinkers, including the what ifs, navigating the unknown, and how to handle the feeling of failure or of having made the wrong decision.

Caregiver's guilt is a reality in our profession. There is a difference between guilt and shame. Guilt is about our behavior and shame is about who we are. Brene Brown, in her study of shame, says, "Recognizing we made a mistake, is far different than believing we are a mistake."

As I navigated George's case, the sinkers did not bring me toward my Ocean of Guilt, but instead to my Ocean of Shame. A painful, lonely place. Because I did not offset the shame with balloon filling, the experience sank me to a dark place on the bottom of my personal ocean floor.

There is another type of sinker to think of and that is moving from the cure mentality to embracing comfort and end of life care. This provides a sinker in a different way. Much of my vet school years had the primary focus on learning prevention of disease and how to treat and cure disease. I received education on pain management control, antiemesis support, surgical approaches, nutrition support, and other approaches to the "maintenance" of disease. However, little was provided to me in developing my resiliency in managing my personal emotional sinkers that these types of cases provided to me. Slowly but surely, as those sinkers developed and I fell more and more into the negative cynical place, I fell into the Name, Blame, Judge way of life. Vilifying the client, I became angry and cynical at the lack of support available to the patient. I started to disconnect and then begin to believe that I was a failure. I started to hate everyone and literally lost my faith in humanity.

Prioritizing Quality of Life

Shifting the idea of "quality of life" versus "cure" was something required of me to help learn to manage the emotional toll these cases took on me. I would fall into the pattern of "research superhero," meaning I would look for every option available and talk to everyone I knew to ensure that I was doing everything I could. I know now that there is no "perfect" way to manage these cases. Forgiving myself that I did not have all the answers, that I did not have the cure, and that sometimes I just made them comfortable, was an effort of acceptance. Shifting from "cure" to "comfort" meant recognizing that my value as a veterinarian was not defined by how long the pet lived. It was defined by the connection I made with the client and pet, and then the support I provided in navigating the unknown space as we traveled toward the end of life with the goal of providing a good death. Because that is the reality of it, death is the end but we can raise our purpose and meaning with the goal of providing a good death for the pet. Hard to hear, but in truth that is where much comfort started. My value is not in keeping things alive, it is in allowing the connection and transition between life and death to occur as best it can in the current moment.

I recognized that the pet's death was not my fault and I also accept euthanasia in my professional career. That doesn't mean the sinkers don't present themselves along the way. Recognizing the sinkers and embracing them was the first step in finding the path to resiliency. In order to embrace the sinkers, I found it required self-forgiveness. Please do not get me wrong, I challenged myself in every case and I am not suggesting we do not do that in this profession. What I am suggesting is not letting each case like George's define our worth. Learn how to prevent the sinkers from taking you to the place of Name, Blame, and Judge.

For each of us it is an individualized journey, and for each of us we will have our own sinkers. I like to call it managing through our tunnels of experiences and developing personalized wounds as we each navigate these tunnels. Same tunnels, yet we each come out with different wounds. Therefore, what may sink me to the bottom of my shame ocean could have minimal to no effect on someone else. Name, Blame, Judge shows up when we compare ours or other responses to the tunnel we navigate through. There is no right or wrong way in how the sinkers affect us. This is why I note that the first step is to embrace the sinkers. Recognizing that we are normal and moving away from the need to "suck it up." These sinkers have an effect on us and the first step is recognizing that we are not robots, but in fact humans who can withstand only so many sinkers for only so long.

Filling Our Well-Being Balloons

How do we offset the sinkers? No matter how hard you try to turn a blind eye or ignore them, the sinkers present themselves every day to each of us in this profession. This is where our wellness balloons come in. As mentioned at the start of this chapter, these balloons are what keep us from sinking in our Ocean of Shame. They are broken down into emotional, spiritual, mental, and physical balloons. Just as only we know our own sinkers, only we know how to fill our own personal wellness balloons.

In choosing a career in veterinary medicine, the human–animal bond is a strong force and has a direct effect on the accumulation of sinkers and on our balloon filling. Every day we are going to be presented with perceived threats and the deeper we are in our shame ocean, the more difficult it is to manage those threats. Taking the time to determine how to fill *our* wellness balloons is critical to our survival in this profession. We cannot stop the sinkers from coming. However, when we stop filling our wellness balloons is when we allow the sinkers to take us to the bottom of the ocean.

The Brown Gauze Moment

Now we are going to take the time to define a perceived threat. This is something that we believe is happening where our amygdala is telling us we are in danger. This will often elicit a physiological response and cause the fight, freeze, or flight reaction. To help provide an understanding of what a perceived threat is, I am going to share my "brown gauze moment." This moment helps to describe the struggle of managing perceived threats while beginning to sink in the ocean, yet helps to normalize the fact that I can only do so much and I am a human being with only so much to give. We all have had these moments, and talking about them helps to provide recognition that we are not alone and normal.

At the time, I was working in a busy corporate general medicine focused practice. Working primarily by myself, seeing about 40–50 patients a day. For anyone in a GP practice, I think you can already assume I was busy, in fact the hospital was so busy and had grown so quickly that we had stopped taking new clients for six months and still continued to grow in revenue. Some may say a good problem to have, yet it was becoming harder and harder to manage the demand.

This day starts out as the day that we all know and hate. Three technicians called in sick and my dental machine broke down. I had three procedures that I didn't expect to come in: one was a hit by a car, nothing major, but still took my time to stabilize and send off to a referral hospital; the next a diabetic, not in ketoacidotic crisis, but again still took significant time to talk the owners through their new normal for their pet; etc.

All day I heard: "Dr. Pope, can you look at this blood work?" and "Dr. Pope, so and so is on line four," and "Dr. Pope, those people that you just talked to for 30 minutes are going on vacation, they can't do anything that you just told them to do," and "Dr. Pope, they can't give oral meds," and "Dr. Pope, the X-ray light is broken," and "Dr. Pope, can you now talk to the husband?"

I think you can get the theme of the day; my name rang through the hospital about every 30 seconds with the demands of my decision making and the fact of being the only veterinarian in the building. Almost every decision was coming down to me, and there were many. This was the no-pee, no-drink, no-eat 10–12-hour day. I am at the end of that day, that beautiful moment where no more of those questions/requests will come my way. I still get to enjoy four hours of doing my records, but I get to be left alone and do them in solitude.

What led up to my "brown gauze moment" is that I stopped filling any balloons because I felt the pressure of all these perceived threats building throughout the day. Every single one of them was a sinker pulling me into my shame ocean. At this point, all I had left to do was a bandage change in room four. It was a routine bandage change. In fact, they had already checked the patient out. The cat was super easy, the clients were amazing; it was a dream last appointment.

Normally I would have just done an exam, touched base with the owners, and then my technician would have come in to do the bandage change. However, I did not have a registered technician there that evening because they called in sick; I had to change the bandage myself. I asked my assistant to get my bandage tote and I prepared myself to enter the room.

Typically, we would use brown gauze in this type of bandage. We specified brown gauze for a number of things in the hospital, including securing endotracheal tubes, e-collar support, etc. Brown gauze is a staple supply to our day-to-day activities in the hospital. However, it was Friday and the order did not come until Tuesday. Being a part of a corporate practice, we do not have substitutes for my core products. You guessed it – there was no brown gauze in the tote! I told my assistant to get the brown gauze and they said; "We don't have brown gauze." An immediate frown came to my face as I asked them to check again.

With their next response, I walked to the treatment area and opened every cabinet, every drawer, even the syringe drawers. I literally pulled everything out. After my mad search for brown gauze, the hospital looked like a tornado had hit it. I was not cussing, swearing, or throwing things, but I was having a moment. I sank to the bottom of my shame ocean in an instant. As I was drowning, I was looking to grab on to anything to cut the sinker. Everything I supported up to that point in my career and my value to the human–animal bond was worth nothing, because I did not have brown gauze to perform the bandage change on that cat in that moment. I was a horrible veterinarian because I could not do the bandage the "right way" and I was a horrible lead doctor because I could not keep my hospital properly stocked. That sinker took me to Name, Blame, Judge. Who does the order? How does this happen? Looking to point the finger where ever I could, because I needed to blame someone for my sinker.

I turned around and saw what I have done and could not believe it. Somehow, I had managed to perform the bandage change without brown gauze!

Going forward, when my team saw that I was getting riled up and needed to go fill a wellness balloon, they would put a little brown gauze next to my computer station. In doing so, they gave me permission to take care of myself – to go fill a balloon.

We must find permission to allow ourselves to fill our own balloons. We must stop going to Name, Blame, Judge and start the journey to Recognize, Embrace, Connect. People do not judge me for that day and can often think of their own brown gauze moment. If they did not judge me, why did I judge myself?

The brown gauze moment helps to simplify and understand the effects of sinkers and provide visibility into how balloons are our lifeline to sustainability. We cannot stop the sinkers and it is easy to have the pressure take us to a place to justify in stopping to fill our balloons. Name, Blame, Judge allows us to be a victim and point the finger on everything else around us.

The goal of this chapter is to be the bridge to start to help each of us recognize that we have the permission to recognize our sinkers, embrace our emotions, and connect with our balloons and passion. We are all just working to move forward in this career and in life. Finding our individualized path to that sustainable authentic career is our unique path. In the end, we are normal and we are not alone.

Mindfulness

Have things around you to remind you to fill a balloon in the moment of a heavy sinker. The things might be jewelry (wedding ring, for example), pictures of places, people, pets you have saved, smells that connect with emotions, quotes, tattoos, or a piece of brown gauze. Whatever speaks to you.

Make time to offset your sinkers by filling your wellness balloons. Mindfulness, positive psychology, religion, exercise, yoga, meditation, spending time in nature, bonding with a family for the lifetime care of their pet, watching your children learn the value of life, spending time with friends, whatever fills your balloon you have permission to fill them.

Summary

We make the decision to connect with life and with the lives around us every day. At the end of the day we each have control over our actions, we create our environment, we have a right to our emotions, and in the end, self-forgiveness is the foundation to a career in veterinary medicine. My brown gauze moment and the George case do not define my worth as a veterinarian or as a human being.

This profession is hard! Making a commitment to managing end of life cases puts an added pressure to the sinkers. Choosing a path to resiliency is not easy, yet the path of falling into Name, Blame, and Judge is not working for us. Find the path to Recognize, Embrace, and Connect. We are all One Life Connected. Let us all make the commitment to find the path away from Name, Blame, Judge and start moving towards Recognize, Embrace, Connect.

You, the veterinarian who works in this space of end of life, should recognize that when you feel sinkers pulling you into the Ocean of Shame, you are not alone and you are normal. Now, you will give yourself permission to find your individualized journey, while counteracting the "sinkers" that will inevitably arise by filling your "well-being balloons." You will be able to maintain that sustainable authentic career you desired when you entered into veterinary medicine and when you chose a path that includes end of life care.

Appendix 1: Specific Tumor Protocols

SKIN CANCER
Mast Cell Cancer

Dx	Sx	RTx	CTx
• FNA all tumors prior to Sx to rule out MCT. • Recently diagnosed MCT is generally confined to the skin in dogs (dermoepidermal); therefore, aspirates of spleen, liver, and bone marrow are generally negative in dogs. • Buffy coat smears are considered useless in early canine disease. • For more prognostic information, order the "MCT Panel." It stains for KIT, Ki-67, PCNA, Agnors, and IDT mutation analysis. It is available from Michigan State University and the Animal Medical Center laboratories. • It is acceptable to proceed with CTx when indicated without complete staging.	• If narrow or dirty margins at first Sx, a second Sx is indicated. • Follow the soft tissue sarcoma protocol for wide and deep excision of all grade II and higher grade cases. At least 2 cm lateral margins and one deep tissue plane below the mass is desired. Prefer more aggressive margins (3 cm) for grade III tumors. • Sx for stage I–II mast cell tumors with histologic grade I and II (excluding scrotal, muzzle, and distal extremities) that yielded 2 cm lateral clean margins and clean deep margins of one fascial plane provided 90% cure rates (Fulcher, R.P., et al. 2015. *JAVMA* 228 (2):210–215). • PREMEDICATE DOGS WTH BENADRYL BEFORE SURGERY. • Electrochemotherapy (ECT)/Electroporation (EP) of small lesions bleomycin given at 15 U/m² IV, and wait 7 minutes prior to ECT/EP or bleomycin given intralesional just prior to ECT/EP as per Chapter 6.	• RTx or CTx provides 90% cure rate when used for stage I–II mast cell tumors with histologic grade I and II. • RTx and/or CTx recommended for patients with high grade II and grade III MCT with narrow or dirty margins and unresectable lesions. Evaluation of local nodes, spleen, liver, and bone marrow is recommended for staging if elected. NOTE: Intralesional injections have been very successful in reducing MCTs. Use patient serum mixed with equal volume of dexamethasone SP. Distribute the solution evenly into the tumor weekly × 4 then q 14 d × 4. Triamcinolone is also used IL q 21 d.	• Pepcid® (famotidine) 0.5 mg kg PO SID or BID on an empty stomach OR cimetidine at 5–10 mg/kg PO TID. • Prednisone 40–50 mg/m² PO SID × 7 days, then 20–25 mg/m² q 48 hours for 6 months. • Leukeran® (chlorambucil): Dogs: 0.2 mg/kg or 6 mg/m² (dogs) q 48 hours. Cats: 2 mg q 48–72 hours or 20 mg/m² q 14 days. • Grade III or resistant cases: Dogs: Lomustine 40–90 mg/m² over 4–5 days q 21 days. Cats: 10 mg over 4–5 days q 30–42 days. CBC before each dose. • Metronomic CTx also effective. • Vinblastine IV at 1.45–2 mg/m². • Toceranib at 2.5 mg/kg MWF to start, dose escalate to 3.25 mg. • Expect recurrence within 6–7 months in high grade II–III. Unresectable grade III with metastases have poor Px without treatment. Some treated cases may respond or stabilize.

Canine and Feline Geriatric Oncology: Honoring the Human–Animal Bond. Second Edition. Alice Villalobos with Laurie Kaplan.
© 2018 John Wiley & Sons, Inc. Published 2018 by John Wiley & Sons, Inc.

SKIN CANCER (*Continued*)
Solar-Induced Squamous Cell Carcinoma

Sx	RTx	CTx
• Cryotherapy is excellent for carcinoma in situ lesions, eyelid lesions, etc. • Excisional biopsy with clean margins is often curative: nosectomy, pinnectomy, resection of bulky lesions, and so forth. • Sx is used for reconstruction and grafting after curative Sx. • Electrochemotherapy/electroporation is an excellent option for deep lesions. See Chapter 6.	• Used as primary treatment to spare structures such as nasal planum and eyes. Not used for pinnae lesions. • Strontium 90 probe is helpful in focal superficial lesions such as Bowen's disease. • Remind clients to use sunscreen and/or shelter the pet from the sun between 10:00 a.m. and 2:00 p.m.	• Imiquimod (Aldara®) topical ointment BID for in situ lesions in cats and dogs. • Systemic CTx is rarely used. May try carboplatin and mitoxantrone (as RTx enhancer) for cats. • Capecitabine (Xeloda®) PO at 250 mg/m²/day in dogs only may help (NEVER in cats!). • Retinoids may be helpful in some cases. • Bleomycin or IL cisplatin for electroporation

Cutaneous Hemangiosarcoma

Sx	RTx	CTx
• Initial superficial multifocal macular lesions are well controlled with cryosurgery. • Excisional biopsy with clean margins is often curative for resection of larger, deeper blood-filled lesions. NOTE: These may metastasize!	No information. Lesions are often too numerous and superficial for external beam approach. • Strontium 90 probe may be helpful. • Remind client to use sunscreen and/or shelter pet from sun between 10:00 a.m. and 2:00 p.m.	Not used when tumor is in superficial stages. • Adriamycin or VAC protocol or carboplatin may help cases with metastatic disease.

MAMMARY CANCER

Sx	RTx	CTx
Sx is generally the best treatment unless there are cutaneous inflammatory lesions radiating outward. • In dogs, perform simple, regional, or unilateral mastectomy. Try to acquire deep and wide margins equal to tumor diameter. Send to Innogenics for detailed Dx, and Tx advice. • In cats, remove the involved mammary chain first and follow with excision of the remaining mammary chain in 3–4 weeks. Histopathology will determine the extent of lymph node involvement. • Esophageal feeding tube if cat is anorectic.	RTx of any type is seldom used for mammary tumors in canine and feline patients. It may increase tumor-free intervals and reduce local recurrence in difficult cases. • Immunocidin™ has been approved for intralesional immunotherapy (ImTx) of mammary tumors in dogs. • Check on availability of novel therapies.	CTx is indicated for solid, inflammatory, metastatic, and high grade tumors. Use the carcinoma protocols suggested in Chapter 6. • Mitoxantrone at 5–6 mg/m² is preferred over Adriamycin at 30 mg/m² in dogs and 1 mg/kg in cats/small dogs q 21 days. • Carboplatin at 300 mg/m² in dogs and at 10 mg/kg or 180 mg/m² q 21 days for cats. • Gemzar® at 200–830 mg/m² start low and use dose escalation. • Xeloda (dogs only) at 250 mg/50 BID × 10 days q 21 days, or metronomic 250 mg/m²/day.

SOFT TISSUE SARCOMAS

Sx	RTx	CTx
• Excisional biopsy should have at least 2 cm (optimally 3 cm) margins around the mass and at least 1–2 fascial planes on all deep margins. • If margins are dirty, expect recurrence • CT or MRI for ambiguous and fixed masses prior to Sx. Send Bx for Enlight™ Assay. • Mass can be debulked and tumor bed treated with ECT/Electroporation (EP) bleomycin 15 U/m² IV, wait 7 minutes prior to ECT/EP or give bleomycin IL just prior to delivering impulse as per last section Chapter 6.	• As first line therapy for inoperable masses. • Used as palliation. • Used prior to Sx to shrink tumors to increase tumor-free interval. • Used intraoperatively to kill residual cells. • Used following Sx delivered to a wide field to sterilize tumor beds, especially if resection was inadequate or residual disease remains. • Stereotactic radiation is an excellent option that can deliver the definitive dose in 1–3 fractions for difficult to access masses.	• Carboplatin and/or Adriamycin are helpful at doses discussed above. • Piroxicam, Metacam, and other NSAIDs for their antiangiogenesis action. • Metronomic lomustine at 4 mg/m²/day. • Antiangiogenic agents: AngioStop protocol. • Tyrosine kinase inhibitors: masitinib or toceranib in combination with above PO Rx. • Ifosfamide IV with mesna-diuresis q 21 days. • Check for new small molecule drugs, novel therapies, and ImTx vaccines such as IFx.

CUTANEOUS LYMPHOMA (MYCOSIS FUNGOIDES, MF)

Sx	RTx	CTx
Sx is rarely helpful if lesions are in the oral cavity and mucocutaneous junctions. Sx used for diagnostic purposes. Cryotherapy for multiple lesions and selected lesions in lips and gingiva may help. Electrochemotherapy/electroporation of lesions bleomycin IV at 15 U/m², wait 7 minutes prior to ECT/EP procedure to treat multiple lesions. See ECT/EP in last section of Chapter 6.	RTx may be helpful in solitary lesions and for palliation. Half-body irradiation may theoretically help but is unproven.	CTx is the primary treatment for MF. • Dogs: prednisone 0.5–1 mg/number on days that oil is given (see * below) and lomustine 40–90 mg/m² divided over 4–7 days. Repeat every 21–30 days if CBC allows. Monitor patients for oral and mucocutaneous lesions. • Cats: prednisone at 5 mg BID and lomustine at 10 mg (divided over 4 days) every 4–6 weeks if CBC allows. • NOTE: Metronomic lomustine may be used. • Tanovea® 1 mg/kg IV in 30 min q 21 days. • High % safflower oil is helpful. – Dogs: 3 ml/kg high % linoleic e-sutras safflower oil, fed on 3 consecutive days/week. www.esutras.com. *Cats: 3–4 capsules of oil of evening primrose, twice daily for linolenic acid.

LYMPHOMA

	Rescue
CTx with (CHOP) Adriamycin-based protocols yields the longest survival data observed in dogs (14 months). Consider a permanent maintenance protocol well into the second year. One-third of responding patients may survive 2+ years. Tanovea™ is a new drug that may be used as first line or as rescue.	Repeat above induction protocols or use rescue protocols in Section C of Table 6.2. Tanovea™ 1 mg/kg IV q 21 days

Protocol

Use modified Wisconsin or CHOP-based protocols (see Tables A.1 and 6.2). Phenotyping (T- versus B-cell) with: IH stains, PARR, flow cytometry, Enlight Assay™.

For T-cell lymphomas, mitoxantrone may be more effective than Adriamycin. Metformin starting at 25 mg/m^2 and increasing to 500 mg/m^2 BID may reduce CTx resistance.

Maintenance

Start maintenance protocol with a 2-week interval for dogs and 10-day interval for cats and all dogs that presented with a high tumor burden or organomegaly. Rotate Oncovin®, Cytoxan, Oncovin, Leukeran, Oncovin, Cytoxan, Oncovin, chlorambucil (Leukeran), etc., for 2 years. Theoretically, the last tumor cell cannot be killed using low-toxicity CTx preferred for geriatric pets. This is the rationale for permanent maintenance CTx.

- Use Leukeran at 1.4 mg/kg divided PO over 2 days or at 10 mg/m^2 PO on 2 consecutive days only: as on the rotation schedule.
- If oral Cytoxan causes GI signs or hemorrhagic cystitis, Leukeran is used in its place.
- To increase visit intervals:
  – Use Leukeran and then Cytoxan in a 10- to 14-day rotation between Oncovin treatments.
  – Give Oncovin IV.
  – 2 weeks later give Leukeran PO.
  – 2 weeks after that give Cytoxan PO with 20 mg/m^2 prednisone and large bowl of broth in the morning before walk to encourage urination.
  – The recheck visit and CBC for Oncovin follows in 2 weeks.
- Each drug is rotated at 2-week intervals. To taper this schedule further, intervals between drugs may be increased to $2\frac{1}{2}$ to 3 weeks apart. Other effective PO drugs: lomustine, melphalan, procarbazine, may be rotated into the schedule to extend the interval between recheck visits. Need CBC q 4–6 weeks.

Table A.1. Dr. Villalobos's Modified Madison/Wisconsin Protocol for Lymphoma for Large/Giant Geriatric Dogs, Featuring "Split Dose" Administration of Adriamycin

Day	Drug	Canine Dosage	Feline Dosage
Day 1	Oncovin®	0.7 mg/m² IV diluted, slow bolus	0.025 mg/kg or 0.5 mg/m² IV diluted, slowly
	L-Asparaginase® (use pretreatment)	10,000–30,000 IU/m² IM in 2 locations	400 IU/kg or 2,000 IU SQ
	Prednisone crushed in food in a.m.	30 mg/m² daily × 7 days, all in a.m.	5 mg BID PO (forever)
Day 8 (week 2)	Cytoxan® (give in morning with prednisone and broth, 20–30 min before urination)	100 mg/m² PO with broth in a.m. before walking dog to encourage urination	25 mg tablet PO with 6 ml water chaser
Day 9	Cytoxan® (give in morning with prednisone and broth, 20–30 min before urination)	100 mg/m² PO with broth in a.m. before walking dog to encourage urination	25 mg tablet PO with 6 ml water chaser
	Prednisone (use gastroprotective medication)	20 mg/m² daily × 7 days in the morning	Continue 5 mg BID for one year
Day 15* Start of week 3	Adriamycin® (with pretreatment) 15–20 minute slow IV infusion for dogs	Small or frail dogs: <9 kg: 1 mg/kg IV Dogs up to 25 kg: 30 mg/m² IV once *Large/giant: 20 mg/m² IV first dose	1 mg/kg IV over 7–10 min (pretreat with 0.1 ml dexamethasone)
	Use extreme caution, vasosclerotic!		
	Prednisone (use gastroprotective medication)	10 mg/m² daily × 7 days (dogs), then discontinue: give on Cytoxan days	Continue 5 mg BID PO for one year
Day 20 or 22	Adriamycin at 20 mg/m² (with pretreatment) Second split dose for large dogs >25 kg	Repeat day 15 for large/giant dogs Second dose on split dose protocol	No treatment but continue prednisone BID
Day 22 week 4	Oncovin®	0.7 mg/m² IV diluted, slow bolus	0.025 mg/kg or 0.5 mg/m² IV diluted, slowly
Day 29	Cytoxan® (give in morning with prednisone and broth, 20–30 min before urination)	100 mg/m² PO with broth in a.m. before walking dog to encourage urination	25 mg tablet PO with 6 ml water chaser
Day 30	Cytoxan® (give in morning with prednisone and broth, 20–30 min before urination)	100 mg/m² PO with broth in a.m. before walking dog to encourage urination	25 mg tablet PO with 6 ml water chaser
Day 36	Adriamycin (with pretreatment)	Repeat as day 15 for <10, <25, >25 kg	1 mg/kg IV slow 7–10 min. PreTx as above
Day 41 or 43	Adriamycin at 20 mg/m² (with pretreatment) Second split dose for large dogs >25 kg	Repeat day 15 for large/giant dogs Second dose on split dose protocol	No treatment but continue prednisone BID
Day 43 week 7	Oncovin®	0.7 mg/m² IV diluted, slow bolus	0.025 mg/kg or 0.5 mg/m² IV diluted, slowly
Day 58 and 59	Cytoxan® repeat 2 days q 30 days maintenance	100 mg/m² PO with broth in a.m.	25 mg tablet PO, repeat 2 days monthly
Day 72 week 11	Oncovin® repeat monthly as maintenance	0.7 mg/m² IV slow bolus, monthly	Maintenance for cats: oncovin or Adria q 30 days
Day 86 and 87	Chlorambucil PO repeat divided dose monthly	1.4 mg/kg divided over 2 days PO	1.4 mg/kg PO divided over 2 days q 30 days
Maintenance a	Recheck monthly: Oncovin IV, rotate PO Rx	Chlorambucil or cytoxan 2 weeks later with	Similar maintenance for cats with lymphoma
Maintenance b	Recheck q 6 weeks Oncovin IV follow in 14 days	Chlorambucil, and Cytoxan in 14 days	Then recheck in 14 days. Continue sequence.

HEAD AND NECK TUMORS

	Sx	RTx	CTx ± Immunotherapy (ImTx)
Canine Oral Cancer Malignant melanoma (MM): 30–40% Most (67%) are pigmented and appear on gingiva, lips, buccal mucosa 57% involve bone Up to 92% metastasize to local nodes and lungs Squamous cell carcinoma (SCC) 17–25% incidence Most appear on rostral mandible but can be located anywhere 77% involve bone Tonsillar SCC: rare but aggressive Fibrosarcoma (FSA); 8–25% Most appear in maxillary gingiva, hard palate, buccal mucosa 60–72% involve bone Acanthomatous Epulis (AE): 5% 80–100% involve bone (from Table 21-1, *SACO*, 4th edn, P. 456)	MRI or CT scan to determine extent of disease prior to Sx and or RTx is highly recommended. Mandibulectomy or maxillectomy with clean margins of at least 2 cm is first choice therapy for oral tumors if margins are possible. Electrochemotherapy (ECT)/electroporation (EP) of large difficult to remove oral tumors may be very helpful. Bleomycin 15 U/m² IV, wait 7 minutes prior to ECT/EP or bleomycin given intralesional just prior to ECT/EP per Chapter 6 Cryotherapy may control some AEs that are under 2 cm.	RTx to the primary tumor bed and draining neck nodes is indicated. Intralesional CTx and intraoperative RTx may provide additional local tumor control. Stereotactic radiation therapy	Chest X-rays recommended q 4–6 months for malignant melanoma. Carboplatin at 300 mg/m² in dogs every 3 weeks yielded 68% objective response in MM at UCD as per Dr. Carlos Rodriguez (*VCS Proceedings*, October 1992, p. 59). MM is highly metastatic. Follow Sx and RTx with systemic treatment and/or immunotherapy. Merial's Oncept is a xenogenic human tyrosinase vaccine that is USDA approved for malignant melanoma in dogs. Best after complete excision. Tumor tissue can be harvested from all oral tumors at Sx and submitted for IFx vaccine production.
Feline Mandibular SCC Prepare carers to expect a poor Px. However, cats with rostral lesions may have long-term survival with: Sx, RTx, CTx combo	Sx mandibulectomy (Mdx) and esophageal feeding tube ECT/EP is a non-invasive option as described above and as per the last section of Chapter 6.	RTx follow-up post-Mdx to include primary site and neck nodes.	CTx with carboplatin or use mitoxantrone as a radiation sensitizer. Zoledronate and meloxicam combo may reduce bone invasion.
Feline Lingual SCC Proliferative ulcerated lesions appear on the tongue, pharynx, and tonsils Very poor Px, 90 days ST	Sx for esophageal feeding tube to offset starvation and wasting No consistent treatment has extended life for affected cats.	Poor response	CTx not effective. Use pain control! Piroxicam: 1 mg PO q 48 hours or Metacam: 1–2 drops q 24–48 hours. Buprenorphine PO, pain patches, Nalbuphine at 0.1 ml diluted to l ml, give 0.1 ml SQ q 6–8 hours.

HEAD AND NECK TUMORS (*Continued*)

	Sx	RTx	CTx ± Immunotherapy (ImTx)
Feline Maxillary SCC Prepare carers to expect a poor Px. However, cats with rostral lesions may have long-term survival with a combination of Sx, RTx, and CTx.	Sx with aggressive maxillectomy may help some cases with more rostral location, but wide margins are difficult in cats and recurrence is common. ECT/EP is a non-invasive option as described above.	RTx with palliative protocols using mitoxantrone enhancement may occasionally yield excellent but temporary results. Monthly palliative booster RTx may extend survival times in some cases. Stereotactic radiation may be an excellent option.	CTx may yield some stable or partial clinical responses with a rotation of carboplatin/Adriamycin or carboplatin/mitoxantrone every 2–4 weeks. Monitor CBC, BUN, and creatinine and SDMA™. • Mitoxantrone at 5–5.5 mg/m² is preferred over Adriamycin. • Carboplatin at 10 mg/kg or 180 mg/m² IV q 21 days. • Gemzar at 200–800 mg/m² IV q 14 days: dose escalate if well. • Check on availability of novel and ImTx vaccine therapies.
Palliative Radiation Therapy for Advanced or Disseminated Head/Neck Cancer		RTx palliation helps cats with nasal planum, facial or oral squamous cell carcinoma and dogs with bulky oral tumors. RTx is given as a short course of 3–4 high dose fractions. The goal is to achieve relief from ulceration and pain in a rapid, effective way. High dose 800–1,000 cGy fractions are delivered on days 0, 7, 21, and 42 and some patients benefit from monthly fractions. Consider stereotactic radiation.	CTx enhancement and/or adjunct IL CTx given prior to RTx may improve tumor control for MM, SCC, FSA, nasal tumors, tonsillar SCC, OSA, etc. Some patients do well with a monthly follow-up using IL CTx and a palliative high-dose RTx fraction. Published data using palliative RTx alone shows 74% of dogs experience pain relief and 25% benefit with extended QoL (VMTH, Guelph, *JVIM* 8, 1994).

HEAD AND NECK TUMORS (*Continued*)

	Sx	RTx	CTx ± Immunotherapy (ImTx)
Nasal Passage Tumors in Dogs No treatment yields 5–7 month survival time.	Sx is used for diagnostic purposes following proper imaging. Rhinotomy alone may reduce survival time. Post-RTx, Sx to remove residual disease is helpful in some cases.	RTx with orthovoltage after rhinotomy yielded 40–45% 1-year survival time (ST). Megavoltage RTx protocols forego rhinotomy using cobalt, linear accelerators, IMRT, etc., for 43–60% 1 year and 11–44% 2 year ST. Stereotactic RTx is an excellent option that may increase survival.	If RTx is declined, recommend a palliation Pawspice program. Treat pain pre-emptively with NSAIDs, etc., to improve QoL. • Use carboplatin for CSA and OSA. For carcinoma, use IV mitoxantrone, carboplatin, Gemzar, or Adriamycin in rotation q 21 days to evaluate for best response. • Xeloda at 250 mg/m² daily PO (do not use Xeloda in cats). • CTx may reduce stridor and nasal discharge.
Nasal Passage Tumors in Cats Most common types: Nasal Respiratory CA, SCC, LSA	Sx is not beneficial.	RTx is indicated for respiratory carcinoma, SCC, and for nasal lymphomas that are presumed to be solitary.	CTx is an excellent option for management of nasal passage tumors in cats. Adriamycin-based protocols are best since lymphoma is often considered a systemic disease by many oncologists. Rotate mitoxantrone, carboplatin, Gemzar, and Adriamycin for carcinomas at doses given in Chapter 6. Look for the best response and then continue the therapy every 21–30 days. Use piroxicam at l mg q 48 hours or meloxicam at 1 drop/4/day for pain control and the anticancer effect of NSAIDs.

HEAD AND NECK TUMORS (*Continued*)

	Sx	RTx	CTx ± Immunotherapy (ImTx)
Brain Tumors Treat symptomatically to control seizures, circling, wandering, disorientation, headache pain, etc.	• Sx is helpful for selected peripheral tumors if MRI or CT scan confirm accessibility. • Meningiomas are most amenable, especially in cats. • Consultation with a neurologist, surgeon, and radiation oncologist is advised if considering specialized brain tumor biopsy procedures.	RTx is helpful for some cases (pituitary macroadenoma, astrocytoma, meningioma), yielding excellent remissions lasting 1 year plus. Stereotactic RTx may be the best option as it can deliver precisely-targeted radiation in fewer high-dose fractions than traditional RTx, which can help preserve healthy brain tissue.	CTx is palliative and may gain responses for lymphoma. Metronomic lomustine: 4 mg/m^2/day or • For dogs: use lomustine at 60 mg/m^2 PO q 21 days divided over 4–5 days, and give high % linoleic eSutras safflower oil at 3 ml/kg on 3 consecutive days per week. www.esutras.com. • For cats: give 3–4 oil of evening primrose capsules (538 mg linolenic) PO q 12 hours and lomustine 2.5 mg daily × 4 days PO q 4–6 weeks. Monitor CBC. • Prednisone at 0.5–1 mg/kg PO q 12–24 hours for relief of CNS edema and inflammation. Dexamethasone PO or SQ may alleviate CNS signs over prednisone for some patients. Must give gastroprotective Rx!

CHEST TUMORS

	Sx	RTx	CTx
Primary Chest Cavity Tumors **Thymoma** **Heart Base Tumors** **Primary Pulmonary Carcinoma** **Tracheal and Esophageal Tumors**	• Lobectomy is helpful if the mass is removed intact and if local nodes are negative. Survival for thymoma may be good if entirely removed. Bronchogenic carcinoma patients may survive 1 year following lobectomy if lymph nodes are negative. Resection of localized esophageal and tracheal tumors may be helpful.	RTx is useful to reduce anterior mediastinal lymphoma and heart base tumors. Stereotactic RTx (SRS) is a good option for localized tumors and heart base tumors.	CTx is palliative in most cases other than granulomatous lymphoma and lymphoma. The use of metronomic (mCTx) lomustine, chlorambucil, cyclophosphamide, toceranib, masitinib, piroxicam, etc., for antiangiogenic effect may help. AngioStop and asparagus: $^1/_2$–1 cap/m^2 q 12 hours: Revivin $^1/_2$–1 cap/m^2/day may extend ST.

CHEST TUMORS (*Continued*)

	Sx	RTx	CTx
Chest Cavity Secondary Tumors (metastases)	• Metastasectomy may be helpful in a subgroup of selected cases where metastatic tumors are limited and amenable to excision.	RTx is generally not used. SRS may be used if metastatic lesion(s) are discrete.	CTx is palliative and occasionally achieves a remission. CTx is individualized for each case. • Carboplatin for its wide range of action against carcinomas and sarcomas and its low toxicity. • Adriamycin, mitoxantrone, Gemzar, Xeloda for carcinoma. • Antiangiogenic Rx as above.

ABDOMINAL TUMORS

	Sx	RTx	CTx
Hemangiosarcoma (HSA) **Splenic Tumors in Dogs** **Common Emergency due to** **Acute Hemoabdomen. Only** **10–15% 1 year ST** **Nodular Hyperplasia** NOTE: 60% of spleens removed from dogs at the University of Minnesota were diagnosed with benign disease.	Sx is used for diagnostics, debulking, and resection of abdominal tumors following appropriate imaging. Splenectomy is commonly performed due to hemoab-domen. If HSA is suspected: • Inform client of poor Px prior to electing Sx. 89 day ST. It is appropriate to stabilize the patient with supportive care and a belly wrap to allow resorption of blood. Some families decline Sx, yet are reluctant to euthanize. They appreciate the option for a home hospice vigil.	• Not used	Use protocols for sarcoma or carcinoma in Chapter 6. Yunnan Baiyo for coagulation action as needed. Check www.modianolab.com for "Liquid Biopsy" early detection test and e-BAT 50 µg/kg for HSA. • For carcinoma: Xeloda at metronomic (mCTx) dose 250 mg/m^2/day PO (dogs only! Not cats!) • Antiangiogenic protocols with mCTx and AngioStop protocol. • Cytoxan at 10 mg/m^2/day. Watch for Cytoxan-induced cystitis. Give with extra fluids (broth) 20–30 min before morning urination. • Chlorambucil at 4 mg/m^2/day or • Lomustine at 4 mg/m^2/day • Masitinib at 12.5 mg/kg BID or • Toceranib at 2–2.5 mg/kg Monday, Wednesday, Friday.

ABDOMINAL TUMORS (*Continued*)

	Sx	RTx	CTx
Mast Cell Tumor (MCT) in cats may be visceral in the spleen or intestine. Up to 26% of splenic dz. in cats is due to MCT. MCT may metastasize to the spleen in dogs with advanced MCT.	• Cats respond well to splenectomy and CTx. • Poor Px for intestinal MCT post Sx.	No information on RTx option for cats with splenic or intestinal MCT. RTx is generally not used for metastatic MCT in abdomen. Consultation with radiation oncologist to determine if RTx can be helpful for an individual patient. Stereotactic RTx may be an excellent option for inoperable localized tumors	• Post MCT Sx cats: prednisone 5 mg q 12 hours • Metronomic Lomustine 3–4 mg/m²/day • Metastatic MCT requires multimodal CTx • Vinblastine at 2 mg/m² IV weekly × 4–6 weeks • Prednisone 40–50 mg/m²/day × 7 days, then 20–25 mg/day × 7 days then q 48 hours • Metronomic (mCTx) and antiangiogenic protocols for carcinomas as described above: – Xeloda at 250 mg/m²/day (Not for cats!) – Cytoxan at 10–12.5 mg/m²/day PO – Piroxicam 10 mg/60 PO or 0.3 mg/kg daily in dogs and 1 mg q 48 hours in cats • Check for updates for novel therapy and HDAC inhibitors (valproic acid, SAHA, and others) for antitumor effect and CTx enhancement.
Renal, Adrenal, Pancreatic Carcinomas	Abdominal ultrasound and CT or MRI imaging to determine extent. Exploratory laparotomy to excise mass when possible or debulk. Tumor tissue may be submitted for vaccine production such as IFx.		

Bladder Cancer

	Sx	CTx
Transitional cell carcinoma (TCC) Use the CADET™ free catch urine assay for early or definitive diagnosis.	Sx is seldom helpful due to extent of mucosal involvement. If mass is apical and confined, Sx may be helpful. Ureteral and or urethral stent placement may be helpful to relieve obstruction. IMRT or stereotactic RTx also called stereotactic radiosurgery (SRS) or Cyber Knife may be helpful.	• Piroxicam provides anti-inflammatory and anticancer benefits in TCC. • Use piroxicam at 0.3 mg/kg daily or 10 mg/60 daily PO for dogs. • For cats: use piroxicam at 1 mg/cat PO q 48 hours. • Use gastroprotective drugs such as famotidine or cimetidine. • Tyrosine kinase inhibitors may help: masitinib and/or toceranib. • Following 4–6 treatments with mitoxantrone, patients may be maintained on: • Xeloda at mCTx dose of 250 mg/m²/day or • Melphalan at 6–8 mg/m² PO for 5 days, repeated every 21 days, may help. • CTx with mitoxantrone 5 mg/m² escalating up to 6.5 mg/m² IV q 21–30 days. Use with piroxicam as above. Benefit provided is 50% response and some patients go into complete remission. May gain one year ST.

ABDOMINAL TUMORS (Continued)

	Sx	RTx	CTx
Prostate Tumors	Sx (prostatectomy) can benefit selected dogs when neoplastic tissue is confined within the capsule if minimal to no urethral involvement. Imaging technology and exploratory surgery can determine operability.	RTx should be a carefully considered option. Responders may survive up to 1 year. • SRS and brachytherapy are more finely targeted than external beam RTx.	Protocols used for TCC are appropriate with the addition of xeloda for dogs. The carcinoma protocols described in Chapter 6 and above may be helpful in cases resistant to mitoxantrone/piroxicam/xeloda.
Hepatic Tumors	• Sx may benefit dogs with massive hepatocellular carcinomas localized to the left liver lobe. Lobectomy improves survival over medical management. • Choledochal senting.	Liver-directed IMRT or SRS incorporating multimodality therapy may help. Image-guided IL Y-90 implants may help. IsoPetSolutions.com	• CTx may be helpful using Carboplatin/Gemzar rotation. • Use Xeloda at mCTx dose PO IN DOGS ONLY. • Appropriate supplements and nutrition may be supportive. • Antiangiogenic protocols as described above.
Gastrointestinal Tract Tumors **Stomach** **Intestines** **Anal sac tumors are associated with hypercalcemia.**	Sx resection with wide margins is the Tx of choice. • Presurgical imaging and FNA or biopsy for diagnosis of GI tumors will assist the surgeon in planning and postoperative recovery. • Sx for cytoreduction can be very helpful for patients with hormone producing tumors such as gastrinomas, insulinomas, adrenal tumors, and metastatic anal sac tumors associated with hypercalcemia (dogs). • Sx plans that include second-look celiotomy may improve management of residual disease and recurrent abdominal masses.	• IMRT or SRS RTx to the sublumbar (iliac) lymph nodes for metastatic anal sac carcinoma may be beneficial.	• CTx using drugs such as gemzar, carboplatin, mitoxantrone, and Adriamycin combined with small molecule therapy is indicated for treating pancreatic, adrenal, and renal carcinomas. • Use xeloda PO (dogs only, do not use in cats). • Supportive care with appropriate supplements and nutrition may also be helpful.

BONE CANCER
Osteosarcoma (OSA)

Sx	RTx	CTx	ImTx
Sx generally involves amputation, limb sparing, rib resection, etc. Poor Px if located in vertebrae. Poor Px associated with elevated serum alkaline phosphatase. Poor Px if metastasis is noted at diagnosis. Chondrosarcomas generally yield better Px and ST. IV Immunotherapy with a vaccine made from *Listeria monocytogenes*, genetically modified to express HER-2/neu, which is found in canine OSA. www.aratana.com	• May be used for palliation in non-amputated cases. • High megadose fraction RTx may be used intraoperatively to kill osteoclasts. • Stereotactic radiation therapy or radiosurgrey (SRS) may alleviate inoperable lesions.	CTx addresses the high potential for metastasis. • For dogs, use carboplatin 300 mg/m^2 IV or in combination with Adriamycin (use precautions from the modified lymphoma protocol above) q 21–30 days and piroxicam 3 mg/kg PO daily. CTx is generally not needed in cats with OSA due to low rate of metastasis. • Consider novel therapies as they become available including the use of HDAC inhibitors such as valproic acid, SAHA, etc.	Immunotherapy with a vaccine made from *Listeria monocytogenes*, genetically modified to express HER-2/neu, which is found in canine OSA. www.aratana.com

Multiple Myeloma

CTx
• Alkeran® (melphalan) 2–4 mg/m^2 q 24 hours × 7 days, then q 48 hours or it may be also used at 6–8 mg/m^2 PO for 5 days q 21 days. • An alternate choice would be Leukeran (chlorambucil) 4–6 mg/m^2 q 48 hours. • Prednisone 40–50 mg/m^2 PO for 7 days, then 30 mg/m^2 for 7 days, then 20 mg/m^2 q 48 hours for 18 months or as needed. • Tanovea® (rabacfosadine) 1 mg/kg IV over 30 min q 21 days. • If hypercalcemia is present, patients must receive saline diuresis or bisphosphonates. Use antibiotics if febrile or septic, and treat symptomatically. • Monitor serum and urine proteins for a 50% reduction over 30–60 days.

MISCELLANEOUS TUMORS

Histiocytosis

	Sx	RTx	CTx
Histiocytic Tumors **Bernese Mt. Dogs most affected** A perplexing group of tumors that are often difficult to differentiate. • Request tumor cell markers to identify cell of origin such as dendritic cell origin (monocyte/macrophage/Langerhans cell lineages), T-cell, B-cell, or mesynchymal origin. • Innogenics Enlight Assay™ may help differentiate and suggest Tx.	Sx used for diagnosis. Wide and deep complete excision should be attempted if the mass is localized. • Splenectomy is very helpful in grade I and II diseases, while grade III disease is very aggressive with metastases to lungs, lymph nodes, omentum, and organs.	Rarely used but may be beneficial for localized tumors. Stereotactic radiation therapy or SRS may be beneficial to reduce localized masses.	• Some responses with steroids and combination chemotherapy. • Cyclosporine and leflunomide are helpful as potent inhibitors of T-cell activation. • Ifosfamide may have a role in treatment for this disease.

Appendix 2: Handouts for Clients

Canine and Feline Geriatric Oncology: Honoring the Human–Animal Bond, Second Edition. Alice Villalobos with Laurie Kaplan.
© 2018 John Wiley & Sons, Inc. Published 2018 by John Wiley & Sons, Inc.

Guidelines for Feeding and Supplements

Enhancing your geriatric pet's nutritional and immune system during the battle against cancer is an important aspect of our total health care approach. You may be given supplements from our immunonutrition protocol that are in the form of powders, liquids, capsules, and tablets. Administering supplements, especially to cats and geriatric pets, may be challenging and perhaps at times very frustrating. Some pets have no qualms about eating anything. Then there are those pets that are simply not going to accept some or any of the supplements. On occasion, some pets develop loose stools, diarrhea, or nausea from a particular item. You should suspect that a pet feels nausea if he/she looks at food but will not eat. Nausea may result from chemotherapy but it may also be induced by a distasteful supplement. If giving a particular supplement causes stress and mistrust, it will defeat the healthy positive goal of the immunonutrition protocol. It is best to develop a positive reinforcement technique for administering at least the most important supplements successfully.

If your pet refuses to eat food containing the supplements, then we suggest another approach. We do not want to cause food aversion and mistrust or put stress on the human–animal bond that you share with your pet. Try to determine which item has the offending taste, and then omit that one while serving the others with regular feedings. See if your pet will accept at least one or two items in the meal. The most important suggestion is to remove the offending taste from your pet's regular food. You can mix the less tasteful supplements into a delicious treat. This makes feeding the supplements a more pleasant experience and something that your pet looks forward to. Try the different methods listed below for a successful technique.

- Hotdog method. Most dogs will accept pills or capsules stuffed in a hotdog.
- Broth method. Some pets are eager to lap up anything placed in a broth or gravy. Empty capsules, crush pills, and add powders to a beef or chicken broth or gravy mixture.
- Meatball method. Some pets will eagerly eat anything disguised into a meatball type of treat. Also try lunchmeat (turkey or roast beef), liverwurst, bratwurst. Flatten the meat on a counter then place powders, capsules, and pills into the middle of the selected meat. Roll up the meat until you have the supplements hidden deeply inside.
- Peanut butter or cream cheese method. Some pets accept pills, capsules, and powders disguised in a ball of peanut butter or cream cheese. Do not use peanut butter that contains xylitol sweetener. Dogs get sick from xylitol kidney toxicity.
- Syringe method. Mix all supplements into a gravy or liquid made from a canned recovery diet. Use a feeding ssyringe and squirt small amounts of the liquid into the back part of the mouth with gentle coaxing. Be sure to maintain an upbeat, encouraging attitude during the feedings.

Feeding

As your pet undergoes cancer therapy, you might find that the normal diet has less appeal. This can be expected. When people or pets feel sick, the normal diet may not seem appetizing. It may be necessary to offer your pet different, more appealing foods as treatment progresses. Following are some suggested food items to try if your pet develops an aversion to the regular diet. Also included are diets for good health, diets for gastrointestinal discomfort, and healthy snack suggestions.

- Available diets For overall healthy cancer patients, we suggest feeding a low-carbohydrate diet. This minimizes sugar, which cancer cells easily utilize. The idea is to feed the patient and starve the cancer. This theory is the basis for feeding cancer patients the Hill's prescription n/d® diet. This concept is also incorporated in the ketogenic diet. For more information: www.ketopetsanctuary.com. For regular store-bought foods we suggest feeding a high-quality canned food diet.

- Homemade diet. You can put the ingredients together and cook once a week and freeze in portions for future feedings. Avoid high-glycemic foods such as fruit and vegetables like carrots, corn, rice, and potatoes. Lightly steam green veggies in broth. Use asparagus, broccoli, kale, Brussel sprouts, green beans. spinach, etc. (no peas or starchy veggies). Put in a blender and store the blended veggies in a glass container to add to meals. Instructions for a good homemade diet can be found in the book *Help Your Dog Fight Cancer*, by Laurie Kaplan and Alice Villalobos (2016, JanGen Press, 272 pp.).

- Gastrointestinal diets. For pets that experience vomiting, diarrhea, or nausea a temporary bland diet is recommended. Some pets need to stay on special diets such as Hill's i/d® continuously. Suggested foods include boiled hamburger, chicken, or turkey, with boiled barley, canned pumpkin, and cottage cheese. Proportions should be equal. Feed the same amount as you would feed canned food. Add vitamins and calcium to home-cooked diets being fed continuously.

- Snacks. Keep your pet on the low-carbohydrate diet. This includes selecting snacks. Use frozen fish fillets (not breaded), turkey, and other lunchmeat slices, meatballs, cooked meat strips kept frozen, veggies.

These are only suggestions for enhancing the well-being and nutritional status of pets with cancer. However, if your pet loves carrots and declines other suggested items, then give the carrots. The main priority is quality of life including fun at feeding and treat time.

Exercise

With a few specific exceptions, most pets being treated for cancer should be allowed to perform all the activities of enjoyment, especially when it comes to exercise. However, it is important to be attentive. If your dog wants to go for a walk, jog, or hike then go for it. However, if your pet seems reluctant, more sluggish, or less enthusiastic on a particular day, then you should skip that day's exercise or modify it to accommodate your pet's level of energy. If your pet has trouble breathing, stop immediately. If unexpected lethargy persists, be sure to take the temperature to rule out a fever. If the temperature is over 102.5 give the antibiotics in your Cancer Care Package. It may be best to see your veterinarian as soon as possible.

Most importantly give your pet as much time as you can for love and enjoyment. Most pets being treated for cancer are actually giving their family and friends an extended and happy farewell. The majority of our clients are amazed and comment that their pet cancer patient feels healthier and more energetic on the improved diet and immunonutrition. As a team, we are striving to achieve the best quality of life for the rest of your pet's life.

CHEMOTHERAPY DISCHARGE INSTRUCTIONS FOR HOME CARE

Care facility name: _____

Contact Information: _____

Client name: _____ Patient name: _____

Date: _____

Chemotherapy agent administered: _____ Route: _____

A chemotherapy agent was administered to your pet today. If complications develop, please notify our office, your local veterinarian, or your local emergency hospital. Your pet may need medical care to treat or offset a serious adverse event. Below are some answers to common questions regarding chemotherapy, home care, and decision making.

NORMAL AND ABNORMAL SIGNS

IV Administration

1. If the injection site or injection leg becomes swollen or red, this is abnormal and should be reported immediately to our office or to your local doctor.
2. Nausea and/or vomiting may occur within the first 72 hours after treatment. This problem is to be expected from some chemotherapy treatments. If your pet is vomiting or has nausea, administer the ondansetron or maropitant (Cerenia®) or metoclopramide (Reglan®) sent home in your "Chemo Care Package." Offer your pet only small amounts of water at a time and restrict food to only small amounts. If there is excessive vomiting (more than four episodes in 24 hours), see your family veterinarian or take your pet to an emergency clinic for injectable antivomiting medications, subcutaneous fluids, and assistance.
3. Diarrhea may result following some chemotherapy agents. It may occur within the first 72 hours and contain a small amount of mucous or blood. Do not panic if there are two or three loose movements a day, but if your pet has over three episodes of loose stool in a 24-hour period with little or no control, dehydration may result. Use the metronidazole or sulfasalazine tablets that may be part of your "Chemo Care Package" at the first sign. Start your pet on a bland diet of chicken or boiled hamburger, cottage cheese, and boiled barley or brown rice. Continue this diet for 3 days after the diarrhea is resolved. If diarrhea persists beyond 48 hours with no improvement, be sure to call us or see your family veterinarian for other medications to soothe the gut and control the diarrhea.
4. A body temperature above 102.5 degrees or below 99.5 degrees is considered abnormal. Do not give any fever-reducing medications without first talking to your veterinarian. Temperatures above 102.5 degrees may indicate infection. Take your pet to your local or emergency veterinarian for an evaluation for sepsis.
5. Your pet may experience some lethargy for the first 72 hours. If lethargy persists beyond 24 hours, take the temperature. See your local doctor if you detect a fever.

After Intralesional Administration of Chemotherapy

1. After an intralesional injection of chemotherapy, the injection site may be mildly swollen or red as an expected side effect. If ulcerated, provide wound care.
2. If your pet is licking occasionally at the injection site, don't worry. If your pet is licking excessively at the injection site, this can cause irritation or infection. Get an E-collar or bandage to protect the lesion from self-trauma.
3. Nausea, vomiting, and diarrhea are rarely seen with intralesional injections.
4. A body temperature above 102.5 degrees or below 99.5 degrees is considered abnormal. Do not give any fever-reducing medications without first talking to your veterinarian. Temperatures above 102.5 degrees with lethargy should prompt a visit to your local or emergency veterinarian for a complete blood count (CBC).

After Subcutaneous Administration of Chemotherapy

1. The injection site should not become swollen or red or painful. If you detect one of these adverse effects, please call us, and see your local doctor.
2. If your pet is licking at the injection site, there may be a problem with local reaction or an abscess. If your pet is licking excessively at the injection site, this may cause irritation or infection. Use a bandage or E-collar to provide protection.
3. Nausea, vomiting, diarrhea, and fever are rare following subcutaneous injections. If your pet becomes ill, do contact us and follow the precautions recommended.
4. Take your pet's temperature. If above 102.5 degrees or below 99.5 degrees, it is abnormal. If the temperature is high, give the antibiotics in your Cancer Care Package and recheck temperature in 6-8 hours. If it is still high, call us.
5. Your pet may experience some mild lethargy for the first 72 hours. If the lethargy is profound or persists beyond 72 hours, be sure to see your veterinarian for help.

EMERGENCY SIGNS

1. If your pet's gums are pale, light gray, or bluish in color.
2. If your pet is having difficulty breathing or is wheezing or gasping for air.
3. If the rectal temperature is 99.5 degrees or below or 103.5 degrees or above. (Normal temperature ranges between 100.5 and 102.5 for dogs and cats.)
4. If your pet vomits excessively (more than four times in 24 hours) or vomits blood.
5. If your pet has liquid stool, or blood in the stool, or has poor control of eliminations for more than twice daily, dehydration may develop.
6. If your pet has seizures or is profoundly listless for several hours or refuses to eat or drink for more than 24 hours.

**IF YOU HAVE CONCERNS OR IF YOUR PET IS EXPERIENCING
AN EMERGENCY, CALL YOUR LOCAL VETERINARIAN
OR LOCAL EMERGENCY ANIMAL HOSPITAL IMMEDIATELY!**

Cancer Pain Management and Your Pet

Cancer pain is the most distressful aspect of managing pets with cancer. Cancer pain and inflammation may be the symptom that initially alerts you to the problem. Your pet's cancer pain needs to be properly controlled to enjoy a good quality of life. The suggestions in this handout are only guidelines. You need to be alert and empathetic to be able to understand when your pet is in pain. Your veterinarian definitely needs your input regarding how your pet feels. The problem with trying to interpret pain in animals is that a lot of their pain goes unnoticed and undertreated. The solution is for all caregivers to agree that certain pre-existing conditions (arthritis and dental disease), and many cancers, cause pain. We should further agree on a strategy to treat for anticipated pain. Since pain of any sort is immunosuppressive and counterproductive to quality of life and survival, this approach results in healthier and happier cancer patients during their Pawspice.

Cancer causes pain in many ways. Dogs with bone cancer have throbbing pain. They show their pain by limping; however, because the nature of dogs is to remain cheerful, many pet owners don't understand the magnitude of their dog's bone pain.

For bone cancer dogs not receiving amputation, the pain may very difficult to manage. Pamidronate and zoledronate have a dual purpose to reduce bone cancer pain and slow down the action of the bone cancer cells. Pamidronate is given monthly as a 1–2 mg/kg IV one hour drip with saline. Another option for pain control for bone pain and other ulcerative or bulky tumors is palliative radiation therapy. Ask your doctor about this.

Cancer pain may be caused by inflammation and infection at the tumor site. Oral tumors are traumatized by teeth and infected with gingivitis organisms. Nail bed tumors can be very painful and infected. Tumors that put pressure on nerves or invade and obstruct organs or tubes such as the intestines, ureters, and urethra (urine outflow from the kidneys and bladder) may cause abdominal or visceral discomfort, nausea, vomiting, constipation, diarrhea, ataxia, lethargy, and pain. We can well imagine that pets with brain tumors have headaches. A pet's behavior changes, loss of motor control, and seizures must cause fear, anxiety, and pain. However, we, as caregivers, can only guess at the magnitude of their feelings and emotions.

Animals have a strong survival instinct that masks pain very well. This trait exists even in our most domesticated house pets. Pets with chronic, steady pain still follow family members (their pack) from room to room despite intense, chronic pain from hidden cancers in the abdomen and chest.

We need to eliminate, minimize, and control pain for our geriatric cancer pets. Many are suffering from arthritis and dental pain before the diagnosis of cancer, which makes them feel worse. Your veterinarian may prescribe a single drug for pain control. A single drug may be effective; however, cancer patients often need more than one drug to achieve good cancer pain control. Each drug would be selected to act upon a particular pain pathway so that the combination will properly alleviate the pain. We must examine combinations. For instance, grapiprant (Galliprant®) may be used to target arthritis pain, but it cannot be used along with other NSAIDs and steroids. It is best to check for contraindications with medications that your pet is receiving before the cancer diagnosis.

Check the graduated scale for pain control from the World Health Organization and information and guidelines from the International Veterinary Academy of Pain Management and the AAHA/AAFP Pain Management Guidelines for Dogs and Cats. Various pain scales are used to measure factors such as heart rate, vocalization, restlessness, cramping, crying, hunching, thrashing, and agitation. Sadly, we still have a huge deficit in recognition of chronic cancer pain in our companion animals.

The Duragesic® pain patch may be prescribed for your pet. It releases the opioid, fentanyl, through the skin into the circulatory system over a 3-day period. It may take up to 24 hours for the full analgesic effect in dogs, whereas 70% of cats may experience the full effect by 6–8 hours. Therefore, if the patch is being used for surgery, the timing of placement is important, or the pet will need supplemental injections for pain control. We may recommend a follow-up pain patch 72 hours from the initial patch. Doses vary, but 1 mgc per pound seems to be effective for most pets. For smaller cats, we expose half of the 25 mgc pain patch membrane for the first 3 days and expose the other half for the second 3 days. Leave the pain patch on until suture removal so that staff may remove the patch painlessly and dispose of it properly. Earlier removal of the patch seems to hurt and may cause an ulcer at the membrane contact site.

Postsurgical pain control is important. Pets should be monitored overnight by family, if going home, or by caring nurses who are trained to assess pain. Look for increased panting and heart rate, crying, restlessness, and, in cats, crouching and holding the head down. At times, you may be the nurse!

Tissue opioid receptors are upregulated in inflamed tissues and respond for up to 48 hours if given intraoperative morphine at low doses. Epidural blocks and local nerve blocks eliminate pain. Local infusion of long-acting local anesthetics along nerves and on to the surgery site prevents anticipated postsurgical pain.

All postop cancer patients need pain control for home care. Commonly used medications for mild pain are non-steroidal anti-inflammatory drugs (NSAIDs) such as: meloxicam, carprofen, firocoxib, etc. Acetaminophen may be used in dogs but NEVER give it to cats. Cats respond well to meloxicam, robenacoxib, oral buprenorphine, and gabapentin. Dogs do well with gabapentin amantadine, and tramadol or trazodone (GAT protocol) in combination with an NSAID each are given at specified intervals. Follow your doctor's advice. *NEVER USE ASPIRIN OR ACETAMINOPHEN IN CATS.*

If your pet has anxiety in the car or during visits to the hospital, use medications to relieve stress such as Zylkene®, pheromones, and gentle sedatives. Anxiety is a form of emotional pain and should be treated as such. The FEAR FREE™ Initiative wants to "take the pet out of petrified" using positive, gentle handling and relaxing agents.

Some cancer patients will be given piroxicam, an NSAID that has dual action against pain and cancer. Piroxicam or another NSAID may be prescribed for bone, bladder, and skin cancer, and some sarcomas. Avoid using steroids with NSAIDs because ulceration of the stomach and intestines is a predictable adverse effect. Pepcid® or another agent may be needed for protection of the intestinal mucosa to prevent ulcers.

Cancer patients who are nearing the end of life generally need special routes of delivery for their pain control. The steady use of a pain patch every 3 days can be very helpful during the hospice phase of their Pawspice.

Good pain management is good medicine. It allows pet caregivers to fully enjoy the human–animal bond shared with their pet during a difficult time. We want to be reassured knowing that our geriatric cancer patient is having a happy, comfortable, good quality of life during the beginning, middle, and last phase of their Pawspice.

The H5M2 Quality of Life Scale for Cats

Feline Quality of Life Scale

Feline caregivers can use this scale to evaluate the success of their Pawspice program. Grading each criterion using a scale of 0 to 10 will help carers determine the Quality of Life of sick cats.

Score	Criterion
0–10	**HURT** Adequate pain control and breathing ability are the first and foremost considerations. Is the cat's pain being successfully managed? Trouble breathing outweighs all other concerns.
0–10	**HUNGER** Is the cat eating enough nutritious food? Does coaxing and hand feeding help? Does the cat require a feeding tube for nutrition?
0–10	**HYDRATION** Is the cat dehydrated, hypovolemic? For cats not drinking or eating enough food that contains water, provide subcutaneous fluids once or twice daily to supplement fluid intake.
0–10	**HYGIENE** The cat should be kept brushed, cleaned, parasite free. This is paramount for cats with oral cancer. Check the body for soiling after elimination. Avoid pressure sores and keep all wounds clean.
0–10	**HAPPINESS** Does the cat express joy and interest? Is the cat responsive to surroundings (family, toys, etc.)? Does the cat purr when scratched or petted? Is the cat depressed, lonely, anxious, bored, afraid? Can the cat's bed be near the kitchen and moved near family activities so as not to be isolated?
0–10	**MOBILITY** Can the cat use a litter box without help? Is the cat ataxic, stumbling or having seizures? Some caregivers feel euthanasia is preferable to a definitive surgery, yet cats are resilient. Cats with limited mobility may still be alert and responsive and can have a good quality of life if the family is committed to providing quality care.
0–10	**MORE GOOD DAYS THAN BAD** When bad days outnumber good days, quality of life for the declining cat might be too compromised. When a healthy human–animal bond is no longer possible, caregivers must be made aware that their duty is to protect their cat from pointless pain and frustration by making the final call for the gift of euthanasia. The decision needs to be made if the cat has unresponsive suffering. If death comes peacefully and painlessly at home, that is okay.
*Total =	*A total score >35 is acceptable Quality of Life for maintaining a good Feline Pawspice.**

Quality of Life Scale (The H5M2 Scale)

Pet caregivers can use this Quality of Life Scale to determine the success of Pawspice care. Score patients using a scale of 0 to 10 (10 being ideal).

Score	Criterion
0–10	**HURT** Adequate pain control and breathing ability are of top concern. If the pet can't breathe properly, nothing else matters. Is oxygen supplementation necessary? Is the pet's pain well managed?
0–10	**HUNGER** Is the pet eating enough? Does hand feeding help? Does the pet need a feeding tube?
0–10	**HYDRATION** Is the pet dehydrated? For patients not drinking enough, use subcutaneous fluids daily to supplement fluid intake.
0–10	**HYGIENE** The pet should be brushed and cleaned, particularly after eliminations. Avoid pressure sores with soft bedding and keep all wounds clean.
0–10	**HAPPINESS** Does the pet express joy and interest? Is the pet responsive to family, toys, etc.? Is the pet depressed, lonely, anxious, bored or afraid? Can the pet's bed be moved to be close to family activities?
0-10	**MOBILITY** - Can the pet get up without assistance? Does the pet need human or mechanical help (e.g., a cart)? Does the dog feel like going for a walk? Is the pet having seizures or stumbling? (Some carers feel that euthanasia is preferable to amputation, but an animal with limited mobility yet still alert and responsive, can have a good quality of life as long as the family is committed to helping their pet.)
0–10	**MORE GOOD DAYS THAN BAD** When bad days outnumber good days, quality of life might be too compromised. When a healthy human–animal bond is no longer possible, the carers must be made aware that the end is near. The decision for euthanasia needs to be made if the pet is suffering. It is ideal when a pet's death comes peacefully and painlessly at home. Original concept, *Oncology Outlook*, by Dr. Alice Villalobos, *Quality of Life Scale Helps Make Final Call,* VPN, 09/2004; formatted for *Canine and Feline Geriatric Oncology: Honoring the Human-Animal Bond,* Blackwell Publishing, 2007, and revised for Second Edition, Wiley, 2017.
*TOTAL	*A total over 35 points represents acceptable life quality to continue with pet hospice (Pawspice).

Created by Dr. Alice Villalobos for *Feline Internal Medicine,* Vol. 6, 2010 and adapted from *Canine and Feline Geriatric Oncology: Honoring the Human–Animal Bond*, Table 10.1, January 2007 and revised for Second Edition, 2017. Original concept, *Quality of Life Scale Helps Make Final Call, Oncology Outlook, VPN*, 09/2004.

Electroporation (EP)/Electrochemoherapy (ECT)

EP is technology that allows cancer patients another option when facing aggressive conventional surgery. EP may also serve as an option to radiation therapy for those pet owners who are under financial constraints.

EP is achieved using a special machine that delivers a precise voltage that opens pores (aquaporins) in the membranes of cancer cells. This allows influx of specific chemotherapy agents into the cancer cells. Dr. Peter Agre, who discovered aquaporins, received a Nobel Prize in 2003.

EP opens cancer cell aquaporins to selectively absorb only two chemotherapy agents: bleomycin (1,000 times) and cisplatin (a few dozen times) greater than normal cells. EP is indicated for difficult to remove tumors of the oral cavity, face, trunk, limbs, and digits. EP may require only one treatment for complete resolution of localized tumors. However, larger tumors often require several EP treatments at 2–3 week intervals.

Larger tumors can be excised or "debulked" with conservative margins and the tumor bed can be treated with EP before skin closure or left as an open wound.

EP controls cancer locally and is compatible with other anticancer therapies needed to prevent metastasis.

Treated tumor tissue of any cell type will undergo necrosis and regression over a period of 3–6 weeks. The wounds generally do not develop infections but need standard wound care post-EP. Healing is excellent in most cases.

EP also provides a special bonus. The body generates an immune reaction to the cancer cells. This occurs with necrosis and antigen release during healing and shrinkage as the body cleans the area (autophagy).

Please note that EP requires that patients be under anesthesia. There is a muscular reflex generated with the delivery of each electrical impulse.

Call us if you have questions. You received this information because your pet's tumor might be controlled with the electroporation (EP) procedure.

Antiangiogenic Protocol

By Dr. Alice Villalobos, Fellow Emeritus National Academies of Practice

Cancer cells accomplish their fatal agenda because of uncontrollable growth and invasion of vital structures. One approach in the battle against cancer is to target common pathways. All types of cancers (sarcomas, carcinomas, and adenocarcinomas) except blood cancers (leukemia and lymphoma) recruit tiny blood vessels to grow. The process is called angiogenesis. If we reduce or cut off the recruitment of cancer's blood supply (antiangiogenesis), we may win more quality time for our pet cancer patients.

Antiangiogenic agents inhibit the growth of tiny blood vessels so cancer cells are less able to grow. In a series of 600 animal cancer patients, 60% responded with their tumors stabilized or reduced. We place our cancer patients on a special combination of antiangiogenic agents (some holistic and some Rx) tailored to the particular type of cancer. In addition, we use kinder, gentler chemotherapy known as "metronomic" chemotherapy (mCTx). It is the use of low doses on a daily basis and it is proven to have antiangiogenic action. Since using antiangiogenic agents at our Pawspice and Animal Oncology practices we have seen good results.

Integrative Antiangiogenesis Protocol for Cancer Patients

1. AngioStop (sea cucumber): $1/2$ capsule per 60 pounds 2–3 × daily
2. Asparagus extract: $1/2$ capsule per 60 pounds 2–3 × daily

3. Revivin: $^1/_2$ capsule per 60 pounds once daily
4. +/- Myomin: $^1/_2$ capsule per 60 pounds 2–3 × daily (use if pet is obese)

Rx with Proven Anticancer and Antiangiogenesis Action

1. Metronomic chemotherapy: low continuous daily dose Rx for cancer type
2. NSAIDs aspirin type Rx: piroxicam or meloxicam (with Pepcid)
3. Metformin: an antidiabetic drug with proven anticancer action

Immunonutrition Supplements (Improve Nutritional Status; Immunity)

1. Agaricus Bio: 600 mg cap 2 × daily (stimulates macrophage and NK cell action)
2. OncoSupport: 1 scoop for dogs >50 pounds 2 × daily (multiple supportive actions)
3. IP-6: 1 cap per 10–20 pounds 2 × daily (antioxidant, best on empty stomach)
4. Platinum performance: start with 25%; increase to 1 TBS/60 pounds/day (for joints)
5. Vitality: 1 cap/20 pounds up to 3 in the a.m. and 3 by 2:00 p.m. (promotes mitochondria)
6. Primal dose: bovine bolostrum (promotes immune health, gut function)

   Cancer patients may need other Rx and items from each category depending upon cancer type, body condition, and age of the patient. Items can be given separately, mixed in meals, or blended into a liquid elixir and given orally 2–3 times a day as directed.

Appendix 3: Canine and Feline Anatomy

CLIENT'S NAME _____   DIAGNOSIS _____   DATE _____

PATIENT'S NAME _____   AGE _____   BREED _____   SEX _____

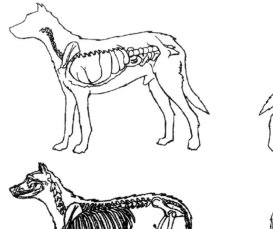
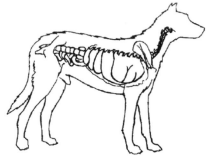
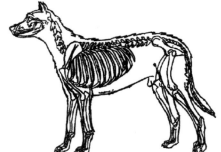
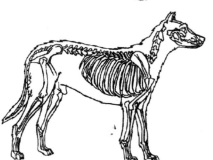

CLIENT'S NAME _____   DIAGNOSIS _____   DATE _____

PATIENT'S NAME _____   AGE _____   BREED _____   SEX _____

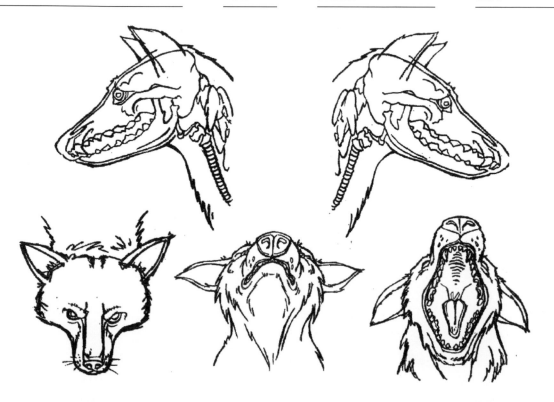

CLIENT'S NAME

DIAGNOSIS

DATE

PATIENT'S NAME

AGE   BREED

SEX

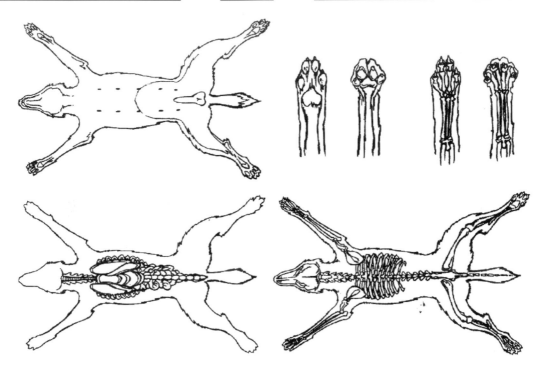

CLIENT'S NAME

DIAGNOSIS

DATE

PATIENT'S NAME

AGE   BREED

SEX

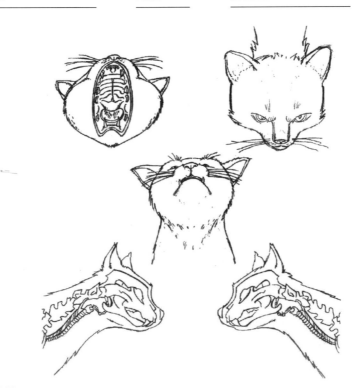

CLIENT'S NAME

PATIENT'S NAME

DIAGNOSIS

AGE   BREED

DATE

SEX

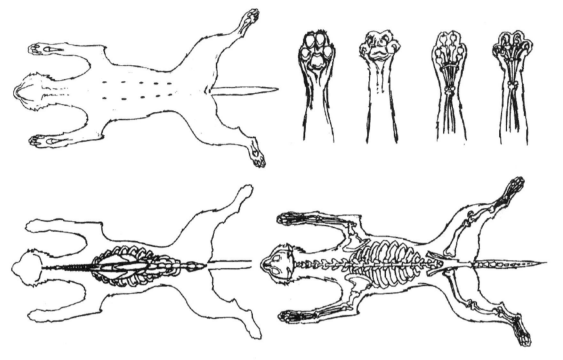

CLIENT'S NAME

PATIENT'S NAME

DIAGNOSIS

AGE   BREED

DATE

SEX

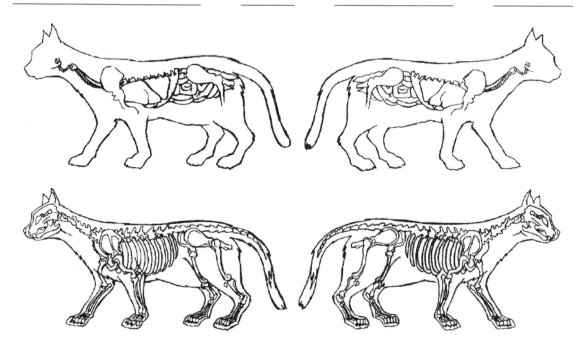

CLIENT'S NAME _____   DIAGNOSIS _____   DATE _____

PATIENT'S NAME _____   AGE _____ BREED _____   SEX _____

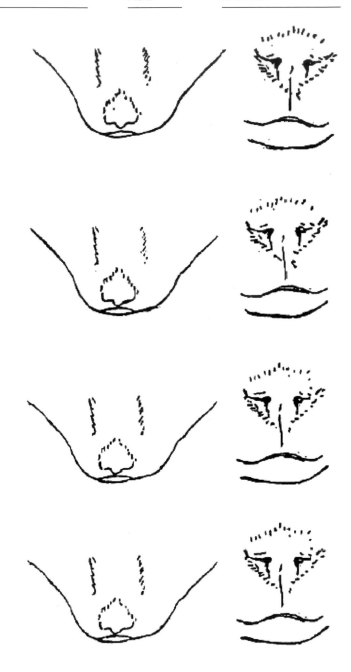

CLIENT'S NAME   DIAGNOSIS   DATE

PATIENT'S NAME   AGE   BREED   SEX

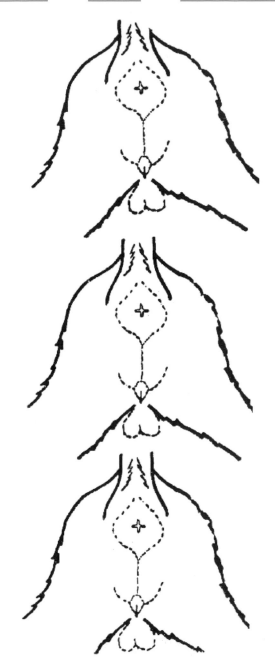

Index

abdominal tumors, 71, 130, 165, 460–462
Accutane, 63–64
Acepromazine, 275
Acetaminophen, 282, 472
Ackerman, L.V., 53
acquired immune deficiency syndrome (AIDS), 8
acupuncture, 286
Adams, Cathy, 399
adenocarcinomas (AC), 17, 103–104
Adriamycin
   aggressive/fractious patients and, 275
   cost restraints and, 322
   Doberman Pinschers and, 346
   extravasation and, 199–200
   mammary cancer and, 332
   sedation and, 199
   split dosage of, 360
Advanced Protection Formula (APF) Drops, 229
advanced/recurrent cancer
   Aesculapian authority and, 310
   anal sac carcinomas and, 333–335
   anemia and, 316–317
   caregiver lifestyle and, 307–310
   chemoprevention and, 337–338
   chemotherapy and, 359–360
   conflict of interest and, 304–306
   cost-saving protocols and, 322–323
   decision-making framework for, 307
   decision-making role and, 312–313
   diagnosing, 317–318
   ethical/economic issues and, 303–304
   expecting recurrence and, 313–314
   family practice skills and, 302–303
   frail/cachectic patients and, 316
   geriatric syndromes and, 317
   hemangiosarcoma and, 328–329
   immunonutrition and, 337–338
   integrative medicine and, 336–337
   lymphoma and, 320–321
   mammary tumors and, 332
   mast cell tumors and, 327–328
   metronomic chemotherapy and, 324–325
   monitoring for, 318–320
   MOPP rescue and, 322
   multiple primary malignancies and, 335–336
   nasal cancer and, 335
   nutrigenomics and, 337
   OSA lesions and, 331
   osteosarcoma and, 329
   patriarchal practitioners and, 306–307
   physical performance assessment and, 314
   pulmonarymetastatectomy and, 330–331
   re-evaluating attitudes toward, 325–326
   softtissue sarcomas and, 325–327
   targeted therapy drugs and, 324
Aesculapian authority, 310
Agaricus, 349
ageism, 22
aging, 5–6
   bond effects of, 33–35
   cancer studies and, 310
   chemotherapy and, 171
   complexity increase and, 29–33
   medical conditions and, 301
   pet population and, 25
aging variability, 22–23